# Percutaneous Treatment of Left Side Cardiac Valves

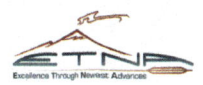

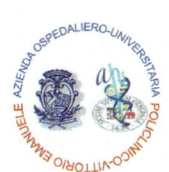

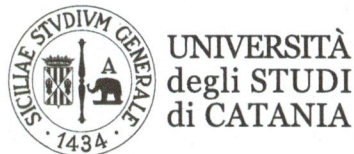

Corrado Tamburino · Marco Barbanti
Davide Capodanno

Editors

# Percutaneous Treatment of Left Side Cardiac Valves

A Practical Guide for the Interventional Cardiologist

Third Edition

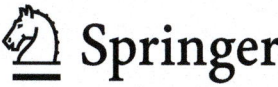 Springer

*Editors*
Corrado Tamburino
Ferrarotto Hospital
University of Catania
Catania, Italy

Marco Barbanti
Ferrarotto Hospital
University of Catania
Catania, Italy

Davide Capodanno
Ferrarotto Hospital
University of Catania
Catania, Italy

The previous editions of this book were edited by Corrado Tamburino and Gian Paolo Ussia

ISBN 978-3-030-09645-8        ISBN 978-3-319-59620-4    (eBook)
https://doi.org/10.1007/978-3-319-59620-4

This Springer imprint is published by Springer Nature
The registered company is Springer International Publishing AG
The registered company address is: Gewerbestrasse 11, 6330 Cham, Switzerland

# Preface

The field of transcatheter therapies for valvular heart disease is a never-ending source of technical and device innovation, novel indications and new treatment solutions. The interest of the scientific community in this sub-discipline of interventional cardiology is demonstrated by the extraordinary volume of literature on the field, as well as the variety of national and international meetings, symposia and teaching courses focusing on this topic. This book – now at its third edition – represents a practical guide addressing the rapidly expanding and innovative field of transcatheter therapies for left-side valvular heart disease. The table of contents has been uniquely built to update the reader with the latest practical and scientific advances in the field.

The first section is dedicated to mitral valve disease, with a focus on the latest interventional strategies of mitral valve repair and replacement. The subsequent section is dedicated to aortic interventions, including a step-by-step guide to newer-generation devices for transcatheter aortic valve implantation. Special attention has been paid to the devices that carry the most interesting novel elements in the field. Each section includes a number of authoritative review articles and accompanying illustrations dealing with various aspects of valvular heart disease, from anatomy to pathophysiology, from pre-procedural planning to in-lab technique.

This third edition would not have been possible without the enthusiastic participation and support of many extraordinary colleagues and friends who have shared their knowledge and experience with us all.

February 2018
Catania, Italy

Corrado Tamburino
Davide Capodanno
Marco Barbanti

# Preface to the Second Edition

At the time of publication of this handbook, percutaneous treatment of left side cardiac valves represented just an exciting and promising opportunity. The lack of outcome data at medium and long term, however, required some caution, since there were still too many unknowns related to a minimally invasive treatment of valvular heart disease, including durability of acute results, long-term impact of procedural complications, patient selection, and so on. After two years since our first publication, the literature has produced substantial data supporting particularly transcatheter aortic valve implantation, in parallel with a considerable increase of the procedures around the world, as well as operators' experience and procedural success. These data allow now to consider these procedures not only a promise for the future, but a solid reality of our present. Not surprisingly, the enthusiasm for these achievements has prompted the industry to continuously improve their own devices. The scenario has therefore changed dramatically in recent years, necessitating a substantial update of the first edition of this volume. Once again, the goal of this practical handbook is to give interventional cardiologists an advanced understanding and the current state of the art of the percutaneous treatment of left side cardiac valves.

April 2012
Catania, Italy

Corrado Tamburino
Gian Paolo Ussia

# Preface to the First Edition

Transcatheter therapy of cardiac valve diseases is a rediscovery by interventional cardiologists. Treating cardiac valve diseases with alternative techniques to cardiac surgery using prosthetic devices has rekindled interest in the field of hemodynamics, which has been neglected in recent years. Within this framework, two sectors can be distinguished: valvuloplasty techniques using a balloon alone to treat mitral, aortic, and pulmonary stenoses, and those using prosthetic heart valves or repair devices. Valvuloplasty techniques should be considered as palliative, as the duration of their effectiveness varies from just a few weeks, as in the case of aortic valvuloplasty for degenerative stenoses, to years, as in the case of mitral and pulmonary valvuloplasty. By contrast, transcatheter implantation of biological prosthetic valves or repair techniques using dedicated devices aim to provide a definitive therapeutic solution or at least a solution offering results that are equal to or just as good as those of cardiac surgery. The advent of devices for the percutaneous treatment of left chamber valve diseases is one of the greatest breakthroughs in interventional cardiology. The goal of this handbook is to give interventional cardiologists the means to understand the context of the percutaneous treatment of valve diseases and the state of the art of the techniques and procedures currently available.

April 2010                                                                 Corrado Tamburino
Catania, Italy                                                            Gian Paolo Ussia

# Contents

# Contributors

**Adrian Attinger-Toller, M.D.** Center for Heart Valve Innovation, St Paul's Hospital, Vancouver, BC, Canada

**Marco Barbanti, M.D.** Ferrarotto Hospital, University of Catania, Catania, Italy

**Giovanni Bartoloni, M.D.** Postgraduate School of Cardiology, University of Catania, Catania, Italy

**Philipp Blanke, M.D.** Department of Radiology, Centre for Heart Valve Innovation St Paul's Hospital, University of British Columbia, Vancouver, BC, Canada

**Vera Bottari, M.D.** Ferrarotto Hospital, University of Catania, Catania, Italy

**Sergio Buccheri, M.D.** Department of General Surgery and Medical-Surgical Specialties, University of Catania, Catania, Italy

**Stefano Cannata, M.D.** Ferrarotto Hospital, University of Catania, Catania, Italy

**Davide Capodanno, M.D.** Ferrarotto Hospital, University of Catania, Catania, Italy

**Piera Capranzano, M.D.** Ferrarotto Hospital, University of Catania, Catania, Italy

**Chekrallah Chamandi, M.D.** Quebec Heart and Lung Institute, Laval University, Quebec City, QC, Canada

**Anson Cheung, M.D.** Center for Heart Valve Innovation, St Paul's Hospital, Vancouver, BC, Canada

**Marta Chiarandà, M.D.** Ferrarotto Hospital, University of Catania, Catania, Italy

**Silvio Gianluca Cosentino, M.D.** Bachelor of Science, University of Catania, Catania, Italy

**Wanda Deste, M.D.** Division of Cardiology, Ferrarotto Hospital, University of Catania, Catania, Italy

**Alessio di Landro, M.D.** Ferrarotto Hospital, University of Catania, Catania, Italy

**Maria Elena Di Salvo, M.D.** Ferrarotto Hospital, University of Catania, Catania, Italy

**Ted Feldman, MD, FESC, FACC, MSCAI** Cardiology Division, Evanston Hospital, Evanston, IL, USA

NorthShore University HealthSystem, Evanston, IL, USA

**Sandra Giaquinta, M.D.** Ferrarotto Hospital, University of Catania, Catania, Italy

**Carmelo Grasso, M.D.** Cardiology Division, Structural Heart Disease, Coronary and Peripheral Intervention Laboratory, Ferrarotto Hospital, Catania, Italy

**Romi Grover, M.D.** Department of Radiology, Centre for Heart Valve Innovation St Paul's Hospital, University of British Columbia, Vancouver, BC, Canada

**Rominder Grover, M.B.B.S.** Department of Radiology, University of British Columbia, Vancouver, BC, Canada

**Mayra Guerrero, M.D., F.A.C.C., F.S.C.A.I.** NorthShore University HealthSystem, Evanston, IL, USA

**Simona Gulino, M.D.** Ferrarotto Hospital, University of Catania, Catania, Italy

**Sebastiano Immè, M.D.** Ferrarotto Hospital, University of Catania, Catania, Italy

**Antonino Indelicato, M.D.** Ferrarotto Hospital, University of Catania, Catania, Italy

**Francesca Indorato, M.D.** Postgraduate School of Legal Medicine, University of Catania, Catania, Italy

**Shaw-Hua Kueh, M.B.Ch.B.** Department of Radiology, University of British Columbia, Vancouver, BC, Canada

**Alessio La Manna, M.D.** Ferrarotto Hospital, University of Catania, Catania, Italy

**Ketty La Spina, M.D.** Ferrarotto Hospital, University of Catania, Catania, Italy

**Jonathon A. Leipsic, M.D.** Department of Radiology, Centre for Heart Valve Innovation St Paul's Hospital, University of British Columbia, Vancouver, BC, Canada

**Justin P. Levisay, M.D., F.A.C.C., F.S.C.A.I.** NorthShore University HealthSystem, Evanston, IL, USA

**Sarah Mangiafico, M.D.** Ferrarotto Hospital, University of Catania, Catania, Italy

**Ines Monte, M.D.** Ferrarotto Hospital, University of Catania, Catania, Italy

**John Mooney, M.D.** Department of Radiology, Centre for Heart Valve Innovation St Paul's Hospital, University of British Columbia, Vancouver, BC, Canada

**Mickaël Ohana, M.D.** Department of Radiology, Centre for Heart Valve Innovation St Paul's Hospital, University of British Columbia, Vancouver, BC, Canada

**Martina Patanè, M.D.** Ferrarotto Hospital, University of Catania, Catania, Italy

**Nicolò Piazza, M.D., Ph.D.** Interventional Cardiology Department, McGill University Health Center, Glen Hospital/Royal Victoria Hospital, Montréal, QC, Canada

**Gerlando Pilato, M.D.** Ferrarotto Hospital, University of Catania, Catania, Italy

**Josep Rodés-Cabau, M.D.** Quebec Heart and Lung Institute, Laval University, Quebec City, QC, Canada

**Giuseppe Ronsivalle, M.D.** Ferrarotto Hospital, University of Catania, Catania, Italy

**Antonio Popolo Rubbio, M.D.** Ferrarotto Hospital, University of Catania, Catania, Italy

**Michael H. Salinger, M.D., F.A.C.C., F.S.C.A.I.** NorthShore University HealthSystem, Evanston, IL, USA

**Salvatore Scandura, M.D.** Ferrarotto Hospital, University of Catania, Catania, Italy

**Stephanie Sellers, M.Sc.** Department of Radiology, University of British Columbia, Vancouver, BC, Canada

**Carmelo Sgroi, M.D.** Ferrarotto Hospital, University of Catania, Catania, Italy

**Anthony Shaw, M.D.** Department of Radiology, Centre for Heart Valve Innovation St Paul's Hospital, University of British Columbia, Vancouver, BC, Canada

**Rita Sicuso, M.D.** Ferrarotto Hospital, University of Catania, Catania, Italy

**Claudia Ina Tamburino, M.D.** Ferrarotto Hospital, University of Catania, Catania, Italy

**Corrado Tamburino, M.D., Ph.D.** Ferrarotto Hospital, University of Catania, Catania, Italy

**Pascal Thériault-Lauzier, M.D.** Interventional Cardiology Department, McGill University Health Center, Glen Hospital/Royal Victoria Hospital, Montréal, QC, Canada

**Denise Todaro, M.D.** Division of Cardiology, Ferrarotto Hospital, University of Catania, Catania, Italy

**Lennart van Gils, M.D.** Department of Interventional Cardiology, Thoraxcenter, Erasmus Medical Center, Rotterdam, Netherlands

**Nicolas M. Van Mieghem, M.D., Ph.D.** Department of Interventional Cardiology, Thoraxcenter, Erasmus Medical Center, Rotterdam, Netherlands

**John G. Webb, M.D.** Center for Heart Valve Innovation, St Paul's Hospital, Vancouver, BC, Canada

# Part I

# Mitral Valve Disease

# Anatomy of the Mitral Apparatus

1

Francesca Indorato, Silvio Gianluca Cosentino, and Giovanni Bartoloni

The mitral valve had its name by Andreas Vesalius (*De Humani Corporis Fabrica*, 1543) due to its shape similar to the bishop's hat (*miter*).

The mitral valve lies in the floor of the left atrium, separating the inflow from the outflow tract of the left ventricle (Fig. 1.1).

The mitral valve is part of the left ventricular outflow tract and of the aortic root; it facilitates the accommodation of blood, eventually followed by its rapid, efficient, and forceful ejection through the left ventricular outflow tract into the aortic root [1, 2].

The mitral valve apparatus and the left ventricle are so interdependent that there is no mitral valve defect that does not affect the left ventricle in some way, and, in turn, there is no morphological or functional alteration of the left ventricle that has no consequence, to a greater or lesser extent, for the mitral valve. Therefore, the mitral valve is not a passive structure that moves solely as a result of the forces generated by cardiac activity, but rather a structure with its own sphincteric activity concentrated mainly in the annulus, which contributes to the ventricle's contractility and, in turn, is heavily affected by it.

The mitral valve apparatus comprises the annulus and portion of myocardium located above and below it, the leaflets, the *chordae tendineae*, and the papillary muscles (Figs. 1.2 and 1.3).

F. Indorato (✉)
Postgraduate School of Legal Medicine, University of Catania, Catania, Italy
e-mail: fra.indorato@gmail.com

S.G. Cosentino
University of Catania, Catania, Italy
e-mail: silvio.cosentino@gmail.com

G. Bartoloni
Professor of Anatomic Pathology - Postgraduate School of Cardiology,
University of Catania, Catania, Italy
e-mail: gbartolo@unict.it

© Springer International Publishing AG 2018
C. Tamburino et al. (eds.), *Percutaneous Treatment of Left Side Cardiac Valves*,
https://doi.org/10.1007/978-3-319-59620-4_1

**Fig. 1.1** Short-axis view of the cardiac basis after section of atrial cavities showing the mitral valve (*MV*), the aortic root (*AoR*), the pulmonary valve (*PV*), and the tricuspid valve (*TV*)

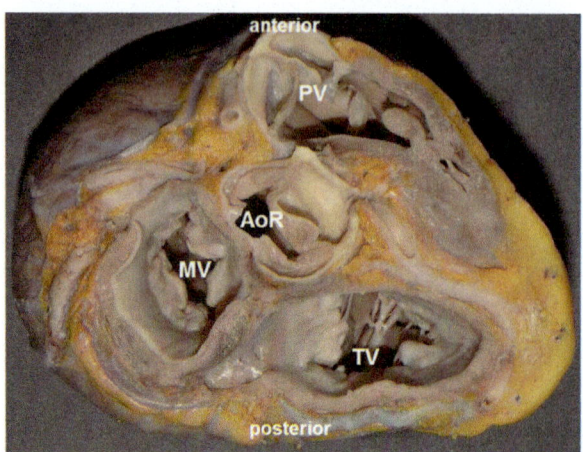

**Fig. 1.2** Atrial view of the mitral valve: anterior (*A*) and posterior (*P*) leaflets

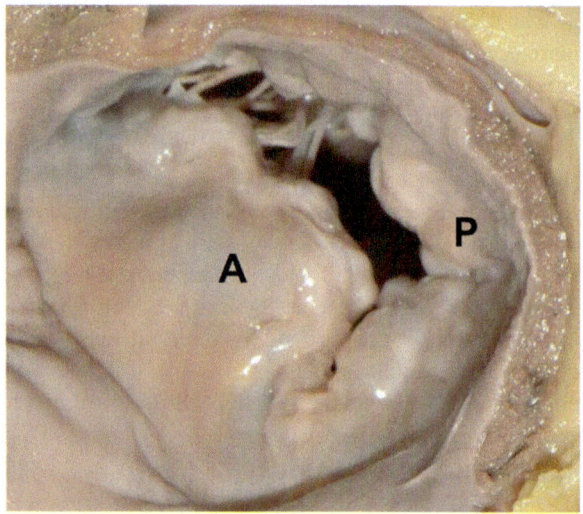

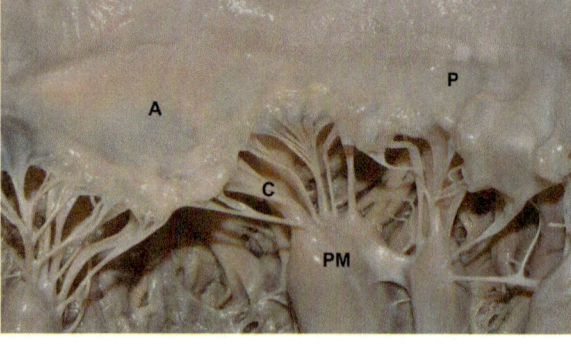

**Fig. 1.3** Gross image of the mitral apparatus showing the anterior (*A*) and posterior (*P*) leaflets, *chordae tendineae* (C) and papillary muscles (*PM*)

## 1.1   The Annulus

The mitral annulus can be described as the junctional zone which separates the left atrium and left ventricle, at the hinge point of the leaflets. From a histological point of view, the mitral annulus is made of a fibrous support and a muscular portion.

The mitral annulus has a mean area of about 7.6 cm², ranging between 5 and 11 cm² [3]. As already described, the annular perimeter of the posterior leaflet is larger than that of the anterior leaflet by a ratio of about 2:1 (Fig. 1.4).

The normal mitral annulus is a dynamic structure that undergoes area changes throughout the cardiac cycle of roughly 23–40% [4], reaching a maximum in late diastole (7.1 ± 1.8 cm²) and a minimum in late systole (5.2 ± 1.6 cm²), thus facilitating both left ventricular filling and competent valve closure. Two-thirds of the reduction in annulus dimensions occurs during atrial systole, i.e., during ventricular presystole, and it is less when the PR interval is reduced, while it is absent in the presence of atrial fibrillation or ventricular pacing.

In a healthy heart the annulus has an almost elliptical shape, which becomes more eccentric during systole compared to diastole [3, 5–8]. In this elliptical configuration, the ratio between the smaller and larger diameters of the annulus amounts to about 0.75 [5–7].

The mitral annulus moves vertically inside the cardiac chambers, according to the phase of the cardiac cycle. During diastole, the annulus moves toward the left atrium, while during systole it moves toward the apex of the heart. The duration and extent of the vertical movement are directly correlated with the state of filling of the left atrium [6, 7, 9, 10]. The systolic motion toward the apex is extremely important for atrial filling; it is also present in cases of atrial fibrillation, and it is correlated with the degree of end-systolic ventricular emptying [6, 7, 10].

During diastole, the mitral annulus moves back toward the left atrium, increasing the velocity of transmitral flow during diastole by about 20% [10, 11].

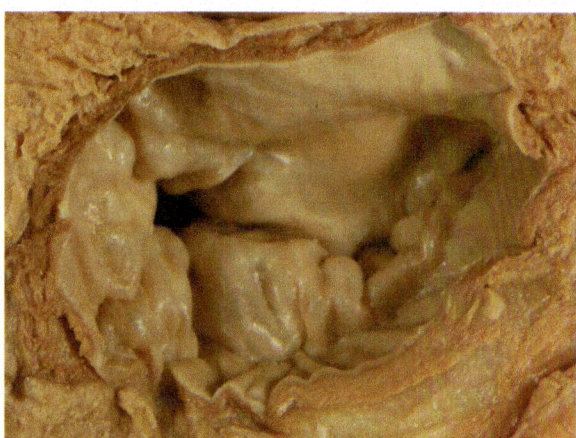

**Fig. 1.4** Anatomical view: the mitral annulus

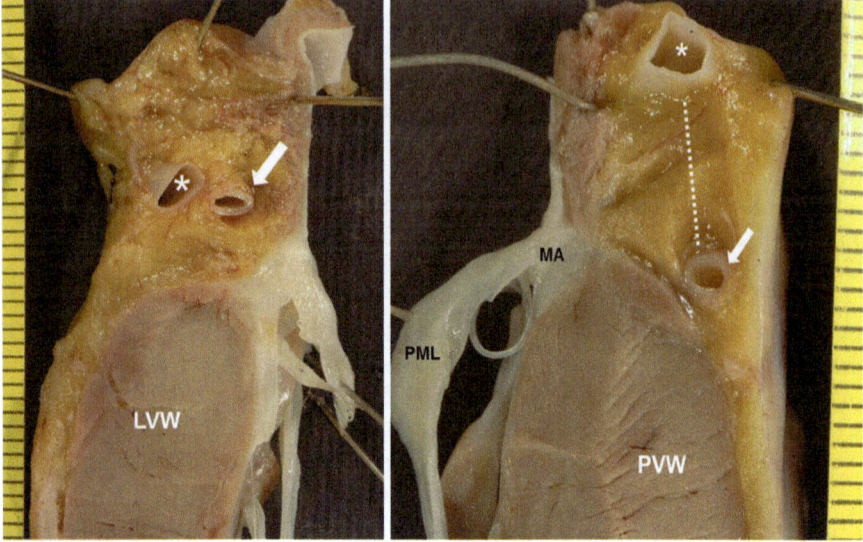

**Fig. 1.5** *Left*, lateral left ventricular wall (*LVW*): the coronary sinus (*asterisk*) is very close to the circumflex coronary artery (*white arrow*). *Right*, posterior left ventricular wall (*PML*): the longer distance (*white dotted line*) between the circumflex coronary artery (*white arrow*) and the coronary sinus (*asterisk*). *MA* mitral annulus, *PML* posterior mitral leaflet

From an interventional cardiology perspective, it was clear from early on that intervention in the mitral annulus was easy to perform in an aggressive manner, because of its anatomical interface with the coronary sinus (Fig. 1.5).

The coronary sinus runs behind the posterior region of the mitral annulus at an average of 10 mm above the mitral annulus. In subjects affected by dilated cardiopathy associated with moderate or severe mitral regurgitation, it has been reported that it runs at about 8 mm above the annulus [12]. The circumflex artery also interacts with the coronary sinus, as it is located right below it (Fig. 1.5). In 80% of the population, the two vessels cross at an average distance of 78 mm from the coronary sinus ostium, and the mean distance between the circumflex artery and coronary sinus at the point of intersection is about 8 mm [12]. This favorable anatomical picture has allowed for the creation of metal devices for transjugular placement, which, once inside the coronary sinus, exert a force capable of remodeling the mitral annulus and reducing the anteroposterior diameter, and subsequently the degree of mitral failure.

## 1.2 Mitral Leaflets

Traditionally, the mitral valve has been presumed to have two leaflets (hence its alternative title of bicuspid valve) usually identified as anterior and posterior, even if it would be more correct to define them anterosuperior and infero-posterior, according to a more appropriate description of their real orientation (Fig. 1.3) [13].

**Fig. 1.6** Photomicrograph of a mitral valve leaflet

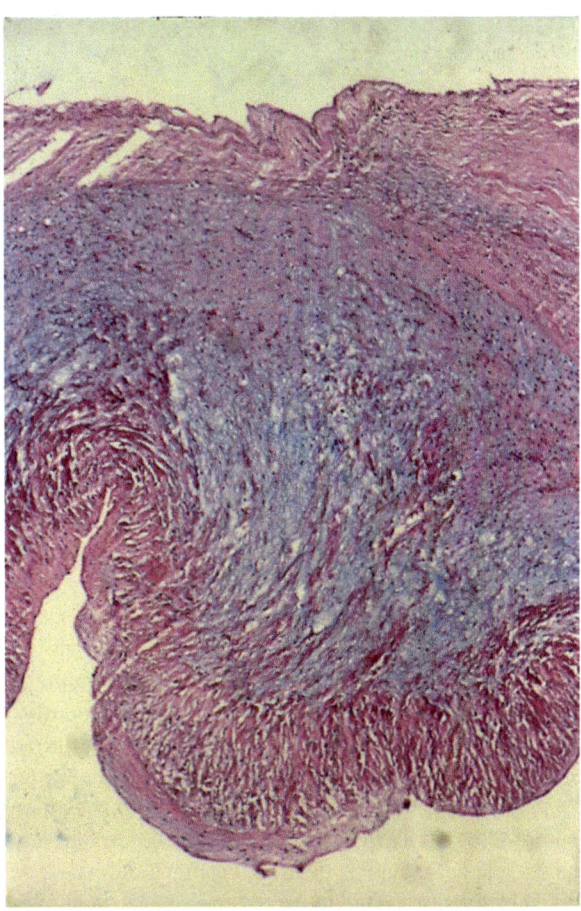

The anterosuperior leaflet is the larger of the two, also called the "large leaflet"; the infero-posterior leaflet is smaller than the other, and it is also called the "small leaflet."

They were firstly described by Vesalius who called them aortic (anterior) and mural (posterior). The thickness of normal leaflets is about 1–2 mm, without any change age-related, and anyway it has to be considered normal up to 4–5 mm.

From a histological viewpoint, the mitral leaflets are formed by a triple layer of tissue (Fig. 1.6):

- A *fibrous layer*, namely, the solid collagen core in direct continuity with the *chordae tendineae*.
- A *spongy layer*, located on the atrial side and forming the contact margins of the leaflets.
- A *fibroelastic layer*, completely covering the leaflets. On the atrial side, this layer is especially rich in elastic fibers, while on the ventricular side, it is thinner and located especially on the anterior leaflet.

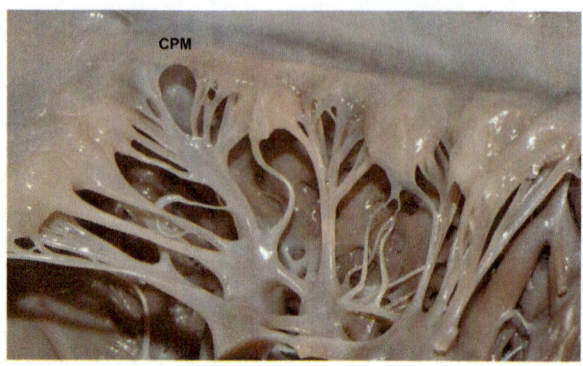

**Fig. 1.7** Gross view of the posteromedial commissure (*CPM*)

From a strictly anatomical view point, the mitral valve is a monoleaflet valve. The valve veil encircles the entire circumference of the annulus [5–7, 11, 14–20]. Two large indentations split the valve veil into an anteromedial leaflet and a posterolateral leaflet. These indentations (posteromedial and anterolateral) take the name of "commissures" (Fig. 1.7).

The aortic leaflet is a compact, semicircular structure. It is positioned anterosuperiorly in the left ventricle. The reason for this name is its fibrous continuity with the left and non-coronary leaflets of the aortic valve. Indeed, unlike the tricuspid valve which is separated by muscle from its counterpart, the mitral valve is immediately adjacent to the aortic valve. The insertion of the aortic leaflet guards about 35–40% of the annular circumference, and it is fibrous with some scarce muscular intrusions. The anterior leaflet is longer than the posterior [5–7, 11, 14–20].

The posterior leaflet is almost always split into three parts by secondary commissures called "scallops" named from the anterolateral to the posterolateral commissures, respectively: P1, P2, and P3 (Fig. 1.8).

This division is due to prolapsing of each scallop into the left atrium regardless of the others, requiring different intervention strategies. At times, even more than three scallops can be found. The anterior leaflet is generally a single veil, but alterations involving only a part of it (ruptured *chordae tendineae*, erosion, etc.) may also be encountered. Therefore, the anterior leaflet is also divided into three parts (A1, A2, A3), corresponding to the posterior leaflet scallops [5–7, 11, 14–20].

The two leaflets meet in an area defined as the "apposition zone," which stretches a few millimeters from the free margin of the leaflets toward the body. The mitral tissue is actually redundant compared to the annular area that it must cover. Leaflet coaptation in the apposition zone greatly reduces the pressure that the valve must bear during systole, as it is simultaneously distributed on all the leaflets facing one another and hence dissipated. The ventricular surface of the leaflets corresponding to the apposition zone is the portion that most of the *chordae tendineae* insert into, hence its name "rough zone" (Fig. 1.9).

The aortic leaflet participates passively in the mechanism of closure of the valve. In fact, its insertion includes all the fibrous tissue of the mitral annulus, which does not participate to the change of the mitral area during the cardiac cycle [21]. On the contrary the posterior leaflet is the key structure in the closure of the valve.

**Fig. 1.8** An atrial view of the mitral valve showing the posterior (mural) leaflet divided in three scallops ($P_1$, $P_2$, $P_3$), the aortic valve (*Ao*) and the aortic leaflet (*AoL*)

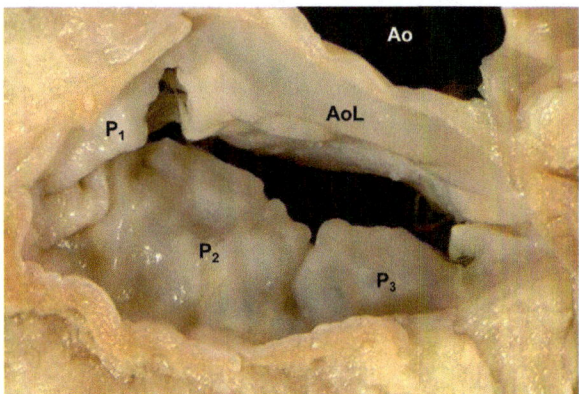

**Fig. 1.9** Ventricular side of the anterior mitral leaflet. Note the "rough zone" (*asterisk*)

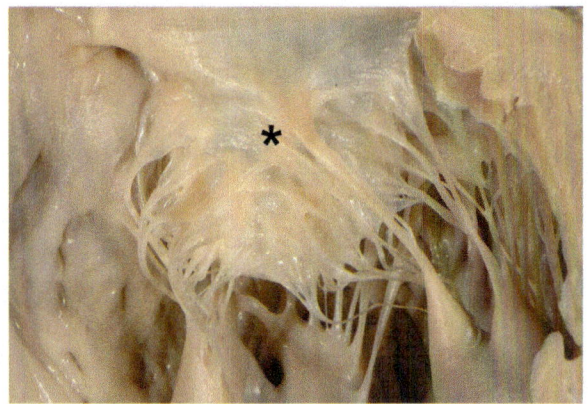

When the posterior annulus contracts, first the scallops coapt together, then the leaflet, moving toward the anterior one, coordinates the valve closure process. This mechanism determines the complete closure (coaptation) and correct apposition (symmetrical overlap) of both leaflets that are essential in preventing regurgitation [1].

During systole, both valve leaflets are concave when observed from the left ventricle, but their shape is actually much more complex. The anterior leaflet is convex toward the ventricle in the regions closest to the free margin, thus giving a sigmoid shape to the leaflets taken as a whole [22, 23]. The valve does not open from the free margin, but from the center of the leaflets, which, starting from a concave configuration, first flatten out and then become convex toward the left ventricle. All this takes place while the extremities are still in contact with one another [22, 24, 25].

Then the free margins separate and move inside the left ventricle. Once they reach their maximum degree of opening, the leaflets show a slow "back-and-forth" movement like that a flag blowing in the wind. Then there is another slight opening pulse triggered by atrial systole. The valve closes, starting with the movements of the leaflets toward the left atrium. The speed at which both leaflets move is different, as the anterior leaflet is about twice the size of the posterior one. This allows the free margin of both leaflets to reach the closing point at the same time [26].

## 1.3     The *Chordae Tendineae* and Papillary Muscles

The papillary muscles originate in the distal third of the ventricular wall and have a variable morphology, although the posteromedial papillary muscle is generally smaller than the anterolateral one. The epicardial fibers in the left ventricle run from the base of the heart to the apex, where they contribute to forming the two papillary muscles, which are marked by a vertical arrangement of the myocardial fibers [20, 22]. The mitral fibers join the papillary muscles by means of *chordae tendineae*, which also run inside the mitral leaflets. These, in turn, are in continuity with the mitral annulus. The vascularization of the papillary muscles differs though: the posteromedial papillary muscle is usually supplied with blood by the right coronary artery, while the anterolateral papillary muscle is supplied by the left anterior descending and the circumflex arteries [20, 27, 28]. The anterolateral and posteromedial papillary muscles contract simultaneously and are innervated by both the parasympathetic and sympathetic systems [29, 30].

Functionally speaking, the *chordae tendineae* are divided into three groups [20, 31] (Fig. 1.10):

- *The primary chordae tendineae* originate near the extremity of the papillary muscles, progressively split, and insert on the extremities of the valve leaflets; their purpose is to prevent prolapse of the valve leaflets during systole.
- *The secondary chordae tendineae* originate in the same area as the primary ones, are thinner and less numerous, and fit into the junction between the rough zone and the smooth zone; their job is to anchor the valve. They are more present in the anterior leaflet and play a key role in the systolic function of the left ventricle.
- *The tertiary chordae tendineae*, also called the *basal chordae*, directly originate from the ventricular wall and head to the posterior leaflet near the annulus.

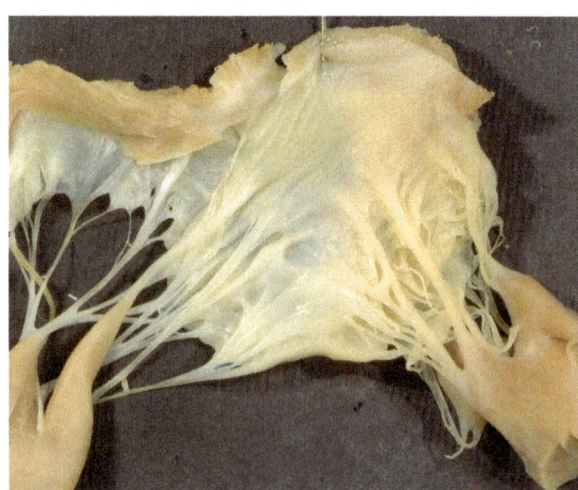

**Fig. 1.10** Ventricular surface of the anterior mitral leaflet: *the chordae tendineae*

The papillary muscles have a major hemodynamic function during the cardiac cycle. During diastole they form a groove allowing inflow into the left ventricle, and during systole they create a route favoring systolic ejection. The shortening and thickening of the papillary muscles with the subsequent increase in volume are associated with a smaller blood content in the left ventricle at the end of systole, and hence an increase in the ejection fraction. The shortening of the papillary muscle during isovolumetric relaxation seems to play a major role in the mechanism that opens the mitral valve, while the stretching in the late diastolic phase seems to favor optimal closing [32].

## References

1. Di Mauro M, Gallina S, D'Amico MA, et al. Functional mitral regurgitation: from normal to pathological anatomy of mitral valve. Int J Cardiol. 2013;163:242–8.
2. Muresian H. The clinical anatomy of the mitral valve. Clin Anat. 2009;22:85–98.
3. Pollick C, Pittman M, Filly K, Fitzgerald PJ, Popp RL. Mitral and aortic valve orifice area in normal subjects and in patients with congestive cardiomyopathy: determination by two dimensional echocardiography. Am J Cardiol. 1982;49:1191–6.
4. van Rijk-Zwikker GL, Delemarre BJ, Huysmans HA. Mitral valve anatomy and morphology: relevance to mitral valve replacement and reconstruction. J Card Surg. 1994;9(2 Suppl):255–61.
5. Silverman ME, Hurst JW. The mitral complex: interaction of the anatomy, physiology, and pathology of the mitral annulus, mitral valve leaflets, chordae tendineae, and papillary muscles. Am Heart J. 1968;76:399.
6. Tsakiris AG, Von Bernuth G, Rastelli GC, et al. Size and motion of the mitral valve annulus in anesthetized intact dogs. J Appl Physiol. 1971;30:611.
7. Ormiston JA, Shah PM, Tei C, et al. Size and motion of the mitral valve annulus in man. I. A two-dimensional echocardiographic method and findings in normal subjects. Circulation. 1981;64:113.
8. Tsakiris AG, Sturm RE, Wood EH. Experimental studies on the mechanisms of closure of cardiac valves with use of roentgen videodensitometry. Am J Cardiol. 1973;32:136–43.
9. Davis PK, Kinmonth JB. The movements of the annulus of the mitral valve. J Cardiovasc Surg. 1963;4:427–31.
10. Keren G, Sonnenblick EH, LeJemtel TH. Mitral annulus motion. Relation to pulmonary venous and transmitral flows in normal subjects and in patients with dilated cardiomyopathy. Circulation. 1988;78:621–9.
11. Toumanidis ST, Sideris DA, Papamichael CM, et al. The role of mitral annulus motion in left ventricular function. Acta Cardiol. 1992;47:331.
12. Choure AJ, Garcia MJ, Hesse B, et al. In vivo analysis of the anatomical relationship of coronary sinus to mitral annulus and left circumflex coronary artery using cardiac multidetector computed tomography: implications for percutaneous coronary sinus mitral annuloplasty. J Am Coll Cardiol. 2006;48:1938–45.
13. Cook AC, Anderson RH. Attitudinally correct nomenclature. Heart. 2002;87:503–6.
14. van Gils FA. The fibrous skeleton in the human heart: embryological and pathogenetic considerations. Virchows Arch A Pathol Anat Histol. 1981;393:61.
15. Davila JC, Palmer TE. The mitral valve: anatomy and pathology for the surgeon. Arch Surg. 1962;84:174.
16. Perloff JK, Roberts WC. The mitral apparatus: functional anatomy of mitral regurgitation. Circulation. 1972;46:227.
17. Fenoglio J Jr, Tuan DP, Wit AL, et al. Canine mitral complex: ultrastructure and electromechanical properties. Circ Res. 1972;31:417.

18. Walmsley R. Anatomy of human mitral valve in adult cadaver and comparative anatomy of the valve. Br Heart J. 1978;40:35.
19. Anderson RH, Wilcox BR. The anatomy of the mitral valve. In: Wells FC, Shapiro LM, editors. Mitral valve disease. Oxford: Butterworth-Heinemann; 1996.
20. Fenster MS, Feldman MD. Mitral regurgitation: an overview. Curr Probl Cardiol. 1995;20:193.
21. Timek TA, Green GR, Tibayan FA, et al. Aorto-mitral annular dynamics. Ann Thorac Surg. 2003;76:1944–50.
22. Karlsson MO, Glasson JR, Bolger AF, Daughters GT, Komeda M, Foppiano LE, Miller DC, Ingels NB Jr. Mitral valve opening in the ovine heart. Am J Physiol. 1998;274:H552–63.
23. Levine RA, Triulzi MO, Harrigan P, Weyman AE. The relationship of mitral annular shape to the diagnosis of mitral valve prolapse. Circulation. 1987;75:756.
24. Sovak M, Lynch PR, Stewart GH. Movement of the mitral valve and its correlation with the first heart sound: selective valvular visualization and high-speed cineradiography in intact dogs. Invest Radiol. 1973;8:150–5.
25. Pohost GM, Dinsmore RE, Rubenstein JJ, et al. The echocardiogram of the anterior leaflet of the mitral valve: correlation with hemodynamic and cineroentgenographic studies in dogs. Circulation. 1975;51:88–97.
26. Tsakiris AG, Gordon DA, Mathieu Y, et al. Motion of both mitral valve leaflets: a cineroentgenographic study in intact dogs. J Appl Physiol. 1975;39:359–66.
27. Luther RR, Meyers SN. Acute mitral insufficiency secondary to ruptured chordae tendineae. Arch Intern Med. 1974;134:568.
28. Voci P, Bilotta F, Caretta Q, Mercanti C, Marino B. Papillary muscle perfusion pattern. A hypothesis for ischemic papillary muscle dysfunction. Circulation. 1995;91:1714–8.
29. Armour JA, Randall WC. Electrical and mechanical activity of papillary muscle. Am J Physiol. 1970;218:1710–7.
30. Cronin R, Armour JA, Randall WC. Function of the in-situ papillary muscle in the canine left ventricle. Circ Res. 1969;25:67–75.
31. Lam JH, Ranganathan N, Wigle ED, Silver MD. Morphology of the human mitral valve. I. Chordae tendineae: a new classification. Circulation. 1970;41:449–58.
32. Marzilli M, Sabbah HN, Lee T, Stein PD. Role of the papillary muscle in opening and closure of the mitral valve. Am J Physiol. 1980;238:H348–54.

# Mitral Stenosis

**2**

Davide Capodanno, Marco Barbanti,
and Corrado Tamburino

## 2.1 Epidemiology

The distribution of mitral stenosis (MS) in the general population is closely associated with rheumatic fever, which is the main cause of MS. Recent data from the World Health Organization (WHO) suggest that acute rheumatic fever and, as a consequence, rheumatic disease affect about 15.6 million people throughout the world. Females are affected more frequently than males, with a ratio ranging between 2:1 and 3:1 [1].

Despite today's drastic reduction in the prevalence of rheumatic fever, MS is still a significant problem in Western countries, where it accounts for about 12% of valvular heart diseases. It is due, in part, to immigration from developing countries [2]. Compared with the past, a change has been observed in the age of onset of the disease, which affects older patients, and most frequently presents with mitral valve calcification [3]. In developing countries, rheumatic fever remains endemic, and MS is a major public health problem.

Patients with severe rheumatic valve damage present with significantly altered hemodynamics, chamber remodeling, and symptoms of heart failure, thereby requiring surgery to replace or, uncommonly, repair the damaged heart valve. If left untreated, subsequent refractory heart failure and/or death is almost inevitable.

It is estimated that rheumatic heart disease causes more than 200,000 deaths annually; predominantly children and young adults living in developing countries [4].

Other causes of MS are severe calcification of valve leaflets, congenital defects of the mitral valve, systemic lupus erythematosus, tumors, left atrial thrombi, vegetations due to endocarditis, and causes linked to prior device implants.

D. Capodanno • M. Barbanti (✉) • C. Tamburino
Ferrarotto Hospital, University of Catania, Via Citelli 6, 95124 Catania, Italy
e-mail: mbarbanti83@gmail.com

© Springer International Publishing AG 2018
C. Tamburino et al. (eds.), *Percutaneous Treatment of Left Side Cardiac Valves*,
https://doi.org/10.1007/978-3-319-59620-4_2

## 2.2    Pathophysiology

MS is an obstruction of blood flow from the left atrium to the left ventricle and is generally caused by rheumatic heart disease [5, 6].

The development of the pathology secondary to rheumatic disease is very slow and manifests clinically after about 20 years.

The cause of rheumatic fever is beta-hemolytic group A streptococcus. Streptococcal antigens react with the human immune system and lead to the formation of antibodies, which, besides destroying the bacterial cells, attack valve tissues, as well, due to cross-reactivity with some heart valve components. The bacterial components involved are hyaluronic acid in the bacterial capsule and the streptococcus M antigen and its peptides [7, 8]. During the chronic phase of rheumatic disease, markers typical of inflammation can be found, and it has been observed that their values have a direct correlation with the severity of valve involvement and the quantity of valve scars [9]. Besides affecting the mitral valve, rheumatic disease can potentially cause pancarditis leading to myocardial, endocardial, and pericardial damage [5, 10]. In most cases (60%), only the mitral valve is affected, followed by the involvement of both the aortic and mitral valves (30%); the involvement of the aortic valve alone is less frequent (10%).

The pathognomonic lesions of rheumatic disease consist of commissural fusion, valve leaflet fibrosis and retraction, and shortening and fusion of the *chordae tendineae* [11] (Fig. 2.1). The *chordae tendineae* can suffer from such a serious shortening that the valve leaflets merge with the papillary muscles. Calcifications are much more common and severe in males, elderly patients, and patients with a higher transvalvular gradient [10]. Calcifications of the mitral annulus may lead to valve sclerosis and stenosis. The anterior mitral leaflet can thicken and become stiff, but the obstruction of ventricular filling is also the result of the calcification of the posterior leaflet.

In patients affected with MS, the diastolic pressure gradient between the left atrium and left ventricle typically rises as stenosis worsens [12–15]. In patients with

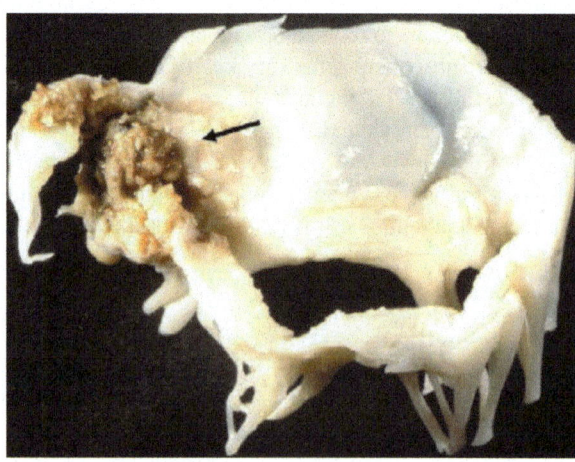

**Fig. 2.1** Surgically resected mitral valve. Note leaflet retraction, *chordae* shortening, and calcific ulceration of the anterolateral commissure (*arrow*)

MS alone, the size of the left ventricle is either normal or reduced, the end-diastole pressure is typically reduced [12, 16, 17], and, hence, the maximum filling flow is reduced as well. Cardiac output is reduced due to the narrowing of the flow into the left ventricle, while the mass of the left ventricle is normal in most patients [16].

Since the mitral transvalvular flow depends on the cardiac output and heart rate, if the latter is high, there is a reduction in ventricular filling time during diastole, leading to an increase in the transvalvular gradient and, consequently, in left atrial pressure [14, 18]. Thus, it is important to monitor the heart rhythm in MS patients. Patients with a normal sinus rhythm have, on average, lower atrial pressures than patients with atrial fibrillation [19, 20]. Sinus rhythm increases the flow through the stenotic valve and helps maintain an adequate cardiac output. The onset of atrial fibrillation is associated with a 20% reduction in cardiac output and, if there is rapid ventricular response, leads to a sharp rise in left atrial pressure and, as a result, dyspnea and pulmonary edema [5, 19, 20].

The chronic rise in left atrial pressure leads to atrial dilation and fibrillation and, together with this, the formation of atrial thrombi. Atrial muscle fiber disarray, abnormal conduction velocity, and inhomogeneous refractory periods are the causes leading to the onset of atrial fibrillation, which is present in about half of the patients affected with MS [10, 17, 21].

In patients with mild or moderate MS, pulmonary arterial pressure is usually normal or slightly elevated at rest, increasing during exercise. In severe MS, there is a rise in pulmonary arterial pressure even at rest, due to elevated left atrial pressure with normal pulmonary vascular resistance ("passive" postcapillary pulmonary hypertension).

When the left atrial pressure exceeds 30 mmHg, plasma oncotic pressure cannot ensure effective elimination of transudate, and this leads to extravasation of fluids in the interstitial and alveolar spaces (pulmonary edema). However, a long-standing increase in left atrial pressure may cause major changes in pulmonary vascular resistance, which results in pulmonary arterial vasoconstriction and remodeling ("reactive" postcapillary pulmonary hypertension). The increase in right ventricular afterload due to pulmonary hypertension leads to right ventricular failure and peripheral congestion [16]. Therefore, the changes occurring in pulmonary circulation in the early phases of MS are aimed at protecting it against pulmonary edema but, in the long run, damage the right ventricle, causing congestive heart failure. Finally, if untreated, MS leads to irreversible changes in the pulmonary vascular bed.

## 2.3  Diagnosis

### 2.3.1  Noninvasive Diagnosis

The first diagnostic approach to patients with MS includes the clinical history, physical examination, electrocardiogram, chest x-ray, and echocardiogram [22, 23].

The symptoms can have varying degrees of severity and are multiple: dyspnea, palpitation, asthenia, abdominal tension, chest pain, and hemoptysis. These are matched by other important circulatory consequences such as the redistribution of pulmonary blood flow (increase in flow in the upper lobes compared with the lower ones) and systemic blood flow (reduction in renal flow) [24]. Patients in an advanced phase of the disease, often with concurrent pulmonary hypertension and right ventricular overload, typically have cyanosis of the lips, nose, and cheekbones (malar flush, mitral facies) and cold and cyanotic hands. In severe forms, arterial pulse is small.

The most important auscultation findings for a diagnosis are accentuated first heart sound ($S_1$), opening snap (OS), low-pitched mid-diastolic rumble, and a presystolic murmur. These signs are perceived in the mitral auscultation area and even better if the patient is resting on the left side. These findings, however, may also be present in patients with nonrheumatic mitral valve obstruction (e.g., left atrial myxoma) and can be absent in the presence of severe pulmonary hypertension, low cardiac output, and a heavily calcified immobile mitral valve. A shorter second heart sound ($S_2$)–OS interval and longer duration of diastolic rumble indicate more severe MS. An $S_2$–OS interval of less than 0.08 s implies severe MS [24].

The electrocardiogram is usually completely normal in mild forms of the disease. In more severe MS, signs of left atrial overload ("mitralic P") (Fig. 2.2) and of hypertrophy and right ventricular overload can be seen when MS is associated with pulmonary hypertension. Evidence of atrial fibrillation is also frequent.

In the anteroposterior (AP) and laterolateral (LL) views, the chest x-ray can be entirely normal or at times show aspecific and indirect signs both in the cardiac silhouette and in the pulmonary fields. In the AP view, the heart may have a roughly triangular shape resulting from an increase in the volume of the atrium and left atrial appendage (LAA), the pulmonary artery, and the right ventricle and atrium. The radiologic picture of the lungs varies with the progression of the mitral disease and hemodynamic impairment (Fig. 2.3).

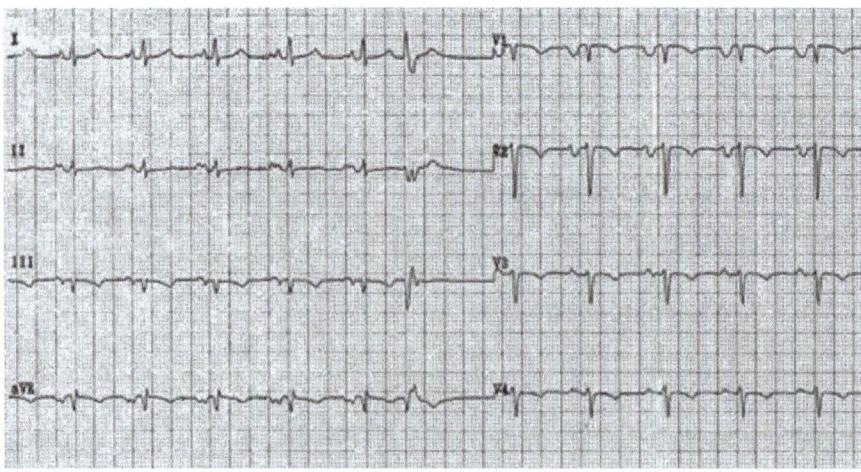

**Fig. 2.2** ECG showing the typical signs of left atrial enlargement (mitral P waves)

**Fig. 2.3** Chest x-ray in anteroposterior view. Modification of cardiac silhouette, increased in volume and with a coarsely triangular shape, with signs of pulmonary venous congestion in both lower lobes

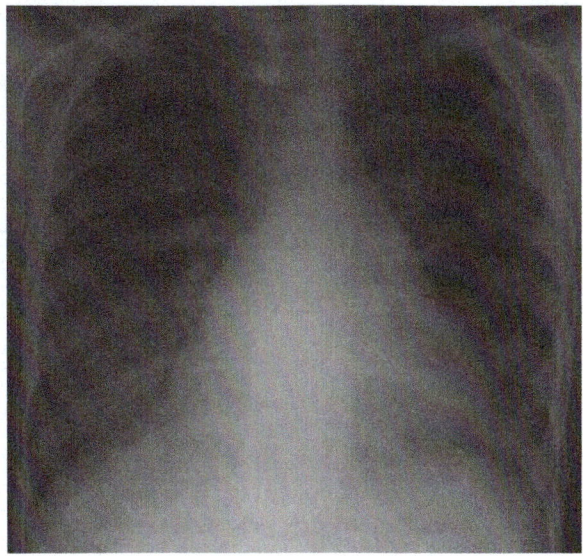

The gold standard for MS diagnosis is 2D echocardiography with Doppler [22–25]. In MS, echocardiography must define:

- The morphology of the valve leaflets and subvalvular apparatus
- The severity of the stenosis
- The dimensions of the left atrium (LA)
- The presence of thrombi in the LA and/or LAA
- Pulmonary artery pressure
- Associated valve defects
- Left and right ventricular function
- The therapeutic indication

The morphological alterations of the leaflets and subvalvular apparatus can be assessed by 2D echocardiography in the parasternal and apical views. The echocardiography elements characterizing MS are thickening, reduced leaflet mobility, and calcification. The narrowing of the diastolic leaflet opening due to "doming" (Fig. 2.4) of the anterior leaflet and reduced or no mobility of the posterior leaflet [25] can be visualized on the parasternal long-axis view, while reduced valve opening with the resulting reduction in the relative valve area can be seen on the parasternal short-axis view (Fig. 2.5). In M-mode, reduced valve opening is indicated by the reduced "EF-slope" of the anterior mitral leaflet and by the movement of the posterior leaflet in accordance with the anterior leaflet. The sensitivity and specificity of 2D echocardiography in assessing mitral valve anatomy are 70% and 100%, respectively, when compared with anatomic and pathologic findings. Sensitivity rises up to 90% if the exam is integrated with transesophageal echocardiogram or real-time three-dimensional (3D) ultrasound [26, 27].

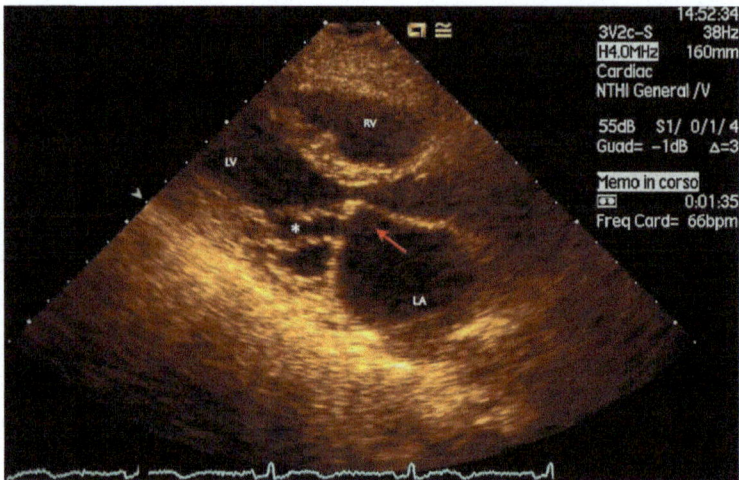

**Fig. 2.4** Transthoracic echocardiogram, parasternal long-axis view; stenotic mitral valve with reduced diastolic excursion, typical diastolic doming shape (*arrow*) and fusion of subvalvular apparatus (*asterisk*). *LA* left atrium, *LV* left ventricle, *RV* right ventricle

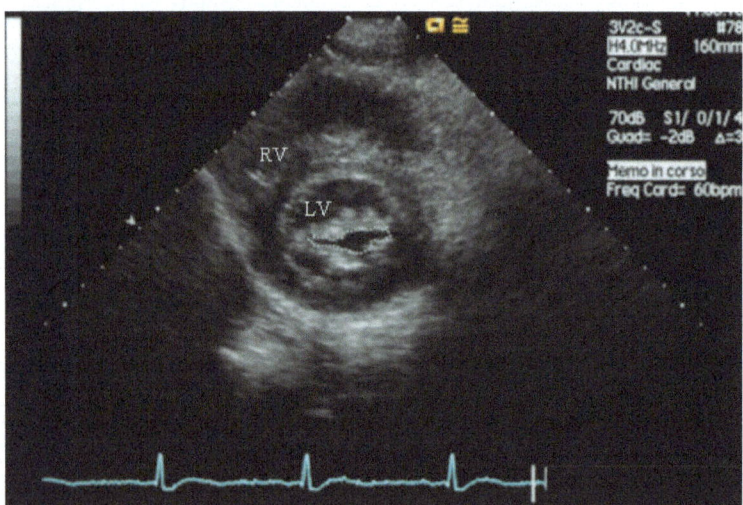

**Fig. 2.5** Transthoracic echocardiogram, parasternal short-axis view, showing planimetric area; stenotic mitral valve orifice (*dotted line*) with typical "fishmouth" shape. *LV* left ventricle, *RV* right ventricle

The description of the morphological alterations in the valvular apparatus in MS is codified in the Wilkins score [28]. It takes into account four parameters (leaflet mobility, leaflet thickening, remodeling of the subvalvular apparatus, and calcifications), and each is given a score of 1–4 (Table 2.1). The single values are summed together to get a score reflecting the severity of valve damage. These characteristics

**Table 2.1** The Wilkins score

| Degree | Mobility | Subvalvular thickening | Leaflet thickening | Calcifications |
|---|---|---|---|---|
| 1 | Extremely mobile valves with reduction in excursions only at the tips of the leaflets | Minimal thickening below mitral leaflets | Leaflets with almost normal thickness (4–5 mm) | Single hyperechogenic zone |
| 2 | Middle and basal portions of the leaflets have normal structure and mobility | Thickening of the *chordae* stretching up to a third of their length | Normal leaflets in central portions, considerable thickening of margins (5–8 mm) | Hyperechogenic multiple areas limited to leaflet margins |
| 3 | Valve continues to move forward during diastole, mainly at its base | Thickening extending up to the distal third of the *chordae* | Thickening extending through the entire leaflet (5–8 mm) | Hyperechogenicity extending in the medial portion of the leaflets |
| 4 | No or minimal forward motion of the leaflets during diastole | Massive thickening and shortening of the *chordae* extending below the papillary muscles | Major thickening of the entire tissue of leaflets (>8–10 mm) | Intense hyperechogenicity covering most of the leaflet tissue |

**Table 2.2** Cormier's anatomical score

| Echocardiography group | Anatomy of the mitral valve |
|---|---|
| 1 | Noncalcified mobile anterior leaflet |
|  | Mild subvalvular disease (thin *chordae* ≥ 10 mm long) |
| 2 | Noncalcified mobile anterior leaflet |
|  | Severe subvalvular disease (thickened *chordae* < 0 mm long) |
| 3 | Calcification of mitral valve of any extent, as assessed by fluoroscopy, whatever the state of the subvalvular apparatus |

are important for the timing and type of intervention to be performed [28–30]. While not the sole one, the Wilkins score is the one most frequently used to assess the degree of damage to the valve apparatus. Other scores used are Cormier's score [31] (Table 2.2) and Reid's score [32] (Table 2.3).

The severity of MS is defined based on the value of the mean transvalvular gradient and mitral valve area (MVA).

The mean transvalvular gradient can be measured accurately and with a high degree of reproducibility by continuous wave (CW) Doppler through the mitral valve using the simplified Bernoulli equation $P = 4v^2$ [26, 33, 34], where $P$ is the mean transvalvular gradient and $v$ is the mitral inflow velocity. If pulsed wave (PW) Doppler is used, the sample volume should be applied at or right after the tip of the leaflets [26]. The mean gradient has a greater correlation with the hemodynamic findings, while the maximum gradient, being derived from the peak mitral inflow

**Table 2.3** Reid's score

|                                                                    | Degree   | Score |
|--------------------------------------------------------------------|----------|-------|
| Leaflet motion: *H/L* ratio[a]                                     |          |       |
| ≥0.45                                                              | Mild     | 0     |
| 0.26–0.44                                                          | Moderate | 1     |
| ≤0.25                                                              | Severe   | 2     |
| Leaflet thickening: mitral valve/aortic wall                       |          |       |
| 1.5–2                                                              | Mild     | 0     |
| 2.1–4.9                                                            | Moderate | 1     |
| ≥5                                                                 | Severe   | 2     |
| Subvalvular disease                                                |          |       |
| Thin, faintly visible *chordae tendineae*                          | –        | 0     |
| Areas of increased density equal to endocardium                    | –        | 1     |
| Areas denser than endocardium with thickened *chordae tendineae*   | –        | 2     |
| Commissural calcium                                                |          |       |
| Homogeneous density of MV orifice                                  | –        | 0     |
| Increased density of anterior/posterior commissure                 | –        | 1     |
| Increased density of both commissures                              | –        | 2     |

[a]*H* (height)/*L* (length) = anterior leaflet excursion

velocity, is affected by LA compliance and left ventricular diastolic function [16] and plays a minor role in determining the severity of MS. Based on the mean gradient values, MS is mild when the gradient is <5 mmHg, moderate when it ranges between 5 and 10 mmHg, and severe when it is >10 mmHg [26] (Fig. 2.6) (Table 2.4). The limitations imposed by the transmitral gradient in determining the severity of stenosis lie in the fact that it is affected by heart rate and by concurrent mitral regurgitation, if present [30].

MVA can be calculated with various methods, each of which offers advantages and disadvantages. Bidimensional planimetry of the mitral orifice offers the benefit of being a direct measurement of MVA and, unlike other methods, is not affected by conditions related to the flow, compliance of the heart chambers, or presence of other associated valve diseases. Two-dimensional planimetric study of MVA has been shown to be better correlated with the anatomical valve area calculated on explanted valves [35]. The planimetric measurements are obtained directly on the mitral orifice in mid-diastole, including the open commissures, in the parasternal short-axis view (Fig. 2.5). However, this method is negatively affected by the quality of the image and cannot be performed accurately in patients with a scarce acoustic window, or in the presence of a severely distorted valve anatomy, often due to the presence of calcifications [26]. Recent studies suggest that 3D real-time echocardiography and 2D-guided biplane imaging are useful in optimizing measurements to improve reproducibility [27]. Based on MVA values, MS is defined as mild when the area is >1.5 cm$^2$, moderate when the area ranges between 1.5 and 1 cm$^2$, and severe when it is <1 cm$^2$ [26] (Table 2.4).

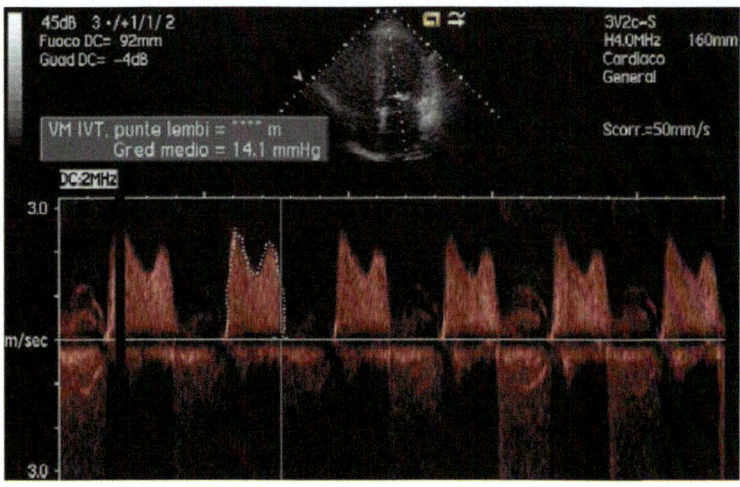

**Fig. 2.6** Severe MS. Transmitral diastolic flow. Continuous wave Doppler gives a mean transvalvular gradient of 14.1 mmHg

**Table 2.4** Criteria for the assessment of MS severity

| Severity of MS | Mean gradient (mmHg) | Mitral valve area (cm$^2$) | Systolic pulmonary artery pressure (mmHg) |
|---|---|---|---|
| Mild | <5 | >1.5 | <30 |
| Moderate | 5–10 | 1.5–1.0 | 30–50 |
| Severe | >10 | <1.0 | >50 |

Another way to determine valve area is by the diastolic pressure half-time (PHT) method, which is based on the hemodynamic principle that the reduction in the gradient between the atrium and ventricle is inversely proportional to the extent of valve stenosis and hence to valve area (Fig. 2.7). MVA is obtained from the following empirical formula [26, 36]:

$$MVA = 220 / PHT$$

PHT is easy to obtain, but is affected by other factors, such as the presence of aortic regurgitation, LA compliance, left ventricular diastolic function [37], or prior mitral valvotomy [38].

MVA can still be calculated with the continuity equation [26, 39], based on the principle of mass conservation, by which the transmitral flow volume should be equal to the systolic output, i.e., the flow through the aorta. By measuring the aortic area, the aortic flow velocity integral, and the integral of the velocity through the mitral valve, the mitral area can be calculated. The continuity equation cannot be used in the case of atrial fibrillation or major mitral or aortic valve failure [26].

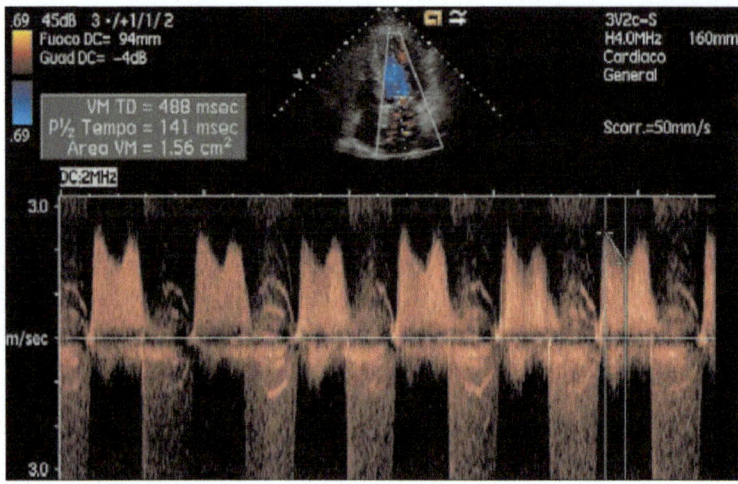

**Fig. 2.7** Severe MS. Transmitral diastolic flow. Mitral valve area (MVA) measured using the pressure half-time (PHT) method

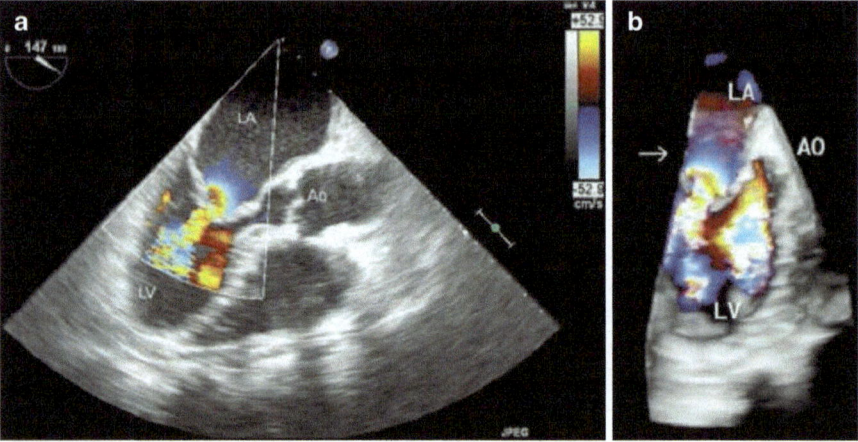

**Fig. 2.8** Transesophageal echocardiogram in a bidimensional long-axis view (147°) (**a**) and three-dimensional full-volume acquisition (**b**), showing a hemispherical convergence area (*arrow*) upon the stenotic mitral leaflets. *LA* left atrium, *LV* left ventricle, *Ao* aorta

Another method to calculate MVA is the proximal isovelocity surface area (PISA). The velocities of a flow approaching a stenotic or diseased orifice gradually rise and spread in a concentric fashion, with an almost hemispherical shape, as shown by color Doppler on the atrial side of the mitral valve (Fig. 2.8). With this method, MVA is obtained from the following formula:

$$\text{MVA} = \mathbf{p}\left(r^2\right)\left(V_{\text{aliasing}}\right) / \text{peak}\, V_{\text{mitral}} \times \alpha / 180°$$

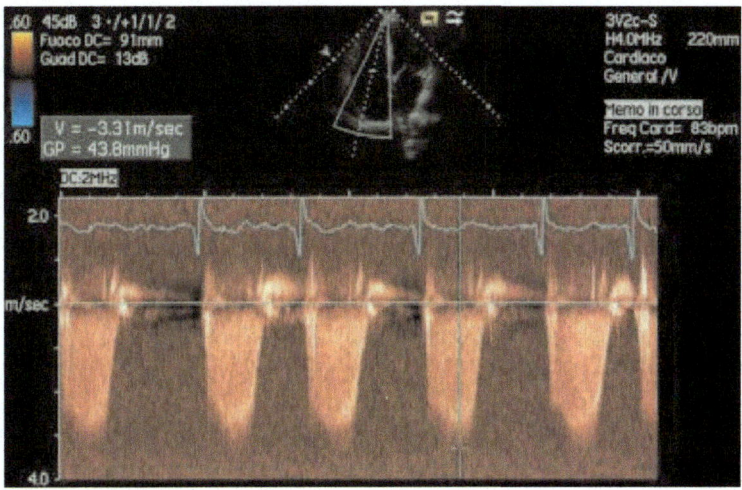

**Fig. 2.9** Measurement of systolic pulmonary artery pressure (sPAP) using continuous wave Doppler across the tricuspid valve in a patient with severe MS

where *r* is the hemispherical convergence radius (cm), $V_{aliasing}$ is the aliasing velocity (cm/s), peak $V_{mitral}$ is the peak CW-Doppler of mitral flow velocity (cm/s), and $\alpha$ is the opening angle of the mitral leaflets compared with the flow direction [40]. This method can also be used in the presence of major mitral failure.

Doppler echocardiography is needed to assess MS patients to determine systolic pulmonary artery pressure (sPAP) from the maximum tricuspid regurgitation velocity [26, 41] (Fig. 2.9). The increase in sPAP is an indicator of hemodynamic impairment. MS classification based on the estimated sPAP values defines MS as mild when sPAP is <30 mmHg, moderate when sPAP is between 30 and 50 mmHg, and severe when sPAP is >50 mmHg [26] (Table 2.4).

Transesophageal echocardiogram (TEE) is not a routine examination unless the quality of the transthoracic echocardiogram (TTE) is unsatisfactory [22]. TEE is recommended before mitral valvuloplasty for [22, 23]:

- Detailed assessment of morphological alterations in the valvular and subvalvular apparatus.
- Search for thrombi, particularly in the interatrial septum (transseptal puncture site) (Fig. 2.10) or on the left atrium roof, as they are absolute contraindications for percutaneous commissurotomy, while the presence of thrombi in the left atrial appendage is considered by some authors as a relative contraindication (Fig. 2.11).
- Morphological characterization of the left atrial appendage, which typically has a "hull's horn" shape, though it can be bilobate or trilobite, with lobes located on different planes. Therefore, the search for thrombi must be done with multiplane probes.

**Fig. 2.10**
Transesophageal echocardiogram, showing a thrombotic formation adherent to the left side of the interatrial septum. *LA* left atrium, *RA* right atrium

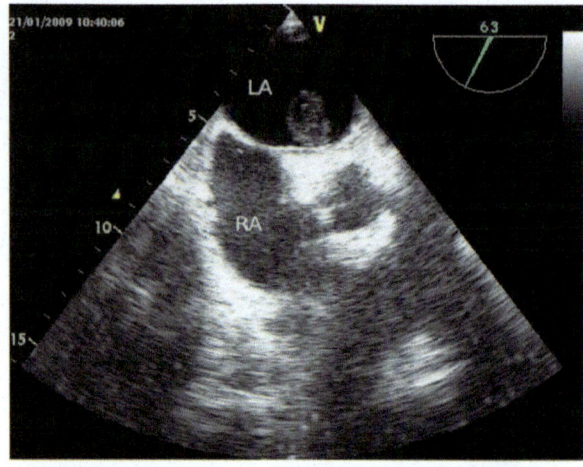

**Fig. 2.11**
Transesophageal echocardiogram, showing a thrombotic formation in the left atrial appendage

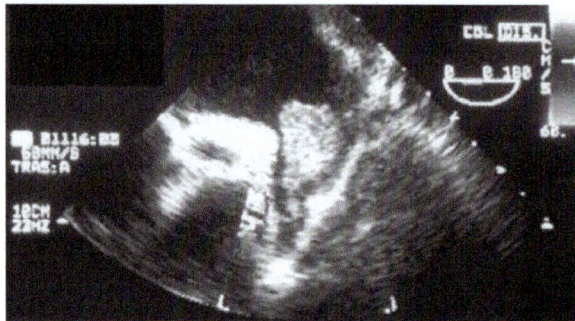

- Assessment of the Doppler velocities in the left atrial appendage; if values are <40 cm/s, there is a correlation with an increased risk of thromboembolism (Fig. 2.12).
- Identification of spontaneous echo contrast, a predictor of an increased risk of thromboembolism (Fig. 2.13).
- More accurate assessment of the severity of the associated mitral regurgitation (Fig. 2.14).

Three-dimensional echocardiography, one of the most significant developments of the last decade in the field of cardiac imaging, provides significant advantages in the noninvasive diagnosis of MS [42]. Three-dimensional reconstruction offers unique orientations of the intracardiac structures that cannot be otherwise obtained with standard 2D views, thereby providing a unique "en face" view and morphologic analysis of the entire mitral valve, including annulus, leaflets, and anatomic relationship to other nearby structures (Fig. 2.15). The ventricular view of a stenotic mitral valve also provides significant additional information, mainly to subvalvular apparatus involvement and in determining the optimal plane of the smallest mitral

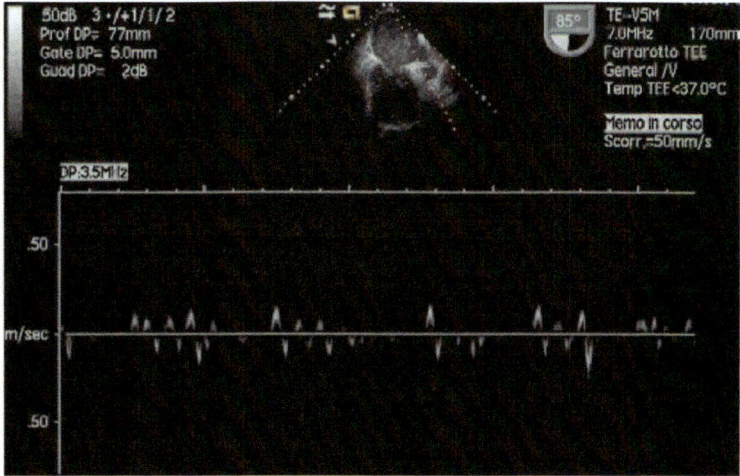

**Fig. 2.12** PW Doppler flow velocity in the left atrial appendage <40 cm/s

**Fig. 2.13** Intense
smokelike effect in the left
atrium (LA)

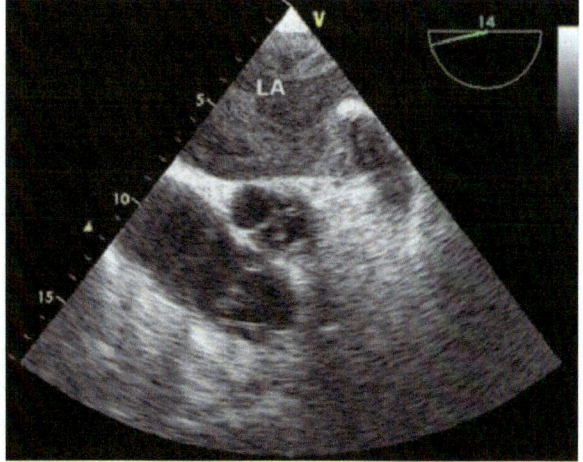

valve orifice area (Fig. 2.16), which helps operators in determining the actual anatomic valve area, especially in cases of funnel-shaped MS. A comparative study of
3D-echo mitral planimetry (Fig. 2.17) versus the invasive measurement of the mitral
valve area, based on the Gorlin formula, has shown a greater accuracy of 3D-echo
planimetry for the assessment of the mitral valve area [43], thereby emphasizing the
additional role that 3D echocardiography can play in determining the severity of
rheumatic MS. 3D echocardiography can also be useful during percutaneous balloon mitral valvuloplasty (commissural splitting and leaflets tears) (Fig. 2.18) and
in determining the Wilkins score [42, 44] (Table 2.5).

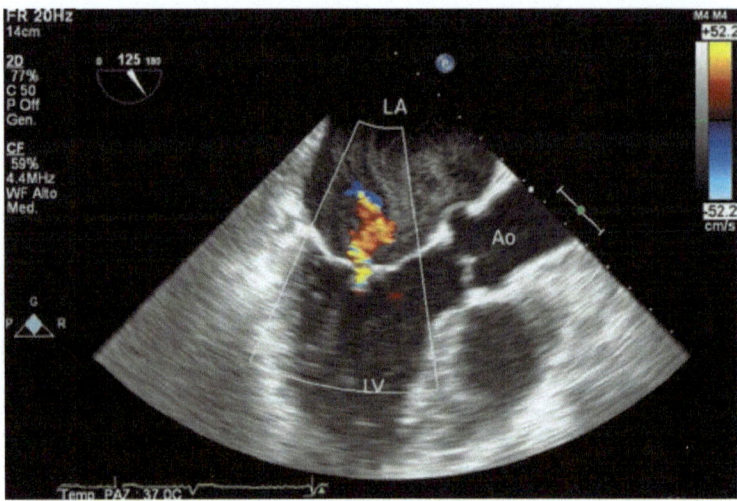

**Fig. 2.14** Transesophageal echocardiogram in a long-axis view (125°) showing a rheumatic MS with associated mild mitral regurgitation. Intense smokelike effect is also evident in the left atrium (*LA*). *LV* left ventricle, *Ao* aorta

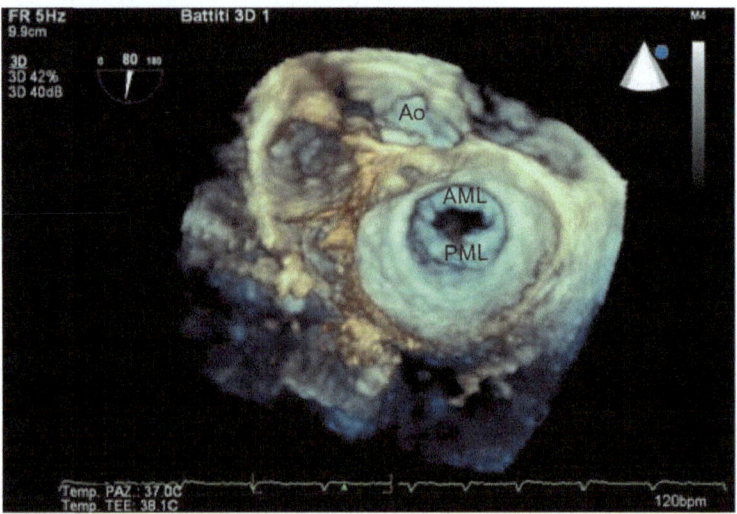

**Fig. 2.15** Three-dimensional transesophageal echocardiogram showing a moderately stenotic mitral valve from an atrial view. *Ao* aorta, *AML* anterior mitral leaflet, *PML* posterior mitral leaflet

Recently, Anwar et al. [45, 46] reported a feasible and reproducible 3D score for predicting outcomes following percutaneous valvuloplasty when assessing MS patients. This score, based on the Wilkins score, and favorably comparable with it, divides each leaflet into three scallops (anterolateral, A1 and P1; middle, A2 and P2; and posteromedial, A3 and P3), which are scored separately. The subvalvular

**Fig. 2.16** Real-time three-dimensional transesophageal echocardiography showing a stenotic mitral valve from a ventricular view. The fibrocalcific involvement of the subvalvular apparatus with thickened *chordae tendineae* is evident. *Ao* aorta, *PML* posterior mitral leaflet

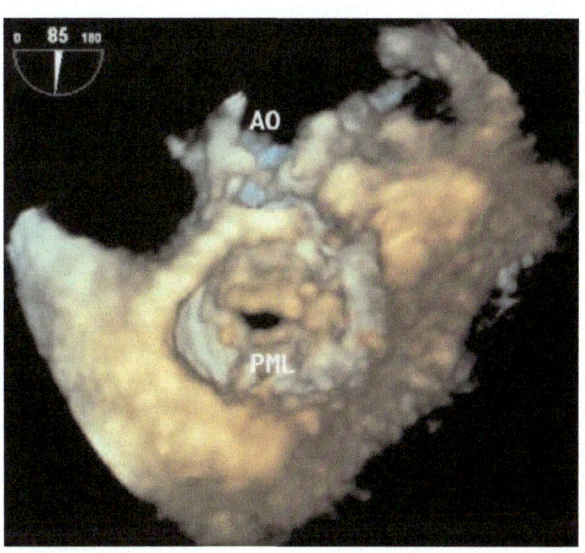

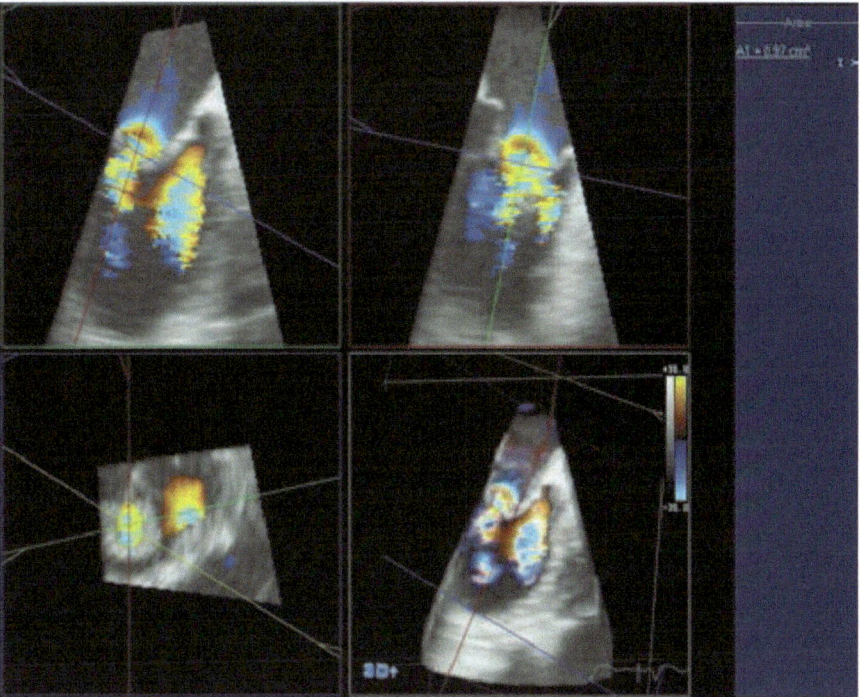

**Fig. 2.17** Mitral valve orifice area calculated with QLab post-processing software (Philips Healthcare, Andover, MA, USA)

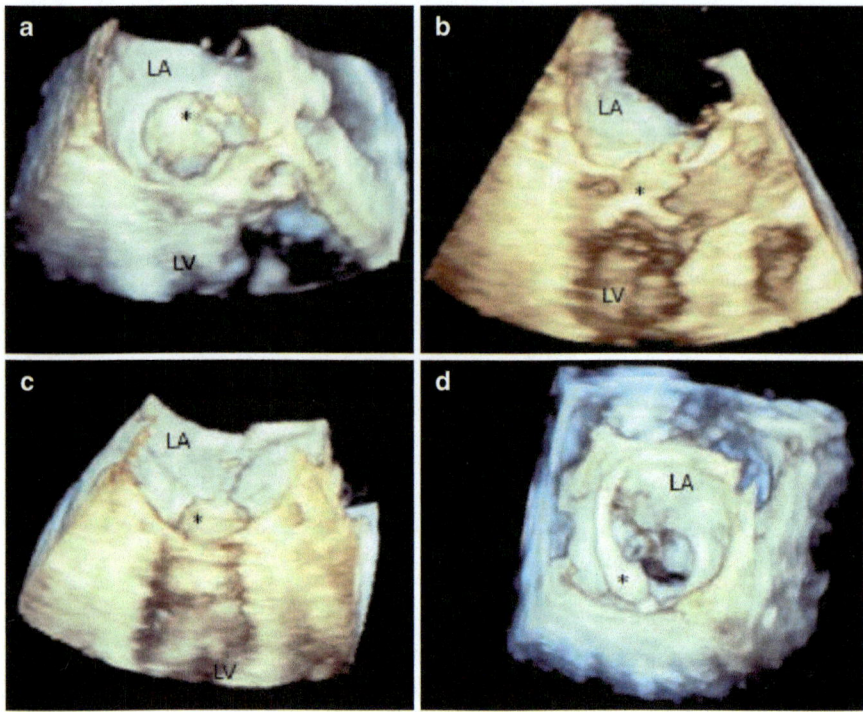

**Fig. 2.18** Real-time three-dimensional transesophageal echocardiography during mitral valvulo-plasty. (**a-c**) Showing Inoue balloon (*asterisk*) inflated across the mitral valve in different echocar-diographic views. (**d**) is during balloon deflation. *LA* left atrium, *LV* left ventricle

**Table 2.5** Advantages and limits of the various methods for determining mitral valve area

| Method | Influence of hemodynamic conditions | Acoustic window needed | Useful after valvuloplasty | Invasive technique |
|---|---|---|---|---|
| 2D planimetry | − | ++ | + | − |
| PHT | ++ | ++ | − | − |
| PISA | + | ++ | + | − |
| RT3D | − | ++ | ++ | − |
| GORLIN | ++ | − | ++ | ++ |

*2D* two-dimensional, *PHT* pressure half-time, *PISA* proximal isovelocity surface area, *RT3D* real-time three-dimensional, − no advantage, + small advantage, ++ great advantage

apparatus is divided into three cut sections of the anterior and posterior *chordae* at three levels: proximal (valve level), middle, and distal (papillary muscle level). Each cut section is scored separately for chordal thickness and separation (Table 2.6). The individual 3D score points of leaflets and subvalvular apparatus are summed to calculate the total 3D score, ranging from 0 to 31 points. A total score of mild MV

**Table 2.6** Three-dimensional echocardiographic score

| | Anterior leaflet | | | Posterior leaflet | | |
|---|---|---|---|---|---|---|
| | A1 | A2 | A3 | P1 | P2 | P3 |
| Thickness (0–6)[a] | 0–1 | 0–1 | 0–1 | 0–1 | 0–1 | 0–1 |
| Mobility (0–6)[b] | 0–1 | 0–1 | 0–1 | 0–1 | 0–1 | 0–1 |
| Calcification (0–10)[c] | 0–2 | 0–1 | 0–2 | 0–2 | 0–1 | 0–2 |
| | Subvalvular apparatus | | | | | |
| | Proximal third | | Middle third | | Distal third | |
| Thickness (0–3)[a] | 0–1 | | 0–1 | | 0–1 | |
| Separation (0–6)[d] | 0, 1, 2 | | 0, 1, 2 | | 0, 1, 2 | |

[a]Thickness: 0 = normal, 1 = thickened
[b]Mobility: 0 = normal, 1 = limited
[c]Calcification: 0 = no, 1–2 = calcified
[d]Separation: 0 = normal, 1 = partial, 2 = no

involvement was defined as <8 points, moderate MV involvement as 8–13 points, and severe MV involvement as ≥14 points [45, 46].

The 3D score has proven to be of significant additional value for a detailed assessment of rheumatic mitral valve stenosis [46]. The single benefits can be summarized as follows:

1. Visualization of leaflets, with regard to the mobility and thickness of each leaflet scallop. 3D echocardiography has proven to be more accurate in the morphological assessment of the posterior leaflet compared with standard 2D echocardiography, as it is often smaller, less mobile, and more retracted compared with the anterior one.
2. Leaflet calcification. Determining leaflet calcification according to the Wilkins score depends on the bright areas and the extension of calcification along the leaflet length. Therefore, 2D echocardiography requires multiple cut planes to determine the calcifications of all the scallops of both leaflets. 3D echocardiography is able to assess the size and distribution of calcifications in the various leaflet subunits in a single view, which is usually the "en face" view of the mitral valve.
3. Subvalvular apparatus. The 3D score provides detailed information on the extent of rheumatic damage of the *chordae tendineae* (thickness and separation) that is not easily obtained by most bidimensional scoring systems, especially for separation.
4. Score applicability. Compared with the Wilkins score, the 3D score is very simple and easy to apply, particularly for less-experienced operators, since the mitral apparatus is analyzed in its single components, which are identified using numbers. This was evident from good interobserver and intraobserver agreements for most of the score components.
5. Score approach. The 3D score can be used during assessment with either TTE or TEE (Fig. 2.19).

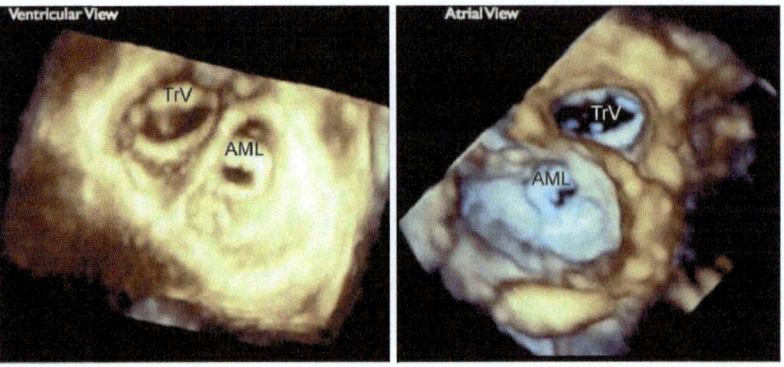

**Fig. 2.19** Three-dimensional transthoracic echocardiography showing a rheumatic stenotic mitral valve. *AML* anterior mitral leaflet, *TrV* tricuspid valve

### 2.3.2 Invasive Diagnosis

Left and right cardiac catheterization plays a major role in determining the severity of MS and assessing the degree of hemodynamic impairment. Unlike echocardiography, catheterization gives direct measurements of pressure in the atrium and left ventricle, which are necessary for obtaining the transmitral gradient [47] and pulmonary artery pressure and estimating pulmonary vascular resistance values, which give an idea of the impact of MS on pulmonary circulation. The Gorlin equation, in which the severity of an obstruction depends on the flow and gradient, allows for the calculation of valve area (*A*) [48]:

$$A = F / k \times (P)^{(1/2)}$$

where $F$ is the flow during the valve opening period, $k$ is a constant = 38 for the mitral valve, and $P$ is the transmitral gradient.

The cardiac catheterization protocol in patients with MS includes the following measurements and calculations:

- Simultaneous left ventricular diastolic pressure, left atrial (or pulmonary capillary wedge) diastolic pressure, heart rate, diastolic filling period, and cardiac output (Fig. 2.20).
- If the transmitral pressure gradient is <5 mmHg, it can present a significant error in calculating the mitral valve orifice. The circulatory measurements should be repeated under circumstances of stress (exercise, reversible increase in preload resulting from passive elevation of the patient's legs, tachycardia induced by pacing) to increase the pressure gradient across the mitral valve.
- Simultaneously, or in close sequence, mean pulmonary arterial pressure, mean left atrial (or pulmonary capillary wedge) pressure, and cardiac output for calculating pulmonary vascular resistance.

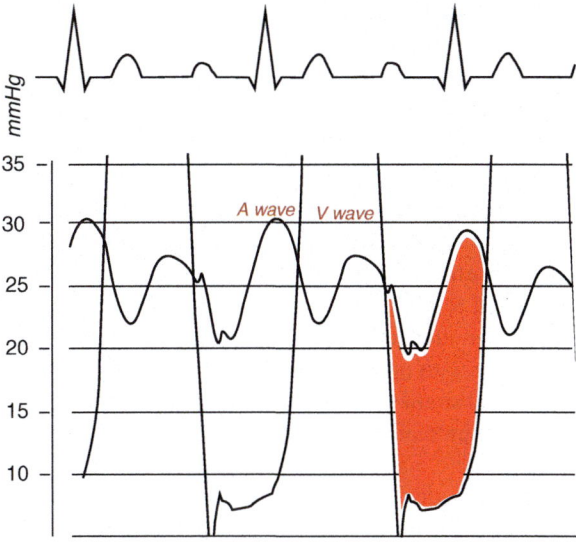

**Fig. 2.20** Simultaneous left ventricular and left atrial pressure traces. The *red area* shows a significant atrioventricular gradient in diastole

- Right ventricular systolic and diastolic pressures for assessing right ventricular function.
- If other lesions are suspected (e.g., mitral regurgitation, aortic valve disease, tricuspid stenosis, left atrial myxoma, atrial septal defect), they too must be evaluated. In this regard, it should be pointed out that certain lesions tend to occur in combination with MS.

According to the current guidelines [22], cardiac catheterization is indicated when noninvasive tests are insufficient or when there is a discrepancy between the hemodynamic data obtained from Doppler echocardiography and the clinical conditions of a symptomatic patient. It is also indicated to determine the causes of severe pulmonary hypertension observed in the echocardiogram when there is a discrepancy with other severity criteria (mean gradient and MVA) and to define the hemodynamic response to exercise when the symptoms and hemodynamics, at rest, contrast. If there are any doubts about the accuracy of the pulmonary capillary wedge pressure, transseptal catheterization can be performed to directly measure left atrial pressure [22].

The invasive tests for the hemodynamic assessment of MS patients also include ventriculography to determine the grade of mitral regurgitation when there is a difference between the mean gradient obtained with Doppler and the valve area; aortic root angiography can be useful to determine the severity of the associated aortic regurgitation, if any. Moreover, a selective coronary angiography is required to assess site, severity, and extension of a concurrent coronary artery disease. It should be performed in patients with angina, reduced left ventricle systolic function, history of coronary artery disease, and the presence of risk factors, including age [22].

## 2.4 Timing of Intervention

The drop in the incidence of rheumatic disease has greatly changed the time of the appearance of the onset symptoms of MS in the general population and the pathology's natural history. The latency between the episode of acute rheumatic fever and the appearance of the symptoms varies greatly and is correlated with the presence of recurrent episodes of streptococcal infection. The transition from the asymptomatic to the symptomatic stage depends on the progression of MS. The onset of dyspnea on effort is generally associated with a one-third reduction in valve area compared to the normal value [49]. Further reductions in area are associated with major hemodynamic impairment and, hence, a progressive worsening of dyspnea, appearing with minimal effort or even at rest.

Several studies were carried out in the 1950s and 1960s [5, 50, 51] on the natural history of untreated MS patients. These showed that MS is a disease with a slow and progressive course, with a first phase possibly lasting even several years, during which the patient is clinically stable and has no or very few symptoms. This phase is followed by a rapid decline with debilitating symptoms [5, 50–52]. In industrialized countries, a long latency of 20–40 years ranging from the first episode of rheumatic fever to the outbreak of symptoms has been observed. It is followed by another long period of about 10 years from the outbreak of the first mild symptoms to the worsening of dyspnea and the functional class [5]. Overall, the 10-year survival of untreated patients presenting with MS is 50–60%, depending on the symptoms at presentation [5, 50]. In the asymptomatic or minimally symptomatic patients, survival is greater than 80% at 10 years, with 60% of patients having no progression of symptoms [50–52]. Patients with an advanced New York Heart Association (NYHA) class have a survival at 10 years ranging from 0 to 15% [5, 50–53]. The onset of severe pulmonary hypertension reduces the survival of untreated MS patients by an average of 3 years [54].

Considering the poor prognosis of symptomatic MS patients, a therapeutic strategy should be considered as soon as the symptoms appear. Therefore, the choice of the type of treatment and the timing of intervention basically depend on two factors: the patient's clinical status and the anatomical and functional characteristics of the stenotic valve [22, 23, 55, 56].

The management strategy for MS patients varies depending on whether they are symptomatic. Once a diagnosis of MS has been confirmed by echocardiography, and the degree of stenosis and the morphology of the diseased valve have been determined, asymptomatic patients with mild MS do not need further diagnostic exams except for clinical and instrumental checks on an annual basis (physical exam, chest x-ray, ECG). Evidence shows that valve disease remains stable for years in these patients [5, 50, 51]. In the case of asymptomatic patients with moderate or severe MS, percutaneous mitral valvotomy (PMV) should be considered. In patients with pliable, noncalcified valves with no or little subvalvular fusion, no calcification in the commissures, and no left atrial thrombus, PMV, which carries a low complication rate, can be performed [22, 23, 55]. High pulmonary artery pressures and pulmonary vascular resistance play a major role in the timing of intervention in asymptomatic patients with moderate/severe MS, as these parameters are significantly correlated with greater hemodynamic impairment. In a patient with moderate pulmonary hypertension (sPAP > 50 mmHg) and a valve anatomy favorable to PMV, percutaneous treatment is recommended by current guidelines, even without symptoms [22, 23, 55]. In asymptomatic patients with a sedentary lifestyle, a hemodynamic exercise test with Doppler echocardiography is useful [55–59]. Objective limitation of exercise tolerance with a rise in transmitral gradient >15 mmHg and a rise in systolic pulmonary artery pressure greater than 60 mmHg can be an indication for percutaneous valvotomy if the MV morphology is suitable [55]. In asymptomatic patients, intervention is also indicated in cases of increased risk of thromboembolism (prior history of embolism, recent episode of paroxysmal atrial fibrillation, left atrial spontaneous echo contrast) [55]. Regarding the subgroup of asymptomatic patients with severe MS and severe pulmonary hypertension (sPAP >75% of systemic pressure either at rest or with exercise), if these patients do not have a valve morphology favorable for PMV or surgical valve repair, there is debate over whether MV replacement should be performed in the absence of symptoms to prevent right ventricular failure, but surgery is generally recommended in such patients [55].

Symptomatic NYHA class II patients with moderate or severe MS must be directly indicated for PMV, if valve morphology allows for it and if there are no thrombi in the left atrium. NYHA class III or IV patients should be considered for intervention with either PMV or surgery [55].

Patients with significantly limiting symptoms but not severe MS should undergo exercise testing or dobutamine stress to distinguish between the symptoms due to valve disease and those due to other causes. Patients who are symptomatic with a pulmonary artery pressure > 60 mmHg, mean transmitral gradient > 15 mmHg, or pulmonary artery wedge pressure > 25 mmHg, during exercise, have hemodynamically significant MS and should be considered for further intervention. Alternatively, patients who do not manifest elevation in either pulmonary artery, pulmonary capillary wedge, or transmitral pressures coincident with development of exertion symptoms would probably not benefit from intervention on the mitral valve [55].

Therefore, it can be concluded that according to current guidelines, in centers with expert operators, PMV (Table 2.7) is the procedure of choice for symptomatic patients with moderate-to-severe MS, with a favorable valve anatomy and without significant mitral regurgitation or thrombi in the left atrium. There is also debate over the role played by PMV in patients with debilitating symptoms and with less favorable valve morphology. In this subgroup, the rationale for PMV is perhaps linked to the clinical and hemodynamic stabilization offered by the percutaneous approach before the patient undergoes surgery [60]. In patients with severe calcifications and a completely altered valve morphology, surgical mitral valve replacement is preferred [55]. For asymptomatic or NYHA class II patients, percutaneous therapy should be considered as the first option, because of the lower degree of invasiveness and the lower morbidity and mortality of PMV compared with surgery [55].

**Table 2.7** Classes of indications for percutaneous mitral commissurotomy in patients with MS and MVA ≤ 1.5 cm², according to the 2017 European Guidelines on the Treatment of Valve Diseases

|  | Code |
|---|---|
| Symptomatic patients with favorable characteristics[a] for PMV | IB |
| Symptomatic patients with contraindication or high risk for surgery | IC |
| As initial treatment in symptomatic patients with unfavorable anatomy but otherwise favorable clinical characteristics[a] | IIaC |
| Asymptomatic patients with favorable characteristics[a] and high thromboembolic risk or high risk of hemodynamic decompensation: |  |
| • Previous history of embolism | IIaC |
| • Dense spontaneous contrast in the LA | IIaC |
| • Recent or paroxysmal AF | IIaC |
| • Systolic pulmonary pressure > 50 mmHg at rest | IIaC |
| • Need for major noncardiac surgery | IIaC |
| • Desire for pregnancy | IIaC |

[a]Favorable characteristics for PMV can be defined by the absence of several of the following: clinical characteristics (advanced age, history of commissurotomy, NYHA class IV, atrial fibrillation, severe pulmonary hypertension) and anatomic characteristics (Wilkins score > 8, Cormier score 3, very small mitral valve area, severe tricuspid regurgitation). *PMV* percutaneous mitral valvotomy, *LA* left atrium, *AF* atrial fibrillation

## 2.5 Percutaneous Therapy

Before the advent of percutaneous therapy, the treatment of MS consisted solely of the surgical option, and the range of techniques included open or closed commissurotomy and replacement with biological or mechanical prostheses [61]. Later, the development of percutaneous devices allowed PMV to become, beginning in the 1980s, not only a valid alternative to surgery but also the procedure of choice for all MS patients with a favorable valve anatomy [22, 23, 62].

PMV is a low-risk and low-cost replicable procedure, which does not require general anesthesia. It is not a contraindication for subsequent surgical valvuloplasty or valve replacement, and does not require permanent anticoagulant therapy, with the exception of a few cases, such as atrial fibrillation, major dilation of the left atrium, or prior episodes of embolism [63].

The main objective of PMV is to separate fused commissures, thus reducing the transmitral pressure gradient, left atrial pressure, and sPAP and increasing the mitral valve area and cardiac output.

In the past, several techniques were used to perform PMV. The major difference between the various techniques described in the literature lies in the route of access (antegrade or retrograde) and in the number of balloon catheters used (single balloon, double balloon; elastic, stiff, or metal material) (Fig. 2.21) [64–69]. Today, PMV is universally performed using the antegrade route via transseptal catheterization [64, 70] and placement of the balloon catheter across the mitral valve following the blood flow [67]. In rare cases, Cribier's metallic valvulotome is used [71].

Currently, in most centers performing PMV, the Inoue catheter is used (Toray Industries, Japan). This is a special device, with a balloon at one end, which is

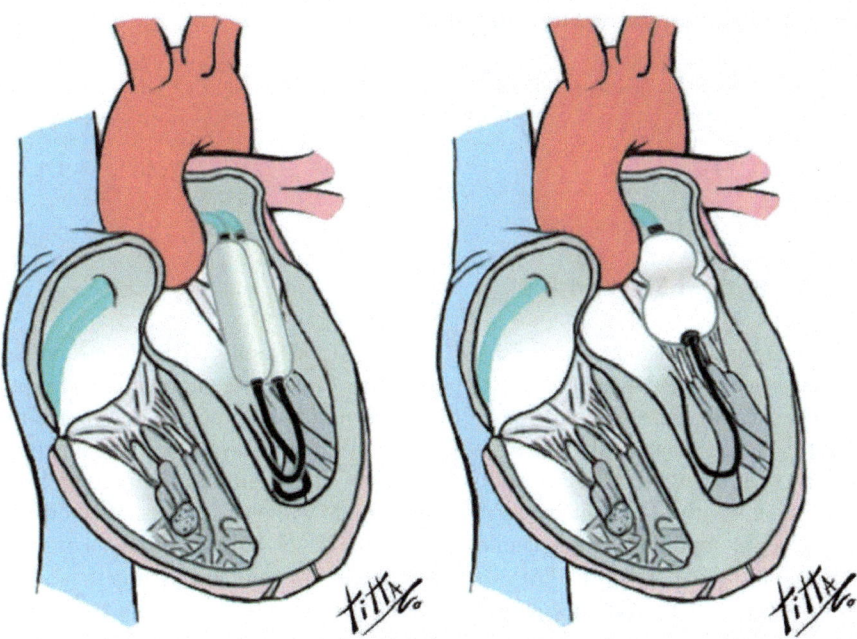

**Fig. 2.21** Percutaneous mitral valvuloplasty using double- and single-balloon technique

anchored on the valve plane and then inflated. The catheter has a 12 Fr diameter with a length of 70 cm; the length of each balloon is 2.5 cm (un-stretched). Two proximally positioned stopcocks achieve balloon inflation and catheter venting. A stainless steel tube is used to stretch and slenderize the balloon prior to insertion, and a 14 Fr tapered dilator enlarges the interatrial opening. The stainless steel stylet and guidewire are employed to guide the catheter inside the heart and blood vessels. The Inoue balloon is made of nylon and a rubber micromesh, and has three different degrees of elasticity, which give sequential expansion, thus allowing optimal and stable placement on the mitral valve [65]. As mentioned earlier, the mechanism by which the valve area is increased consists of "splitting" the fused commissures and mobilizing the valve leaflets. The presence of paracommissural calcifications requires that the technique be performed gradually, namely, by means of progressive inflations, using balloons with smaller diameters compared to those normally used based on the body surface. The Inoue catheter ensures stability during inflation, thanks to its hourglass shape, with the narrower portion placed on the valve and the wider portions located upstream and downstream of it. It also ensures minor trauma, and, above all, it offers various inflation diameters without any need for changing the catheter [66, 67, 71]. The reference diameters for the Inoue balloon are normally chosen based on the patient's weight and height, surface area, degree of valve apparatus damage, and mitral valve area, as measured by cardiac catheterization and/or with noninvasive methods, and vary between 22 and 30 mm (Table 2.8). Patient age and gender can be factors affecting the choice of the balloon.

**Table 2.8** Reference diameters for Inoue balloon

| Cat. no. | Balloon dilation available range (mm) | Diameter maximum (mm) | Patient weight (kg) | Patient height (cm) | Surface area (m²) |
|---|---|---|---|---|---|
| PTMC-30 | 26–30 | 30 | ≥70 | ≥180 cm | ≥1.9 |
| PTMC-28 | 24–28 | 28 | 45–70 | 160–180 cm | 1.6–1.9 |
| PTMC-26 | 22–26 | 26 | ≤45 | ≤160 | ≤1.6 |

## 2.5.1 Patient Selection

The determining factors for the short- and long-term results of PMV are proper patient selection and the possibility of performing PMV in a center with good experience and procedure skills. Briefly, PMV is currently the procedure of choice for symptomatic patients with moderate-to-severe MS, with a favorable valve anatomy and no significant mitral regurgitation or thrombi in the left atrium. In asymptomatic patients with a favorable valve morphology, PMV should be considered only in the presence of proven hemodynamic impairment [22, 23, 55]. This does not exclude the possibility of performing PMV on patients with low cardiac output or those who have undergone prior cardiac surgery, including surgical mitral commissurotomy, and who have subsequently developed restenosis due to commissural refusion [72]. In rare cases, PMV can also be performed on stenotic biological prostheses [73, 74]. PMV is also an important therapeutic strategy in pregnant women, as the procedure has few complications and low fetal mortality, thanks to lead shielding of the abdomen [22, 23, 55, 75, 76]. Pregnant women with severe cardiac failure due to MS have a high morbidity rate, and there is an unfavorable effect on the fetus [77]. Compared with surgical open commissurotomy, PMV has shown fewer fetal complications, with a lower neonatal and fetal mortality rate and excellent long-term results [70, 78]. The procedure can also be performed as a bridge to surgery in patients in extremely poor clinical conditions, with an unfavorable valve anatomy, to allow for clinical and hemodynamic stabilization and better functional recovery in the workup to intervention [60].

When screening MS patients to undergo PMV, special attention must be paid to possible contraindications [23, 79] (Table 2.9). Absolute contraindications for PMV include floating thrombus in the left atrium or interatrial septum, while a left atrial appendage thrombus is not an absolute contraindication. In these cases, PMV can be preceded by adequate anticoagulation therapy and monitoring by TEE [80, 81]. Atriomegaly and atrial fibrillation are not a contraindication to PMV.

Another critical factor in patient selection is echocardiographic assessment aimed, in particular, at studying the anatomy and functions of the mitral apparatus, and quantifying alterations using the Wilkins score, as described earlier (Table 2.1). Values ≤8 indicate a favorable anatomy and are generally associated with excellent post-PMV final results. However, patients with a Wilkins score >8 and, hence, an unfavorable anatomy, in whom results will be partial and temporary, cannot a priori be excluded as candidates for percutaneous treatment. In these cases, comorbidities

**Table 2.9** Contraindications (absolute/relative) for percutaneous mitral valvuloplasty

Related to valve
- Mitral valve area $\geq 1.5$ cm$^2$
- Left atrial thrombus
- Mitral regurgitation $\geq 2+$
- Severe or bicommissural calcification
- Absence of commissural fusion
- Mild MS

Related to medical center
- Lack of appropriate procedural skill and experience
- Concomitant valvulopathy and need for open heart surgery
- Severe concomitant aortic valve disease
- Severe concomitant tricuspid regurgitation or tricuspid stenosis
- Concomitant coronary artery disease requiring bypass surgery
- Concomitant aorta disease requiring surgery

Procedural difficulties related to transseptal puncture
- Severe tricuspid regurgitation
- Huge right atrium
- Distorted/displaced atrial septum
- Femoral-iliac veins obstructed or thrombosed
- Inferior vena cava, obstructed or thrombosed; drainage into azygos vein
- Severe kyphoscoliosis (thoracic/abdominal)

and the presence of any other valve diseases or multiple significant coronary stenoses should be assessed in order to choose between surgical treatment and palliative PMV [64].

Other score-based models have been proposed, among which Reid's score [82] (Table 2.3) and Fatkin's score [64], by which post-PMV commissural splitting, examined by echocardiography in parasternal short-axis view, is the major determinant of procedural success.

## 2.5.2 Procedure and Technical Aspects

The percutaneous procedure is performed using the antegrade approach and requires access through the femoral vein and transseptal puncture with the Brockenbrough needle. Echocardiographic monitoring is needed at times during the procedure (Fig. 2.22). A Mullins dilator is then placed, and a catheter is inserted through it into the left atrium (Fig. 2.23). When an intraprocedural echocardiogram is not available, a small quantity of contrast medium is injected to confirm that the catheter is in the right position. The operator then measures the pressure in the left atrium and left ventricle to confirm the hemodynamic gradient generated by the stenosis. A 0.6 mm guidewire is then inserted up to the left atrium and the Mullins dilator is removed. The next step consists of dilating the orifice in the femoral vein and the interatrial septum using a special 14 Fr dilator; the dilator is then run through the

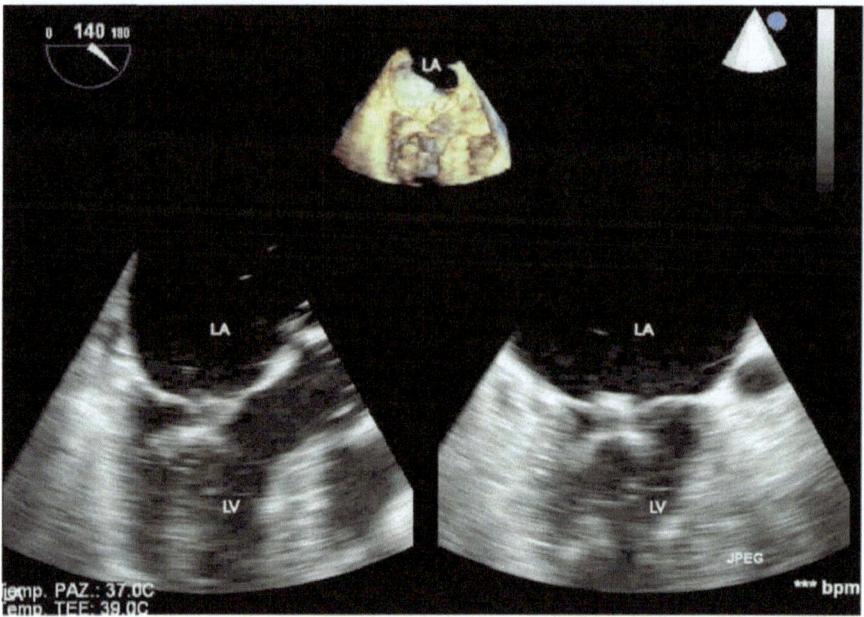

**Fig. 2.22** Transesophageal echocardiographic guidance during mitral valvuloplasty. *LA* left atrium, *LV* left ventricle

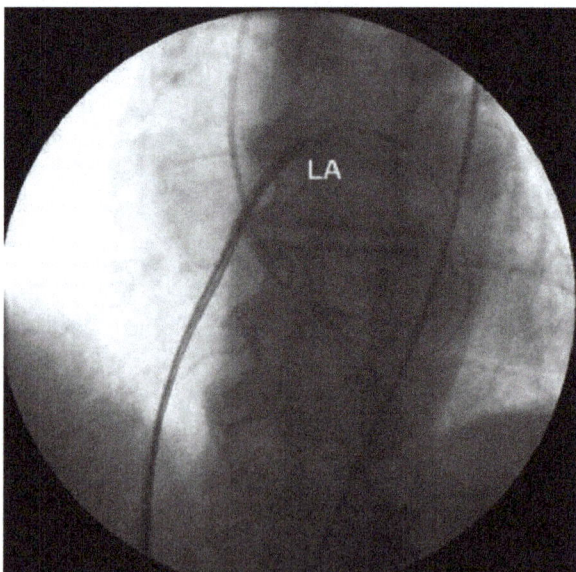

**Fig. 2.23** Transseptal placement of 14 Fr dilator on guidewire positioned in the left atrium (*LA*)

guidewire previously placed. At this point, the Inoue balloon is prepared, tested, and inserted through the guidewire up to the left atrium. After advancing the Inoue balloon inside the left ventricle and making sure that it does not interfere with the *chordae tendineae*, the distal end of the balloon is inflated (Fig. 2.24). The catheter is pulled back to position the device on the stenotic valve, and the balloon is sequentially expanded from the distal to the proximal portion (Fig. 2.25). Each time it is

**Fig. 2.24** Distal end of the balloon inflated in the left ventricle. The partially inflated balloon is pulled back toward the left atrium and anchored to the stenotic valve orifice

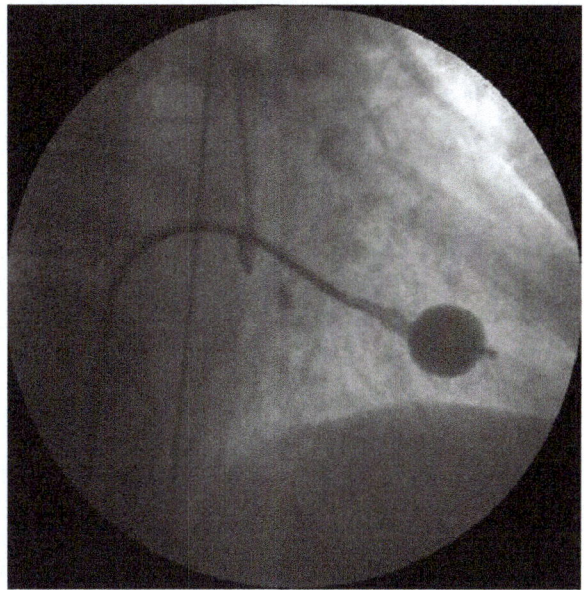

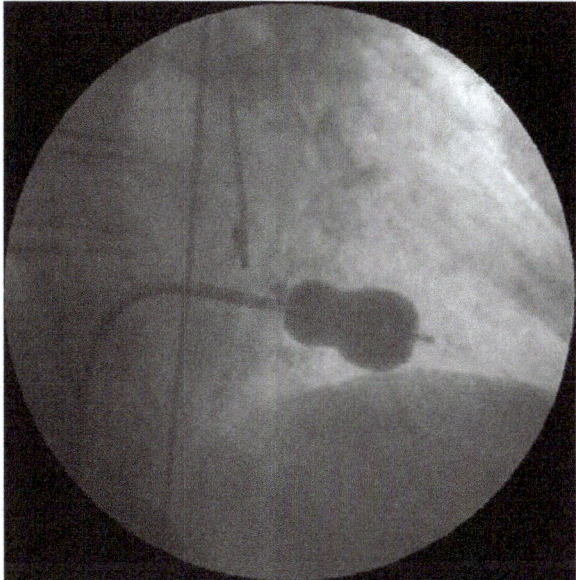

**Fig. 2.25** Inflation of the proximal portion of the balloon, which takes the shape of a "dog bone"; the incisure corresponds to the mitral valve plane

**Fig. 2.26** Completion of balloon inflation, with opening of commissures

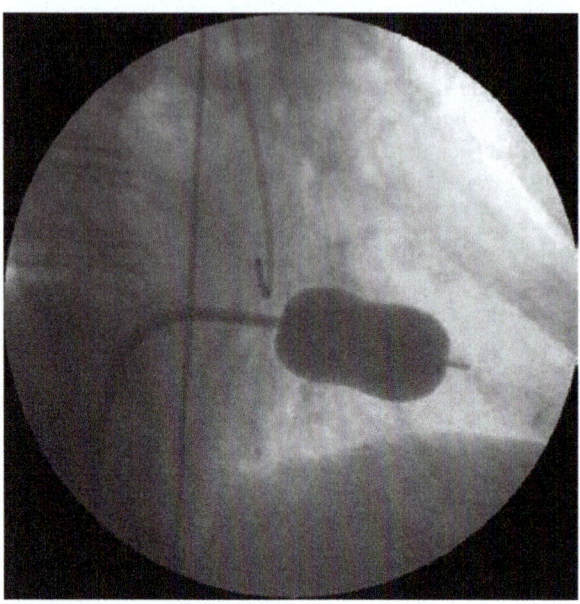

expanded, the transmitral gradient and any damage generated is assessed. Dilations will be continued until the desired result is achieved (Fig. 2.26). If an acceptable transvalvular gradient is not reached, dilation can be continued using Inoue devices that are 1 or 2 mm larger [82].

This technique also envisages right and left catheterization with cineangiography both before and after the procedure, ventriculography in 30° right anterior oblique projection, and, in the case of mitral regurgitation, also in laterolateral projection. Cardiac output and MVA are also measured using the Gorlin formula. If effective, there is an increase in MVA by at least 25% and a sudden drop in left atrial pressure, pressure gradient, and sPAP. There can also be an increase in left ventricular end-diastolic pressure due to the greater transmitral diastolic flow and an increase in cardiac output. Pulmonary resistance values can behave inconsistently. The rise in resistance is, above all, the result of the increased difference between the mean pulmonary artery pressure and left atrial pressure following the sudden drop in the latter, which is greater than the concurrent drop in sPAP. In the case of pulmonary hypertension, the return to normal pulmonary vascular pressures and resistance values can either be immediate or slow and gradual.

Echocardiographic guidance in the catheterization laboratory is useful for transseptal puncture, placement of the balloon at the commissures, assessment of the immediate result, and early detection of any complication. Echocardiographic guidance is usually performed by TTE, while TEE is seldom used during PMV, as it may not be easily tolerated by the conscious patient lying on the catheterization laboratory table for the entire time of the procedure. TEE is especially useful in pregnant women, as it reduces exposure to x-rays. Echocardiography allows for real-time

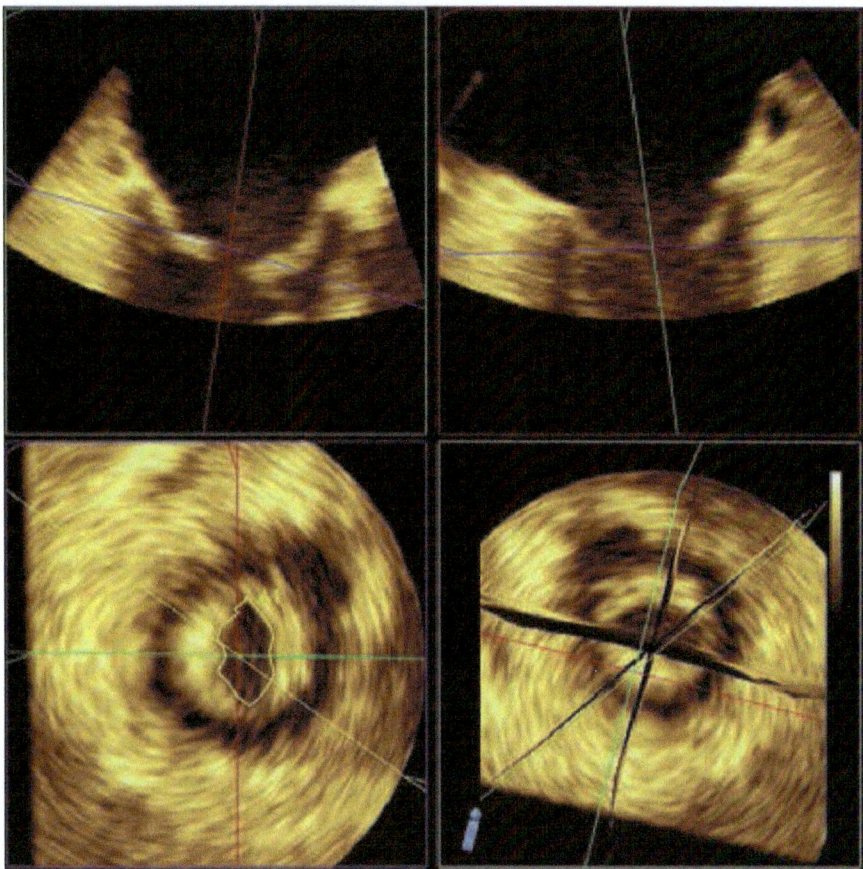

**Fig. 2.27** Residual mitral valve orifice area after balloon valvuloplasty. The measurement is calculated by the QLab software (Philips Healthcare, Andover, MA, USA)

measurement of MVA, pressure gradient, commissure opening, leaflet mobility, leaflet tears, and the degree of residual mitral regurgitation. Area calculation by PHT is not reliable in the catheterization laboratory, because this method cannot be applied due to sudden changes in compliance, such as those occurring during valve dilation. However, the use of 3D echocardiography provides an immediate estimate of the residual post-valvuloplasty mitral valve orifice area (Fig. 2.27).

PMV performed in patients with a Wilkins score of ≤8 has a success rate of 85–90% [28]. In patients with a score of 9–12, the procedure is successful in 80–85% of cases [28, 63]. An optimal result is an area of ≥1.5 cm$^2$, an increase by at least 25% compared with the initial area in the absence of mitral regurgitation ≥2/4+; a suboptimal result is an MVA increase of less than 25% or a final area of <1.5 cm$^2$; the procedure fails when there is no increase in MVA or the onset of MR ≥3/4+. Mortality is very low (<1%) [63].

### 2.5.3 Complications

The most frequent complication in PMV is the increase and/or the new onset of significant mitral regurgitation (2–3%) [30, 68, 82]. Usually, this is the result of the tearing of the valve leaflets or the placement of the balloon at too short a distance between the fused *chordae tendineae,* thus tearing them. By contrast, mild and transient mitral insufficiency, or a slight worsening of it, is due to the temporary dysfunction of the mitral subvalvular apparatus immediately after balloon inflations. It is normally solved within the next 24 h. However, the new onset of mild mitral regurgitation or worsening in the degree of preexisting mitral insufficiency is usually well tolerated in patients with enlarged atrial chambers and pulmonary vessels used to high venous pressures. Another complication is the onset of a major atrial septal defect (ASD) with a left-right shunt volume of >1.5 (<5% of cases if PMV is performed using the Inoue technique). The frequency of iatrogenic ASD caused by transseptal puncture and catheter placement varies between 30 and 53%. However, in most cases, the ratio between pulmonary output and systemic output is <1.5 and, thus, negligible; in any event, ASD tends to close spontaneously over time. Its persistence is usually linked to the sharp drop in left atrial pressure, which is almost always a sign of inadequate valve dilation. Other complications are rather rare and almost always reported during the early phases of application of the procedure; these include peripheral embolism (0.3–1%), left ventricular perforation followed by cardiac tamponade (2–5%), and interventricular septum perforation or severe mitral regurgitation requiring emergency surgery (2–6%) [30, 63, 83]. A study of several case histories has shown that the procedure-related complications are directly related to operator experience; it has been noted that at the centers with highest number of procedures, complications are much fewer than those of centers with a low number of procedures [82].

### 2.5.4 Results

Many studies have shown the short- and long-term efficacy of PMV [29, 31, 84–87] (Table 2.10). These studies show quite satisfactory results for this technique. A study by Iung et al. [29] on 528 patients who successfully underwent percutaneous mitral commissurotomy (dilation was performed using a single balloon in 13 patients, a double balloon in 349, and the Inoue balloon in 166) reports a survival rate for patients in NYHA functional class I or II, with no cardiac-related deaths or

**Table 2.10** Long-term follow-up in patients who underwent balloon mitral valvuloplasty

| Author [Reference] | Patients | Mean age (years) | Follow-up (months) | Survival (%) | Freedom from surgery (%) |
|---|---|---|---|---|---|
| Palacios [85] | 327 | 54 | 48 | 90 | 79 |
| Cohen [79] | 146 | 59 | 60 | 76 | 51 |
| Pan [86] | 350 | 46 | 60 | 94 | 91 |
| Iung [29, 31] | 606 | 46 | 60 | 94 | 74 |
| NHLBI [84] | 736 | 54 | 48 | 84 | 66 |

need for mitral surgery or repeat dilation, of 76 ± 6% at 5 years. On multivariate analysis, the independent predictors of good functional results were echocardiography group, functional class, and cardiothoracic index before the procedure and valve area after the procedure.

The National Heart, Lung, and Blood Institute (NHLBI) Balloon Valvuloplasty Registry reported multicenter results in 736 patients older than 18 years who were monitored for 4 years [84]. The actuarial survival rates at 1, 2, 3, and 4 years were 93%, 90%, 87%, and 84%, respectively. The rates of event-free survival (freedom from death, mitral valve surgery, or repeat balloon valvuloplasty) at 1, 2, 3, and 4 years were 80%, 71%, 66%, and 62%, respectively. Multivariate predictions of mortality were NYHA functional class IV, Wilkins score > 12, post-procedure sPAP > 40 mmHg, and left ventricular end-diastolic pressure > 15 mmHg.

Restenosis, defined as a loss of 50% of the result obtained and a reduction of MVA to <1.5 $cm^2$, has been seen in younger populations in 2–10% of cases with a 37-month follow-up and among older patients in about 22% of cases with a follow-up of 13 months [87, 88]. The main predictor of restenosis, as reported by Thomas et al. [89], is a high Wilkins score; different results are likely due to use of the same technique: commissural splitting is most common in patients with low Wilkins score and carries a low risk of restenosis, whereas valve stretching is frequent in those patients with high Wilkins score and high restenosis rate. However, re-PMV can be performed in the case of restenosis. Encouraging results have been obtained by Iung et al. [90] in 53 cases of restenosis, with a doubling of the mitral area, and a 5-year survival of 69% in NYHA class I or II.

## References

1. Carapetis JR, Steer AC, Mulholland EK, et al. The global burden of group a streptococcal diseases. Lancet Infect Dis. 2005;5:685–94.
2. Iung B, Baron G, Butchart EG, et al. A prospective survey of patients with valvular heart disease in Europe: the Euro heart survey on valvular heart disease. Eur Heart J. 2003;24:1231–43.
3. Messika-Zeitoun D, Iung B, Brochet E, et al. Evaluation of mitral stenosis in 2008. Arch Cardiovasc Dis. 2008;101:653–63.
4. Sliwa K, Carrington M, Mayosi BM, et al. Incidence and characteristics of newly diagnosed rheumatic heart disease in urban African adults: insights from the heart of Soweto study. Eur Heart J. 2010;31:719–27.
5. Wood P. An appreciation of mitral stenosis. Clinical features. Br Med J. 1954;4870:1051–63.
6. Essop MR, Nkomo VT. Rheumatic and nonrheumatic valvular heart disease: epidemiology, management, and prevention in Africa. Circulation. 2005;112:3584–91.
7. Burge DJ, DeHoratious RJ. Acute rheumatic fever. Cardiovasc Clin. 1993;23:3–23.
8. Guilherme L, Cury P, Demarchi LM, et al. Rheumatic heart disease: proinflammatory cytokines play a role in the progression and maintenance of valvular lesions. Am J Pathol. 2004;165:1583–1.
9. Davutoglu V, Celik A, Aksoy M. Contribution of selected serum inflammatory mediators to the progression of chronic rheumatic valve disease, subsequent valve calcification and NYHA functional class. J Heart Valve Dis. 2005;14:251–6.
10. Roberts WC. Morphologic aspects of cardiac valve dysfunction. Am Heart J. 1992;123: 1610–32.

11. Spencer FC. A plea for early, open mitral commissurotomy. Am Heart J. 1978;95:668–70.
12. Carabello BA. Timing of surgery in mitral and aortic stenosis. Cardiol Clin. 1991;9:229–38.
13. Hygenholtz PG, Ryan TJ, Stein SW, et al. The spectrum of pure mitral stenosis. Hemodynamic studies in relation to clinical disability. Am J Cardiol. 1962;10:773–84.
14. Arani DT, Carleton RA. The deleterious role of tachycardia in mitral stenosis. Circulation. 1967;36:511–6.
15. Schofield PM. Invasive investigation of the mitral valve. In: Wells FC, Shapiro LM, editors. Mitral valve disease. Oxford: Butterworth-Heineman; 1996. p. 84.
16. Kennedy JW, Yarnall SR, Murray JA, et al. Quantitative angiocardiography. IV. Relationships of left atrial and ventricular pressure and volume in mitral valve disease. Circulation. 1970;41:817–24.
17. Choi BW, Bacharach SL, Barcour DJ, et al. Left ventricular systolic dysfunction: diastolic filling characteristics and exercise cardiac reserve in mitral stenosis. Am J Cardiol. 1995;75:526–9.
18. Braunwald E, Turi ZG. Pathophysiology of mitral valve disease. In: Wells FC, Shapiro LM, editors. Mitral valve disease. Oxford: Butterworth-Heineman; 1996. p. 16.
19. Thompson ME, Shaver JA, Leon DF. Effect of tachycardia on atrial transport in mitral stenosis. Am Heart J. 1977;94:297–306.
20. Stott DK, Marpole DGF, Bristow JD, et al. The role of left atrial transport in aortic and mitral stenosis. Circulation. 1970;41:1031–41.
21. Diker E, Aydogdu S, Ozdemir M, et al. Prevalence and predictors of atrial fibrillation in rheumatic valvular heart disease. Am J Cardiol. 1996;77:96–8.
22. American College of Cardiology, American Heart Association Task Force on Practice Guidelines (Writing Committee to revise the 1998 guidelines for the management of patients with valvular heart disease), Society of Cardiovascular Anesthesiologists, Bonow RO, Carabello BA, Chatterjee K, et al. ACC/AHA 2006 guidelines for the management of patients with valvular heart disease: a report of the American College of Cardiology/American Heart Association Task Force on Practice Guidelines (writing Committee to Revise the 1998 guidelines for the management of patients with valvular heart disease) developed in collaboration with the Society of Cardiovascular Anesthesiologists endorsed by the Society for Cardiovascular Angiography and Interventions and the Society of Thoracic Surgeons. J Am Coll Cardiol. 2006;48:1–148.
23. Vahanian A, Baumgartner H, Bax J, et al. Task force on the Management of Valvular Heart Disease of the European Society of Cardiology ESC Committee for Practice Guidelines. Guidelines on the management of valvular heart disease: the Task Force on the Management of Valvular Heart Disease of the European Society of Cardiology. Eur Heart J. 2007;28:230–68.
24. Braundwald E. Valvular heart disease. In: Braundwald E, editor. Heart disease. Philadelphia: W.B. Saunders; 1984. p. 1063–135.
25. Nichol PM, Gilbert BW, Kisslo JA. Two-dimensional echocardiographic assessment of mitral stenosis. Circulation. 1977;55:120–8.
26. Baumgartner H, Hung J, Bermejo J, et al. Echocardiographic assessment of valve stenosis: EAE/ASE recommendations for clinical practice. J Am Soc Echocardiogr. 2009;22:1–23.
27. Messika-Zeitoun D, Brochet E, Holmin C, et al. Three-dimensional evaluation of the mitral valve area and commissural opening before and after percutaneous mitral commissurotomy in patients with mitral stenosis. Eur Heart J. 2007;28:72–9.
28. Wilkins GT, Weyman AE, Abascal VM, et al. Percutaneous balloon dilatation of the mitral valve: an analysis of echocardiographic variables related to outcome and the mechanism of dilatation. Br Heart J. 1988;60:299–308.
29. Iung B, Cormier B, Ducimetiere P, et al. Functional results 5 years after successful percutaneous mitral commissurotomy in a series of 528 patients and analysis of predictive factors. J Am Coll Cardiol. 1996;27:407–14.
30. Rahimtoola SH, Durairaj A, Mehra A, et al. Current evaluation and management of patients with mitral stenosis. Circulation. 2002;106:1183–8.
31. Iung B, Cormier B, Ducimetiere P, et al. Immediate results of percutaneous mitral commissurotomy. Circulation. 1996;94:2124–30.

32. Reid CL, McKay CR, Chandraratna PA, et al. Mechanisms of increase in mitral valve area and influence of anatomic features in double-balloon, catheter balloon valvuloplasty in adults with rheumatic mitral stenosis: a Doppler and two-dimensional echocardiographic study. Circulation. 1987;76:628–36.
33. Nishimura RA, Rihal CS, Tajik AJ, et al. Accurate measurement of the transmitral gradient in patients with mitral stenosis: a simultaneous catheterization and Doppler echocardiographic study. J Am Coll Cardiol. 1994;24:152–8.
34. Thomas JD, Newell JB, Choong CY, et al. Physical and physiological determinants of transmitral velocity: numerical analysis. Am J Physiol. 1991;260:1718–31.
35. Faletra F, Pezzano A Jr, Fusco R, et al. Measurement of mitral valve area in mitral stenosis: four echocardiographic methods compared with direct measurement of anatomic orifices. J Am Coll Cardiol. 1996;28:1190–7.
36. Thomas JD, Weyman AE. Doppler mitral pressure half-time: a clinical tool in search of theoretical justification. J Am Coll Cardiol. 1987;10:923–9.
37. Schwammenthai E, Vered Z, Agranat O, et al. Impact of atrioventricular compliance on pulmonary artery pressure in mitral stenosis: an exercise echocardiographic study. Circulation. 2000;102:2378–84.
38. Thomas JD, Wilkins GT, Choong CY, et al. Inaccuracy of mitral pressure half-time immediately after percutaneous mitral valvotomy. Dependence on transmitral gradient and left atrial and ventricular compliance. Circulation. 1988;78:980–93.
39. Nakatani S, Masuyama T, Kodama K, et al. Value and limitations of Doppler echocardiography in the quantification of stenotic mitral valve area: comparison of the pressure halftime and the continuity equation methods. Circulation. 1988;77:78–85.
40. Messika-Zeitoun D, Fung Yiu S, Cormier B, et al. Sequential assessment of mitral valve area during diastole using colour M-mode flow convergence analysis: new insights into mitral stenosis physiology. Eur Heart J. 2003;24:1244–53.
41. Currie PJ, Seward JB, Chan KL, et al. Continuous wave Doppler determination of right ventricular pressure: a simultaneous Doppler catheterization study in 127 patients. J Am Coll Cardiol. 1985;6:750–6.
42. de Agustin JA, Nanda NC, Gill EA, et al. The use of three-dimensional echocardiography for the evaluation of and treatment of mitral stenosis. Cardiol Clin. 2007;25:311–8.
43. Pérez de Isla L, Casanova C, Almerìa C, et al. Which method should be the reference method to evaluate the severity of rheumatic mitral stenosis? Gorlin's method versus 3D-echo. Eur J Echocardiogr. 2007;8:470–3.
44. Applebaum RM, Kasliwal RR, Kanojia A, et al. Utility of three-dimensional echocardiography during balloon mitral valvuloplasty. J Am Coll Cardiol. 1998;32:1405–9.
45. Anwar AM, Attia WM, Nosir YF, et al. Validation of a new score for the assessment of mitral stenosis using real-time three-dimensional echocardiography. J Am Soc Echocardiogr. 2010;23:13–22.
46. Soliman OI, Anwar AM, Metawei AK, et al. New scores for the assessment of mitral stenosis using real-time three-dimensional echocardiography. Curr Cardiovasc Imaging Rep. 2011;4:370–7.
47. Braunwald E, Moscovitz HL, Mram SS, et al. The hemodynamics of the left side of the heart as studied by simultaneous left atrial, left ventricular and aortic pressures; particular reference to mitral stenosis. Circulation. 1955;12:69–81.
48. Gorlin R, Gorlin SG. Hydraulic formula for calculation of the area of the stenotic mitral valve, other cardiac valves, and central circulatory shunts. Am Heart J. 1951;41:1–29.
49. Hugenholtz PG, Ryan TJ, Stein SW, et al. The spectrum of pure mitral stenosis: hemodynamic studies in relation to clinical disability. Am J Cardiol. 1962;10:773–84.
50. Rowe JC, Bland EF, Sprague HB, et al. The course of mitral stenosis without surgery: ten and twenty-year perspectives. Ann Intern Med. 1960;52:741–9.
51. Olesen KH. The natural history of 271 patients with mitral stenosis under medical treatment. Br Heart J. 1962;24:349–57.
52. Selzer A, Cohn KE. Natural history of mitral stenosis: a review. Circulation. 1972;45:878–90.

53. Munoz S, Gallardo J, Diaz-Gorrin JR, et al. Influence of surgery on the natural history of rheumatic mitral and aortic valve disease. Am J Cardiol. 1975;35:234–42.
54. Ward C, Hancock BW. Extreme pulmonary hypertension caused by mitral valve disease: natural history and results of surgery. Br Heart J. 1975;37:74–8.
55. Bonow RO, Carabello BA, Chatterjee K, et al. American College of Cardiology/American Heart Association Task Force on Practice Guidelines. 2008 focused update incorporated into the ACC/AHA 2006 guidelines for the management of patients with valvular heart disease: a report of the American College of Cardiology/American Heart Association Task Force on Practice Guidelines (Writing Committee to revise the 1998 guidelines for the management of patients with valvular heart disease): endorsed by the Society of Cardiovascular Anesthesiologists, Society for Cardiovascular Angiography and Interventions, and Society of Thoracic Surgeons. Circulation. 2008;118:523–661.
56. Himelman RB, Stulbarg M, Kircher B, et al. Noninvasive evaluation of pulmonary artery pressure during exercise by saline-enhanced Doppler echocardiography in chronic pulmonary disease. Circulation. 1989;79:863–71.
57. Tamai J, Nagata S, Akaike M, et al. Improvement in mitral flow dynamics during exercise after percutaneous transvenous mitral commissurotomy: noninvasive evaluation using continuous wave Doppler technique. Circulation. 1990;81:46–51.
58. Leavitt JI, Coats MH, Falk RH. Effects of exercise on transmitral gradient and pulmonary artery pressure in patients with mitral stenosis or a prosthetic mitral valve: a Doppler echocardiographic study. J Am Coll Cardiol. 1991;17:1520–6.
59. Cheriex EC, Pieters FA, Janssen JH, et al. Value of exercise Doppler-echocardiography in patients with mitral stenosis. Int J Cardiol. 1994;45:219–26.
60. Tamburino C, Russo G, Di Paola G, et al. La valvuloplastica percutanea nella stenosi mitralica. Cardiologia. 1993;38:7–17.
61. Palacios IF. Farewell to surgical mitral commissurotomy for many patients. Circulation. 1998;97:223–6.
62. Davidson MJ, Baim DS. Percutaneous catheter-based mitral valve repair. In: Cohn LH, editor. Cardiac surgery in the adult. New York: McGraw-Hill; 2008. p. 1101–8.
63. Marsocci G, Neri M, Natale N. Cardiopatie valvolari. Il Pensiero Scientifico Editore. 2004. p. 73–103.
64. Fatkin D, Roy P, Morgan JJ, et al. Percutaneous balloon mitral valvotomy with the Inoue single-balloon catheter: commissural morphology as a determinant of outcome. J Am Coll Cardiol. 1993;21:390–7.
65. Inoue K. Percutaneous transvenous mitral commissurotomy using the Inoue balloon. Eur Heart J. 1991;12:99–108.
66. Vahanian A, Acar J. Mitral valvuloplasty: the French experience. In: Topol EJ, editor. Textbook of interventional cardiology. Philadelphia: WB Saunders; 1994. p. 1206–25.
67. Block PC, Palacios IF. Aortic and mitral balloon valvuloplasty: the United States experience. In: Topol EJ, editor. Textbook of interventional cardiology. Philadelphia: WB Saunders; 1994. p. 1189–205.
68. Inoue K, Hungs JS. Percutaneous transvenous mitral commissurotomy (PTMC): the Far East experience. In: Topol EJ, editor. Textbook of interventional cardiology. Philadelphia: WB Saunders; 1994. p. 1226–42.
69. Tamburino C, Russo G, Calvi V, et al. La valvuloplastica mitralica: risultati immediati e followup a 2 anni. Cardiologia. 1993;38:367–75.
70. Ross J Jr. Catheterization of the left heart through the interatrial septum: a new technique and its experimental evaluation. Surg Forum. 1959;9:297–301.
71. Inoue K, Owaki T, Nakamura T, et al. Clinical application of transvenous mitral commissurotomy by a new balloon catheter. J Thorac Cardiovasc Surg. 1984;87:394–402.
72. Iung B, Garbarz E, Michaud P, et al. Percutaneous mitral commissurotomy for restenosis after surgical commissurotomy: late efficacy and implications for patient selection. J Am Coll Cardiol. 2000;35:1295–302.

73. Lip G, Wasfi M, Hamil M, et al. Percutaneous balloon valvuloplasty of stenosed mitral bioprosthesis. Int J Cardiol. 1997;59:97–100.
74. Lin PJ, Chang JP, Chang CH. Balloon valvuloplasty is contraindicated in stenotic mitral bioprosthesis. Am Heart J. 1994;127:724–6.
75. Gupta A, Lokhandwala YY, Satoskar PR, et al. Balloon mitral valvotomy in pregnancy: maternal and fetal outcomes. J Am Coll Surg. 1998;187:409–15.
76. Fawzy ME, Kinsara AJ, Stefadouros M, et al. Long-term outcome of mitral balloon valvotomy in pregnant women. J Heart Valve Dis. 2001;10:153–7.
77. Hameed A, Karaalp IS, Tummala PP, et al. The effect of valvular heart disease on maternal and fetal outcome of pregnancy. J Am Coll Cardiol. 2001;37:893–9.
78. de Souza JA, Martinez EE Jr, Ambrose JA, et al. Percutaneous balloon mitral valvuloplasty in comparison with open mitral valve commissurotomy for mitral stenosis during pregnancy. J Am Coll Cardiol. 2001;37:900–3.
79. Cohen DJ, Kuntz RE, Gordon SP, et al. Predictors of long-term outcome after percutaneous balloon mitral valvuloplasty. N Engl J Med. 1992;327:1329–35.
80. Kamalesh M, Burger AJ, Shubrooks SJ. The use of transesophageal echocardiography to avoid left atrial thrombus during percutaneous mitral valvuloplasty. Cathet Cardiovasc Diagn. 1993;28:320–2.
81. Tsai LM, Hung JS, Chen JH, et al. Resolution of left atrial appendage thrombus in mitral stenosis after warfarin therapy. Am Heart J. 1991;121:1232–4.
82. Grossman W, Baim DS. Grossman's cardiac catheterization, angiography and intervention. 7th ed. Baltimore: Lippincott Williams and Wilkins; 2006.
83. Vahanian A, Palacios IF. Percutaneous approaches to valvular disease. Circulation. 2004;109:1572–9.
84. Dean LS, Mickel M, Bonan R, et al. Four-years follow up of patients undergoing percutaneous balloon mitral commissurotomy. A report from the National Heart, Lung, and Blood Institute Balloon Valvuloplasty Registry. J Am Coll Cardiol. 1996;28:1452–7.
85. Palacios IF, Tuzuc ME, Weyman AE, et al. Clinical Follow-up of patients undergoing percutaneous mitral balloon valvotomy. Circulation. 1995;91:671–6.
86. Pan M, Medina A, Lezo JJ, et al. Factors determining late success after mitral balloon valvulotomy. Am J Cardiol. 1993;71:1181–6.
87. Arora R, Kalra GS, Murty GS, et al. Percutaneous transatrial mitral commissurotomy: immediate and intermediate results. J Am Coll Cardiol. 1994;23:1327–32.
88. Palacios IF, Block PC, Wilkins GT, Weyman AE. Follow-up of patients undergoing percutaneous mitral balloon valvotomy. Analysis of factors determining restenosis. Circulation. 1989;79:573–9.
89. Thomas MR, Monaghan MJ, Michalis LK, et al. Echocardiographic restenosis after successful balloon dilatation of the mitral valve with the Inoue balloon: experience of a United Kingdom centre. Br Heart J. 1993;69:418–23.
90. Iung B, Garbarz E, Michaud P, et al. Immediate and midterm results of repeat percutaneous mitral commissurotomy for restenosis following earlier percutaneous mitral commissurotomy. Eur Heart J. 2000;21:1683–9.

# Mitral Regurgitation: Epidemiology, Etiology and Physiopathology

**3**

Salvatore Scandura, Sarah Mangiafico, and Sandra Giaquinta

## 3.1    Epidemiology

In industrialized countries, mitral regurgitation (MR) ranks second among valve diseases, after aortic stenosis, and affects 9.3% of the population over 75 years of age. Epidemiological studies have shown that the prevalence of moderate or severe MR increases with age, with over 2–2.5 million patients in the United States in 2000, and is expected to double by 2030 due to the increase in life expectancy. In the United States, the prevalence of valve diseases is growing at a rate of 0.7% in patients aged between 18 and 44 years and 13.3% in patients over 75 years of age [1]. In Europe, the situation is similar, with a prevalence of mitral regurgitation that is on the rise, despite the reduced incidence of rheumatic disease [2].

At least moderate-to-severe MR is present in 15–20% of patients with heart failure, and in 12% of patients at 30 days from acute myocardial infarction (AMI), while MR of any grade is present in 25–50% of patients after an AMI, whether non-ST segment elevation myocardial infarction (NSTEMI) and ST-segment elevation myocardial infarction (STEMI) [3–5]. In patients with chronic and stable ischemic heart disease associated with left ventricular dysfunction, ischemic MR is even more frequent, exceeding 50% [6, 7]. Therefore, though valve diseases have a lower incidence compared with AMI or heart failure, the association between these conditions, especially between coronary disease and functional MR, underscores how urgent and necessary it is to focus on valve diseases by considering their incidence, the need to treat them, and, especially, recent therapeutic advances [8].

S. Scandura (✉) • S. Mangiafico • S. Giaquinta
Cardio-Thoracic-Vascular Department, Ferrarotto Hospital, Catania, Italy
e-mail: salvatore.scandura@tin.it

© Springer International Publishing AG 2018
C. Tamburino et al. (eds.), *Percutaneous Treatment of Left Side Cardiac Valves*,
https://doi.org/10.1007/978-3-319-59620-4_3

## 3.2    Etiology and Pathophysiology

Inadequate systolic coaptation of the mitral valve leaflets, in addition to changes in the pressure gradient between the atrium and left ventricle, is the cause of mitral valve regurgitation. Coaptation and correct apposition (symmetrical overlap, usually a minimum of 4–5 mm) [9] are essential to prevent regurgitation. MR, however, is the result of various etiological causes and regurgitation mechanisms. Therefore, it is possible to classify MR based on the etiological causes (acute and chronic), regurgitation mechanisms (according to Carpentier's functional classification [10]), and pathophysiology (degenerative/organic or functional causes).

The acute causes [11] include pathologies affecting the mitral annulus, such as infectious endocarditis or traumatic lesions; the leaflets, such as infectious endocarditis (perforation of the leaflet or presence of vegetation preventing the closing of the valve), traumatic lesions, atrial myxoma, and myxomatous degeneration; systemic lupus erythematosus (Libman–Sacks endocarditis); the chordae tendineae, such as myxomatous degeneration (valve prolapse, Marfan syndrome, and Ehlers–Danlos syndrome); infectious endocarditis; acute rheumatic disease and traumas; and the papillary muscles, such as acute coronary disease (rupture, muscle dysfunction), infiltrative diseases (sarcoidosis, amyloidosis), and traumas.

The chronic causes [11] include inflammatory diseases (rheumatic fever, systemic lupus erythematosus, scleroderma); degenerative diseases (Barlow's disease, Marfan syndrome, Ehlers–Danlos syndrome, mitral annulus calcifications) and infectious causes (infectious endocarditis); structural alterations (chordal rupture, rupture or malfunction of the papillary muscles, dilation of the mitral annulus and of the left ventricle); dilated and hypertrophic cardiomyopathy; and congenital abnormalities, such as cleft or fenestrated mitral valve and parachute mitral valve.

Regardless of the cause (Table 3.1), the mechanisms determining mitral regurgitation follow the "physiopathological triad" described by Carpentier [10, 12], who defined these variants to implement the most suitable strategies for surgical repair.

**Table 3.1** Mitral regurgitation: etiology

| Acute | Chronic primary MR |
|---|---|
| Endocarditis | Myxomatous (MVP) |
| Papillary muscle rupture (post-MI) | Rheumatic fever |
| Trauma | Endocarditis (healed) |
| Chordal rupture/leaflet flail (MVP, IE) | Mitral annular calcification |
|  | Congenital (cleft, AV canal)/HOCM with SAM |
|  | Radiation |
|  | Chronic secondary MR |
|  | Ischemic (LV remodeling) |
|  | Dilated cardiomyopathy |

**Key**: *MI* myocardial infarction, *MVP* mitral valve prolapse, *IE* infective endocarditis, *AV Canal* atrioventricular canal defect, *HOCM* hypertrophic obstructive cardiomyopathy, *SAM* systolic anterior motion of the mitral valve, *LV* left ventricular

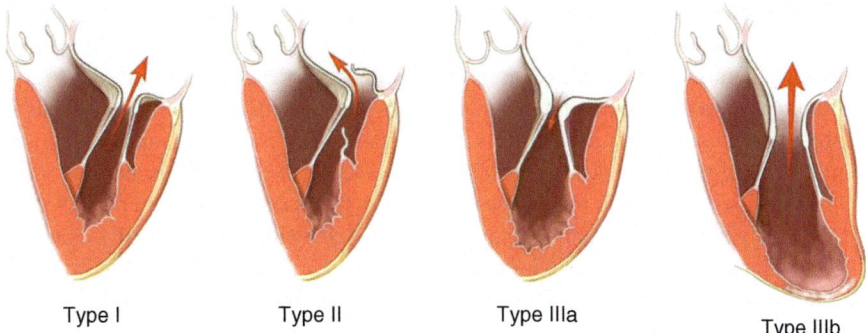

Type I          Type II          Type IIIa          Type IIIb

**Fig. 3.1** Carpentier's functional classification. Type I defines normal leaflet motion; type II, leaflet prolapsed or excessive motion; type III, restricted leaflet motion such as in rheumatic mitral valve disease (type IIIa) or ischemic mitral regurgitation (type IIIb). Adapted by Carpentier [10]

Carpentier's functional classification (Fig. 3.1) identifies three different types of mitral regurgitation, depending on the type of motion of the valve leaflets:

- Type I: Normal leaflet motion
- Type II: Leaflet prolapse
- Type III: Restricted leaflet motion

In type I, mitral regurgitation is secondary to annular dilation due to dilated and ischemic cardiomyopathy. This type also includes leaflet perforation secondary to endocarditis.

The causes of type II comprise prolapse, elongation, or rupture of the chordae tendineae and/or papillary muscles, especially secondary to coronary artery disease.

Type III may be due to rheumatic disease, ischemic heart disease, and dilated cardiomyopathy. It is divided, in turn, into types IIIa and IIIb. Type IIIa is characterized by reduced leaflet motion both during diastole and systole due to chordal shortening or thickened valve leaflets. Type IIIb occurs, instead, when leaflet motion is reduced only during systole. Regurgitation with reduced leaflet motion of ischemic origin is type IIIb. This classification underscores that the different mechanisms do not exclude one another. For example, a type IIIa lesion may also occur in association with type II lesions [13].

From a pathophysiological point of view, there are, instead, two MR categories [9, 14]: organic or degenerative (or primary) and functional (or secondary).

The organic or degenerative form involves intrinsic pathologies of the valve or valve apparatus. The functional form is also generally defined as ischemic, since the valve apparatus remains intact, and regurgitation is secondary to postischemic remodeling of the left ventricle. However, this remodeling also brings about structural changes of the leaflets in time.

Leaflet adaptation consists in both greater thickness and increased stiffness [15]. However, ischemic MR does not necessarily imply the presence of acute myocardial ischemia. It is indeed an abridgment that characterizes a clinical condition corresponding to chronic coronary disease, often associated with a prior history of one or more myocardial infarctions that lead to a progressive overall or regional pathologic remodeling of the left ventricle, usually in the absence of reversible ischemia [16].

In addition to ischemic forms, there are also some nonischemic functional forms in which overall or regional remodeling of the left ventricle is linked to various types of nonischemic cardiomyopathies [17].

Generally speaking, organic forms are the most frequent (60%), followed by those of functional (20%), endocarditic (2–5%), and rheumatic (2–5%) [9] origin. However, these data seem to refer to estimates obtained from patients with an indication for surgical treatment of valve disease and may therefore not reflect the actual prevalence of the various causes in the population. Longer life expectancy and the increasing incidence of heart failure have contributed to an increase in the incidence and prevalence of forms of functional MR, which would become the most frequent form in Western countries [18]. This distinction between organic and functional MR is important because these two forms differ greatly in terms of pathophysiology, treatment, and prognosis.

### 3.2.1 Organic or Degenerative Mitral Regurgitation

Organic or degenerative disease is the most frequent form of MR in the United States [19], and this condition was defined for the first time in studies by Barlow and Bosman [20] in the 1960s. It comprises a range of conditions in which acquired or congenital tissue alterations, either infiltrative or dysplastic, cause chordal elongation or rupture, resulting in a prolapse of the leaflets (most often the median scallop of the rear leaflet), also in association with annular dilation. More in general, it is described as myxomatous degeneration, a condition that leads to a situation called floppy valve, in addition to, as mentioned above, mitral prolapse. It is estimated that about 2% of the general population is affected with mitral degenerative disease [21], while echocardiographic findings show different degrees of mitral prolapse in about 5–6% of the female population alone. Despite the fact that the percentage is greater in women, evidence of severe regurgitation associated with organic MR is, however, more frequent in men [22]. The term "degenerative" covers a range of abnormalities, ranging from situations of fibroelastic deficiency, as in the Marfan and Ehlers–Danlos syndromes, to conditions involving valve tissue in excess, such as Barlow's disease [9, 23].

The term "fibroelastic deficiency" was initially proposed by Carpentier [24]. This condition describes a state of acute loss of mechanical integrity of the valve due to abnormalities of the connective tissue forming the valve apparatus [13]. The valve leaflets are thinned, transparent (pellucid according to Carpentier's definition), with thin and weakened chordae. In some cases, instead, the valve segments

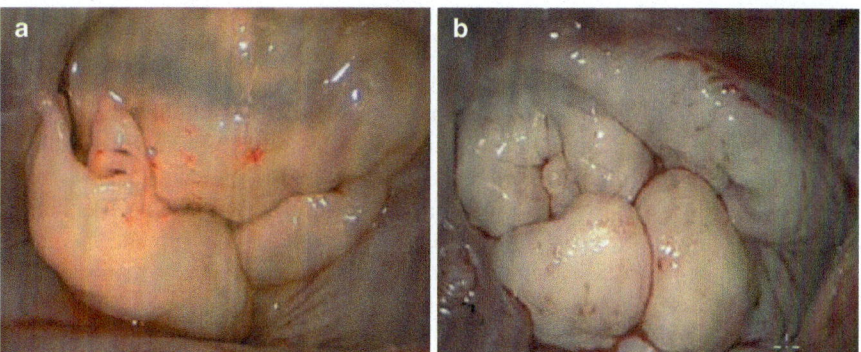

**Fig. 3.2** Intraoperative pictures of a mitral valve with fibroelastic deficiency (**a**) and Barlow's disease (**b**)

are absolutely normal and have a single, very thin chorda tendinea (Fig. 3.2a). MR is most frequently associated with the rupture of a single chorda and the prolapse of a single valve segment, generally P2. If the process progresses to becoming chronic, the prolapsing segment tends to experience an accumulation of mucopolysaccharides in the valve mucosa (through modifications of a biomechanical nature that have not been well characterized). This causes a myxomatous degeneration in which the leaflets become more extended and stiffer [25]. The patients most affected with this form of organic MR are aged >60 years and have a relatively short clinical history of regurgitation [23].

At the other end of the spectrum of degenerative mitral regurgitation, we find Barlow's disease, which is characterized by an excess of tissue, affecting multiple segments of the mitral leaflets following myxoid infiltration of the valve, with structural alterations, involving mainly the collagen (Fig. 3.2b). The valve almost always appears to be enlarged, while the leaflets have thickened and redundant tissue, and are affected by myxomatous degeneration that progresses into what is called "floppy valve," with extended yet thickened leaflets (diastolic thickness > 5 mm). There is also a presence of elongated and thickened chordae that are at risk of rupture [13]. Typically, the dimensions of the valve, based on the surface area of the anterior leaflet, correspond to a mitral annulus measuring ≥36 mm on average. It is also possible to see varying degrees of annular dilation or calcification, also associated with fibrosis and calcification of the papillary muscles, and specifically of the anterolateral muscle. The etiology is unknown; though some cases have a familial component, its distribution is sporadic [26]. Patients with this organic form of MR are often aged 60 years or younger, with a longer clinical history of mitral regurgitation than of fibroelastic deficiency [21]. This disease, which mainly affects women, can be diagnosed at an age of 40 years or younger, with evidence of mid-diastolic click and end-systolic murmur in the mitral area. Patients often remain asymptomatic for a long time. MR severity depends on the number of prolapsing segments.

Though the incidence of rheumatic disease is decreasing [21], it nevertheless remains a common cause of mitral regurgitation (to the extent that rheumatic disease is involved primarily in the genesis of valve stenosis [27]). The prevalence of rheumatic disease is still high in developing countries and would be even higher if these patients were studied by echocardiographic screening [28]. This disease leads to widespread fibrous thickening of the leaflets, also associated with calcific deposits. Chordal shortening, fibrosis of the papillary muscles, and asymmetric annular dilation may also be found [29]. During a first episode of rheumatic disease, a patient may also experience acute mitral regurgitation, mainly linked to the prolapse of the anterior or posterior leaflet [30]. In the event of anterior prolapse, patients respond better to medical treatment, while it has a worse outcome in patients with posterior leaflet prolapse, thus requiring surgical therapy.

Annular calcification is another organic mechanism involved in the onset of MR. Described for the first time in 1908 by Bonninger [31], it is a disorder that mainly affects older populations, aged >60 years, and has a greater incidence among women. The pathogenesis is not exactly known and is believed to play a significant role in the mechanical stress acting on the annulus, as happens in conditions of hypertension [32]. It is well known that annular calcification is more frequent in patients suffering from systemic arterial hypertension, hypertrophic cardiomyopathy, Barlow's disease, chronic kidney failure, and diabetes mellitus. In 50% of cases, it is possible to also document a concomitant presence of aortic stenosis. Due to these changes, the annulus may also develop brittle and massive calcifications, resulting in leaflet deformation and chordal elongation. Regurgitation will hence be the result of a process of displacement or immobilization of the leaflets, which thus hinders correct valve coaptation [33].

The pathophysiology of MR differs depending on whether valve damage is acute or the result of a chronic process. The causes that generally elicit primary acute MR are spontaneous rupture of the chordae tendineae, acute endocarditis, or chest trauma [34–37]. In severe acute MR, the LA and LV receive a sudden volume overload, which, in turn, leads to a rise in left ventricur preload, allowing for a moderate increase in systolic output. However, being an acute form, eccentric hypertrophy, a compensatory mechanism maintaining CO constant, cannot take place. The hemodynamic consequences of the failure of the left heart chambers to adapt to volume overload are large "V" waves in the LA, and pulmonary edema. This serious condition of hemodynamic decompensation requires urgent mitral valve repair or replacement.

In the case of chronic MR, there is plenty of time for LA and LV to make compensatory changes, allowing for increased atrial and pulmonary vein compliance. Therefore, patients do not usually report the symptoms of pulmonary edema for many years. During systole, in the presence of MR, blood is not entirely directed along the outflow tract into the aorta and is pushed in part into the LA. The quantity of blood reflowing into the atrium takes the name of regurgitant volume; the volume is strictly correlated with the square root of the systolic gradient between the LV and LA, the duration of regurgitation, and effective regurgitant orifice (ERO) [34, 38–40]. Regurgitation in the LA leads to an increase in atrial pressure, while reducing the antegrade output. In cases of major regurgitation, LA pressure remains high even during the late diastolic phase. At a ventricular level, MR is the cause of major preload, while afterload is normal or reduced due to the regurgitant volume returning to a low-pressure chamber, thus allowing the ventricle to spend most of its energy in shortening the fibers, rather than generating tension [34, 41]. These reduced wall-stress conditions resulting from low afterload, and associated with high preload, lead to left ventricular remodeling, with an increase in chamber volume, an increase in end-diastolic volume, and preserved antegrade output. As stated above, this type of compensation allows MR to remain asymptomatic for a long period of time [34, 42, 43]. The type of hypertrophy generated is determined by the serial replication of sarcomeres, opposite to increased afterload in which sarcomeres replicate in parallel. After an initial compensation phase, the left ventricular contractility progressively reduces [44, 45]. In this case, left ventricular ejection fraction (LVEF), if taken as an index of left ventricular contractility, can remain within normal range, despite a drop in systolic function [46–48], because of the impact of the regurgitant volume in the measurement of LVEF. Therefore, a LVEF of less than 60% in the presence of severe MR is a sign of left ventricular dysfunction [47]. Other indexes for the assessment of LV function are the end-systolic diameter (LVESD) and end-systolic volume (LVESV), both of which are more independent factors compared with ventricular preload conditions [49–53]. A greater LVESV corresponds to a worsening in left ventricular contractility. It has been noted that preoperative measurements of LVESV and the left ventricular end-systolic volume index (LVESVI) are the best predictors of postoperative left ventricular systolic function [53].

## 3.2.2 Functional or Secondary Mitral Regurgitation

### 3.2.2.1 Ischemic Mitral Regurgitation

The pathophysiology of ischemic mitral regurgitation is much more complex than that of organic MR. It is caused by structural modifications of the left ventricle, following an ischemic process that results in a deficit of functional efficiency of the cardiac pump. Ischemic necrosis, whether acute or subacute, causes an overall or regional remodeling of the left ventricle, which becomes more global and spherical, losing its typical ellipsoidal shape [54]. In the initial stages, MR linked to this etiology is moderate, with mild or barely perceptible systolic murmur. It occurs in 20% of patients with AMI, and in half of these patients who also develop heart failure [55], with increased mortality and morbidity [4]. The relative risk of MR varies from 1.48 to 7.5, with a poor long-term prognosis in patients who present primarily with NSTEMI [56]. Ischemic functional MR should be distinguished from acute complications of myocardial infarction that may determine mitral valve regurgitation, as in the case of rupture or elongation of the papillary muscles (usually a head of the posteromedial muscle). Instead, in ischemic MR we speak of an event that occurs in terms of chronic coronary disease the onset of which generally occurs after approximately 2 weeks, in the absence of intrinsic valve structural alterations [57]. In other words, it is defined as a condition that affects mostly the shape and function of the left ventricle, which shows dyssynchrony of wall muscles, especially in the basal segments, and of the papillary muscles, causing altered contraction of the mitral annulus and reduced cardiac contractility. Moreover, the annulus becomes rounder, losing its typical saddle shape, while the papillary muscles are more displaced [58]. On the mitral valve, this involves reduced closing force, on the one hand, and an increase in tethering forces, on the other. Tethering of the mitral valve is a phenomenon linked to the specific alteration that the papillary muscles experience. They generally undergo a posterolateral displacement at their base, and a displacement toward the apex of the heart. This mechanism results in increased traction on the valve by the chordae tendineae, and this creates an abnormal cuspido-chordal tension that displaces the mitral leaflets and the coaptation point of the leaflets apically. The chordae are, therefore, tauter due to the lack of synergy of the ventricle wall. Due to the tethering forces, it has been observed that over time the valve leaflets may also undergo structural changes, with increased stretching and stiffness [15]. Examined by two-dimensional echocardiography, tethering produces the shape of a tent between the annular plane and the displaced leaflets [59]. Such displacement also results in a characteristic echocardiographic deformity of the anterior leaflet, creating the so-called *seagull sign* [60]. It is thus possible to consider a tenting volume and a tenting area. The tenting volume relates closely to the regurgitant orifice area, while the tenting area, which must be evaluated in mid-systole, is a predictor of surgical repair failure when it is $\geq 1.6$ cm$^2$ [61]. Moreover, the tenting area can be asymmetrical or symmetrical. When infarction occurs in the posterior region, the tenting area is asymmetric due to reduced mobility, especially of the posterior leaflet. When there is an anterior infarction or an infarction that is both anterior and posterior, the left ventricle is more global and spherical, and both papillary muscles are affected by the ischemic process and are therefore displaced. In this case, the tenting area is symmetrical. Echocardiographically, when tethering is symmetrical, the regurgitant jet is central [59]. It will also be important to determine postischemic remodeling of the left ventricle by measuring the ventricular volumes and calculating the sphericity index. Finally, there is also the assessment of the ERO, which may vary during systole, decreasing in mid-systole compared with end-systole. However, it should be pointed out that despite pathogenetic differences, functional MR differs from organic MR also echocardiographically [62]. While one normally speaks of severe organic MR when an ERO of >40 mm$^2$ is estimated, this value is lower, i.e. >20 mm$^2$, in the functional form. These changes are determined by dynamic changes of transmitral pressure, contributing to valve closure. These changes can be better appreciated in exercise Doppler echocardiogram [59]. Exercise- or stress-induced geometric ventricular change increases regurgitant orifice area and volume and may result in dyspnea; it is also associated with a history of acute pulmonary edema [63].

### 3.2.2.2 Nonischemic Mitral Regurgitation

Dilation and increased sphericity of the left ventricle can also be the result of non-ischemic heart diseases, such as dilated cardiomyopathy and heart failure [64]. The suggested mechanisms for the onset of functional MR in patients with dilated cardiomyopathy are the decreased transmitral pressure gradient, geometrical changes in the mitral annulus, papillary muscles, and mitral valve, associated with dyssynchronic left ventricular contractions [65]. In this case, too, however, as in functional ischemic MR, it is believed that leaflet changes make a decisive contribution to the severity of functional MR. Chronic ventricular remodeling (which affects mostly the lateral, posterior, and inferior segments) involves, in this case as well, a displacement of the papillary muscles, the dyssynchrony of which is considered to be an independent predictor of mild or moderate–severe MR [65]. Therefore, this involves a lateralization of the tethering forces, causing incomplete closure of the valve leaflets. Tethering length, understood as the distance from the apex of the papillary muscles to the anterior mitral annulus, is also an independent predictor of MR [66, 67].

Annular dilation and reduced closing forces primarily modify tethering but are not the predominant mechanisms of MR [15]. In the chronically volume-overloaded ventricle, constitutive increases in LV wall stress eventually cause a decrease in contractility [45] and a corresponding reduction in the annular and closing forces that may otherwise lessen MR due to tethering alone. In heart failure patients, the onset of chronic MR complicates ventricular dysfunction and, more often, heart failure. The left ventricle is enlarged, becomes more compliant, and the driving forces are relatively scant. MR-related volume overload contributes to creating a vicious circle: the greater the degree of ventricular remodeling is, the greater the degree of MR; the latter, in turn, further dilates the left ventricle, thereby further increasing the valve defect. The perpetuation of this vicious circle significantly affects left ventricular geometry, thus inducing ventricular sphericity. Although MR reduces impedance and has an unloading effect, left ventricular dilatation increases LV wall stress, thereby impairing its contractile strength [68, 69] (Fig. 3.3).

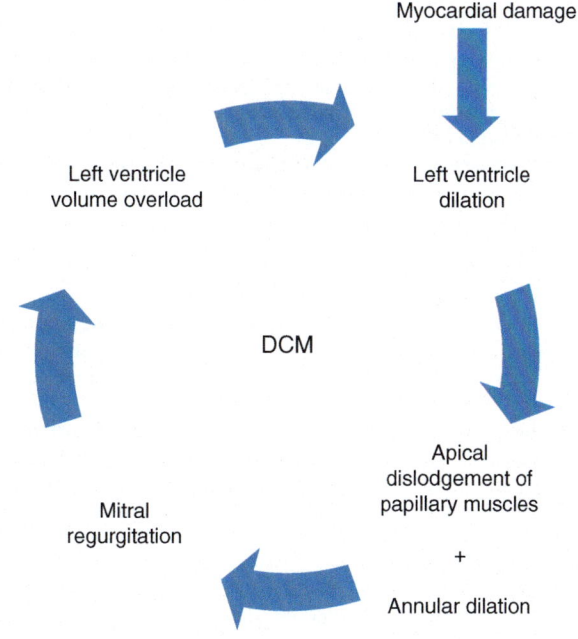

**Fig. 3.3** Vicious circle of the dilated cardiomyopathy (DCM) and mitral regurgitation

The upstream consequences are high LA pressure and pulmonary hypertension. Several authors have emphasized the fact that MR in patients with advanced heart failure and severe LV remodeling is a "ventricular disease" that takes on the manifestation of a valvular disease [66, 68, 70].

As shown by several studies, evidence of functional MR is therefore associated with a reduction in the survival of patients with dilated cardiomyopathy [71] and heart failure of a systolic nature [72]. For this reason, early cardiac resynchronization therapy (CRT) has shown a significant reduction in the incidence of MR in patients with left ventricular heart failure [73], also showing beneficial effects on the severity of any MR [74]. The improvement in ventricular contractility after resynchronization is able to increase the closing force of the mitral valve, reducing early systolic mitral regurgitation [75]. The reduction of left ventricular dyssynchrony and changes of ventricular geometry seem to be able to reduce the degree of MR and, therefore, morbidity and mortality [76], especially in patients with an ejection fraction lower than 35% and left bundle branch block. However, there is still a lack of data to predict which patients can effectively respond to CRT, though it seems that patients with extensive infarction or a tenting area >3.8 cm² would benefit little [77].

## References

1. Nkomo VT, Gardin JM, Skelton TN, Gottdiener JS, Scott CG, Enriquez-Sarano M. Burden of valvular heart diseases: a population-based study. Lancet. 2006;368:1005–11.
2. Stott DK, Marpole DG, Bristow JD, et al. The role of left atrial transport in aortic and mitral stenosis. Circulation. 1970;41:1031–41.
3. Robbins JD, Maniar PB, Cotts W, et al. Prevalence and severity of mitral regurgitation in chronic systolic heart failure. Am J Cardiol. 2003;91:360–2.
4. Bursi F, Enriquez-Sarano M, Nkomo VT, et al. Heart failure and death after myocardial infarction in the community: the emerging role of mitral regurgitation. Circulation. 2005;111:295–301.
5. Pèrez de Isla L, Zamorano J, Quezada M, et al. Functional mitral regurgitation after a first non-ST-segment elevation acute coronary syndrome: contribution to congestive heart failure. Eur Heart J. 2007;28:2866–72.
6. Deja MA, Grayburn PA, Sun B, et al. Influence of mitral regurgitation repair on survival in the surgical treatment for ischemic heart failure trial. Circulation. 2012;125:2639–48. doi:10.1161/CIRCULATIONAHA.111.072256.
7. Rossi A, Dini FL, Faggiano P, et al. Independent prognostic value of functional mitral regurgitation in patients with heart failure. A quantitative analysis of 1256 patients with ischaemic and non-ischaemic dilated cardiomyopathy. Heart. 2011;97:1675–80. doi:10.1136/hrt.2011.225789.
8. Iung B, Baron G, Butchart EG, et al. A prospective survey of patients with valvular heart disease in Europe: the Euro Heart Survey on Valvular Heart Disease. Eur Heart J. 2003;24:1231–43.
9. McCarthy KP, Ring L, Rana BS. Anatomy of the mitral valve: understanding the mitral valve complex in mitral regurgitation. Eur J Echocardiogr. 2010;11:i3–9.
10. Carpentier A. Cardiac valve surgery—the "French correction". J Thorac Cardiovasc Surg. 1983;86:323–37.
11. Otto CM, Bonow RO. Mitral regurgitation. In: Bonow RO, Mann DL, Zipes DP, Libby P, editors. Braunwald's heart disease. 8th ed. Philadelphia: Elsevier, Saunders; 2007. p. 1657–73.

12. Carpentier AF, Lessana A, Relland JY, et al. The "physio-ring", an advanced concept in mitral valve annuloplasty. Ann Thorac Surg. 1995;60:1177–85.
13. Tsang W, Freed BH, Langin RM. Three-dimensional anatomy of the aortic and mitral valves. In: Otto CM, Bonow RO, editors. Valvular heart disease: a companion to Braunwald's heart disease. 4th ed. Philadelphia: Elsevier, Saunders; 2013. p. 14–29.
14. Lancellotti P, Moura L, Pierard L, et al. European Association of Echocardiography recommendations for the assessment of valvular regurgitation. Part 2: mitral and tricuspid regurgitation (native valve disease). Eur J Echocardiogr. 2010;11:307–32.
15. Chaput M, Handschumacher MD, Tournoux F, et al. Mitral leaflet adaptation to ventricular remodelling occurrence and adequacy in patients with functional mitral regurgitation. Circulation. 2008;118:845–52.
16. Levine RA, Schwammenthal E. Ischemic mitral regurgitation on the threshold of a solution: from paradoxes to unifying concepts. Circulation. 2005;112:745–58.
17. Hueb A, BiscegliJatene F, PinhoMoreira L, et al. Ventricular remodeling and mitral valve modifications in dilated cardiomyopathy: new insight from anatomic study. J Thorac Cardiovasc Surg. 2002;124:1216–24.
18. Maisano F, Alamanni F, Alfieri O, et al. Transcatheter treatment of chronic mitral regurgitation with the MitraClip system: an Italian consensus statement. J Cardiovasc Med. 2014;15:173–88.
19. Hayek E, Gring C, Griffin B. Mitral valve prolapse. Lancet. 2005;365:507–18.
20. Barlow J, Bosman C. Aneurysmal protrusion of the posterior leaflet of the mitral valve: an auscultatory-electrocardiographic syndrome. Am Heart J. 1966;71:166–78.
21. Enriquez-Sarano M, Akias CW, Vahanian A. Mitral regurgitation. Lancet. 2009;373:1382–94.
22. Barlow J, Pocock W. Mitral valve prolapse, the specific billowing mitral leaflet syndrome, or an insignificant non-ejection systolic click. Am Heart J. 1979;97:277–85.
23. Adams DH, Rosenhek R, Falk V. Degenerative mitral valve regurgitation: best practice revolution. Eur Heart J. 2010;31:1958–66.
24. Carpentier A, Lacour-Gayet F, Camilleri J. Fibroelastic dysplasia of the mitral valve: an anatomical and clinical entity. Circulation. 1982;3:307.
25. Barber JE, Kasper FK, Ratliff NB, et al. Mechanical properties of myxomatous mitral valves. J Thorac Cardiovasc Surg. 2001;122:955–62.
26. Anyanwu AC, Adams DH. Etiologic classification of degenerative mitral valve disease: Barlow's disease and fibroelastic deficiency. Semin Thorac Cardiovasc Surg. 2007;19:90–6.
27. Iung B, Vahanian A. Epidemiology of valvular heart disease in the adult. Nat Rev Cardiol. 2011;8:162–72.
28. Marijon E, Ou P, Celermajer DS, et al. Prevalence of rheumatic heart disease detected by echocardiographic screening. N Engl J Med. 2007;357:470–6.
29. Waller B, Howard J, Fess S. Pathology of mitral valve stenosis and pure mitral regurgitation, part I. Clin Cardiol. 1994;17:330–6.
30. Kamblock J, N'Guyen L, Pagis B, et al. Acute severe mitral regurgitation during first attacks of rheumatic fever: clinical spectrum, mechanisms and prognostic factors. J Heart Valve Dis. 2005;14:440–6.
31. Fox CS. Mitral annular calcification predicts cardiovascular morbidity and mortality: the Framingham Heart Study. Circulation. 2003;107:1492–6.
32. Boon A, Cheriex E, Lodder J, et al. Cardiac valve calcification: characteristics of patients with calcification of the mitral annulus or aortic valve. Heart. 1997;78:472–4.
33. Korn D, DeSanctis R, Sell S. Massive calcification of the mitral annulus. N Engl J Med. 1962;267:900–9.
34. Fenster MS, Feldman MD. Mitral regurgitation: an overview. Curr Probl Cardiol. 1995;20:193–280.
35. Luther RR, Meyers SN. Acute mitral insufficiency secondary to ruptured chordae tendineae. Arch Intern Med. 1974;134:568–78.
36. Hansen DE, Sarris GE, Niczyporuk MA, et al. Physiologic role of the mitral apparatus in left ventricular regional mechanics, contraction synergy, and global systolic performance. J Thorac Cardiovasc Surg. 1989;97:521–33.

37. Yun KL, Niczyporuk MA, Sarris GE, et al. Importance of mitral subvalvular apparatus in terms of cardiac energetics and systolic mechanics in the ejecting canine heart. J Clin Invest. 1991;87:247–54.
38. Yiu SF, Enriquez-Sarano M, Tribouilloy C, et al. Determinants of the degree of functional mitral regurgitation in patients with systolic left ventricular dysfunction. Circulation. 2000;102:1400–6.
39. Grigioni F, Enriquez-Sarano M, Zehr KJ, et al. Ischemic mitral regurgitation: long-term outcome and prognostic implications with quantitative Doppler assessment. Circulation. 2001;103:1759–64.
40. Enriquez-Sarano M, Avierinos JF, Messika-Zeitoun D, et al. Quantitative determinants of the outcome of asymptomatic mitral regurgitation. N Engl J Med. 2005;352:875–83.
41. Waller BF, Howard J, Fess S. Pathology of mitral valve stenosis and pure mitral regurgitation, part II. Clin Cardiol. 1994;17:395–402.
42. Grossman W. Profiles in valvular heart disease. In: Baim DS, editor. Cardiac catheterization, angiography and intervention. Baltimore: Lippincott Williams and Wilkins; 2006.
43. Ross J Jr. Adaptations of the left ventricle to chronic volume overload. Circ Res. 1974;35:64–70.
44. Yun KL, Rayhill SC, Niczyporuk MA, et al. Left ventricular mechanics and energetics in the dilated canine heart: acute versus chronic mitral regurgitation. J Thorac Cardiovasc Surg. 1992;104:26–39.
45. Carabello BA, Nakano K, Corin W, et al. Left ventricular function in experimental volume overload hypertrophy. Am J Physiol. 1989;256:974–81.
46. Urabe Y, Mann DL, Kent RL, et al. Cellular and ventricular contractile dysfunction in experimental canine mitral regurgitation. Circ Res. 1992;70:131–47.
47. Starling MR, Kirsh MM, Montgomery DG, et al. Impaired left ventricular contractile function in patients with long-term mitral regurgitation and normal ejection fraction. J Am Coll Cardiol. 1993;22:239–50.
48. Nakano K, Swindle MM, Spinale F, et al. Depressed contractile function due to canine mitral regurgitation improves after correction of the volume overload. J Clin Invest. 1991;87:2077–86.
49. Carabello BA, Crawford FA Jr. Valvular heart disease. N Engl J Med. 1997;337:32–41.
50. Carabello BA, Nolan SP, McGuire LB. Assessment of preoperative left ventricular function in patients with mitral regurgitation: value of the end-systolic wall stress-end-systolic volume ratio. Circulation. 1981;64:1212–7.
51. Carabello BA, Williams H, Gash AK, et al. Hemodynamic predictors of outcome in patients undergoing valve replacement. Circulation. 1986;74:1309–16.
52. Grossman W, Braunwald E, Mann T, et al. Contractile state of the left ventricle in man as evaluated from end-systolic pressure-volume relations. Circulation. 1977;56:845.
53. Borow KM, Green LH, Mann T, et al. End-systolic volume as a predictor of postoperative left ventricular performance in volume overload from valvular regurgitation. Am J Med. 1980;68:655–3.
54. Sharp N. Ventricular remodeling following myocardial infarction. Am J Cardiol. 1992;70:20C–6C.
55. Otsuji Y, Levine RA, Takeuchi M, et al. Mechanism of ischemic mitral regurgitation. J Cardiol. 2008;51:145–56.
56. Perez de Isla L, Zamorano J, Quezada M, et al. Prognostic significance of functional mitral regurgitation after a first non-ST-segment elevation acute coronary syndrome. Eur Heart J. 2006;27:2655–60.
57. Marwick TH, Lancellotti P, Pierard L. Ischaemic mitral regurgitation: mechanisms and diagnosis. Heart. 2009;95:1711–8.
58. Sadeghpour A, Abtahi F, Kiavar M, et al. Echocardiographic evaluation of mitral geometry in functional mitral regurgitation. J Cardiothorac Surg. 2008;3:54.
59. Piérard LA, Carabello BA. Ischaemic mitral regurgitation: pathophysiology, outcomes and the conundrum of treatment. Eur Heart J. 2010;31:2996–3005.
60. Messas E, Guerrero JL, Handschumacher MD, et al. Chordal cutting: a new therapeutic approach for ischemic mitral regurgitation. Circulation. 2001;104:1958–63.

61. Kongsaerepong V, Shiota M, Gillinov AM, et al. Echocardiographic predictors of successful versus unsuccessful mitral valve repair in ischemic mitral regurgitation. Am J Cardiol. 2006;98:504–8.
62. O'Gara PT. Randomized trials in moderate ischemic mitral regurgitation: many questions, limited answers. Circulation. 2012;126:2452–5.
63. Salukhe TV, Henein MY, Sutton R. Ischemic mitral regurgitation and its related risk after myocardial infarction. Circulation. 2005;111:254–6.
64. Donal E, De Place C, Kervio G, et al. Mitral regurgitation in dilated cardiomyopathy: value of both regional left ventricular contractility and dyssynchrony. Eur J Echocardiogr. 2009;10:133–8.
65. Tigen K, Karaahmet T, Dundar C, et al. The importance of papillary muscle dyssynchrony in predicting the severity of functional mitral regurgitation in patients with non-ischaemic dilated cardiomyopathy: a two-dimensional speckle-tracking echocardiography study. Eur J Echocardiogr. 2010;11:671–6.
66. Otsuji Y, Handschumacher M, Schwammenthal E, et al. Insights from three-dimensional echocardiography into the mechanism of functional mitral regurgitation direct in vivo demonstration of altered leaflet tethering geometry. Circulation. 1997;96:1999–2008.
67. Karaca O, Avci A, Guler GB, et al. Tenting area reflects disease severity and prognosis in patients with non-ischaemic dilated cardiomyopathy and functional mitral regurgitation. Eur J Heart Fail. 2011;13:284–91.
68. Olson L, Subramanian R, Ackermann D, et al. Surgical pathology of the mitral valve: a study of 712 cases spanning 21 years. Mayo Clin Proc. 1987;62:22–4.
69. Carabello BA. Ischemic mitral regurgitation and ventricular remodelling. J Am Coll Cardiol. 2004;43:384–5.
70. Di Salvo T, Acker MA, Dec GW, et al. Mitral valve surgery in advanced heart failure. J Am Coll Cardiol. 2010;55:271–82.
71. Blondheim D, Jacobs L, Kotler M, et al. Dilated cardiomyopathy with mitral regurgitation: decreased survival despite a low frequency of left ventricular thrombus. Am Heart J. 1991;122:763–71.
72. Schaufelberger M, Swedberg K, Koster M, et al. Decreasing one-year mortality and hospitalization rates for heart failure in Sweden: data from the Swedish Hospital Discharge Registry 1988 to 2000. Eur Heart J. 2004;25:300–7.
73. Porciani M, Macioce R, Demarchi G, et al. Effects of cardiac resynchronization therapy on the mechanisms underlying functional mitral regurgitation in congestive heart failure. Eur J Echocardiogr. 2006;7:31–9.
74. Cleland J, Daubert J, Erdmann E, et al. Cardiac Resynchronization-Heart Failure (CARE-HF) Study Investigators. The effect of cardiac resynchronization therapy on morbidity and mortality in heart failure. N Engl J Med. 2005;352:1539–49.
75. Ypenburg C, Lancellotti P, Tops L, et al. Mechanism of improvement in mitral regurgitation after cardiac resynchronization therapy. Eur Heart J. 2008;29:757–65.
76. Di Biase L, Auricchio A, Mohanty P, et al. Impact of cardiac resynchronization therapy on the severity of mitral regurgitation. Europace. 2011;13:829–38.
77. Sitges M, Vidal B, Delgado V, et al. Long-term effect of cardiac resynchronization therapy on functional mitral valve regurgitation. Am J Cardiol. 2009;104:383–8.

# Mitral Regurgitation: Diagnosis and Timing of Intervention

**4**

Marta Chiarandà, Sarah Mangiafico, and Salvatore Scandura

## 4.1 Noninvasive Diagnosis

The clinical manifestations of mitral regurgitation (MR) are conditioned by the magnitude and rapidity of onset and the ability of the chambers of the heart to adapt from a hemodynamic and neuroendocrine perspective. Patients with MR are often asymptomatic despite a severe degree of valve regurgitation. The major symptom is dyspnea, at first on exertion and then at rest, accompanied by peripheral edemas, marked asthenia, and palpitations. The most serious clinical manifestation is acute pulmonary edema [1]. Echocardiography is the key imaging modality used in the workup of patients with MR.

By favoring the ejection of the left ventricle in a chamber at low pressure, and limiting the transmission of the high-pressure gradient due to MR to pulmonary circulation, the distensibility of the left atrium is the most relevant physiopathological determinant of clinical and hemodynamic tolerance to volume overload.

A thorough clinical history is often essential to have information about the etiology of the valve disease (prior infarctions, episodes of angina pectoris, rheumatic fever, endocarditis) [2].

*Physical examination*: At physical examination, arterial pressure is normal, arterial pulse is rapid, and heart auscultation directs us toward MR in the presence of systolic murmur, often holosystolic, including the first and second heart sound. In the case of prolapse, the murmur is often end systolic, while it is early systolic in the case of functional MR. The murmur is typically very loud and blowing, but it can even be harsh, especially in the case of mitral prolapse. The first sound (S1) is included in the murmur, and is usually normal, but may also be loud in the case of a rheumatic valvulopathy. The second sound (S2) is generally normal too, but may be split if the left ventricle's ejection time is very short. There can also be a third sound (S3), which is

M. Chiarandà • S. Mangiafico • S. Scandura (✉)
Division of Cardiology, Ferrarotto Hospital, University of Catania, Catania, Italy
e-mail: salvatore.scandura@tin.it

© Springer International Publishing AG 2018
C. Tamburino et al. (eds.), *Percutaneous Treatment of Left Side Cardiac Valves*,
https://doi.org/10.1007/978-3-319-59620-4_4

directly correlated with the regurgitant volume. Typically, it becomes louder with exhalation and, in the case of functional or ischemic MR, is often associated with a restrictive ventricular filling pattern. A gallop rhythm (S4) can be detected in the case of MR with a recent onset and functional and/or ischemic MR. MR is often associated with a protodiastolic murmur generated by the increase in mitral flow in diastole. A mid-diastolic click can be heard in the case of prolapse [2].

*Electrocardiogram*: In the case of chronic MR, the electrocardiogram (ECG) shows signs of enlarged left heart chambers, with increased P waves and QRS complexes. When MR is ischemic, there can be ECG signs of recent or prior ischemic damage.

*Chest x-ray*: In chronic MR, the chest x-ray usually shows a dilation of the left chambers, and calcifications can be seen in the mitral annulus in degenerative valvulopathy or near the mitral leaflets in rheumatic valvulopathy.

*Echocardiography*: Echocardiography is still the method of choice for the diagnosis of MR. Both transthoracic echocardiogram (TTE) and transesophageal echocardiography (TEE) make it possible to evaluate the degree of regurgitation and the morphofunctional characteristics of the valve (determining the pathogenetic mechanisms and ventricular function), as well as to determine the best therapeutic strategy [3–5]. One of the major obstacles to a diagnosis of the degree of severity of MR is the lack of a single gold standard method. This is probably due to the great variability of regurgitation, which, in turn, is strongly influenced by the hemodynamic conditions at the time of assessment. An increase or reduction of the preload and/or afterload and changes in heart rate, myocardial contractility, and atrial compliance are all factors that can most affect the regurgitant volume. For this reason, an echocardiographic assessment of multiple parameters is needed to determine the extent and severity of valve regurgitation as reliably as possible [6].

MR can be assumed in the presence of:

- Altered morphology of the valve apparatus (valve prolapse, flail, calcification of the annulus, dysfunction or breakage of the papillary muscles) (Fig. 4.1)
- Dilation of the left atrium
- Atrial septal aneurysm, with convexity toward the right atrium (increased pressure and/or atrial volume) (Fig. 4.2)

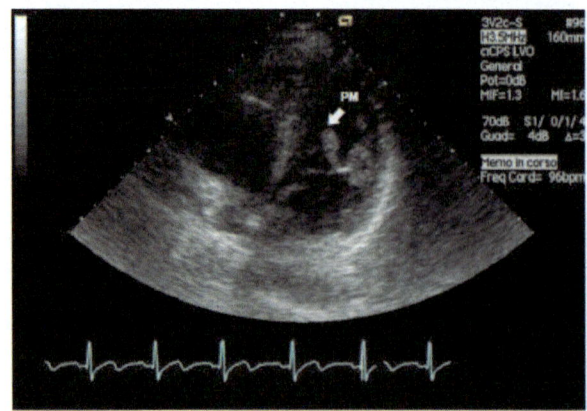

**Fig. 4.1** Transthoracic echocardiogram. Apical four-chamber view. Rupture of the posterolateral papillary muscle (PM), (*arrow*)

- Dilation of the left ventricle (Fig. 4.3)
- Hyperkinesia of the left ventricular walls
- The presence of akinetic/aneurysmal areas in some segments in the case of ischemic MR (Fig. 4.4)
- Clear signs of right ventricular overload (Fig. 4.5).

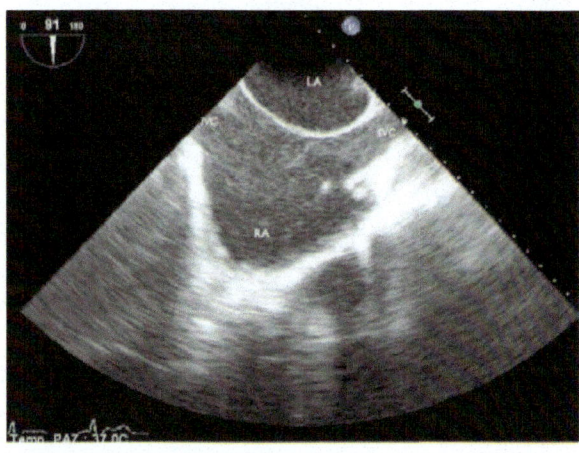

**Fig. 4.2** Transesophageal echocardiogram. Bicaval view (90°). Right convexity of the interatrial septum in a patient with left atrium (LA) volume overload. *RA* right atrium, *IVC* inferior vena cava, *SVC* superior vena cava

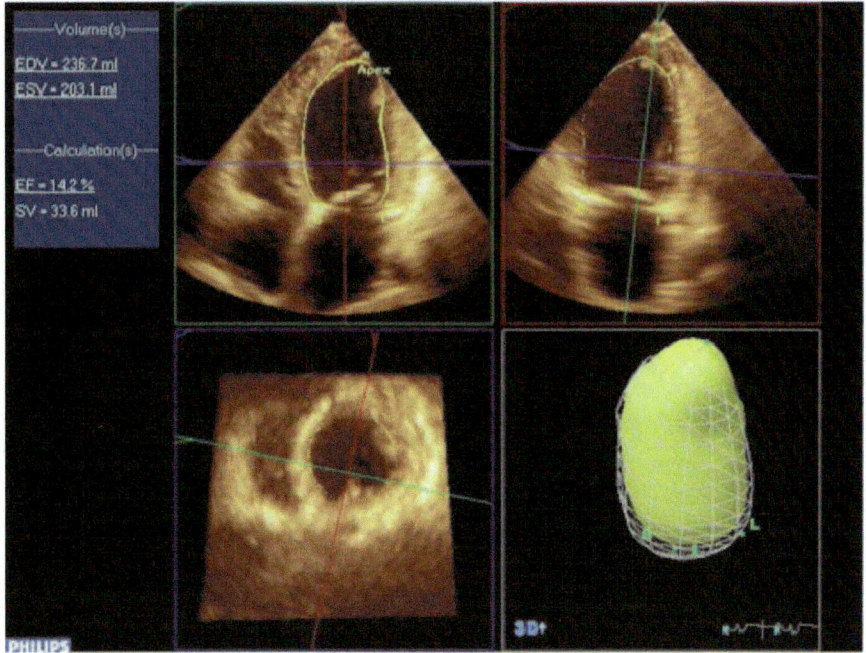

**Fig. 4.3** 3D left ventricle volumes reconstruction using Q-Lab software (Philips Healthcare, Andover, MA, USA). Increase in left ventricular end-diastolic (EDV) and end-systolic (ESV) volumes. Estimated left ventricle ejection fraction (EF) is about 14% and stroke volume (SV) is 34 mL

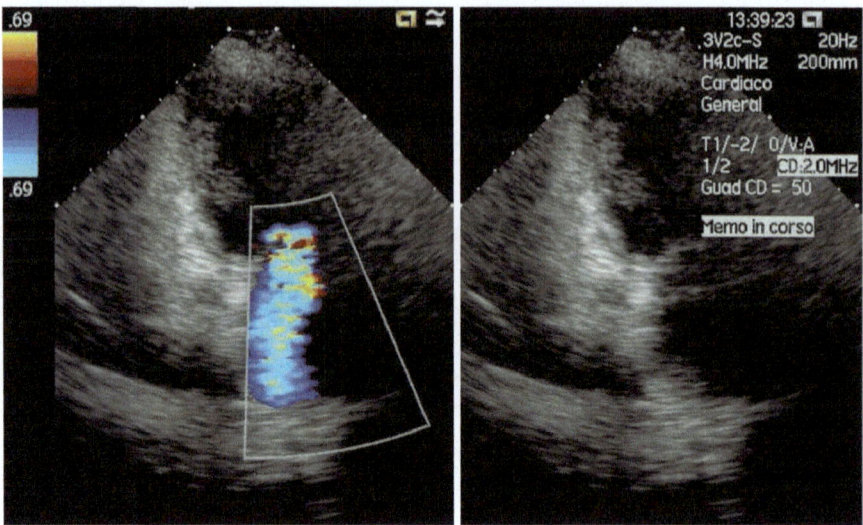

**Fig. 4.4** Transthoracic echocardiogram. Apical two-chamber view. Functional ischemic mitral regurgitation due to posterior leaflet tethering for akinesia of the infero-posterior wall

**Fig. 4.5** Transthoracic echocardiogram. Short-axis view. D-shape of the left ventricle (LV), secondary to right ventricular (RV) overload

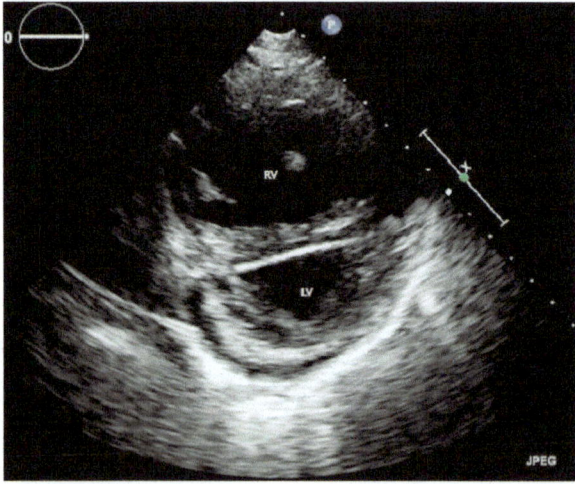

Clearly, the following are indispensable for evaluating leaflet malcoaptation indices and functional abnormalities of the annulus, which, despite a normal anatomy, are responsible for the development of valve regurgitation:

**Fig. 4.6** Chamber transesophageal echocardiogram of left ventricular outflow tract (LVOT). Coaptation gap between the annular plane and coaptation point

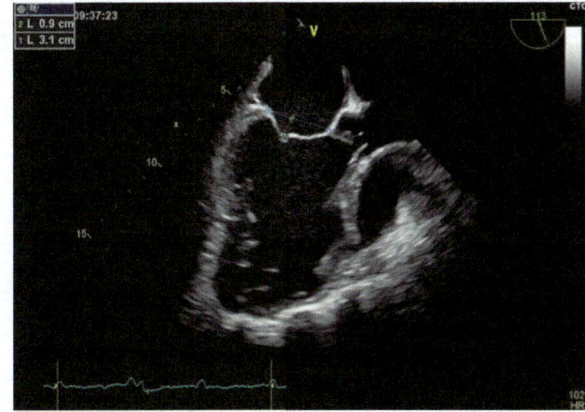

**Fig. 4.7** Chamber transesophageal echocardiogram of left ventricular outflow tract. Tenting area

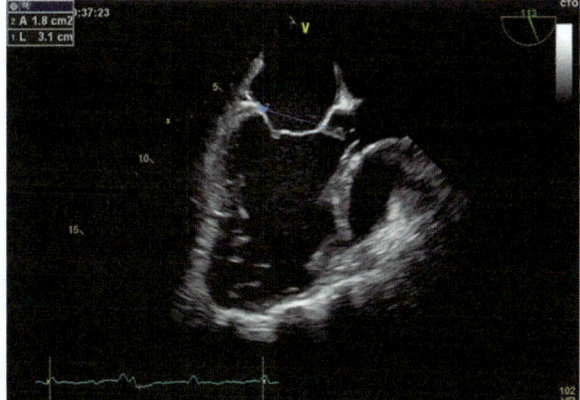

- Coaptation distance between the annular plane and the coaptation point (normal value 0.5 cm) (Fig. 4.6)
- Tenting area determined by the coaptation gap of the leaflets below the annulus plane (normal value 0.8 cm$^2$) (Fig. 4.7)
- Anteroposterior and intercommissural dimensions of the annulus.

In general, flail motion of a leaflet segment, associated with ruptured *chordae tendineae*, can lead to the suspicion of significant regurgitation (Fig. 4.8). In this case, an eccentric jet moving in the direction opposite to that of the prolapsing leaflet should be expected (Fig. 4.9). Severe MR can also be suspected when there is a coaptation gap between the leaflets (Fig. 4.10).

**Fig. 4.8** Posterior leaflet flail (*arrow*) due to *chordae tendineae* rupture observed in bidimensional transthoracic echocardiography and confirmed with the 3D transesophageal reconstruction (atrial view). *Ao* aorta, *PML* posterior mitral leaflet

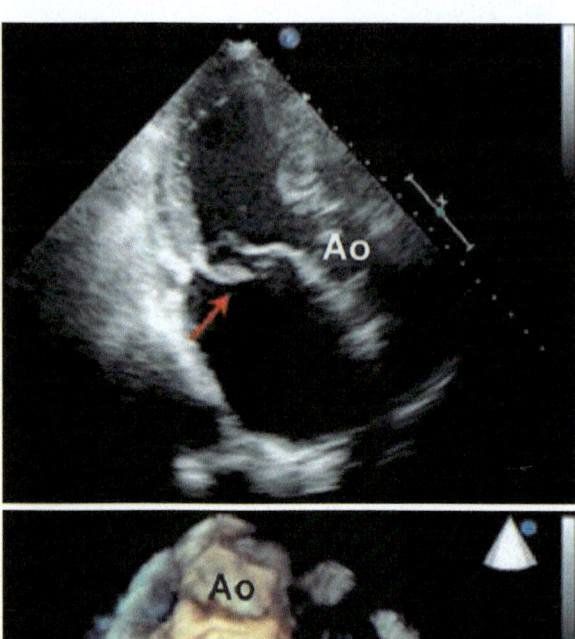

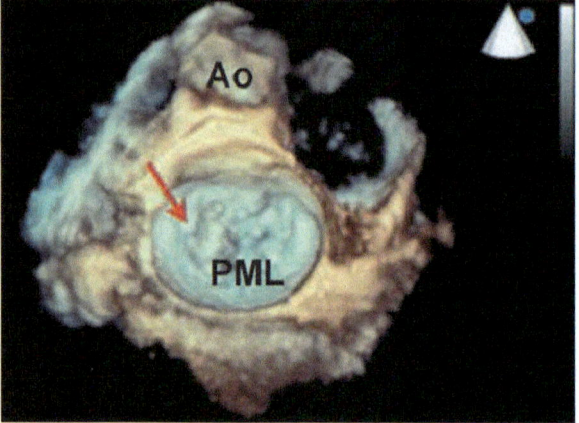

As part of the systolic restrictive motion (Carpentier type IIIb), it is possible to observe two types based on the apposition modes:

1. Asymmetric: prevailing posterior tethering resulting from regional remodeling of the left ventricle
2. Symmetrical: apical tethering of both leaflets, with homogeneous geometry of the coaptation plane resulting from overall remodeling of the left ventricle

Color Doppler flowmetry is useful in evaluating the spatial distribution characteristics of regurgitation, as well as identifying the mechanism responsible for valve regurgitation (Table 4.1). Specifically, in the context of an asymmetric malcoaptation pattern, it is possible to observe a predominantly posteromedial paracommissural jet origin with eccentric direction. Vice versa, in symmetric malcoaptation, the jet has almost a central origin and direction (Fig. 4.11). Multiple jets may occur due to

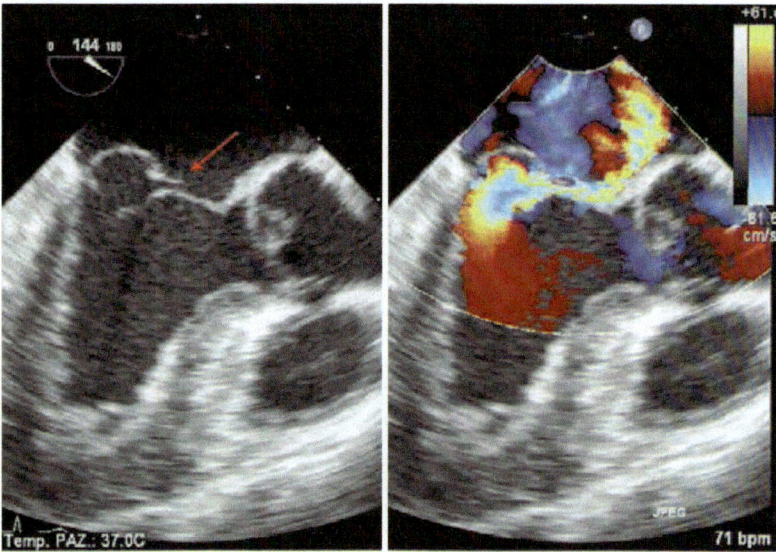

**Fig. 4.9** Transesophageal echocardiogram at 144°. Coaptation gap (*arrow*) due to posterior leaflet prolapse, determining severe eccentric mitral regurgitation

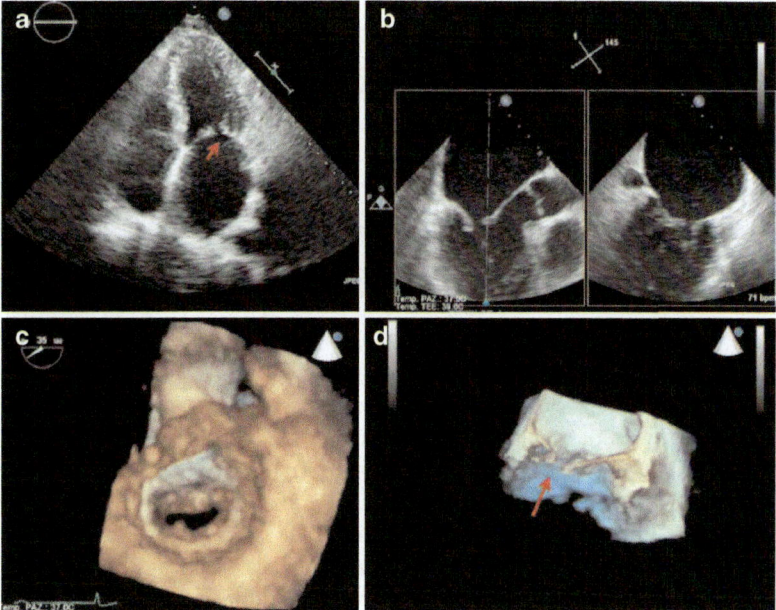

**Fig. 4.10** Significant coaptation gap (*arrow*) between the two mitral valve leaflets because of a prevalent retraction of the posterior leaflet. (**a**) Transthoracic echocardiogram, apical four-chamber view. (**b**) Transesophageal echocardiogram in X-plane orthogonal views (three chambers and two chambers). (**c**) 3D transesophageal echocardiogram showing the mitral valve from a ventricular view. (**d**) 3D transesophageal echocardiogram from a lateral view

**Table 4.1** Mechanism responsible for mitral regurgitation

| Origin | Direction | Mechanism |
| --- | --- | --- |
| Anterior | Lateral | AL prolapse/flail |
|  |  | PL restriction |
| Posterior | Medial | PL prolapse/flail |
|  |  | AL restriction |
| Central | Central | Left ventricle dilation |
|  |  | Annular dilation |
| Commissural | Mediolateral | Commissural prolapse/flail |
|  |  | Commissural restriction |
| Intraleaflet |  | Leaflet perforation |

*AL* anterior leaflet, *PL* posterior leaflet

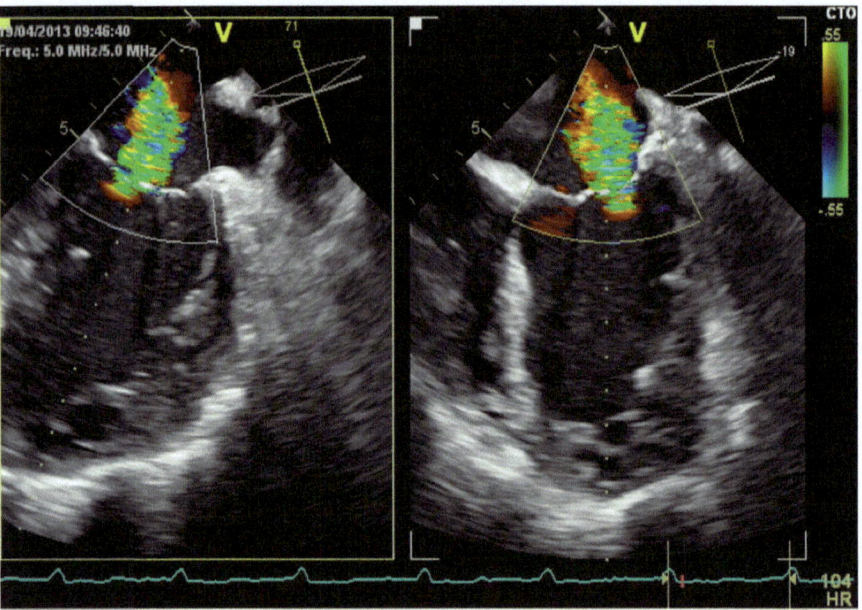

**Fig. 4.11** Transesophageal echocardiogram in X-plane orthogonal views (two chambers and four chambers) showing a single central jet

deformed dilation of the annulus or deformed diastase of the scallops of the posterior mitral leaflet.

In the case of rheumatic mitral regurgitation, the leaflets will exhibit signs of fibrosis, and their reduced motility will result in the shortening of the *chordae tendineae*, and it is not unusual to see concomitant stenosis. Echocardiography can also provide important information in the case of endocarditis concerning the extent of infection by identifying sessile or pedunculated vegetation and valve tissue damage (Fig. 4.12).

M-mode examination can be useful in MR assessment in the search for indirect signs on the ventricular cavities, such as enlarged LA or LV, and in the timing of MR, defined as duration of regurgitation (Fig. 4.13).

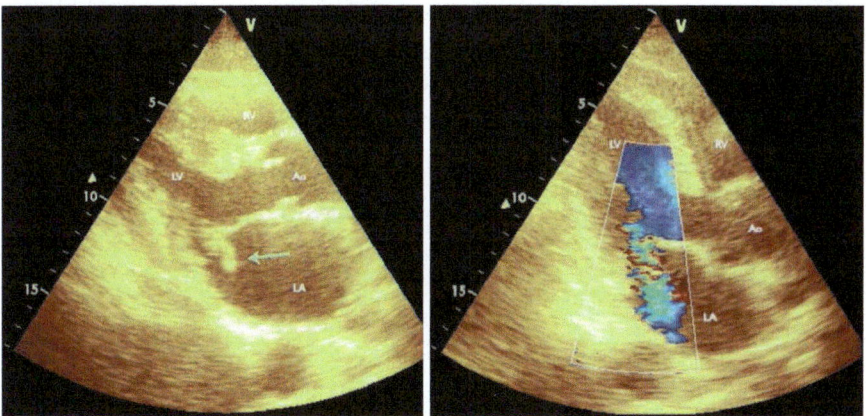

**Fig. 4.12** Transthoracic echocardiogram. Three-chamber apical view showing endocarditic vegetation (*arrow*) on the anterior mitral leaflet causing significant mitral regurgitation. *Ao* aorta, *LA* left atrium, *LV* left ventricle, *RV* right ventricle

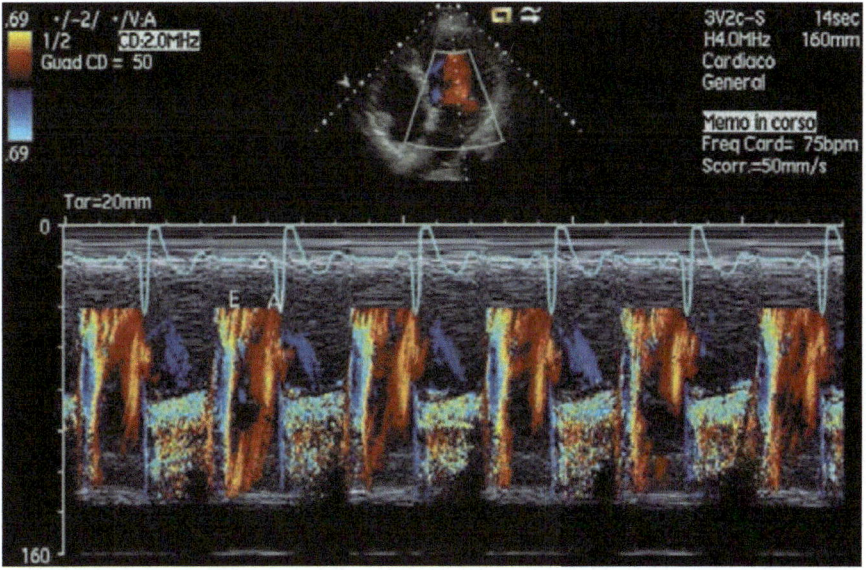

**Fig. 4.13** Transthoracic echocardiogram. Color M-mode, apical four-chamber view. Holosystolic mitral regurgitation

Doppler echocardiography is the technique most commonly used to detect and assess the extent of regurgitation. A review of the literature and clinical practice makes it possible to distinguish the Doppler measurements as parameters derived from regurgitant jet and parameters not derived from regurgitant jet sampling. These are summarized in Table 4.2.

**Table 4.2** Color Doppler parameters to assess the grade of mitral regurgitation

| Parameters | Extent of mitral regurgitation | | | |
|---|---|---|---|---|
| | Mild | Moderate | Medium | Severe |
| Extension of regurgitant jet/LA (%) | <20 | Variable | Variable | >40 |
| Vena contracta (mm) | <3 | Variable | Variable | >7 |
| PISA radius (cm) | Variable | Variable | Variable | >1 |
| ERO (cm²) | <0.20 | 0.20–0.29 | 0.30–0.39 | >0.40 |
| Regurgitant volume (mL) | <30 | 30–44 | 45–59 | >60 |
| Regurgitant fraction | <30 | 30–39 | 40–49 | >50 |
| Pulmonary venous flow | Normal | Normal | Monolateral systolic inversion | Bilateral systolic inversion |
| Transmitral diastolic flow | E/A < 1 | | | E/A > 2 |

*LA* left atrium, *PISA* proximal isovelocity surface area, *ERO* effective regurgitation orifice

There are three areas in the regurgitant jet:

- The pre-orifice convergence area of the velocities (area next to the valve where the flow converges and accelerates before entering the regurgitant orifice)
- Vena contracta (zone where the flow is smallest after the regurgitant orifice)
- Distribution of the regurgitant jet in the left atrium (post-orifice turbulence area)

The following identify just as many methods to quantify mitral regurgitation: the PISA method, vena contracta quantification, and regurgitant jet analysis.

*PISA method*: The flow convergence region proximal to a circular orifice is a laminar field of converging flow lines associated with a family of concentric and hemispherical isovelocity surfaces with decreasing area and increasing velocity (Fig. 4.14). Based on the principle of continuity, the flow (Q) is constant on all iso-velocity surfaces and is equal to the flow to the orifice. This way, the effective regurgitant orifice area (EROA) can be calculated by dividing the regurgitant flow (obtained from the flow convergence region and aliasing velocity) by the maximum velocity through the orifice (obtained by continuous wave Doppler) (Fig. 4.15):

$$\text{Regurgitant flow} = \left(2\pi\, r2 \times Va\right)$$

$$\text{EROA} = \text{Regurgitant flow} / V\text{reg}$$

$$\text{Regurgitant volume} = \text{EROA} \times \text{MR-VTI}$$

where $r$ is the hemispherical convergence radius (cm), $Va$ is the velocity at which aliasing occurs in the flow convergence toward the regurgitant orifice, $Vreg$ is the peak velocity of the regurgitant jet, and MR-VTI is the velocity time integral of the regurgitant jet, determined by continuous wave Doppler.

The PISA method [7], though, has four major limitations, which need to be taken into account [8]:

- Flattening of the isovelocity profile, and hence the loss of its hemispherical shape, which leads to a significant underestimation of regurgitation (this occurs especially when the aliasing velocity exceeds 10% of the flow velocity through the orifice).

**Fig. 4.14** Proximal flow convergence area in case of degenerative (**a**) and functional (**b**) mitral regurgitation, using Nyquist limit of ~20 (**a**) and 50–60 cm/s (**b**), respectively

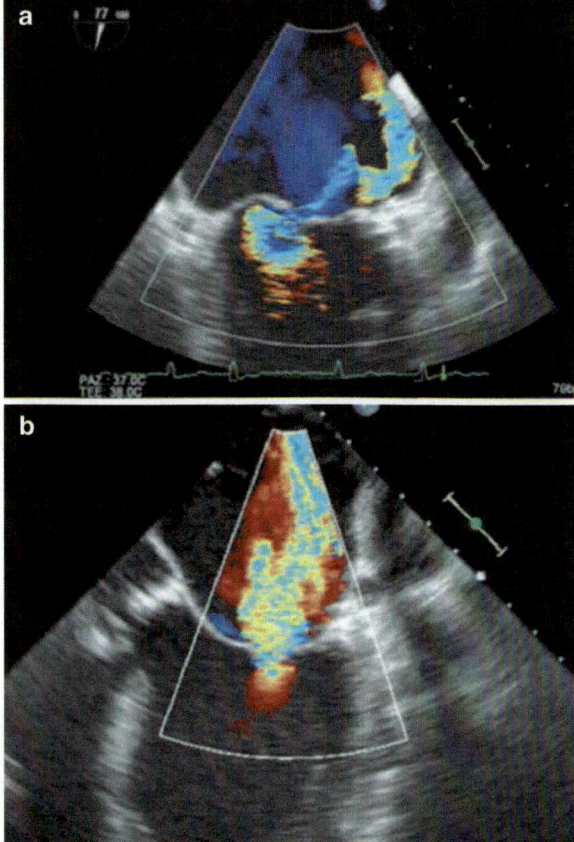

- Containment of the convergence area by adjacent structures hindering its free spatial development (typical of mitral prolapse).
- Difficulty in precisely identifying the orifice site, as the hemisphere's radius is determined based on the orifice's location and the radius is squared.
- In many patients, regurgitation is not constant throughout systole, and the assessment of the degree of regurgitation based on the maximum area of the regurgitant orifice can be misleading.

The PISA method cannot be considered as an absolute quantitative parameter and independent from MR quantization. Therefore, it needs to be integrated with other approaches to estimate regurgitation.

*Vena contracta*: Vena contracta (VC), namely, the narrowest portion of the jet at or immediately below the orifice, is the zone of maximum transformation of the pressure energy of the regurgitant flow into kinetic energy (Fig. 4.16). It is characterized by a laminar flow with the highest velocity [6]. Using VC as a parameter to assess the extent of MR is based on the assumption that its width is correlated with the regurgitant area (Table 4.2): a VC width > 7 mm indicates severe MR; a width of VC < 3 mm indicates mild MR; and VC values of 3–7 mm indicate moderate

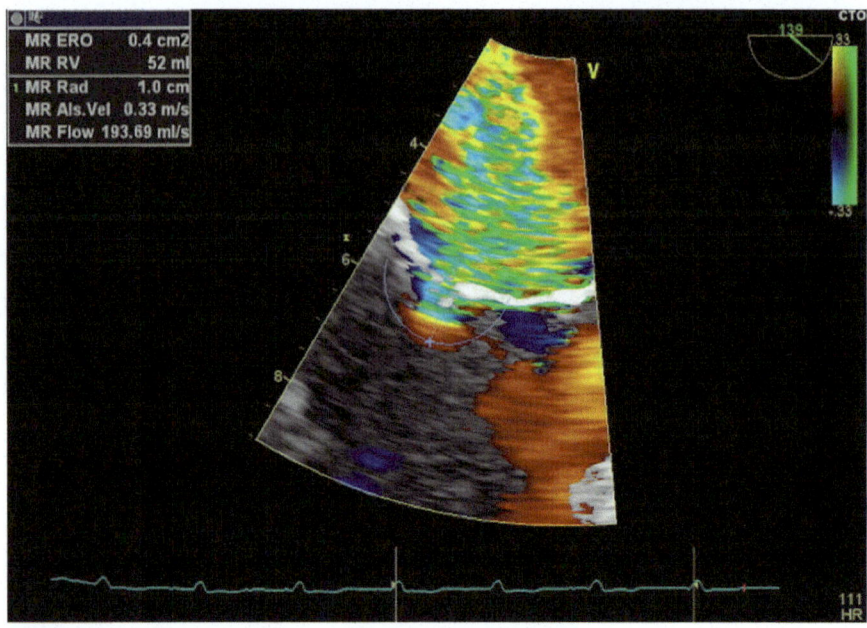

**Fig. 4.15** The hemispherical convergence radius

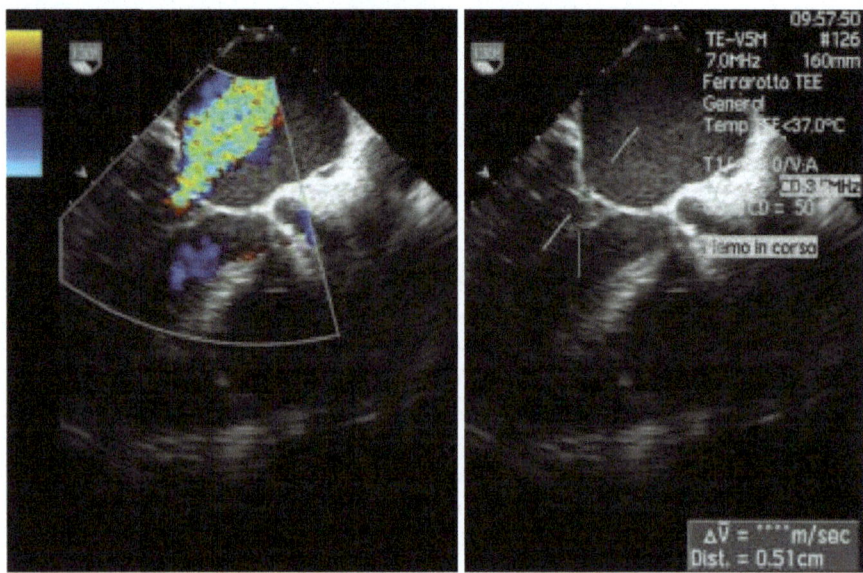

**Fig. 4.16** Transesophageal echocardiogram at 130°. Vena contracta width

MR. VC is measured perpendicularly to the intercommissural coaptation line of the leaflets (parasternal long-axis view or apical long axis) and gives the anteroposterior dimension of the effective regurgitation area. According to some authors, this quantification method is independent of the hemodynamic variables and orifice geometry and appears to be associated with a low interobserver variability [9]. It can be used for single jets, while it poses limits for multiple jets. Sections in which the commissural fissure runs parallel to the scanning plane are to be avoided (e.g., two apical chambers). In these cases, small regurgitations can have a very wide VC. In searching for the VC, a zoom with maximum time resolution and, hence, with a color Doppler angle as narrow as possible should be used (Fig. 4.17). Since the measurement is in millimeters, minor assessment errors lead to great variations in the grading of severity.

*Regurgitant jet analysis*: Turbulence visualized in the LA by color Doppler is not the regurgitant volume but the chromatic representation of the flow direction (red/blue), its velocity (more or less bright color), and type of flow (laminar or turbulent). The spatial dispersion of the regurgitant jet is proportional to the flow's kinetic energy, which is the product of the mass by the velocity, which, in turn, depends on

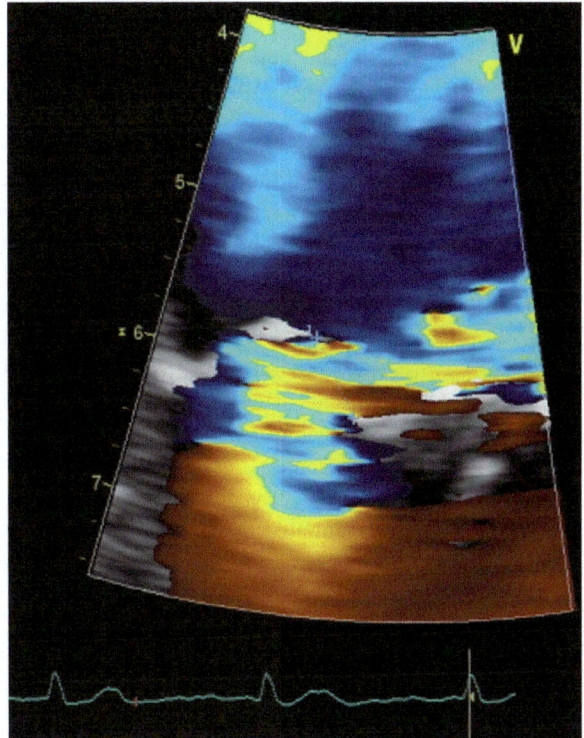

**Fig. 4.17** Color Doppler TEE with zoom, measurement of the vena contracta

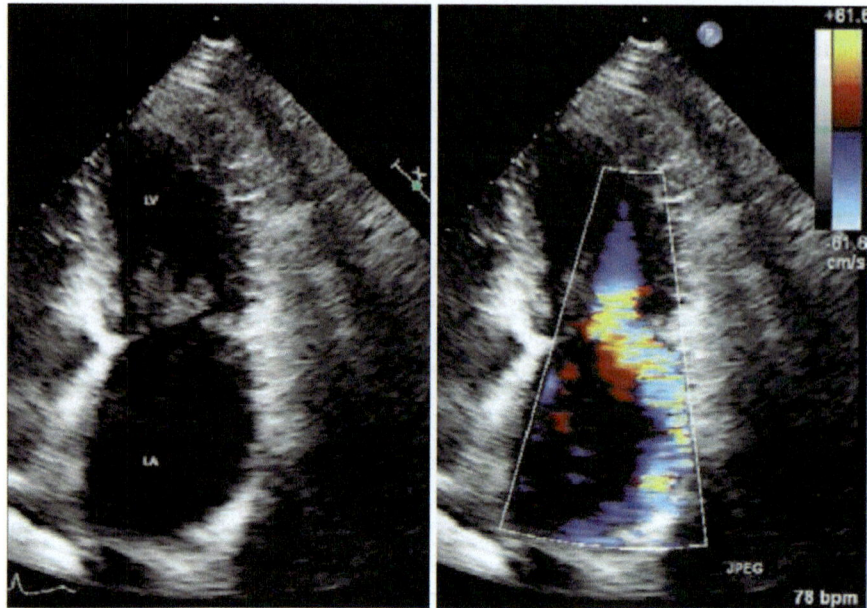

**Fig. 4.18** Transthoracic echocardiogram. Apical four-chamber view with and without color. Severe eccentric mitral regurgitation (Coanda effect). *LV* left ventricle, *LA* left atrium

the pressure gradient. The dimensions of the turbulence area due to MR are hence only partially influenced by regurgitant volume, as they are affected by the conditions modifying the transmitral gradient in systole, as well as by technical aspects more specifically linked to the type of equipment used [10].

The most commonly adopted criterion is the maximum turbulent flow area, either as an absolute value or related to LA area [6]. The cross sections routinely studied are parasternal long-axis view, four-chamber apical view, and two-chamber apical view. The study envisages a thorough assessment of changes throughout systole. Jet dimensions are not always representative of regurgitation severity. One example is given by extremely eccentric regurgitation in which the jet is directed against the atrial walls, thus transferring a part of its kinetic energy (Coanda effect) and leading to underestimated Doppler examination results (Fig. 4.18). Despite its evident limits, regurgitant jet analysis is the most widely used method in the semi-quantitative study of MR severity.

Regurgitation is considered mild when:

- The LA color jet is visible only on the valvular plane and if the wave front is thin (Fig. 4.19).
- The regurgitant jet area is <4 cm$^2$ (absolute value).
- The jet area/LA area ratio is <20%.

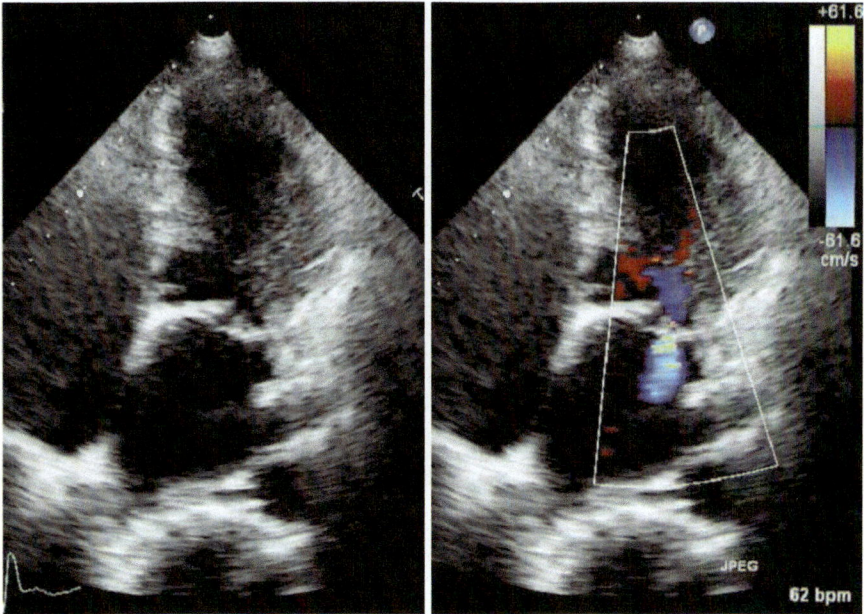

**Fig. 4.19** Transthoracic echocardiogram. Apical four-chamber view with and without color. Mild mitral regurgitation

Regurgitation is considered moderate when:

- The color jet is visible up to the middle of the LA (moderately wide jet).
- The absolute area is between 4 and 8 cm$^2$ (Fig. 4.20).
- The jet area/LA area ratio varies, but it is generally <20–40%.

Regurgitation is considered severe when:

- The color jet propagates in all directions filling the atrial cavity.
- The absolute area is >8 cm$^2$ (Fig. 4.21).
- The jet area/LA area ratio is >40%.

MR assessment correlated with the jet study also includes its spectrum analysis by means of CW Doppler [6] (Fig. 4.22). The velocity does not provide useful data on the severity of the regurgitation, unlike the profile and density of the jet at CW Doppler. A truncated, triangular jet contour with early peaking of the maximal velocity indicates elevated LA pressure or a prominent regurgitant pressure wave in the LA. Jet density is correlated with MR severity. An intense signal indicates severe MR, while an incomplete or faint signal is a sign of mild MR. In the case of eccentric jets, though of some relevance, it can be difficult to fully capture the regurgitation's CW Doppler signal due to the eccentric direction of the flow.

Fig. 4.20 Transthoracic
echocardiogram. Apical
four-chamber view.
Moderate mitral
regurgitation (planimetric
jet area of 4.58 cm²)

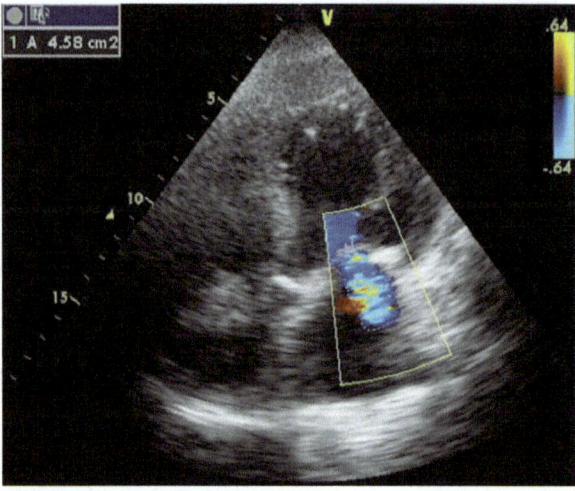

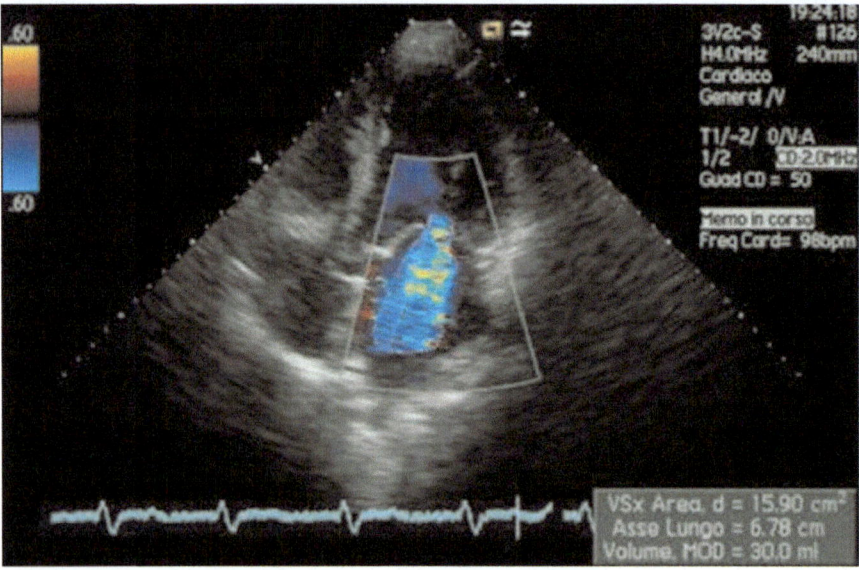

Fig. 4.21 Transthoracic echocardiogram. Apical four-chamber view. Severe mitral regurgitation
(planimetric jet area of 15.90 cm²)

*Parameters not derived from regurgitation jet*: The ideal approach to assessing
MR comprises other parameters as well:

• Regurgitant fraction
• Pulmonary venous flow
• Transmitral diastolic flow

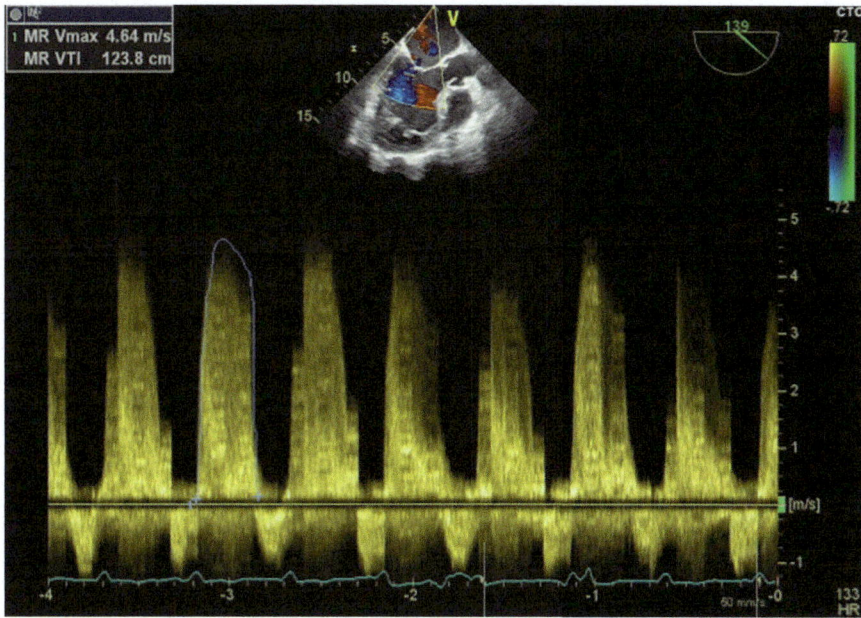

**Fig. 4.22** Transthoracic echocardiogram of left ventricular outflow tract, profile and density of the jet at CW Doppler

*Regurgitant fraction*: The relationship between regurgitant volume and end-systolic left ventricular volume is called the regurgitant fraction (RF). It is calculated by dividing the difference between the mitral output and the aortic valve output by the transmitral output [6]. This method can also be used with multiple and eccentric jets, providing information on jet severity and volume overload. However, this method is not widely used, as it is difficult and has limits [6]:

- Small variations in heart rate or small errors in measuring ventricular diameters and volumes can lead to errors in output calculation.
- There is no standardization based on the body mass index.
- It cannot be used if there is aortic failure or atrial fibrillation.
- Technical difficulties due to annulus calcifications.

The quantification of the degree of MR based on the RF is as follows:

- RF <30% = mild MR
- RF 30–50% = moderate MR
- RF >50% = severe MR

*Pulmonary venous flow*: PW Doppler assessment of pulmonary venous flow (PVF) is useful in determining the hemodynamic consequences of MR. Normal PVF typically has two velocity peaks, systolic and diastolic (the systolic peak is higher than the diastolic one), and a small inverted wave corresponding to atrial contraction.

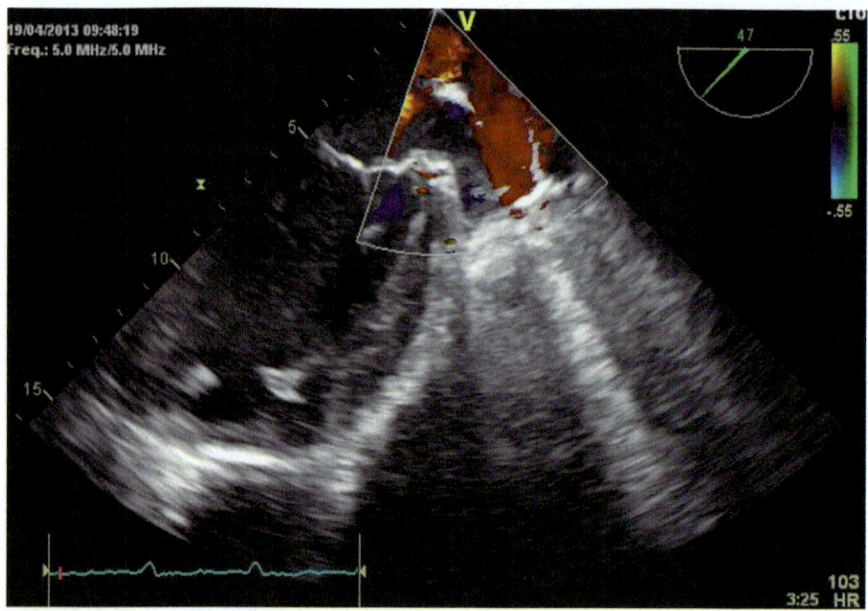

**Fig. 4.23** Pulmonary venous reversal flow in a case of severe mitral regurgitation. PW Doppler in 50° transesophageal two-chamber view

In MR, there is an increase in LA pressure matched by a decrease in systolic velocity. In severe MR, there is total systolic wave inversion (Figs. 4.23 and 4.24) [6]. Due to the anatomical position of the pulmonary veins, this sign is searched for in clinical practice, primarily by using TEE and directing the sample volume at 1–2 cm inside the outlet of the pulmonary veins to the LA by means of PW Doppler.

Since the regurgitant jet is generally directed toward a pulmonary vein, and the systolic flow of that vein is negative, while the others have positive systolic waves, all four pulmonary vessels need to be examined.

This type of assessment of MR is affected by several factors, such as patient age, heart rhythm, jet direction, and LA distensibility. A flow inversion can also occur without any significant MR in patients with high LA pressures or with an eccentric jet [11]. This sign is often unreliable in patients with left ventricular dysfunction with a reduced systolic component.

*Transmitral diastolic flow*: Diastolic mitral flow by PW Doppler, though indicating a prevalence of the atrial component over the early-diastolic one, can be an easy, immediate, and very useful parameter to exclude a diagnosis of severe MR [12]. However, this method depends on the LA pressure and hence can be used if there is no mitral stenosis or other causes leading to an increase in LA pressure. This type of study is recommended for the apical portions. Color Doppler allows for a better analysis of the nature and direction of the flow. In the four-chamber apical view, by applying the sample volume at the apex of the opening valve leaflets, the rapid filling early-diastolic wave (E) and the wave secondary to atrial contraction (A) are recorded in patients with normal sinus rhythm (Fig. 4.25). Once the peak velocity is

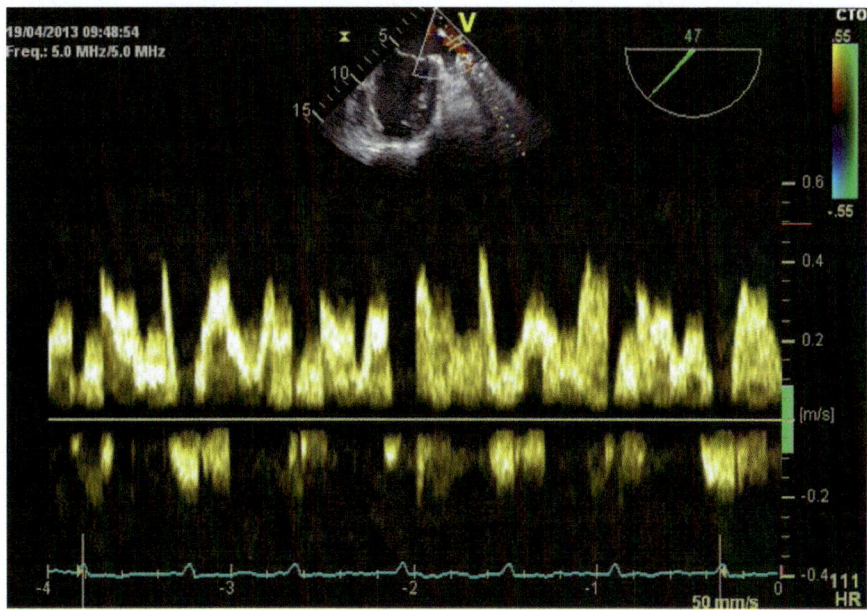

**Fig. 4.24** Pulmonary venous reversal flow in a case of severe mitral regurgitation. PW Doppler in 50° transesophageal two-chamber view

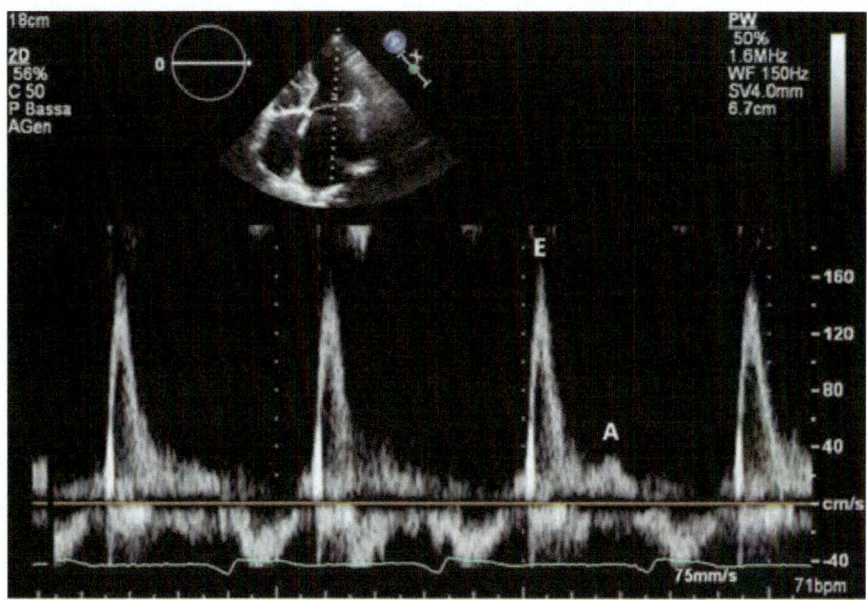

**Fig. 4.25** PW Doppler transmitral flow, showing increased E wave velocity as a sign of rapid protodiastolic filling in severe mitral regurgitation

**Table 4.3** Echocardiography methods to assess the degree of regurgitation

| 2D echo | Color | Pulsed wave Doppler | Continuous wave Doppler |
|---|---|---|---|
| Mitral valve morphology | Jet area | Regurgitant volume | Jet spectral analysis |
| Left atrium volume | Vena contracta | Regurgitant fraction | Systolic pulmonary artery pressure |
| Left ventricle dimension | Convergence area | ERO area | |
| | PISA-ERO area | A wave, E wave Pulmonary venous flow | |

*PISA* proximal isovelocity surface area, *ERO* effective regurgitation orifice

reached, the E wave progressively returns to the baseline value in a period defined "deceleration E-time" (DT). A normal transmitral flow pattern in a middle-aged patient with sinus rhythm is given by a prevalent E wave, with a DT of about 200 ms. An *E/A* ratio < 1 indicates MR without hemodynamic relevance, while, an *E/A* ratio > 2 is an indicator of severe MR (Table 4.3).

Table 4.3 summarizes the various echocardiography methods that are useful for multiparameter assessment of MR and any resulting hemodynamic impairment.

*Exercise echocardiography*: In asymptomatic severe MR, exercise echocardiography may help in identifying patients with unrecognized symptoms or subclinical latent LV dysfunction [13]. Moreover, exercise echocardiography may also be helpful in patients with equivocal symptoms out of proportion of MR severity at rest. Worsening of MR severity, a marked increase in pulmonary arterial pressure, impaired exercise capacity, and the occurrence of symptoms during exercise echocardiography can be useful findings to identify MR patients who may benefit from early surgery despite the absence of symptoms [13, 14].

Exercise echocardiography is useful in patients with functional ischemic MR and chronic LV systolic dysfunction to unmask the dynamic behavior of MR. Dynamic MR is strongly related to exercise-induced changes in systolic tenting area and to intermittent changes in LV synchronicity. Large exercise-induced increases in functional ischemic MR (ERO area $\geq 13$ mm$^2$) are associated with an increased risk of cardiovascular events [13, 15, 16].

In some patients with moderate or severe MR at rest, it is possible to observe a reduction in ERO area during exercise. As previously reported, this effect is usually the result of the LV contractile reserve, especially in the posterobasal segment, and/or the reduction in left intraventricular dyssynchrony [17].

*TEE and 3D echocardiography*: TEE is indicated to evaluate MR severity when TTE does not provide adequate information on MR severity or when TTE is technically limited [3–5, 13, 14]. All the quantitative criteria for estimating MR mentioned above can be used during the TEE. Nevertheless, conventional 2D echocardiography requires multiple views and a mental 3D reconstruction of the mitral valve and its structures (annulus, *chordae tendineae*, and mitral-aortic junction), while 3D echocardiography provides this information by analyzing simultaneously the mitral valve and its components during the same cardiac cycle. Several authors have demonstrated the utility of 3D echocardiography in viewing, locating, and quantifying abnormalities of the mitral valve in MR patients and in displaying the valve scallops and adjacent structures in an excellent way [18, 19] (Fig. 4.26). There are three basic ways to acquire images when using 3D TEE: real-time 3D, 3D zoom, and full-volume acquisition. These are differentiated by sector width, frame rate, and spatial resolution (Figs. 4.27, 4.28, and 4.29). The surgical view (atrial or en face view) of the valves, with the aortic root at 12 o'clock and the left atrial appendage at 9 o'clock (lateral), is widely accepted as the standard modality of real-time 3D TEE [20] and allows better communication between the echocardiographic cardiologist, surgeon, and interventional cardiologist. This view shows the anterolateral commissure on the

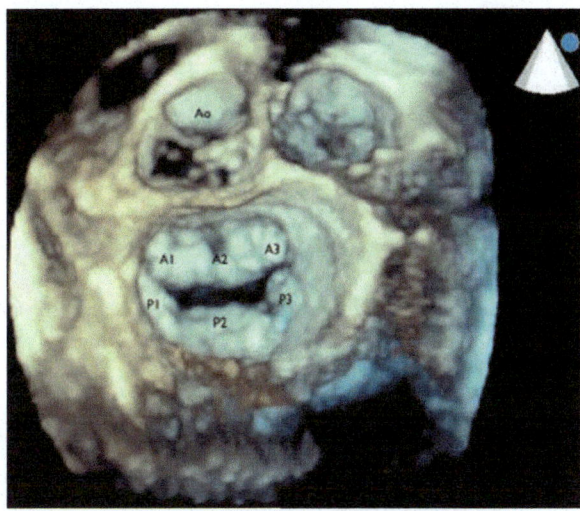

**Fig. 4.26** Real-time 3D echocardiogram showing the atrial view of the mitral valve. The leaflet scallops are identified (*A1, A2, A3, P1, P2, P3*). *Ao* aorta

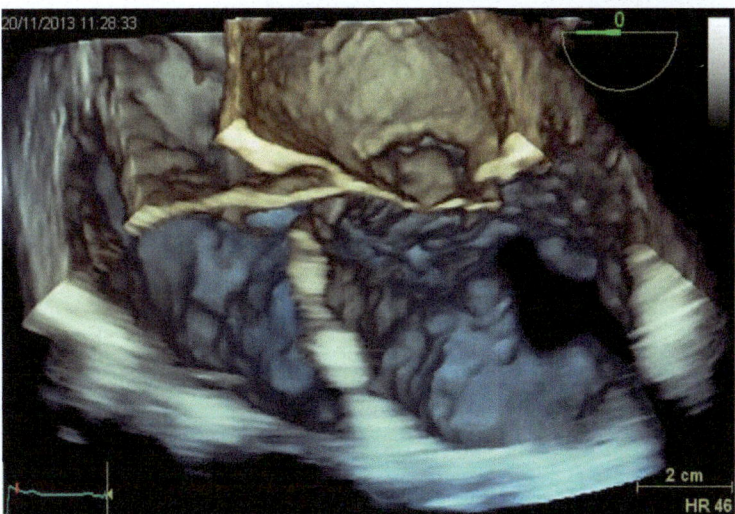

**Fig. 4.27** Transesophageal 3D echocardiography, acquisition in full volume. The right atrium, left atrium, interatrial septum, right ventricle, left ventricle, interventricular septum, mitral valve (repaired with surgical miniband), tricuspid valve, and right atrial appendage are visible

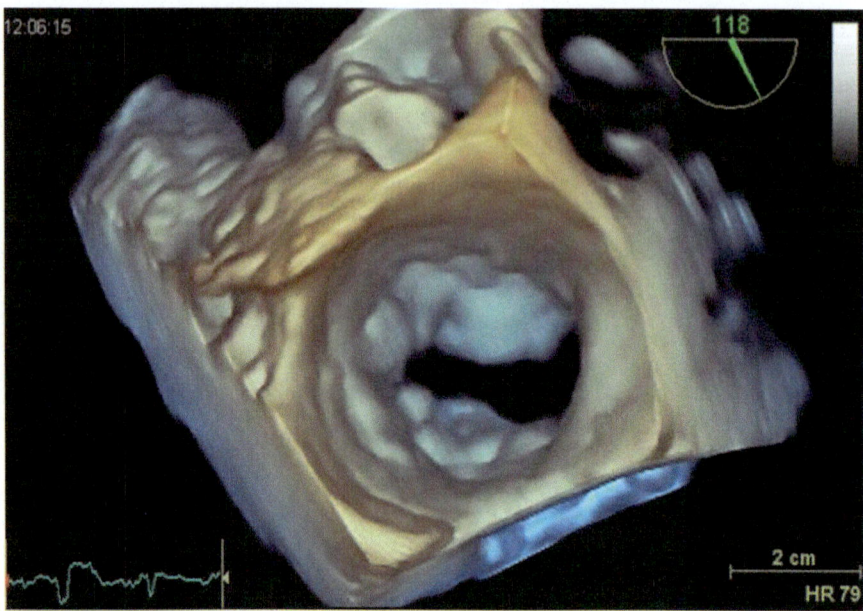

**Fig. 4.28** Zoom 3D atrial view shows mitral valve

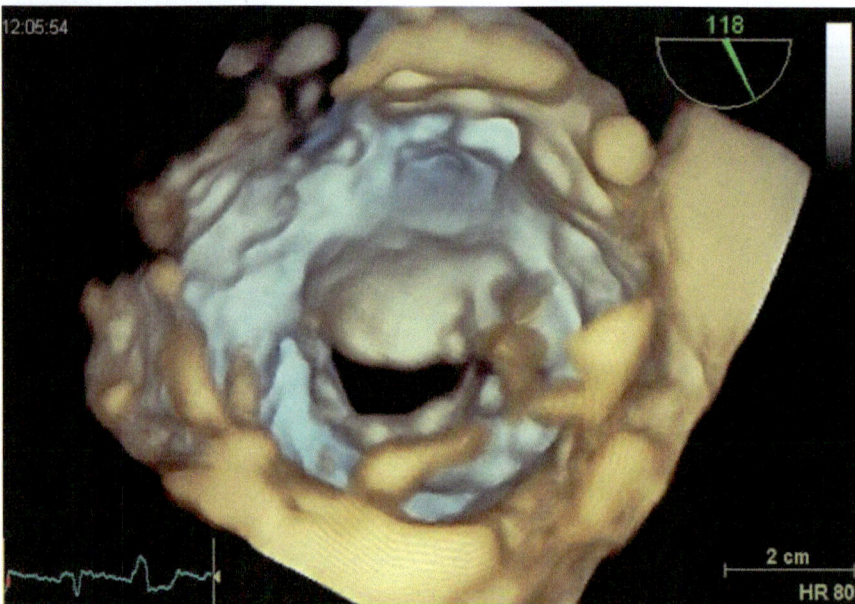

**Fig. 4.29** Zoom 3D ventricular view shows mitral valve

left (laterally) and the posteromedial commissure on the right (medially). The anterior mitral leaflet is, in relation to the aortic root, in the upper part of the image, and the posterior mitral leaflet, on the opposite side, is in the lower part. It is possible to clearly identify the posterior leaflet scallops and the corresponding scallops of the anterior leaflet (Fig. 4.30). During a 3D real-time (RT) study of the mitral valve, a ventricular view of the valve can also be useful, allowing more definitive identification of prolapse or other lesions of individual scallops and segments (Fig. 4.31). 3D

**Fig. 4.30** 3D TEE, extreme tethering of the rear leaflet

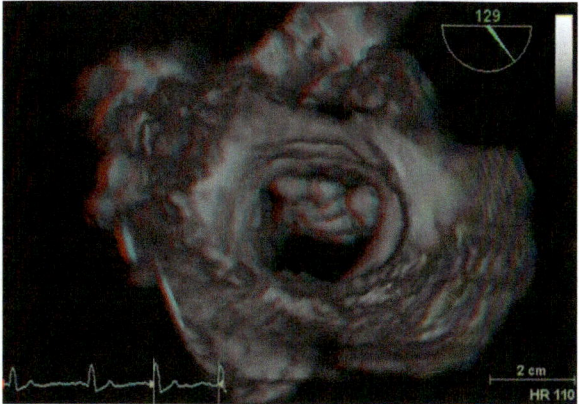

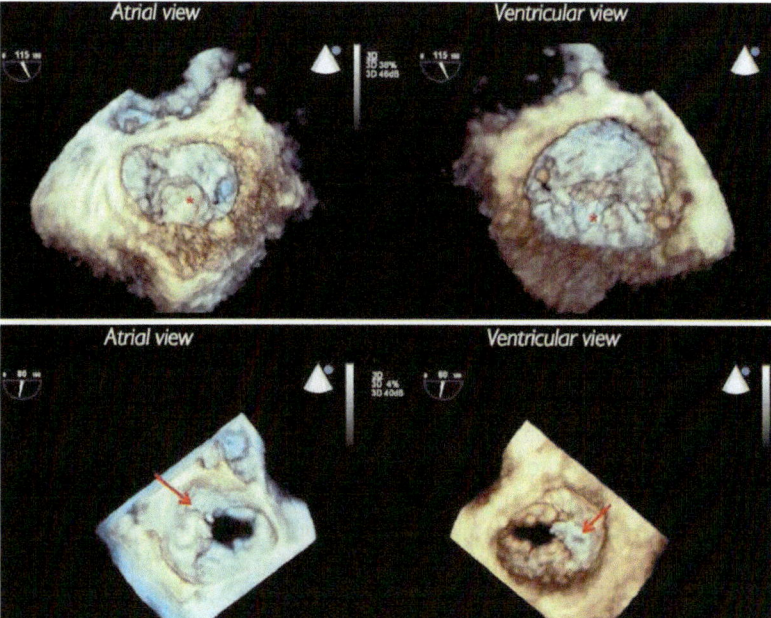

**Fig. 4.31** Real-time 3D echocardiogram showing a large P2 prolapse (*asterisk*) and a P1 flail (*arrow*), from both atrial and ventricular view

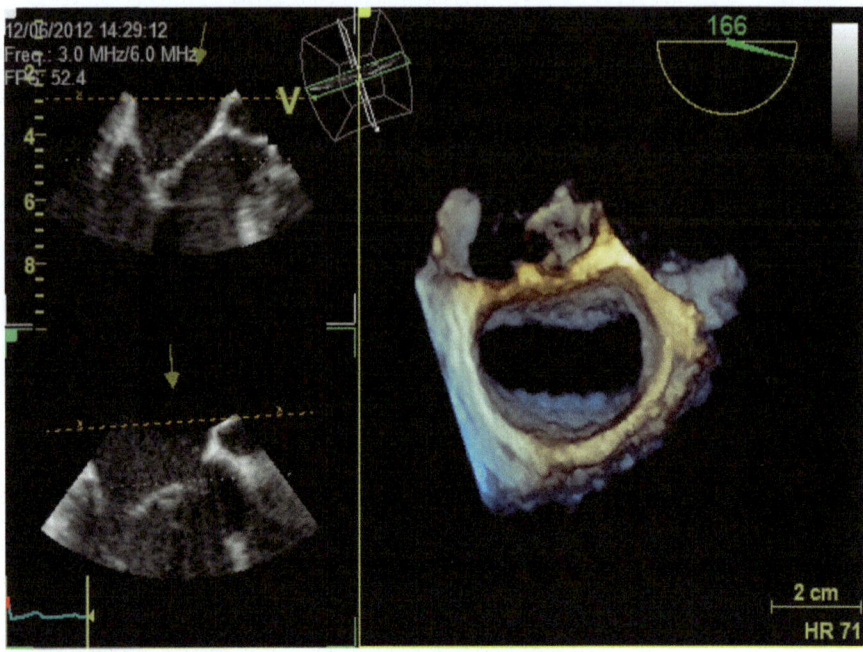

**Fig. 4.32** Zoom 3D showing the mitral annulus

echocardiography also provides important information on the morphology of the
mitral annulus (Fig. 4.32). This structure is saddle-shaped and, hence, difficult to
reproduce spatially using 2D echocardiography, which provides just two measurements: the septolateral and intercommissural distances. A single 3D RT image can
display the shape of the mitral annulus, any pathological alterations (dilatation, loss
of saddle shape, flattening), the relations to the aortic valve, and the motion dynamics
of the leaflets during the cardiac cycle (Fig. 4.33). In addition, 3D TEE mitral valve
quantification function can be used to assess the mitral annulus to confirm the size
and shape of the annulus [21] (Fig. 4.34).

In patients with MR, color Doppler capability, which was initially introduced in
reconstruction 3D systems, then later in real-time 3D transthoracic and real-time 3D
TEE, can provide 3D images of regurgitant flow jets and flow convergence
(Figs. 4.35 and 4.36). The location and size of the flow convergence zone or PISA
can determine the location of the regurgitant orifice and severity of MR [22]
(Fig. 4.37). Such information, especially on the location of the regurgitant orifice, is
critical for selection of an appropriate treatment protocol, such us the edge-to-edge
MitraClip procedure. In addition, 3D color Doppler ultrasound has demonstrated
that in several cases the convergence area does not have a hemispherical shape, due
to the irregular and asymmetrical shape of the orifice, especially in cases of ischemic or functional MR (Fig. 4.38). For this reason, various authors have proposed
more realistic geometrical shapes for the convergence area, as a semiellipse or semi-
ellipsoid to obtain a more accurate measure of the regurgitant volume [23–25]. The
VC is determined by 3D color Doppler: two orthogonal planes of images parallel to

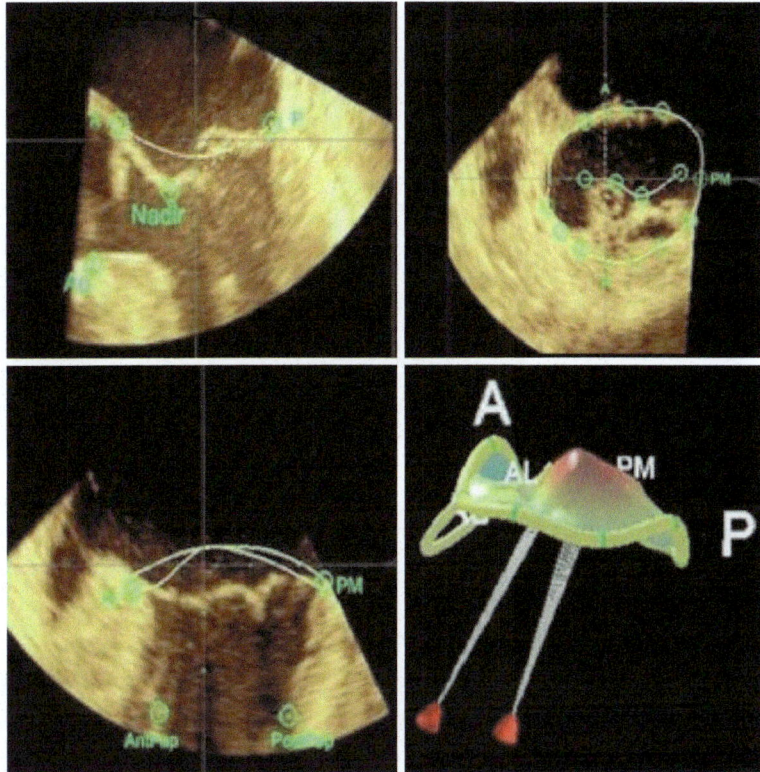

**Fig. 4.33** 3D reconstruction of the mitral valve in a case of P2 prolapse. *A* anterior, *AL* anterolateral, *P* posterior, *PM* posteromedial

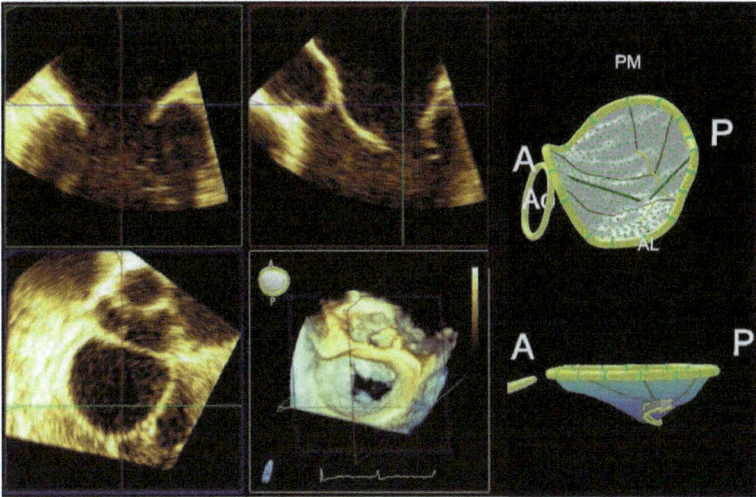

**Fig. 4.34** 3D reconstruction of the mitral valve apparatus, including annulus, leaflets, commissures (*PM* posteromedial, *AL* anterolateral), and relationship with the aortic valve (Ao). *A* anterior, *P* posterior. MVQ software (Philips Healthcare, Andover, MA, USA) was used

Fig. 4.35 3D Color
Doppler (Zoom 3D). Note
the extensive valve
regurgitation along the
entire coaptation orifice
(A1, A2, P1, P2)

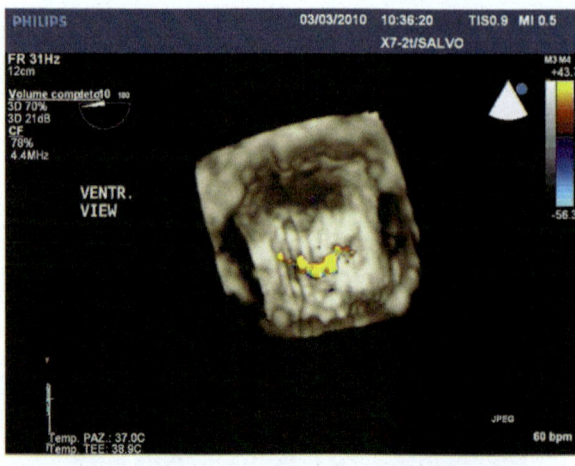

Fig. 4.36 3D
transesophageal
echocardiogram with color.
Ample regurgitant mitral
jet in the left atrium (LA).
*LV* left ventricle

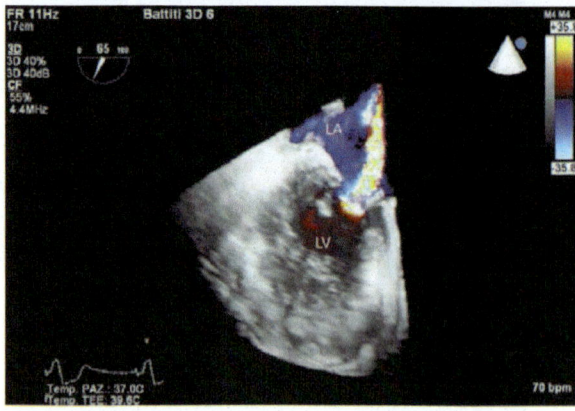

the direction of the regurgitant jet are cut manually on the regurgitant jet. A third
cutting plane, oriented perpendicularly to the direction of the jet, is then moved
along the direction of the jet until the area of the cross section at the level of the VC
is displayed. The frame with the largest vena contract area (VCA) in systole is
blown up, and VCA is measured on the direct plan of the color Doppler flow. In
order to analyze the circularity of the regurgitant orifice, it calculates the ratio
between the VCA long axis and short axis (*L/S* ratio) [26] (Fig. 4.39). The results of
several studies have demonstrated that 3D measurement of the VC correlated well
with the integrative 2D method in assessing the severity of MR. In addition, 3D
VCA has shown a high diagnostic value in distinguishing moderate regurgitation in
all the various forms of valve disease. This is a very important factor to take into
account. In fact, the 2D PISA method tends to underestimate the ROA in patients
with functional MR due to the hemispherical shape of the convergence zone, while
this PISA area most often has a semielliptical shape. The three-dimensional measurement of VCA, which is derived from the direct plan of the regurgitant orifice

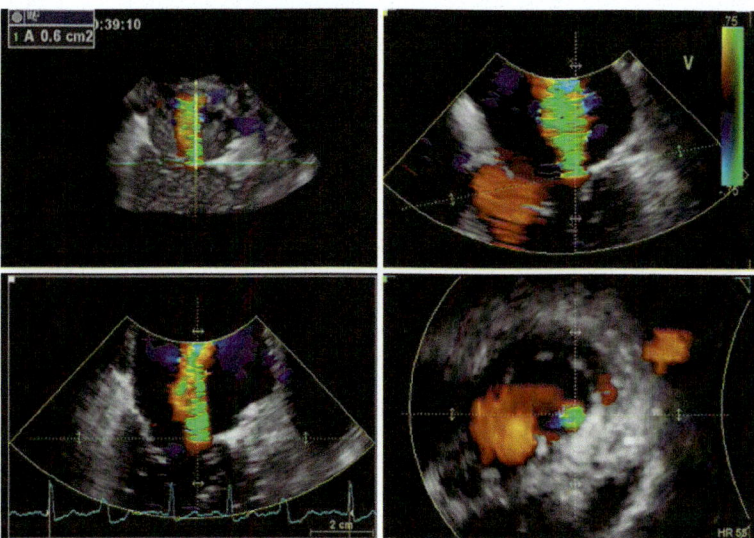

**Fig. 4.37** 3D calculation of the effective regurgitant orifice area

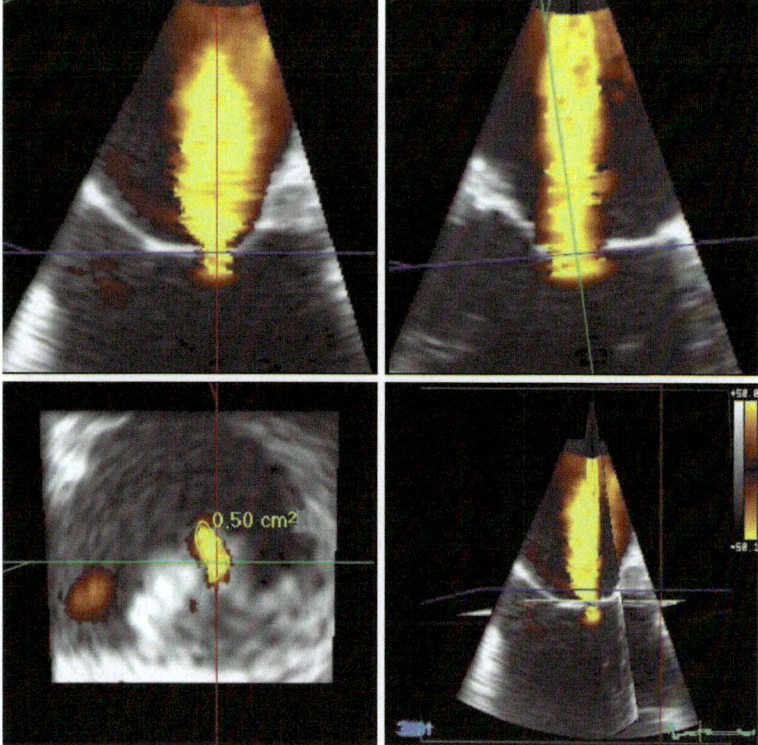

**Fig. 4.38** 3D EROA showing an irregular shape of the regurgitant orifice

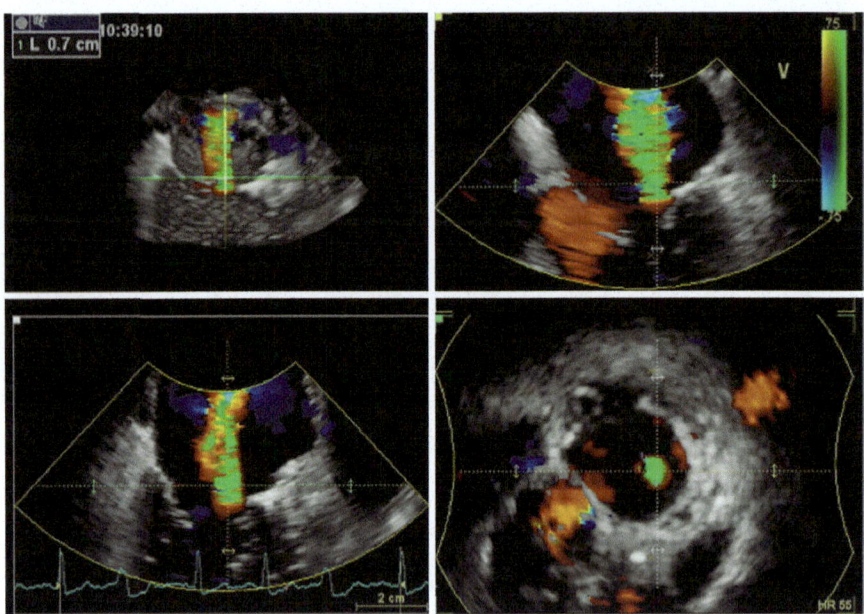

**Fig. 4.39** 3D calculation of the VCA

surface, bypasses this intrinsic limitation of 2D PISA and provides uniform classification and range cutoffs that apply regardless of etiology and shape of the orifice [27].

*Other imaging techniques*: Cardiac magnetic resonance (CMR) is another advanced imaging technique that can be used to study valvular diseases. It requires electrocardiographic gating and breath-held acquisitions. The morphological assessment of valve structures and the identification of any regurgitation jets are carried out through balanced steady-state free precession sequences in short-axis, two-, three-, and four-chamber views. If information about the velocity of flow across the mitral valve is specifically needed, velocity-encoded cine phase-contrast (VENC-PC) images are obtained in a plane perpendicular to mitral blood flow. Post-contrast inversion recovery gradient recalled echo sequences are routinely performed to assess for the presence of late gadolinium myocardial enhancement [26, 28].

Both CMR and CT are not usually recommended in the case of acute MR; however, it can be occasionally diagnosed with a chest x-ray or chest CT in the case of unilateral pulmonary edema localized mainly in the upper lobe of the right lung [29]. In the case of chronic MR, CMR is indicated in patients with chronic primary MR to assess LV and RV volumes, function, or MR severity and when these are not satisfactorily addressed by TTE (Class I B) [14]. Nonetheless, there are typical CMR and CT findings for chronic MR that are specific by etiology [26, 30–33] (Table 4.4). These imaging techniques can also be especially useful for an assessment that integrates conventional echocardiographic diagnostics to quantify the degree of regurgitation by calculating the regurgitant volume and RF (Table 4.5). In

**Table 4.4** Selected imaging findings in chronic mitral regurgitation

| Etiology | Image findings |
|---|---|
| Mitral valve prolapse | Systolic bowing of mitral leaflet >2 mm into left atrium; thickened leaflet (> 5 mm); flail |
| Flail leaflet | Systolic eversion of leaflet tip into left atrium; severe mitral regurgitation |
| Ischemic cardiomyopathy | Left ventricle wall motion abnormality; left ventricle dilatation; annular dilatation; late gadolinium enhancement; mural thinning; coronary artery disease on CT |
| Systolic anterior movement in hypertrophic obstructive cardiomyopathy | Signal defacing in left ventricle outflow tract; posterior jet of mitral regurgitation; signal of myocardial fibrosis on CMR |

*CT* computed tomography, *CMR* cardiac magnetic resonance

**Table 4.5** Mitral regurgitation grading according to regurgitant volume and regurgitant fraction

| | Regurgitant volume (mL/beat) | Regurgitant fraction (%) |
|---|---|---|
| Mild | <30 | <30 |
| Moderate | 30–59 | 30–49 |
| Severe | >60 | >50 |

the case of isolated MR, the regurgitant volume is equal to the difference between the stroke volume of the left ventricle and right ventricle measured by CMR or CT [33], while CMR is to be preferred in the case of multiple valve diseases. In this case, VENC-PC of the ascending aorta can be used to quantify the forward flow volume, which is subtracted from the left ventricle stroke volume (by volumetric calculation) to obtain the regurgitant volume [34]. The RF is then obtained by dividing the regurgitant volume by the stroke volume.

## 4.2 Invasive Diagnosis

The current guidelines recommend hemodynamic and angiographic assessment when there is a major difference between the patient's clinical status and the data resulting from the noninvasive approach. They are recommended if the noninvasive examinations provided incomplete data and left doubts on MR severity, LV contractility, and the indication to treatment [3–5, 14].

The information being sought and that is obtainable from cardiac catheterization is MR severity, pulmonary and systemic hemodynamic impairment, and left ventricle dimensions and contractility. Coronarography should always be performed to search for and rule out the presence of coronary artery disease in patients with risk factors for atherosclerosis [3–5, 14].

*Hemodynamic assessment*: The hemodynamic parameters that are useful in assessing MR severity and hemodynamic impairment are pulmonary artery pressure, pulmonary capillary wedge pressure (PCWP), left ventricular end-diastolic pressure, and $O_2$ saturation in the pulmonary artery and aorta, which allow us to calculate cardiac output using the Fick method [35].

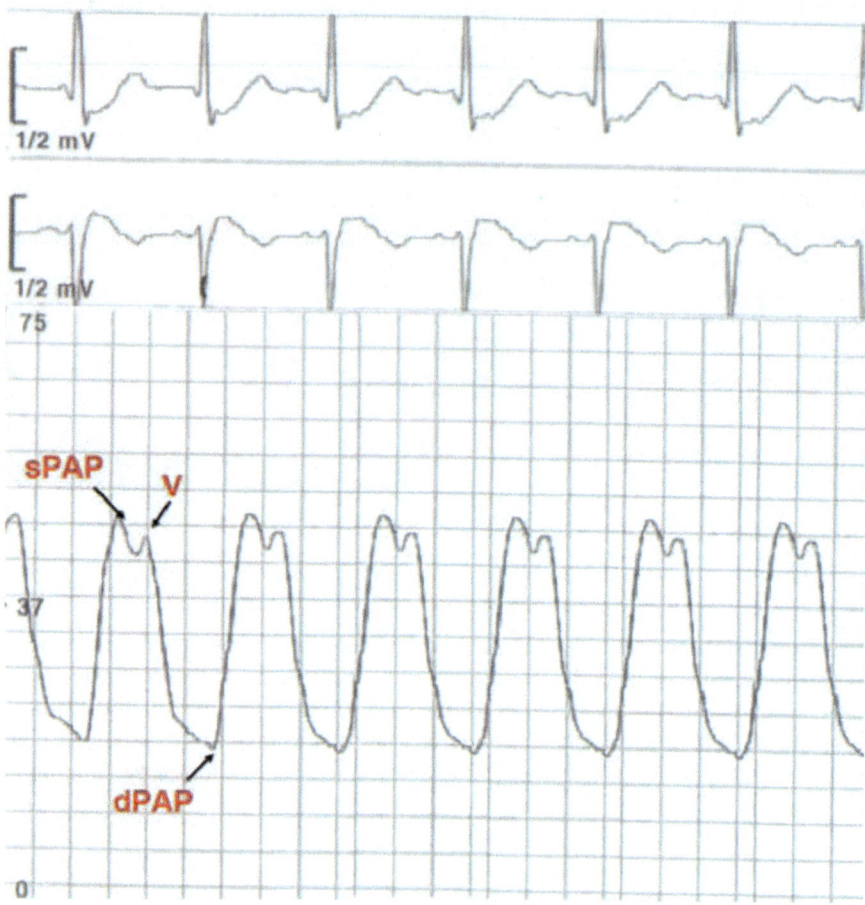

**Fig. 4.40** Pulmonary capillary wedge pressure tracing. V wave inscribed in the dicrotic phase of pulmonary pressure curve. *dPAP* diastolic pulmonary artery pressure, *sPAP* systolic pulmonary artery pressure

When the *v* wave in PCWP tracing gives a value more than double that of the mean PCWP, MR is severe. There are other situations with a high *v* wave without severe MR; these include, for instance, left ventricular failure of any etiology with a small and noncompliant left atrium or, in the case of acute pulmonary hyperflow, postinfarction interventricular defect. By contrast, severe MR does not always have a high *v* wave, as in the case of chronic forms with marked left atrium dilation, since the atrium can receive large regurgitant volumes without increasing the mean PCWP or height of the *v* wave [35, 36]. Severe MR with concurrent left ventricular dysfunction often has a *v* wave inscribed in the dicrotic phase of the pulmonary pressure curve (Fig. 4.40), often with a maximum pressure value equal to the systolic pulmonary pressure. An increased afterload in the presence of MR can increase the regurgitant volume and/or the *v* wave height (e.g., aortic stenosis or systemic blood hypertension).

The dynamic exercise test with supine cycloergometer can sometimes be useful for assessing the severity of MR with normal cardiac output at rest, especially when the patient's symptoms occur with exertion. In this case the increase cardiac output is less than 80% of predicted [35].

*Angiographic assessment*: Left ventriculography is very useful in assessing MR, as it provides important information on MR severity using the qualitative method (Table 4.6), LV dimensions, and ejection fraction (Fig. 4.41). The angiographic assessment of severity of MR consists also, in a quantitative evaluation, of the regurgitant fraction, measuring the total left ventricular stroke volume from the left ventriculogram, and the cardiac output (the forward stroke volume [FSV] by the Fick or the thermodilution technique (Table 4.7).

**Table 4.6** Examination of systolic leakages of contrast from the left ventricle back into the left atrium and the opacification of the left atrium relative to the left ventricle during ventriculography

| Grade | Qualitative assessment criteria |
| --- | --- |
| 1+ (mild) | Regurgitation clears with each beat and never opacifies the entire left atrium |
| 2+ (moderate) | Regurgitation does not clear with one beat and generally does opacify the entire left atrium (though faintly) after several beats; however, opacification of the left atrium does not equal that of the left ventricle |
| 3+ (moderately severe) | Left atrium completely opacified and equal opacification with the left ventricle |
| 4+ (severe) | Opacification of the entire left atrium within one beat, opacification becomes progressively denser with each beat, and contrast material can be seen refluxing into the pulmonary veins during left ventricular systole |

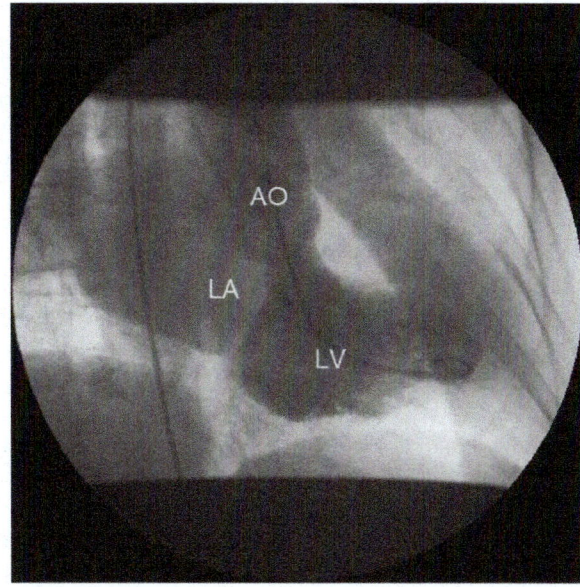

**Fig. 4.41** Left ventriculography. Opacification of the entire left atrium during the systolic phase of the cardiac cycle; this is indicative of severe mitral regurgitation. *AO* aorta, *LA* left atrium, *LV* left ventricle

**Table 4.7** Quantitative estimate of regurgitant fraction by angiographic assessment

| Angiographic measurement | Formula |
|---|---|
| Ventricular stroke volume (VSV) | EDV – ESV |
| Regurgitant stroke volume (RSV) | VSV – FSV |
| Regurgitant fraction (RF) | RSV/VSV |

*EDV* end-diastolic left ventricular volume, *ESV* end-systolic left ventricular volumes, *FSV* forward stroke volume

The accuracy of the calculations is affected by various factors. Since FSV is obtained by dividing the cardiac output by the heart rate, as assessed by mean of Fick or thermodilution methods, it will give a mean stroke volume. Therefore, the beat chosen for left ventriculography to determine the volume must be an average or representative beat. Alternatively, volumes from multiple beats can be calculated and averaged. In patients with atrial fibrillation and ectopic beats during ventriculography, RSV and RF calculation using this method is not recommended due to the great inaccuracy.

FSV quantification should be carried out simultaneously with cardiac output calculation, since, as mentioned above, an increase in arterial pressure can lead to an increase in the degree of MR, with a reduction of forward output. Therefore, if the blood pressure or other hemodynamic variables change significantly between the time of cardiac output determination and left ventriculography, it is useless to calculate regurgitant fraction. Finally, the RF quantifies, at best, the total amount of regurgitation.

Therefore, if a patient has both mitral and aortic regurgitation, the RF gives an assessment of the regurgitation resulting from both lesions combined [35].

## 4.3    Timing of Intervention

Due to greater life expectancy, chronic MR is currently the most frequent valve defect after aortic stenosis. The often advanced age of patients with valve disease and the development of percutaneous techniques and more conservative surgical approaches make the decision-making process rather complex with regard to both the right timing of intervention and the choice of the most appropriate therapeutic strategy. Therefore, the decision to intervene on a patient with valve disease is based on the individual risk–benefit analysis considering the fact that the improvement of the prognosis compared with the pathology's natural history should exceed the risk associated with the intervention and the possible late complications related to it.

The elements to be considered in the risk–benefit analysis are multiple and associated with:

- The pathophysiological and prognostic characteristics of the specific valvulopathy
- The patient's clinical characteristics, especially with regard to comorbidities

Recourse to an evidence-based approach to treat heart valve diseases has been hindered by the lack of rigorous data on clinical outcome predictors.

The natural history of chronic MR is marked by its different forms: organic, functional ischemic, and functional nonischemic MR. In patients with organic MR, clinical outcomes are mostly the consequence of regurgitation through the valve, and the recovery of valve competence is hence the therapeutic rationale. In these patients, the main clinical question is to determine when in the course of the disease's natural history the benefits of valve surgery exceed the related risks.

The high morbidity and mortality rates associated with severe chronic MR and the excellent results of mitral valve repair procedures in the presence of organic disease favor an early intervention, before the onset of symptoms, but with atrial fibrillation, pulmonary hypertension, and early signs of left ventricular dysfunction [37]. It is estimated that the mean time between the diagnosis of mitral valve prolapse and the development of symptoms is approximately 5 years [38], though a certain degree of impairment of left ventricular function occurs before the onset of symptoms.

In the American College of Cardiology and American Heart Association (ACC/AHA) guidelines, the factors that determine the timing for surgery in the case of isolated severe MR include the following symptoms: left ventricular ejection fraction, left ventricular end-systolic diameter, atrial fibrillation, and pulmonary hypertension. Intervention for patients with primary MR consists of either surgical mitral valve repair or mitral valve replacement. Mitral valve repair is preferred over replacement if a successful and durable repair can be achieved. Repair success is dependent on the mitral valve morphology and surgical expertise. Percutaneous mitral valve repair provides a less invasive alternative to surgery, but has not been approved for clinical use in the United States [14]. There is consensus that patients who can undergo surgical repair should be operated on before the onset of signs of LV dysfunction; on the other hand, the negative outcomes associated with mitral valve replacement lead to the statement that asymptomatic patients with severe MR and preserved LV function should not undergo surgery, if the only available option is mitral valve replacement [5, 14]. Recently, the physiological effects of valve competence recovery have been assessed. A reduction in LVEF following valve replacement in the case of MR has been widely described. It had been hypothesized that this event was the inevitable consequence of elimination of the favorable hemodynamic conditions created by MR. Restoring valve competence would reduce the preload and increase the afterload, leading to a reduction in LVEF. Therefore, if LVEF was already reduced, surgery would further reduce it. For this reason, it had to be ruled out in the presence of advanced left ventricular dysfunction before the intervention. However, there is anatomical and functional evidence that this concept is false [39]. Two decades ago, mitral valve surgery consisted of replacing the valve by removing the entire valve apparatus, underestimating its important functional role in maintaining LV shape and contractility. Today it is known that destruction of the subvalvular apparatus, and not the hemodynamic changes following intervention, is the main cause for the reduction in LVEF after mitral surgery [40–42]. This has been proven by the fact that in cases of mitral repair without destroying the apparatus, there has been no or only a slight reduction in LVEF. Considering Laplace's law, as a result of valve repair, the afterload drops instead of rising, as the radius is reduced. Therefore, there are almost no cases of MR that cannot be operated on by an expert, in the absence of other comorbidities, and it makes no difference whether the LVEF is reduced and what the left ventricular end-systolic diameter is, provided that the valve apparatus is preserved during surgery. On the other hand, if the valve and its apparatus cannot be preserved, valve replacement for patients with an LVEF <35% is not recommended [43].

The management of asymptomatic patients is still debated because of the lack of randomized clinical trials. However, the good results of conservative surgery and the preliminary results of recent percutaneous approaches vouch for early treatment. Therefore, current ACC/AHA guidelines recommend that patients in NYHA functional class I and II and with severe MR should be referred for surgery, based on the deterioration of left ventricular function (class I) or the presence of atrial fibrillation or pulmonary hypertension (class IIa).

An independent predictor of mortality and postoperative LV dysfunction in MR patients is the NYHA class [44, 45]. Severe symptoms of congestive heart failure, both transient and persistent, almost invariably suggest the need for early surgery [45]. A stress test could be needed to determine the actual NYHA class and reveal the symptoms in a small subset of seemingly asymptomatic patients [13, 14].

The strongest predictor of the postoperative outcome of chronic MR is preoperative LVEF [45, 46], though in the case of significant MR, LVEF may underestimate the degree of left ventricular dysfunction. ACC/AHA guidelines recommend surgery in patients with severe MR and LVEF <60%, regardless of the presence of symptoms, and suggest that patients with LVEF >60% must be monitored by echocardiography performed on a periodic basis. Recourse to surgery should be made, if there are signs of a progressive deterioration in LVEF [14].

Left ventricular end-systolic diameter (LVESD) and left ventricular end-systolic volume index (LVESVI) are simple, reproducible measurements of LV function that can be obtained noninvasively and are relatively independent of the hemodynamic status. Preoperative LVESD is an independent predictor of outcome after surgeries: LVESD >45 mm is correlated with a high likelihood of developing postoperative left ventricular dysfunction [47]. Preoperative LVESVI is inversely correlated, instead, with postoperative LV function and with survival, as LVESVI values >50 mL/m$^2$ are predictors of persistent postoperative left ventricular dilatation [46]. ACC/AHA guidelines recommend surgery for patients with severe MR and LVESD >40 mm, regardless of the symptoms (class I) [14].

Atrial fibrillation is present in at least one-third of medically treated MR patients [44] and has significant mortality and morbidity rates. Chronic atrial fibrillation occurs almost solely in patients with a left atrial diameter >40 mm, and there is a lower likelihood that sinus rhythm will be restored following surgery compared with intermittent or new-onset atrial fibrillation [48]. This is why ACC/AHA guidelines recommend surgery for MR and atrial fibrillation patients, regardless of left ventricular function and symptoms (class IIa).

Pulmonary hypertension is associated with a significant rise in early postoperative mortality, a poorer functional status, and reduced survival [49]. As an index of severe LV diastolic dysfunction and MR severity, increased pulmonary artery pressure is associated with poor postoperative left ventricular function indices [46, 50]. ACC/AHA guidelines recommend surgery in patients with severe MR and pulmonary artery pressure values >50 mmHg at rest or >60 mmHg during exercise, regardless of left ventricular function and symptoms (class IIa).

Clinical outcomes and therapeutic approaches also depend on the etiology of primary valve dysfunction. For instance, with regard to organic forms of MR, Barlow's disease patients are more likely to remain asymptomatic without developing LV dysfunction, pulmonary hypertension, or atrial fibrillation for a long period of time. Therefore, "watchful waiting" is probably the best strategy for this group of individuals. In contrast, patients with fibroelastic deficiency are more likely to experience adverse events early during follow-up (and more likely to undergo successful valve repair), and a strategy of early mitral valve repair is certainly reasonable [37].

Considering functional MR, despite the fact that both the pathophysiology and clinical consequences of ischemic MR are well defined, there are still doubts on the choice of the most appropriate treatment [51]. This is because it is still unknown whether MR is a mere marker of LV dilatation and dysfunction or whether it is a direct cause of poor prognosis. Briefly, medical therapy is mandatory for all patients; some patients are good candidates for cardiac resynchronization therapy, which can reduce the degree of MR; percutaneous myocardial revascularization is not usually enough to reduce MR; in patients undergoing surgical myocardial revascularization, the role of a combined therapy, including concurrent valve repair, has not been defined.

The appropriateness of mitral surgery in patients with severe MR and advanced heart failure is still controversial [14]. On the one hand, it has been proven that in the presence of irreversible ventricular remodeling and pulmonary hypertension, the reduction of MR in this subset of patients does not yield any benefit [16, 52]; on the other hand, reduced LVEF is of negative prognostic value after mitral repair surgery [45, 46, 53]. Guidelines on the treatment of valvular diseases [3–5, 14] recommend mitral valve surgery in patients with advanced heart failure only if valve replacement or repair is linked to sparing chordal structures for the purpose of preserving already impaired LV systolic function in the postoperative period. In turn, there is, however, evidence by which the treatment of MR in patients with severely impaired left ventricular function is associated with significant left ventricular reverse remodeling (increased LVEF, reduced LV end-systolic and end-diastolic volumes, and reduced sphericity index) and an improvement in the functional class and quality of life [52]. For carefully selected patients with advanced heart failure, mitral valve surgery (particularly mitral valve annuloplasty) appears reasonably safe, with reported 30-day mortality rates in the majority of studies between 1.6 and 5% [52, 54]. The reduction in volume overload due to reduced MR following surgery would reduce the LV wall stress, thereby improving ventricular efficiency and pulmonary hemodynamics and, hence, the patient's clinical status [53, 55]. Finally, the risk–benefit ratio of repair versus mitral valve replacement in patients with severe LV dysfunction is still controversial. Indeed, mitral repair surgery has a lower cardiac surgery risk compared with valve replacement vis-à-vis a higher frequency of resurgence of failure in repair surgery.

Even though it is very likely that these patients have permanent left ventricular dysfunction, it is believed that surgery can improve symptoms and prevent a further deterioration of left ventricular function [14]. For patients at high surgical risk, percutaneous techniques seem to be a valid alternative to treatment according to clinical guidelines [14].

# References

1. Woolley K, Stark P. Pulmonary parenchymal manifestations of mitral valve disease. Radiographics. 1999;19(4):965–72.
2. Rahimtoola SH, Dell'Italia LJ. Mitral valve disease. In: Fuster V, Alexander RW, O'Rourke RA, et al., editors. Hurst's the heart. 11th ed. New York: McGraw-Hill; 2004. p. 1669–95.
3. American College of Cardiology, American Heart Association Task Force on Practice Guidelines (Writing Committee to revise the 1998 guidelines for the management of patients with valvular heart disease), Society of Cardiovascular Anesthesiologists, Bonow RO, Carabello BA, Chatterjee K, et al. ACC/AHA 2006 guidelines for the management of patients with valvular heart disease: a report of the American College of Cardiology/American Heart Association Task Force on Practice Guidelines (writing Committee to Revise the 1998 guidelines for the management of patients with valvular heart disease) developed in collaboration with the Society of Cardiovascular Anesthesiologists endorsed by the Society for Cardiovascular Angiography and Interventions and the Society of Thoracic Surgeons. J Am Coll Cardiol. 2006;48:1–148.
4. Vahanian A, Baumgartner H, Bax J, et al. Task Force on the Management of Valvular Heart Disease of the European Society of Cardiology ESC Committee for Practice Guidelines. Guidelines on the management of valvular heart disease: the Task Force on the Management of Valvular Heart Disease of the European Society of Cardiology. Eur Heart J. 2007;28:230–68.
5. Bonow RO, Carabello BA, Chatterjee K, et al. American College of Cardiology/American Heart Association Task Force on Practice Guidelines. 2008 focused update incorporated into the ACC/AHA 2006 guidelines for the management of patients with valvular heart disease: a report of the American College of Cardiology/American Heart Association Task Force on Practice Guidelines (Writing Committee to revise the 1998 guidelines for the management of patients with valvular heart disease): endorsed by the Society of Cardiovascular Anesthesiologists, Society for Cardiovascular Angiography and Interventions, and Society of Thoracic Surgeons. Circulation. 2008;118:523–661.
6. Zoghbi WA, Eriquez-Sarano M, Foster E, et al. Recommendations for evaluation of the severity of native valvular regurgitation with two-dimensional and doppler echocardiography. J Am Soc Echocardiogr. 2003;16:777–802.
7. Bargiggia GS, Tronconi L, Sahn DJ, et al. A new method for quantitation of mitral regurgitation based on color flow Doppler imaging of flow convergence proximal to regurgitant orifice. Circulation. 1991;84:1481–9.
8. Simpson IA, Shiota T, Gharib M, et al. Current status of flow convergence for clinical applications: is it a leaning tower of "PISA"? J Am Coll Cardiol. 1996;27:504–9.
9. Baumgartner H, Schima H, Kuhn P. Value and limitations of proximal jet dimensions for the quantitation of valvular regurgitation: an in vitro study using Doppler flow imaging. J Am Soc Echocardiogr. 1991;4:57–66.
10. Sahn DJ. Instrumentation and physical factors related to visualization of stenotic and regurgitant jets by Doppler color flow mapping. J Am Coll Cardiol. 1988;12:1354–65.
11. Pu M, Griffin BP, Vandervoort PM, et al. The value of assessing pulmonary venous flow velocity for predicting severity of mitral regurgitation: a quantitative assessment integrating left ventricular function. J Am Soc Echocardiogr. 1999;12:736–43.
12. Thomas L, Foster E, Schiller NB. Peak mitral in flow velocity predicts mitral regurgitation severity. J Am Coll Cardiol. 1998;31:174–9.

13. Lancellotti P, Moura L, Pierard LA, et al. European Association of Echocardiography recommendations for the assessment of valvular regurgitation. Part 2: mitral and tricuspid regurgitation (native valve disease). Eur J Echocardiogr. 2010;11:307–32.

14. Nishimura RA, Otto CM, Bonow RO, Carabello BA, Erwin JP 3rd, Guyton RA, O'Gara PT, Ruiz CE, Skubas NJ, Sorajja P, Sundt TM 3rd, Thomas JD, Anderson JL, Halperin JL, Albert NM, Bozkurt B, Brindis RG, Creager MA, Curtis LH, DeMets D, Guyton RA, Hochman JS, Kovacs RJ, Ohman EM, Pressler SJ, Sellke FW, Shen WK, Stevenson WG, Yancy CW, American College of Cardiology, American College of Cardiology/American Heart Association, American Heart Association. 2014 AHA/ACC guideline for the management of patients with valvular heart disease: a report of the American College of Cardiology/American Heart Association Task Force on Practice Guidelines. J Thorac Cardiovasc Surg. 2014;148(1):e1–32. doi:10.1016/j.jtcvs.2014.05.014. Epub 9 May 2014.

15. Lancellotti P, Gérard P, Piérard LA. Long term outcome of patients with heart failure and dynamic functional mitral regurgitation. Eur Heart J. 2005;26:1528–32.

16. Enriquez-Sarano M, Basmadjian AJ, Rossi A, et al. Progression of mitral regurgitation: a prospective Doppler echocardiographic study. J Am Coll Cardiol. 1999;34:1137–44.

17. Lancellotti P, Lebrun F, Piérard LA. Determinants of exercise-induced changes in mitral regurgitation in patients with coronary artery disease and left ventricular dysfunction. J Am Coll Cardiol. 2003;42:1921–8.

18. Shiota T. Role of modern 3D echocardiography in valvular heart disease. Korean J Intern Med. 2014;29(6):685–702. doi:10.3904/kjim.2014.29.6.685. Epub 31 Oct 2014. Review.

19. Sugeng L, Shernan SK, Salgo IS, et al. Live 3-dimensional transesophageal echocardiography initial experience using the fully-sampled matrix array probe. J Am Coll Cardiol. 2008;52:446–9.

20. Biaggi P, Gruner C, Jedrzkiewicz S, et al. Assessment of mitral valve prolapse by 3D TEE. J Am Coll Cardiol Img. 2011;4:94–7.

21. Quader N, Rigolin VH. Two and three dimensional echocardiography for pre-operative assessment of mitral valve regurgitation. Cardiovasc Ultrasound. 2014;12:42. doi:10.1186/1476-7120-12-42.

22. Altiok E, Hamada S, van Hall S, et al. Comparison of direct planimetry of mitral valve regurgitation orifice area by three-dimensional transesophageal echocardiography to effective regurgitant orifice area obtained by proximal flow convergence method and vena contracta area determined by color Doppler echocardiography. Am J Cardiol. 2011;107:452–8.

23. Yosefy C, Levine RA, Solis J, Vaturi M, Handschumacher MD, Hung J. Proximal flow convergence region as assessed by real-time 3-dimensional echocardiography: challenging the hemispheric assumption. J Am Soc Echocardiogr. 2007;20:389–96.

24. Matsumura Y, Saracino G, Sugioka K, et al. Determination of regurgitant orifice area with the use of a new three-dimensional flow convergence geometric assumption in functional mitral regurgitation. J Am Soc Echocardiogr. 2008;21:1251–6.

25. Hopmeyer J, He S, Thorvig KM, et al. Estimation of mitral regurgitation with a hemielliptic curve-fitting algorithm: in vitro experiments with native mitral valves. J Am Soc Echocardiogr. 1998;11:322–31.

26. Morris M, Araoz P. Advanced imaging of mitral valve disease. US Cardiol. 2011;8:24–9.

27. Zeng X, Levine RA, Hua L, Morris EL, Kang Y, Flaherty M, Morgan NV, Hung J. Diagnostic value of vena contracta area in the quantification of mitral regurgitation severity by color Doppler 3D echocardiography. Circ Cardiovasc Imaging. 2011;4(5):506–13. doi:10.1161/CIRCIMAGING.110.961649. Epub 5 Jul 2011.

28. Glockner JF, Johnston DL, McGee KP. Evaluation of cardiac valvular disease with MR imaging: qualitative and quantitative techniques. Radiographics. 2003;23:9.

29. Schnyder PA, Sarraj AM, Duvoisin BE, et al. Pulmonary edema associated with mitral regurgitation: prevalence of predominant involvement of the right upper lobe. AJR Am J Roentgenol. 1993;161:33–6.

30. Hayek E, Gring CN, Griffin BP. Mitral valve prolapse. Lancet. 2005;365:507–18.

31. D'Ancona G, Mamone G, Marrone G, et al. Ischemic mitral valve regurgitation: the new challenge for magnetic resonance imaging. Eur J Cardiothorac Surg. 2007;32:475–80.

32. Rubinshtein R, Glockner JF, Ommen SR, et al. Characteristics and clinical significance of late gadolinium enhancement by contrast-enhanced magnetic resonance imaging in patients with hypertrophic cardiomyopathy. Circ Heart Fail. 2010;3:51–8.

33. Guo YK, Yang ZG, Ning G, et al. Isolated mitral regurgitation: quantitative assessment with 64-section multidetector CT—comparison with MR imaging and echocardiography. Radiology. 2009;252:369–76.
34. Gelfand EV, Hughes S, Hauser TH, et al. Severity of mitral and aortic regurgitation as assessed by cardiovascular magnetic resonance: optimizing correlation with Doppler echocardiography. J Cardiovasc Magn Reson. 2006;8:503–7.
35. Grossman W, Baim DS. Grossman's cardiac catheterization, angiography and intervention. 7th ed. Baltimore: Lippincott Williams and Wilkins; 2006.
36. Braunwald E, Awe W. The syndrome of severe mitral regurgitation with normal left atrial pressure. Circulation. 1963;27:29–35.
37. Chikwe J, Adams DH. State of the art: degenerative mitral valve disease. Heart Lung Circ. 2009;18:319–29.
38. Delahaye JP, Gare JP, Viguier E, et al. Natural history of severe mitral regurgitation. Eur Heart J. 1991;12:5–9.
39. Enriquez-Sarano M, Freeman WK, Tribouilloy CM, et al. Functional anatomy of mitral regurgitation: accuracy and outcome implications of TEE. J Am Coll Cardiol. 1999;34:1129–36.
40. Thamilarasan M, Griffin B. Choosing the most appropriate valve operation and prosthesis. Cleve Clin J Med. 2002;69:668–703.
41. Lee EM, Shapiro LM, Wells FC. Superiority of mitral valve repair in surgery for degenerative mitral regurgitation. Eur Heart J. 1997;18:655–63.
42. Enriquez-Sarano M, Schaff HV, Orszulak TA, et al. Valve repair improves the outcome of surgery for mitral regurgitation. A multivariate analysis. Circulation. 1995;91:1022–228.
43. Trichon BH, Felker GM, Shaw LK, et al. Relation of frequency and severity of mitral regurgitation to survival among patients with left ventricular systolic dysfunction and heart failure. Am J Cardiol. 2003;91:538–43.
44. Ling LH, Enriquez-Sarano M, Seward JB, et al. Clinical outcome of mitral regurgitation due to flail leaflet. N Engl J Med. 1996;335:1417–23.
45. Tribouilloy CM, Enriquez-Sarano M, Schaff HV, et al. Impact of preoperative symptoms on survival after surgical correction of organic mitral regurgitation: rationale for optimizing surgical implications. Circulation. 1999;99:400–5.
46. Crawford MH, Souchek J, Oprian CA, et al. Determinants of survival and left ventricular performance after mitral valve replacement. Department of Veterans Affairs Cooperative Study on Valvular Heart Disease. Circulation. 1990;81:1173–81.
47. Enriquez-Sarano M, Tajik AJ, Schaff HV, et al. Echocardiographic prediction of left ventricular function after correction of mitral regurgitation: results and clinical implications. J Am Coll Cardiol. 1994;24:1536–43.
48. Sherrid MV, Clark RD, Cohn K. Echocardiographic analysis of left atrial size before and after operation in mitral valve disease. Am J Cardiol. 1979;43:171–8.
49. Nashef SA, Roques F, Michel P, et al. European system for cardiac operative risk evaluation (EuroSCORE). Eur J Cardiothorac Surg. 1999;16:9–13.
50. Enriquez-Sarano M, Rossi A, Seward JB, et al. Determinants of pulmonary hypertension in left ventricular dysfunction. J Am Coll Cardiol. 1997;29:153–9.
51. Carabello BA. The current therapy for mitral regurgitation. J Am Coll Cardiol. 2008;52:319–26.
52. DiSalvo T, Acker MA, Dec GW, et al. Mitral valve surgery in advanced heart failure. J Am Coll Cardiol. 2010;55:271–82.
53. Bishay ES, McCarthy PM, Cosgrove DM, et al. Mitral valve surgery in patients with severe left ventricular dysfunction. Eur J Cardiothorac Surg. 2000;17:213–21.
54. Wu AH, Aaronson KD, Bolling SF, et al. Impact of mitral valve annuloplasty on mortality risk in patients with mitral regurgitation and left ventricular systolic dysfunction. J Am Coll Cardiol. 2005;45:381–7.
55. Gaasch WH, Meyer TE. Left ventricular response to mitral regurgitation: implications for management. Circulation. 2008;118:2298–303.

# Computed Tomography Imaging for Mitral Valve Regurgitation

**5**

Rominder Grover, Philipp Blanke, Shaw-Hua Kueh, Stephanie Sellers, and Jonathon A. Leipsic

## 5.1 Introduction

The clinical utility of coronary computed tomography angiography for the evaluation of coronary artery disease is well established in routine cardiology practice. Advances in multidetector computed tomography (MDCT) technology over the past decade have seen dramatic improvements in both spatial and temporal resolution, which has permitted acquisition of high-quality images despite the challenges presented by cardiac motion. Above and beyond allowing for the comprehensive assessment of the epicardial coronary vessels, cardiac chamber contrast opacification with new-generation MDCT scanners also enables accurate and detailed segmentation of the left-sided cardiac valves. Traditional two-dimensional (2D) echocardiography has long been the reference standard for the diagnosis and evaluation of valvular pathology; however, transthoracic echocardiography (TTE) is operator dependent and can be limited in patients with poor acoustic windows, and transesophageal echocardiography (TEE) is invasive. Both approaches limit acquisition to a restricted number of planes/projections, which cannot be subsequently manipulated. In contrast, three-dimensional (3D) imaging techniques such as MDCT permit rapid acquisition of volumetric datasets with unlimited 2D planar reconstruction post-processing capability. This recent development in MDCT technology has fortunately paralleled the rapid expansion of percutaneous valvular repair strategies for patients with symptomatic severe valvular heart disease who are deemed inoperable.

R. Grover, M.B.B.S. • P. Blanke, M.D. • S.-H. Kueh, M.B.Ch.B. • S. Sellers, M.Sc.
J.A. Leipsic, M.D. (✉)
Department of Radiology, University of British Columbia, Vancouver, BC, Canada
e-mail: jleipsic@providencehealth.bc.ca

© Springer International Publishing AG 2018
C. Tamburino et al. (eds.), *Percutaneous Treatment of Left Side Cardiac Valves*,
https://doi.org/10.1007/978-3-319-59620-4_5

Mitral regurgitation (MR) and aortic stenosis are the two most frequent valvular cardiac pathologies, and together they represent a major health burden in the context of an aging population [1, 2]. Surgical valve repair or replacement has long been considered standard therapy for these patients, though many elderly patients who otherwise meet guideline-directed criteria for such therapy are precluded from this option due to unacceptably prohibitive surgical risk [3, 4]. The development of percutaneous- or transcatheter-based therapies has seen exponential growth in an attempt to address this important clinical dilemma in high-risk populations.

Transcatheter aortic valve replacement (TAVR) has become well embedded within the therapeutic armamentarium for patients with inoperable aortic stenosis following the results of sentinel trials such as the PARTNER trial [5].

In the context of MR, traditional surgical mitral valve replacement confers a decreased recurrence risk. However, there is data to support the notion that overall clinical outcomes are superior with repair strategies that preserve the integrity of the subvalvular mitral apparatus [6]. Transcatheter mitral valve implantation (TMVI) aims to both replace the valve and simultaneously spare the subvalvular chordal structures and has been developed using a similar conceptual paradigm as TAVR, with promising early results [7–12].

Imaging is a vital component of transcatheter valvular interventions. Invasive cardiothoracic surgery permits direct intraoperative visualization of the diseased valve. However decisions regarding patient suitability, prosthesis selection, and access planning for transcatheter approaches are critically dependent on pre-procedural imaging of the valves and their anatomical relationships to surrounding cardiac structures [13]. In contrast to, and building on, the experience with TAVR, advanced imaging has undergone much earlier integration in TMVI [14]. Indeed the role of imaging is possibly even more vital in the TMVI domain given the complex 3D structure and functional dynamics of the mitral valve, with its nonplanar annulus; lack of a circular, fibrous annular structure; variability of leaflet and subvalvular apparatus anatomy; as well as the proximity of the mitral valve to the left ventricular outflow tract.

MDCT analysis of the mitral valve has led to novel insights into the underlying mechanisms of various etiologies of MR and emerged as a powerful tool in the multimodality imaging assessment of mitral valvular pathology in the context of TMVI. This chapter aims to describe these advances in detail and is divided into the following four major parts:

1. Technical aspects of cardiac computed tomographic image acquisition for the purposes of mitral valvular assessment
2. Incremental role of MDCT for the assessment of the mitral valve and MR in the context of TMVI
3. The role of MDCT in determination of TMVI feasibility and safety
4. MDCT assessment of prosthetic heart valves, valvular masses, and infective endocarditis

## 5.2    Part 1: Technical Aspects of 3D Imaging with MDCT for Mitral Valve Analysis

Cardiac MDCT is a relatively more technically demanding examination to perform compared with the majority of routine body CT scanning protocols. Optimal image quality is highly dependent on a number of variables, including hardware, software, and technologist expertise, with wide variation in protocols among different hardware vendors and centers. Compliance with guideline-directed minimum standards for the acquisition, post-processing, and interpretation of cardiac MDCT is imperative both to maximize diagnostic yield while minimizing patient risk from unnecessary or excessive exposure to radiation and contrast media.

### 5.2.1   Scanner Requirements

The inherent efficacy of any cardiac imaging modality is defined by its ability to acquire images of high anatomical quality and detail (spatial resolution) in the shortest window of time possible (temporal resolution). Employing current generation scanners, with a minimum of 64-slice technology, is critical in the context of MDCT analysis of the cardiac valves, which exhibit a high degree of rapid and dynamic motion. These scanners expediently acquire large 3D volumetric datasets, with sufficient spatial and temporal resolution [13]. Latest-generation scanners are able to image a 16 cm slab within one gantry rotation and hence provide whole-heart coverage within a single R-R interval [13]. State-of-the-art dual-energy source CT scanners are now capable of imaging at a temporal resolution of 67 ms and a gantry rotation of 250 ms. Spatial resolution with current generation scanners is submillimeter ($0.5 \times 0.5$ mm in the axial plane with a minimum slice thickness of 0.5–0.75 mm) [13]. With these specifications, the resulting 3D volumetric dataset is isotropic, which enables post-processing reconstruction along unlimited imaging planes for the detailed evaluation of cardiac structure and function, without degradation of spatial resolution [15]. The orientation of the 3D dataset is prespecified and standardized by the position of the patient on the CT scanner table. Hence these reconstructed planes can be formatted with respect to the standard anatomical body axes in exact fluoroscopic angle coordinates (LAO/RAO-cranial/caudal) [15].

### 5.2.2   ECG Gating and Radiation Exposure

Synchronization to the cardiac cycle (ECG gating) is a requirement for cardiovascular CT, with two techniques most commonly employed depending on the clinical indication: prospective ECG triggering and retrospective gating. Each technique entails prespecification of the image acquisition window within the cardiac cycle (systolic and/or diastolic phase). The beginning and end of every individual cardiac cycle is defined by an R-wave, as detected by the scanner from the patient's

ECG-trace. A phase is a specific time point in the cardiac cycle and is defined as a percentage relative to its position in the R-R interval.

(a) Prospective ECG triggering: When X-ray exposure and, hence, data acquisition only occur during a specific phase of the cardiac cycle. This mode is typically employed for coronary artery analysis, with data usually only acquired during a narrow diastolic window (typically 70–80% of the R-R interval). The major advantage of this mode is the low radiation dosage. The disadvantages include restriction to static rather than dynamic image acquisition and susceptibility to poor gating and artifact due to arrhythmias and elevated heart rates.

(b) Retrospective ECG gating: This scans throughout the entire R-R interval and allows image reconstruction at multiple phases during the cardiac cycle [16–18]. This allows for dynamic time-resolved four-dimensional (4D) cine analysis of cardiac and valvular motion, which is essential in the context of MDCT imaging for transcatheter valvular interventions [13, 15]. The other relative advantage of this technique includes its lack of susceptibility to arrhythmia. In this mode, X-rays are continuously exposed throughout the cardiac cycle, hence retrospective ECG gating obviously results in significantly higher radiation exposure compared with prospective gating. However, it is important to carefully assess the relative risk-to-benefit ratio in any individual patient of this radiation exposure with respect to the desired diagnostic yield and accuracy of the scan, especially in the context of transcatheter valvular intervention. Dose modulation techniques (e.g., lowered tube voltage and/or current as determined by the patient's BMI) should be utilized because image quality does not need to be of the same standard as required for coronary CT [14].

Typical retrospectively ECG-synchronized acquisition protocols for mitral valve analysis involve radiation doses of between 7 and 15 mSv depending on the scanner (reduced doses with more recent technology), the degree of tube current modulation used, and patient variables (reduced doses with lower BMI and lower heart rates).

### 5.2.3   Iodine Contrast Media Injection

In addition to radiation exposure, the other major procedural consideration with MDCT is the requirement for iodine-based contrast media. Timing of the iodine contrast bolus is critically important to optimize cardiac chamber attenuation for the desired clinical indication. Sufficient contrast opacification of the left-sided cardiac chambers is mandatory for high-quality depiction of mitral valvular morphology. This in turn is dependent on the use of high-concentration iodinated contrast medium and subsequent data acquisition in the arterial phase at the correct time interval postinjection. Volumes of approximately 1 mL/kg of iodinated contrast medium of at least 350 mg/mL concentration are required in general, though doses should be adjusted to an individual's renal function. The standard contraindications to the administration of iodinated contrast material include severe renal impairment (defined as an estimated glomerular filtration rate of $<30$ mL/min/1.73m$^2$) and previous anaphylaxis. Large-bore intravenous access is required to accommodate a high injection rate of iodinated contrast (usually 5–7 mL/s) administered via an automated power injector and followed by a saline chaser bolus. A bolus-tracking technique is then employed to monitor the progressive circulation of contrast medium, using serially repeated axial slices through the ascending aorta to track in real time the progressive arterial contrast inflow, until a predefined attenuation threshold (usually 100–250 Hounsfield units) is reached and triggers the acquisition. This monophasic injection protocol is typically employed for MDCT analysis of the coronary arteries and left-sided cardiac chambers and valves. In this setting, the right-sided cardiac chambers are non-opacified, precluding analysis of the right-sided valves. A biphasic injection protocol ensures right-sided opacification, which enables evaluation of all four cardiac valves and chambers. If such a biphasic injection protocol is followed in conjunction with a retrospectively ECG-gated study, it is possible to quantitate biventricular volumes and systolic function [19].

### 5.2.4  Image Post-processing and Analysis

Following completion of the acquisition protocol, review of the raw axial dataset by the supervising CT physician is mandatory prior to offloading the patient from the scanner table. This is to ensure that all necessary images have been obtained and are of appropriate diagnostic quality. Source CT datasets are then typically post-processed offline using advanced 3D software packages to accurately and optimally define valvular morphology. A number of post-processing tools are employed including:

(a) *Multiplanar reconstruction (MPR)* analysis, which represents the derivation of thin 2D planes using the 3D volumetric dataset, including the reproduction of standardized views obtained on echocardiography and angiography. Except for annular measurements, the mitral apparatus is best evaluated with MPR views mimicking the commissural, three-chamber, four-chamber, and short-axis echocardiographic windows as depicted in Fig. 5.1 [14].

(b) *Volume rendering (VR)*, which is designed to accurately depict 3D anatomical relationships using color display shading algorithms based on the varying voxel densities of different tissues. Cardiac VR requires suppression of adjacent thoracic structures, including the ribcage and lungs. VR enables true 3D depiction of valvular surfaces, including prosthetic valves.

(c) *Maximum intensity projection (MIP)* is a specific type of volume rendering that projects the voxels with the highest attenuation value on every view throughout a 3D dataset onto a 2D image. This method highlights contrast-opacified vascular and bony structures. MIP is more appropriate for analysis of the vascular tree.

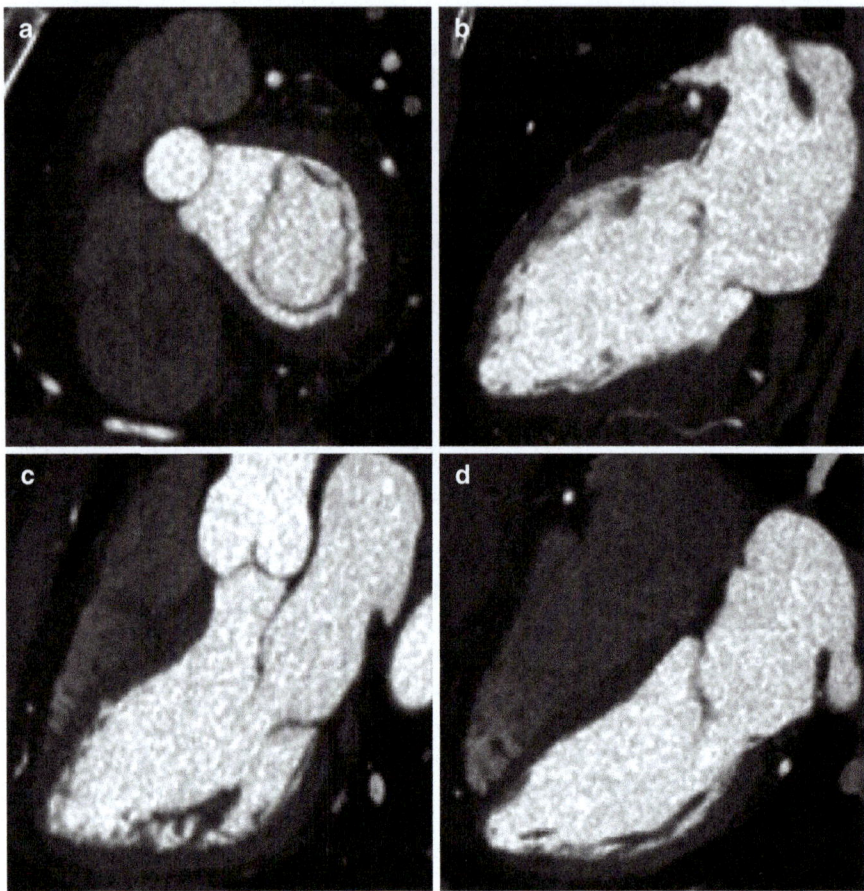

**Fig. 5.1** Multiplanar reformats of a cardiac CT aangiogram in standard cardiac projections: Short axis (**a**), 2-chamber/vertical long axis (**b**), 3-chamber (**c**), and 4 chamber (**d**)

Findings on both VR- and MIP-derived images should be correlated with the source-acquired axial dataset and MPRs.

Quantitative analysis involves both length measurements (e.g., mitral leaflet length) and segmentation-based measurements (e.g., planimetry of mitral valvular orifice area) from the MPRs, as described in further detail in the following sections.

## 5.3    Part 2: Incremental Role of MDCT in the Assessment of the Mitral Valve and Mitral Regurgitation

### 5.3.1    Multimodality Imaging

The etiologies of MR have been extensively discussed elsewhere in this textbook but in brief can be divided into two major subcategories: degenerative (primary) and functional (secondary). Comprehensive structural and functional valvular assessment, including accurate identification of the etiology and severity of regurgitation, is of paramount importance in guiding therapy. Transthoracic and transesophageal echocardiography are the first-line imaging investigations in this context, with 3D techniques now well established as the preferred method for echocardiographic mitral valvular evaluation [20]. However, both clinician- and patient-dependent technical variables exist that are well-recognized limitations of echocardiography, necessitating the use of complementary 3D imaging modalities for the purposes of mitral assessment, especially in the context of planning for TMVI. MDCT acquired 3D volumetric datasets, with their relatively higher spatial resolution compared with both echocardiography and cardiac MRI provides detailed illustration of the anatomy, geometry, and spatial relationships of the mitral valve complex. Qualitative and quantitative information can also be obtained, which is of critical importance in the context of pre-procedural planning and candidate selection for TMVI.

### 5.3.2    Validation of MDCT-Acquired Data for the Assessment of MR with Echocardiography and Cardiac MRI

The hallmark imaging manifestation of MR on MDCT is systolic mal-coaptation of the mitral valve leaflets resulting in a regurgitant orifice. MDCT data reconstructed with more (e.g., 5%) phase intervals throughout the cardiac cycle provide improved temporal resolution imaging, allowing better isolation of the systolic frame of maximal mitral leaflet coaptation failure. Oblique short-axis images of the mitral valve can be derived via MPR analysis, and from these images, the inner contour of the regurgitant orifice can be traced using a planimetric technique to derive the anatomical regurgitant orifice area. Studies have confirmed excellent correlation between MDCT- and echocardiography-derived effective regurgitant orifice area, which is used to stratify the severity of MR [21, 22].

Thin-section MPR allows direct visualization of the mitral leaflets, annulus, and subvalvular apparatus, and studies have demonstrated good correlation with 3D TEE with respect to quantitative assessment of mitral valve geometry, including leaflet lengths and angles [23].

As discussed in Sect. 5.2.3, if a biphasic MDCT contrast-injection protocol is followed in conjunction with a retrospectively ECG-gated study, it is possible to quantitate biventricular volumes and systolic function. End-diastolic and end-systolic ventricular chamber dimensions can be obtained with contour-detection algorithms and manual correction if necessary. In the setting of MR, comparison of the left- and right-ventricular stroke volumes as derived from such quantitative analysis can be used to calculate the mitral regurgitant volume and regurgitant fraction assuming there is no other significant valvular regurgitation or intracardiac shunt. MDCT-derived regurgitant volume calculations have demonstrated good correlation with CMR-derived quantification, which is considered the gold standard for biventricular volumetric analysis [24].

### 5.3.3 Mechanism of MR

Correct assessment of the underlying etiology of MR is an essential first step for determining the appropriate treatment strategies for the management of MR. Traditionally, surgical options for primary or valvular MR require valve repair or replacement, and secondary or functional MR typically requires annuloplasty if optimal therapy of the underlying cause of left ventricular dysfunction fails [25].

However, complete resolution of MR is often unattainable with these surgical methods. TMVI has the potential to treat a broader range of mitral pathologies compared with surgical techniques. Comprehensive anatomical assessment of the mitral valvular and subvalvular apparatus with MDCT is of tremendous potential benefit in understanding the underlying mechanisms contributing to MR in any individual patient so as to ensure appropriate candidate selection and periprocedural planning.

MDCT can accurately differentiate between primary and secondary causes of MR, and numerous studies have not only highlighted this with respect to echocardiography but also enhanced our understanding of the unique anatomical repercussions involved with both of these subcategories of pathology to help in developing novel approaches to TMVI.

MDCT has been shown to have a strong diagnostic accuracy in the identification of mitral valve prolapse as evaluated in a multicenter study including 112 patients [26]. MPR views mimicking the traditional echocardiographic three- and two-chamber views were the most reliable planes for identifying a patient with mitral valve prolapse, as depicted in Fig. 5.2. The accuracy of CT compared with TTE was excellent, with a sensitivity of 96%, specificity of 93%, positive predictive value of 93%, and negative predictive value of 96%. In addition to allowing for precise localization of the prolapsed leaflet scallop, the high spatial and temporal resolution of MDCT was able to discriminate between flail segments vs. bowing/billowing leaflets. Mitral leaflet thickening (defined as maximum leaflet thickness > 2 mm) was also used to define myxomatous and degenerative pathological manifestations of MVP. Disjunction between the posterior mitral valve leaflet insertion and the atrioventricular junction is also characteristic of mitral valve prolapse and can be readily appreciated on MDCT, as depicted in Fig. 5.3b. In contrast, basal myocardial remodeling in functional MR leads to the formation of an atrioventricular shelf, which can also be depicted on MDCT (see Fig. 5.3c).

Mitral valve geometrical analysis including measurement of the tenting heights (coaptation depth) and leaflet angles can also be done with high accuracy and reproducibility in patients with functional MR [27]. Delgado et al. evaluated the mitral valve geometry and subvalvular anatomy in a series of 151 patients, including 67 heart failure (HF) patients of whom 29 had significant (moderate-to-severe) functional MR. In the majority of patients, the subvalvular apparatus showed highly variable anatomy, which was attributable to the multiple heads and insertions of the posterior papillary muscle compared with the anterior papillary muscle, which tends to have a single insertion. Patients with moderate-to-severe functional MR had asymmetrical deformation of the mitral valve leaflets, with significantly increased posterior leaflet angles and mitral valve tenting heights at the central and posteromedial levels compared with patients with heart failure without functional MR. The mitral

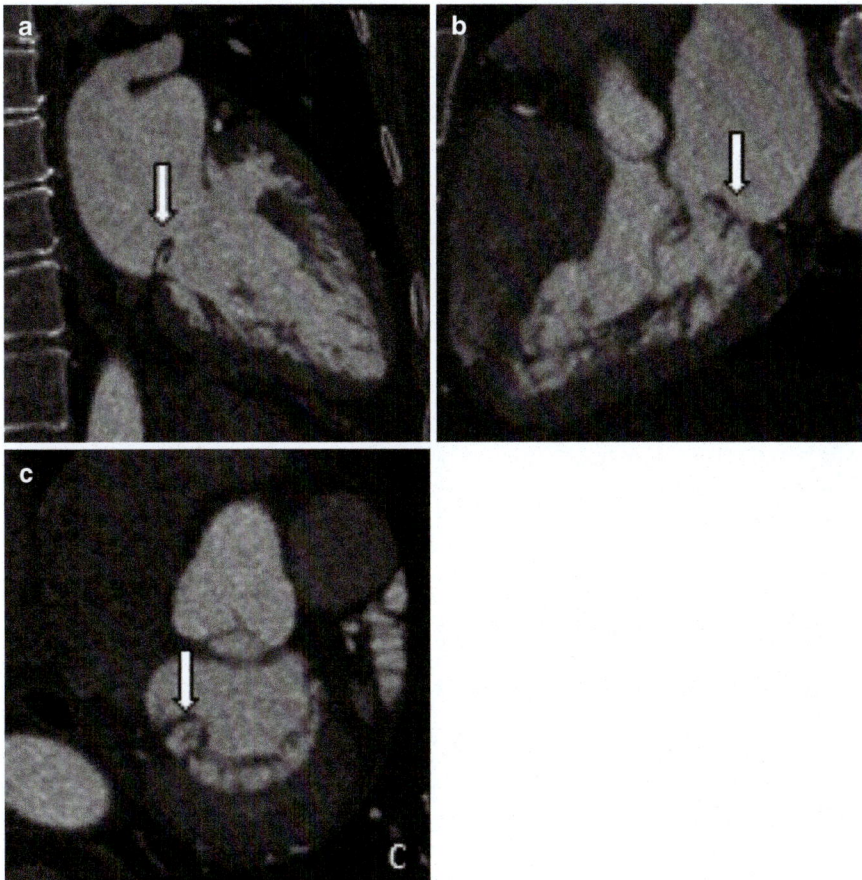

**Fig. 5.2** 2 Chamber (**a**), 3 chamber (**b**), and enface (**c**) projection in a patient with severe mitral regurgitation owing to Posterior leaflet (P1) prolapse (*arrows*)

valve sphericity index was also calculated as a measure of papillary muscle displacement and was defined as the ratio of the distance between the papillary muscle basis and the distance from this level to the mitral annulus. In the HF patients with significant MR, more outward displacement of the papillary muscles (higher sphericity indices) was noted compared with the HF patients without functional MR. Both the mitral valve tenting height at the central level and the mitral valve sphericity index correlated with the severity of MR, as determined on echocardiography.

Further study by Beaudoin et al. [28] provides additional insights into the role of mitral valve leaflet adaptation in the pathophysiology of functional MR. MDCT-derived measurements of the mitral valve leaflet, closure, and annular areas were first validated against 3D echocardiography, showing high intra- and interobserver reproducibility and good correlation with echocardiography-derived mitral valvular measurements. The above MDCT mitral valvular parameters were then quantified in HF patients, both those with and without functional MR. The study found that

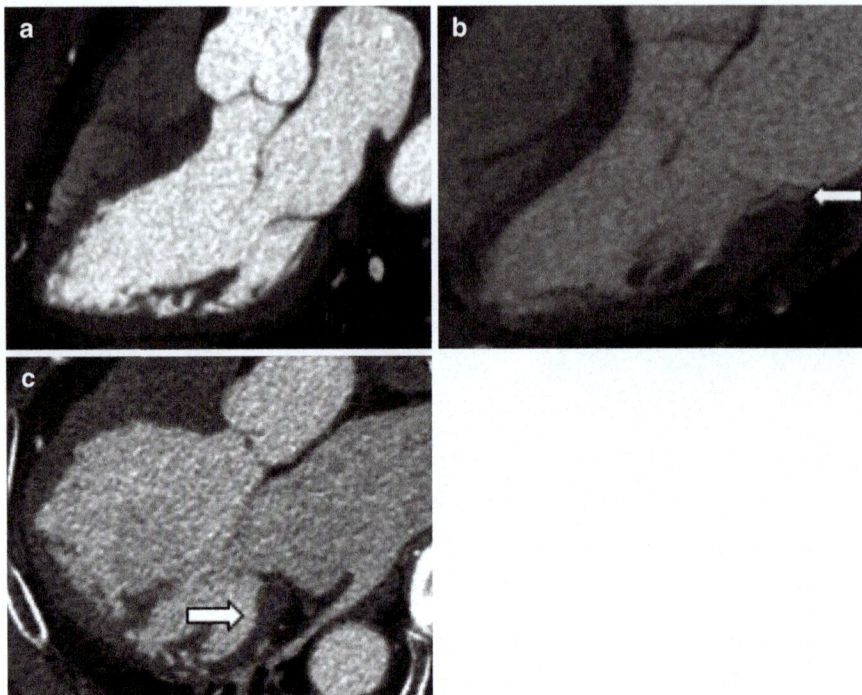

**Fig. 5.3** Three chamber projection CT angiograms highlighting normal anatomical relationship of the posterior annulus insertion (**a**), mitral annular dysjunction (*arrow*) in mitral valve prolapse (**b**), and the posterior shelf (*arrow*) that is a hallmark of FMR (**c**)

total mitral leaflet area increases in the context of cardiomyopathy and left ventricular dilatation, consistent with compensatory mitral valvular enlargement. Patients without functional MR had larger mitral valvular areas, which remained proportional to left ventricular size. Conversely, patients with functional MR had insufficient mitral valvular enlargement to match the left ventricular dilatation. The findings from this study are commensurate with previous 3D echocardiography and animal studies, which have also suggested that MV size is not fixed but, rather, can enlarge in an adaptive attempt to minimize the development of functional MR in patients with left ventricular dilatation and dysfunction.

### 5.3.4 Mitral Annular Assessment for TMVI

Optimal hemodynamic outcomes in the context of transcatheter valve implantation are critically dependent on accurate assessment of the native valvular annulus. This in turn allows appropriate sizing of the prosthetic valve to ensure that it conforms to and anchors securely within the native annulus. Assessment of the native mitral annulus can be challenging in the context of its relatively complex geometry. Compared with the aortic valve, the mitral annulus is a nonplanar, 3D saddle-shaped structure with an anterior and posterior peak, with the former being continuous with the aortic valvular complex and the latter formed by the insertion of the posterior mitral leaflet (PML), with the nadirs located at the level of the fibrous trigones [29].

Both the major and minor 2D mitral annular diameters can be derived from the commissural/two-chamber and long axis/three-chamber views, respectively, on both echocardiography and MDCT. However these 2D measurements may be over-simplified in their representation of the complex 3D geometry of the mitral annulus, and their applicability is limited especially in the context of planning for TMVI. 3D segmentation of the mitral annular contour overcomes these limitations and is read-ily performed with MDCT [14].

Our group has proposed a simplified D-shaped model of the mitral annulus to facilitate MDCT-based assessment prior to TMVI. This model involves truncation of the saddle-shaped mitral annular contour at a virtual inter-connecting line between both fibrous trigones, referred to as the trigone-to-trigone (TT) distance [29]. This is based on the observation that the anterior horn of the saddle-shaped contour would otherwise protrude into the left ventricular outflow tract (LVOT), whereas the more planar D-shaped mitral annulus does not. The TT distance repre-sents an anterior border, which if passed by a device signifies encroachment upon the native LVOT. Like the entire mitral valve complex, the aorto-mitral junction is a highly dynamic structure, with the potential for systolic bulging into the D-shaped contour and diastolic motion toward the LVOT [14].

This segmentation approach firstly requires derivation of MPRs in the long and short axis in alignment with the left ventricular long axis by placing seeding points for the cubic spline along the PML insertion (see Fig. 5.4). Segmentation of the anterior horn is performed by placing seeding points along the insertion of the non-coronary and right coronary aortic cusps into the intervalvular fibrosa. Following identification of the trigones (see Fig. 5.6), the D-shaped annulus is then formed via truncation

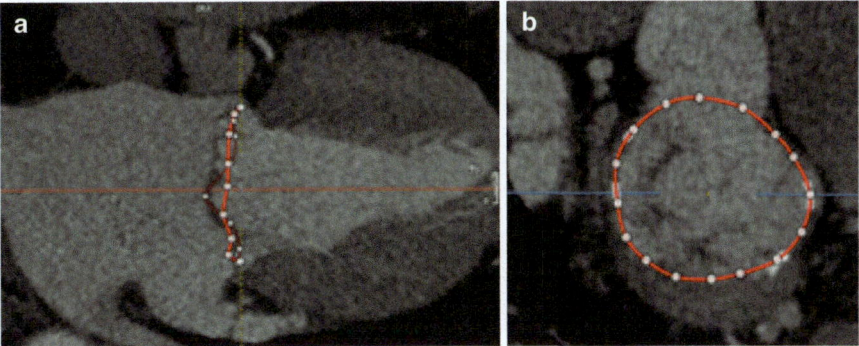

**Fig. 5.4** CT angiogram reconstructions in an oblique (**a**) and en face (**b**) fashion highlighting the 16 point seeding process involved in the segmentation of the mitral annulus

along the TT distance (see Fig. 5.5) [30]. Post-processing derives the annular area and perimeter. The total D-shaped perimeter comprises the posterior annular perimeter annulus (P.Pe as indicated in Fig. 5.5) and the TT distance. Mitral annular geometry is further quantified by measurement of the septal-to-lateral (SL) distance (A2-to-P2 distance), which represents the minor annular diameter, and the intercommissural (IC) distance, which represents the major annular diameter (Fig. 5.6).

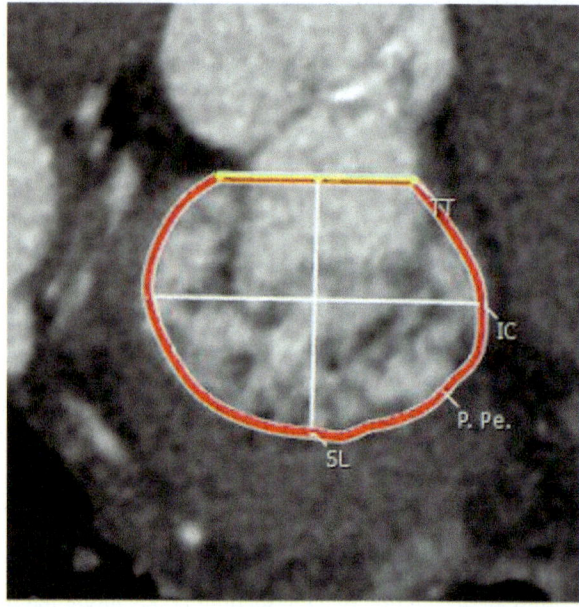

**Fig. 5.5** En face projection of the D shaped mitral annulus (*TT* Trigone -Trigone line); (*IC* Intercommissural distance); *SL* Septal to lateral distance; *P. Pe* Posterior Perimeter

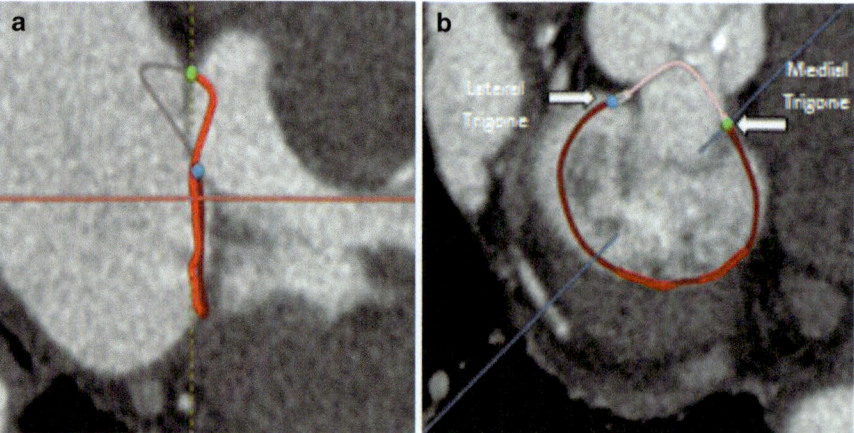

**Fig. 5.6** Vertical long axis (**a**) and enface (**b**) projections of the saddle shaped annulus with the medial and lateral trigones which define the nadir of the annulus annotated

### 5.3.5   Assessment of Annular and Landing Zone Geometry for TMVI

There is wide variation in normative data on mitral annular dimensions. This is primarily due to discrepancies among different imaging modalities and segmentation methodology, especially with respect to the anterior horn. Relatively smaller annular areas were obtained in normal patients on previous 2D echocardiographic studies [31]. This is in contrast to more recent 3D echocardiographic studies, which report mean annular areas ranging between 8.4 and 11.8 cm$^2$ [32–34] with comparable values also published for control cohorts in studies utilizing cardiac CT [28, 34–36]. A recent investigation by our group found a mean D-shaped mitral annular area of $9.0 \pm 1.5$ cm$^2$ in normal patients without valvular abnormalities, with significant interindividual variation [37]. In the TMVI population, overall mean mitral annular dimensions are larger, with further differences noted according to the etiology of MR: increased annular dimensions are observed in MVP compared with FMR [14]. There is a unique reduction in the saddle height in FMR, with a subsequently more planar saddle-shaped annular contour [32]; however, this has no impact on the already more planar D-shaped annular segmentation [29]. Interestingly, with respect to in-plane geometry, there is a relatively greater increase in the SL compared with the IC distance seen in both FMR and MVP patients [27, 28, 37].

Important differences in landing zone anatomy exist between FMR and MVP, which is of particular relevance to TMVI planning. Regional wall motion abnormalities and/or left ventricular dilation in FMR result in marked mitral leaflet tethering and annular dilation, which account for the characteristic structural findings, including increased leaflet tenting height, reduced coaptation length, and basal myocardial remodeling with fashioning of an atrioventricular "myocardial shelf" identifiable on both echocardiography and MDCT [37] (see Fig. 5.3c).

Two subcategories of primary degenerative mitral valve disease are recognized, including fibroelastic deficiency (FED), which is defined by isolated single-scallop prolapse with normal architecture of the other scallops, and diffuse myxomatous degeneration (DMD), in which generalized valvular thickening is observed along with leaflet redundancy and chordal elongation [14]. In both forms of disease, the insertion of the mitral valve leaflet may be displaced into the left atrium, referred to as mitral annular disjunction [38, 39]. A posterior myocardial shelf is not characteristically seen in either form unless the left ventricle is severely dilated. In contrast, the eccentric left ventricular hypertrophy and hyperdynamic systolic function resulting from MR often result in bulging of the basal myocardium into the left ventricular cavity [14].

### 5.3.6   Mitral Annular Dynamics

Mitral annular measurements can be made at multiple points in the cardiac cycle using both MDCT and echocardiography, allowing a more comprehensive assessment of the dynamism of the entire mitral valve complex [14]. The annulus exhibits a dynamic "sphincteric" function or "annular folding," with systolic contraction and deepening of the saddle shape, thus facilitating leaflet coaptation to ensure mitral valvular competency [40]. Early systolic mitral annular dimensions are the smallest increasing toward late systole. Interestingly, annular dynamics are impacted to varying degrees according to the etiology of MR. MDCT studies of mitral annular shape, size, and motion in patients with cardiomyopathy have found that the extent of dynamism is generally blunted in functional MR [35, 41, 42]. Significantly abnormal dynamics have been described in primary or degenerative MR [40, 41], with failure of systolic area contraction, as well as a pronounced increase in annular area from early to late systole. Within the category of degenerative MR, relevant differences exist between the two phenotypes—FED and DMD, described in Sect. 5.3.5. Though both exhibit increased mitral annular dimensions, abnormal dynamics are only observed in DMD [43]. This variation in mitral annular dimensions throughout the cardiac cycles underscores the importance of dynamic imaging with derivation of multiple serial annular measurements to ensure optimal outcomes for TMVI.

### 5.3.7   Annular Calcification

MDCT is superior to both echocardiography and MRI for the assessment of calcification. Degenerative mitral annular calcification (MAC) is commonly seen in the elderly population and present in approximately 6% of the general population [44]. MR and MAC as individual entities have a high prevalence, and, hence, both may coexist without necessarily bearing any causal relationship [14]. MAC is most frequently limited to the posterior annular rim; however, its extent can vary from mild to severe circular involvement of the entire annulus. Caseous annular calcification is a rare variant of MAC that typically manifests along the posterior annulus as large-volume, space-occupying lesions [45–47]. On echocardiography, caseous MAC appears less echodense than typical MAC and can even contain zones of echolucency. On contrast-enhanced CT, caseous MAC can show focal areas of similar attenuation to the blood pool, but these lesions can be readily differentiated on non-contrast-enhanced sequences [48]. Severe MAC is a contraindication to TMVI in the majority of current feasibility studies due to the expected interference with the apposition of the self-expandable TMVI systems [14].

### 5.4   Part 3: The Role of MDCT in Determining TMVI Feasibility and Safety

Derivation of mitral valvular geometrical data parameters with MDCT is of great potential value in guiding TMVI. MDCT enables accurate 3D visualization of the mitral leaflets and detailed evaluation of the various device-specific anatomic criteria to aid with optimal pre-procedural planning and can result in a significant shortening of fluoroscopy and procedure timings.

### 5.4.1  Anatomical Factors

TMVI devices have a diverse range of anchoring mechanisms and, hence, have different anatomical requirements, which should be assessed with MDCT. TMVI devices require accurate mitral annular sizing and thorough assessment of the landing zone. Annular dimensions should be assessed at multiple time points throughout the cardiac cycle, as mentioned in Sect. 5.3.6 in the context of mitral valvular dynamism. Excessive MAC and bulky subvalvular calcification should be noted because of the potential for interference with proper device apposition.

Assessment of the structural suitability for device-specific anchoring mechanisms is critical. For devices which anchor via paddles grasping onto the leaflets [11], e.g., at A2-P2, sufficient leaflet length should be documented via accurate measurement. Mitral valve prolapse and annular disjunction at P2 should also be excluded as these are factors which could possibly interfere with stable device deployment.

The anatomy of the subvalvular apparatus is well visualized on MDCT. The papillary muscles and chordae should be thoroughly assessed to exclude anomalies that may also interfere with device deployment, such as false bands and directly inserting papillary muscles (see Sect. 5.3.7). It is imperative to document the persistence of a myocardial shelf throughout the cardiac cycle for devices that anchor via tabs in the basal infero-lateral myocardium [10]. Basal myocardial hypertrophy or heavy annular calcification can interfere with the anchoring mechanism in these devices. Leaflet length and pathology are of minimal consequence for TMVI devices that anchor via an apical tether [9]. A common theme relevant to all TMVI devices is the requirement that the basal LV cavity be capable of accommodating the device, which can be an issue in the context of a small-sized left ventricular cavity, especially with concomitant hyperdynamic systolic function [14].

### 5.4.2  Predicting LVOT Obstruction

LVOT obstruction (LVOTO) is a serious and potentially lethal complication post-TMVI. TMVI devices currently being validated in early feasibility studies include circumferentially covered stent struts [10, 11, 49], which can protrude into the left ventricular cavity and potentially interfere with the anterior mitral leaflet (AML) and encroach upon the LVOT. In the context of this protrusion, our group has proposed the concept of the "neo-LVOT," which is fashioned by the device itself along with both the AML and interventricular septum [50]. Theoretically, LVOTO can refer to either narrowing of the native LVOT above the level of the TT distance or formation of a narrow neo-LVOT below the level of the TT distance toward the left ventricle [50].

Both anatomical- and device-related factors predispose to LVOTO. There is significant interindividual variability in LVOT anatomy with the major structural

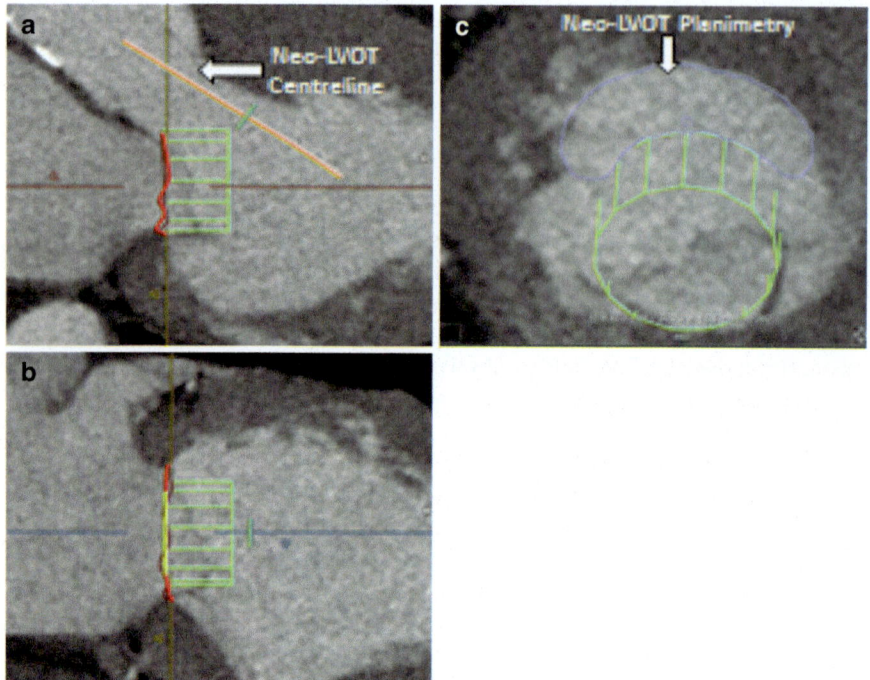

**Fig. 5.7** 3 chamber (**a**), 2 chamber (**b**) and orthogonal projection to the Neo LVOT (**c**) highlighting the method for adjudicating the risk of LVOT obstruction. A virtual implantation is performed and then a centreline is drawn along the path of the neo-lvot. An orthogonal projection is then created to assess the residual Neo-LVOT size in diastole and systole to assess the adequacy of the patient specific anatomy to accomodate the implanted device

determinants, including the interventricular septum, left ventricular cavity size, and the aorto-mitral angulation. Of these, the LVOT and neo-LVOT cross-sectional areas are most negatively influenced by a hypertrophied, protuberant interventricular septum [14]. Device protrusion and flaring are the major device-related factors.

MDCT is of tremendous potential value in this setting because post-TMVI neo-LVOT geometry can be partially predicted by TMVI simulation, e.g., by embedding a cylindrical or device-specific contour into the CT dataset, followed by segmentation and planimetrical assessment of the neo-LVOT cross-sectional area [14], as depicted in Figs. 5.7 and 5.8.

### 5.4.3  Prediction of Fluoroscopic Angulations and Coronary Sinus Location with MDCT

TMVI deployment is performed under fluoroscopic guidance, and coplanar fluoroscopic projections are important to ensure coaxial device deployment. In a fashion analogous to TAVR, MDCT provides these projection angulations based on the

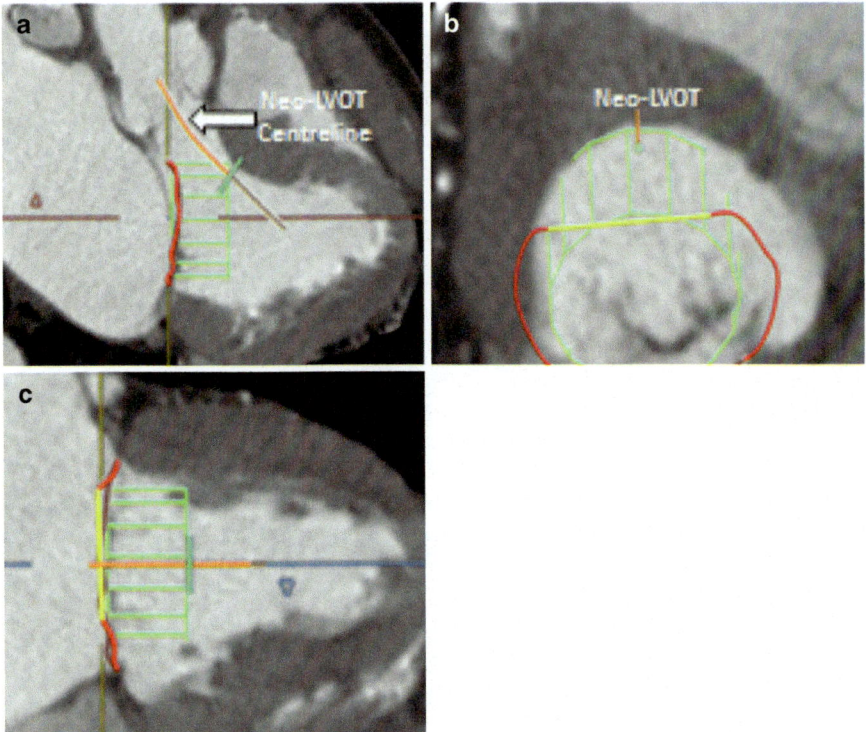

**Fig. 5.8** Multiplanar reconstructions of a patient being considered for Transcatheter mitral valve implantation. A virtual device was implanted with the neo-lvot centreline segmented resulting in no residual space with the virtual device contacting the septum on all three reconstructed images

mitral annular plane, yielding an optimal viewing curve and displaying the corresponding cranial/caudal angulation for any given LAO/RAO angulation. Due to the relatively vertical orientation of the mitral annulus, these optimal curves exhibit a steep slope with dramatic changes in cranial/caudal angulation for any given change in LAO or RAO angulation. C-arm projections for TMVI have to be both orthogonal to the mitral annulus and also aligned with defined anatomical structures to permit visualization of anchoring elements during deployment. Given the asymmetric mitral annulus, two views are considered relevant: a septal-to-lateral view parallel to the SL-line (A2-P2 view) and the TT-view parallel to the TT-line. However, projection angulations are limited by physical restraints of the C-arm, and suitable access is a procedural prerequisite. The SL-view can be derived with projected angulations, which are generally in the practical range of C-arm working angles, as opposed to angulations for the TT-view, which are generally not [51]. Alternatively, a compromise view between the TT-view and SL-view has been derived and shown efficacy in the context of device deployment [51], as depicted in Fig. 5.9.

Unlike TAVR, pre-procedural angiography is not routinely performed prior to TMVI, and a fluoroscopically identifiable structural landmark is absent in the

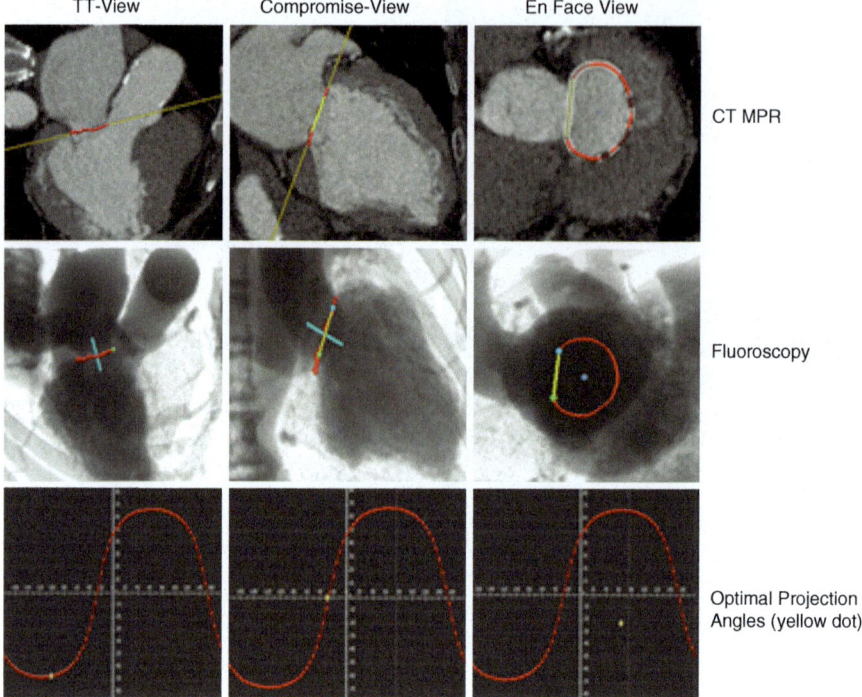

**Fig. 5.9** CT MPR (multiplanar reformats), Virtual Fluoroscopic images, and then optimal projection angles aligned to the T-T (trigone-trigone) view, the Compromise view which is intended to be an angle on the optimal projection angle in between the TT and septal to lateral projection, and an En face projection which can be used to help provide guidance to the interventionalist to ensure a perpendicular deployment

context of a non-calcified mitral annulus. An indirect landmark can be created by placing a guide wire in the coronary sinus [51]. MDCT provides the capability of coronary sinus segmentation in advance of TMVI, providing valuable information in light of the significant interindividual variability in the anatomical relationship between the coronary sinus and the mitral annulus.

Combining the axial views and 3D volume renderings, MDCT assessment of these variable relationships between the mitral annulus, coronary sinus, and also the left circumflex artery not only promotes a more individualized approach as to the requirement for a landmark guidewire but also enhances assessment of both the suitability and safety of coronary sinus-based percutaneous mitral annuloplasty procedures [52].

Tops et al. [53] assessed these specific anatomical relationships in 105 patients undergoing MDCT. The coronary sinus was superior to the mitral valve annulus in 90% of patients, with a distance ranging between 1.4 and 16.8 mm. Compared with controls, this distance was also found to be significantly higher in patients with heart failure. Poor pressure transmission from the sinus to the annulus and increased risk of procedural failure are predicted by a wide angle between the two structures, as depicted on MDCT, which highlights the value of pre-procedural acquisition of this information. Furthermore, variability in left circumflex coronary artery anatomy was also found in this MDCT study, with the vessel coursing between the coronary sinus and the mitral annulus in 68% of patients, indicating an increased risk of arterial impingement during percutaneous coronary sinus-based annuloplasty.

## 5.5   Part 4: MDCT Assessment of Prosthetic Valves, Valvular Masses, and Infective Endocarditis

### 5.5.1   Prosthetic Heart Valve (PHV) Dysfunction

PHV imaging is a common and important, yet often challenging, clinical dilemma. Increasing evidence supports the role of MDCT as a valuable modality for this indication in conjunction with TTE, TEE, and fluoroscopy, which are the current first- and second-line modalities, respectively. MDCT allows full 3D depiction of the PHV and paravalvular region, without the metal-composition-related reverberation artifacts commonly seen with mechanical PHVs on echocardiography. MDCT also enables dynamic 4-D cine loop evaluation of leaflet motion to further assess the etiology and mechanism of elevated transvalvular pressure gradients on echocardiography. A number of smaller studies have demonstrated the high accuracy of MDCT compared with echocardiography and surgery for the detection of PHV thrombus/pannus, suture loosening and paravalvular leak, and pseudoaneurysm [54, 55]. A recent large multicenter registry confirmed these findings and included a balanced number of mechanical and bioprosthetic valves in both the aortic and mitral positions [56]. In this registry, the overall sensitivity and specificity of MDCT for the diagnosis of PHV dysfunction compared with surgery were 94.0% and 98.5% per lesion, respectively. MDCT exhibited superior performance to TEE for the assessment of paravalvular pseudoaneurysms and dehiscence (see Fig. 5.10). The findings from this registry support the utility of MDCT in the multimodality imaging assessment of suspected PHV dysfunction.

### 5.5.2   Valvular Masses

Echocardiography is often unable to accurately differentiate between the etiology of valvular masses, including tumors, thrombi, vegetations, and calcification, which all appear hyperechogenic on echo. MDCT is able to clearly distinguish hyperdense calcium from hypodense soft tissue masses, such as vegetations, tumor, or thrombi, which can also be further differentiated based on post-contrast attenuation [19, 57].

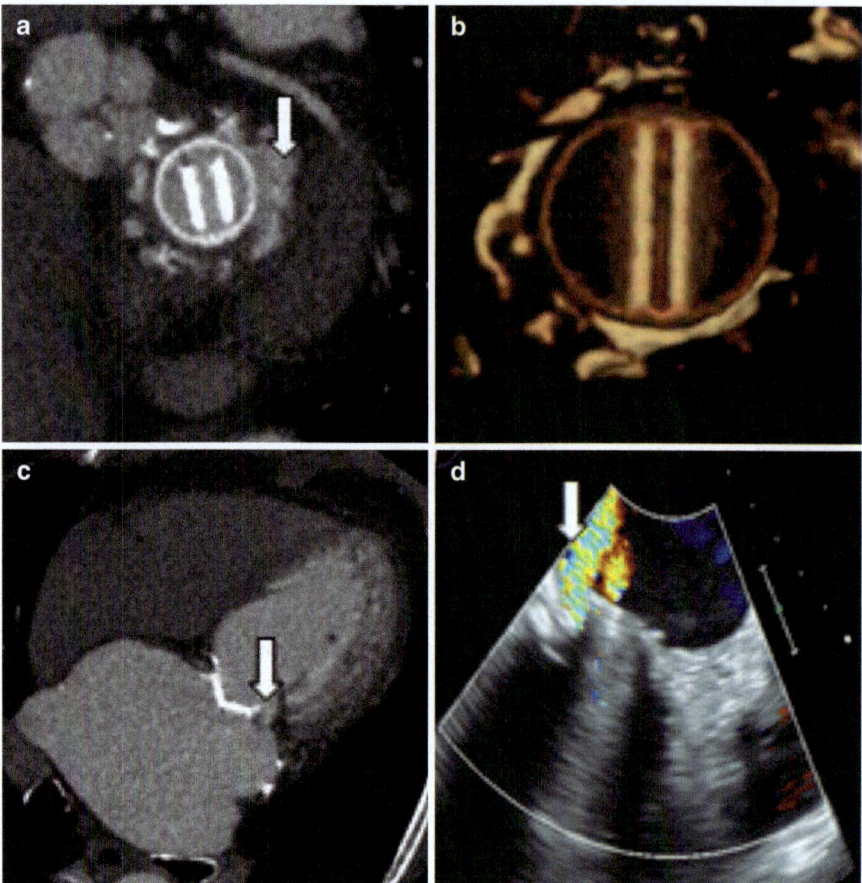

**Fig. 5.10** Short axis multiplanar reformat (**a**), volume rendered (**b**), 4 chamber (**c**) and echocardiographic (**d**) assessment of a patient with dehiscence a mechanical mitral valve posteriorly. The arrows on CT highlight the detachment posteriorly with the arrow on the echocardiographic image highlighting the resultant paravalvular regurgitation

### 5.5.3    Infective Endocarditis

A preliminary study by Feuchtner et al. [58] demonstrated the diagnostic value of MDCT for the assessment of valvular abnormalities associated with infective endocarditis (IE). They assessed 37 patients with suspected IE, of whom 29 (14 cases involving the mitral valve either native or prosthetic) had subsequently confirmed IE and underwent surgery. MDCT had a sensitivity of 97% and specificity of 88% for the diagnosis of IE compared with TEE and/or intraoperative specimen, with a good correlation for the detection of specific valvular lesions. Additional MDCT findings included abscess formation, leaflet perforation, and fistula between chambers and/or great vessels. Furthermore, the use of 4D cine imaging loops allowed for documentation of vegetation mobility in 96% of patients. Large perforations were detected, but leaflet perforations of <2 mm were missed.

The added benefit of MDCT in the clinical context of PHV dysfunction and infective endocarditis is that it allows concurrent noninvasive coronary artery assessment, which is necessary preoperatively in surgical candidates. This is of particular benefit in patients with vegetations/masses for whom invasive coronary angiography carries a higher risk due to the possibility of embolization. It also allows comprehensive visualization of the retrosternal anatomy in patients undergoing redo sternotomy.

### Conclusion

Cardiac MDCT enables high-quality detailed assessment of the complex anatomy of the mitral valvular and subvalvular apparatus, which is of significant value in the context of evaluation of MR and, in particular, pre-procedural planning for TMVI.

## References

1. Nkomo VT, Gardin JM, Skelton TN, Gottdiener JS, Scott CG, Enriquez-Sarano M. Burden of valvular heart diseases: a population-based study. Lancet. 2006;368:1005–11.
2. Iung B, Baron G, Butchart EG, Delahaye F, GohlkeBärwolf C, Levang OW, Tornos P, Vanoverschelde JL, Vermeer F, Boersma E, Ravaud P, Vahanian A. A prospective survey of patients with valvular heart disease in Europe: the Euro Heart Survey on Valvular Heart Disease. Eur Heart J. 2003;24:1231–43.
3. Mehta RH, Eagle KA, Coombs LP, Peterson ED, Edwards FH, Pagani FD, Deeb GM, Bolling SF, Prager RL, Society of Thoracic Surgeons National Cardiac Registry. Influence of age on outcomes in patients undergoing mitral valve replacement. Ann Thorac Surg. 2002;74:1459–67.
4. Nishimura RA, Otto CM, Bonow RO, Carabello BA, Erwin JP 3rd, Guyton RA, O'Gara PT, Ruiz CE, Skubas NJ, Sorajja P, Sundt TM 3rd, Thomas JD, ACC/AHA Task Force Members. 2014 AHA/ACC Guideline for the Management of Patients with Valvular Heart Disease: a report of the American College of Cardiology/American Heart Association Task Force on Practice Guidelines. Circulation. 2014;129:e521–643.
5. Leon MB, Smith CR, Mack M, et al. Transcatheter aortic-valve implantation for aortic stenosis in patients who cannot undergo surgery. N Engl J Med. 2010;363:1597–607.
6. Acker MA, Parides MK, Perrault LP, Moskowitz AJ, Gelijns AC, Voisine P, et al. Mitral-valve repair versus replacement for severe ischemic mitral regurgitation. N Engl J Med. 2014;370:23–32.
7. Feldman T, Young A. Percutaneous approaches to valve repair for mitral regurgitation. J Am Coll Cardiol. 2014;63:2057–68.
8. Herrmann HC, Maisano F. Transcatheter therapy of mitral regurgitation. Circulation. 2014;130:1712–22.
9. Moat N, Duncan A, Lindsay AC, et al. Transcatheter mitral valve implantation for the treatment of mitral regurgitation: in hospital outcomes of first-in-man experience with an apically tethered device. J Am Coll Cardiol. 2015;2;65(21):2352–3. doi: 10.1016/j.jacc.2015.01.066.
10. Cheung A, Webb J, Verheye S, et al. Short-term results of transapical transcatheter mitral valve implantation for mitral regurgitation. J Am Coll Cardiol. 2014;64:1814–9.
11. Bapat V, Buellesfeld L, Peterson MD, et al. Transcatheter mitral valve implantation (TMVI) using the Edwards FORTIS device. EuroIntervention. 2014;10 Suppl U:U120–8.

12. Sondergaard L, Brooks M, Ihlemann N, et al. Transcatheter mitral valve implantation via transapical approach: an early experience. Eur J Cardiothorac Surg. 2015;48(6):873–7.
13. Schoenhagen P, Numburi U, Halliburton SS. Three-dimensional imaging in the context of minimally invasive and transcatheter cardiovascular interventions using multi-detector computed tomography: from pre-operative planning to intra-operative guidance. Eur Heart J. 2010;31:2727–40.
14. Blanke P, Naoum C, Webb J, Dvir D, Hahn R, Grayburn P, Moss R, Reisman M, Piazza N, Leipsic J. Multimodality imaging in the context of transcatheter mitral valve replacement: establishing consensus among modalities and disciplines. JACC Cardiovasc Imaging. 2015;8:1191–208.
15. Natarajan N, Patel P, Bartel T, et al. Peri-procedural imaging for transcatheter mitral valve replacement. Cardiovasc Diagn Ther. 2016;6(2):144–59.
16. Abbara S, Arbab-Zadeh A, Callister TQ, et al. SCCT guidelines for performance of coronary computed tomographic angiography: a report of the Society of Cardiovascular Computed Tomography Guidelines Committee. J Cardiovasc Comput Tomogr. 2009;3(3):190–204.
17. Machida H, Tanaka I, Fukui R, et al. Current and novel imaging techniques in coronary CT. Radiographics. 2015;35(4):991–1010. A review publication of the Radiological Society of North America, Inc.
18. Halliburton SS, Abbara S, Chen MY, et al. SCCT guidelines on radiation dose and dose-optimization strategies in cardiovascular CT. J Cardiovasc Comput Tomogr. 2011;5(4):198–224.
19. Feuchtner G. Imaging of cardiac valves by computed tomography. Scientifica (Cairo). 2013;2013:270579.
20. Van de Heyning CM, Magne J, Vrints CJ, Piérard L, Lancellotti P. The role of multi-imaging modality in primary mitral regurgitation. Eur Heart J Cardiovasc Imaging. 2012;13:139–51.
21. Alkadhi H, Wildermuth S, Bettex DA, et al. Mitral regurgitation: quantification with 16-detector row CT—initial experience. Radiology. 2006;238:463.
22. Vural M, Ucar O, Celebi OO, et al. Evaluation of effective regurgitant orifice area of mitral valvular regurgitation by multislice cardiac computed tomography. J Cardiol. 2010;56:236–9.
23. Shanks M, Delgado V, Ng AC, et al. Mitral valve morphology assessment: three-dimensional transesophageal echocardiography versus computed tomography. Ann Thorac Surg. 2010;90:1922–9.
24. Guo YK, Yang ZG, Ning G, et al. Isolated mitral regurgitation: quantitative assessment with 64-section multidetector CT—comparison with MR imaging and echocardiography. Radiology. 2009;252(2):369–76.
25. Killeen RP, Arnous S, Martos R, Abbara S, Quinn M, Dodd JD. Chronic mitral regurgitation detected on cardiac MDCT: differentiation between functional and valvular aetiologies. Eur Radiol. 2010;20:1886–95.
26. Feuchtner GM, Alkadhi H, Karlo C, et al. Cardiac CT angiography for the diagnosis of mitral valve prolapse: comparison with echocardiography. Radiology. 2010;254(2):374–83.
27. Delgado V, Tops LF, Schuijf JD, et al. Assessment of mitral valve anatomy and geometry with multislice computed tomography. JACC Cardiovasc Imaging. 2009;2:556–65.
28. Beaudoin J, Thai WT, Wai B, et al. Assessment of mitral valve adaptation with gated cardiac computed tomography: validation with three-dimensional echocardiography and mechanistic insight to functional mitral regurgitation. Circ Cardiovasc Imaging. 2013;6:784–9.
29. Blanke P, Dvir D, Cheung A, et al. A simplified D-shaped model of the mitral annulus to facilitate CT-based sizing before transcatheter mitral valve implantation. J Cardiovasc Comput Tomogr. 2014;8:459–67.
30. Blanke P, Dvir D, Cheung A, et al. Mitral annular evaluation with computed tomography in the context of transcatheter mitral valve implantation. JACC Cardiovasc Imaging. 2015;8(5):612–5.
31. Ormiston JA, Shah PM, Tei C, Wong M. Size and motion of the mitral valve annulus in man. I. A two-dimensional echocardiographic method and findings in normal subjects. Circulation. 1981;64:113–20.

32. Flachskampf FA, Chandra S, Gaddipatti A, et al. Analysis of shape and motion of the mitral annulus in subjects with and without cardiomyopathy by echocardiographic 3-dimensional reconstruction. J Am Soc Echocardiogr. 2000;13:277–87.
33. Mihaila S, Muraru D, Piasentini E, et al. Quantitative analysis of mitral annular geometry and function in healthy volunteers using transthoracic three-dimensional echocardiography. J Am Soc Echocardiogr. 2014;27:846–57.
34. Sonne C, Sugeng L, Watanabe N, et al. Age and body surface area dependency of mitral valve and papillary apparatus parameters: assessment by real-time three-dimensional echocardiography. Eur J Echocardiogr. 2009;10:287–94. The journal of the Working Group on Echocardiography of the European Society of Cardiology.
35. Alkadhi H, Desbiolles L, Stolzmann P, et al. Mitral annular shape, size, and motion in normals and in patients with cardiomyopathy: evaluation with computed tomography. Invest Radiol. 2009;44:218–25.
36. Gordic S, Nguyen-Kim TD, Manka R, et al. Sizing the mitral annulus in healthy subjects and patients with mitral regurgitation: 2D versus 3D measurements from cardiac CT. Int J Cardiovasc Imaging. 2014;30:389–98.
37. Naoum C, Leipsic J, Cheung A, et al. Mitral annular dimensions and geometry in patients with functional mitral regurgitation and mitral valve prolapse: implications for transcatheter mitral valve implantation. JACC Cardiovasc Imaging. 2016;9(3):269–80.
38. Carmo P, Andrade MJ, Aguiar C, Rodrigues R, Gouveia R, Silva JA. Mitral annular disjunction in myxomatous mitral valve disease: a relevant abnormality recognizable by transthoracic echocardiography. Cardiovasc Ultrasound. 2010;8:53.
39. Hutchins GM, Moore GW, Skoog DK. The association of floppy mitral valve with disjunction of the mitral annulus fibrosus. N Engl J Med. 1986;314:535–40.
40. Grewal J, Suri R, Mankad S, et al. Mitral annular dynamics in myxomatous valve disease: new insights with real-time 3-dimensional echocardiography. Circulation. 2010;121:1423–31.
41. Levack MM, Jassar AS, Shang EK, et al. Three-dimensional echocardiographic analysis of mitral annular dynamics: implication for annuloplasty selection. Circulation. 2012;126: S183–8.
42. Kaplan SR, Bashein G, Sheehan FH, et al. Three-dimensional echocardiographic assessment of annular shape changes in the normal and regurgitant mitral valve. Am Heart J. 2000;139: 378–87.
43. Clavel MA, Mantovani F, Malouf J, et al. Dynamic phenotypes of degenerative myxomatous mitral valve disease: quantitative 3-dimensional echocardiographic study. Circ Cardiovasc Imaging. 2015;8(5). pii: e002989. doi: 10.1161/CIRCIMAGING.114.002989. PMID: 25956922.
44. Savage DD, Garrison RJ, Castelli WP, et al. Prevalence of submitral (anular) calcium and its correlates in a general population-based sample (the Framingham Study). Am J Cardiol. 1983;51:1375–8.
45. Fox CS, Vasan RS, Parise H, et al. Mitral annular calcification predicts cardiovascular morbidity and mortality: the Framingham Heart Study. Circulation. 2003;107:1492–6.
46. Maher ER, Young G, Smyth-Walsh B, Pugh S, Curtis JR. Aortic and mitral valve calcification in patients with end-stage renal disease. Lancet. 1987;2:875–7.
47. Deluca G, Correale M, Ieva R, Del Salvatore B, Gramenzi S, Di Biase M. The incidence and clinical course of caseous calcification of the mitral annulus: a prospective echocardiographic study. J Am Soc Echocardiogr. 2008;21:828–33.
48. Plank F, Al-Hassan D, Nguyen G, et al. Caseous calcification of the mitral annulus. Cardiovasc Diagn Ther. 2013;3:E1–3.
49. Lutter G, Lozonschi L, Ebner A, et al. First-in-human off-pump transcatheter mitral valve replacement. JACC Cardiovasc Interv. 2014;7:1077–8.
50. Blanke P, Naoum C, Dvir D, et al. Predicting LVOT obstruction in transcatheter mitral valve implantation: concept of the neo-LVOT. JACC Cardiovasc Imaging. 2017;10(4):482–5.
51. Blanke P, Dvir D, Naoum C, et al. Prediction of fluoroscopic angulation and coronary sinus location by CT in the context of transcatheter mitral valve implantation. J Cardiovasc Comput Tomogr. 2015;9:183–92.

52. Ewe SH, Klautz RJ, Schalij MJ, Delgado V. Role of computed tomography imaging for trans-catheter valvular repair/insertion. Int J Cardiovasc Imaging. 2011;27:1179–93.
53. Tops LF, Van de Veire NR, Schuijf JD, et al. Noninvasive evaluation of coronary sinus anatomy and its relation to the mitral valve annulus: implications for percutaneous mitral annuloplasty. Circulation. 2007;115:1426–32.
54. Habets J, Mali WP, Budde RP. Multidetector CT angiography in evaluation of prosthetic heart valve dysfunction. Radiographics. 2012;32:1893–905.
55. Tsai I-C, Lin Y-K, Chang Y, et al. Correctness of multidetector-row computed tomography for diagnosing mechanical prosthetic heart valve disorders using operative findings as a gold standard. Eur Radiol. 2009;19:857–67.
56. Feuchtner G, Plank F, Mueller S, et al. Cardiac computed tomography angiography for evaluation of prosthetic valve dysfunction: a multicenter study in comparison with surgery. Abstract presented at European Society of Cardiology Annual Scientific Meeting. 2016.
57. Taylor AJ, Cerqueira M, Hodgson JM. ACCF/SCCT/ACR/AHA/ASE/ASNC/NASCI/SCAI/SCMR 2010 appropriate use criteria for cardiac computed tomography: a report of the American College of Cardiology Foundation Appropriate Use Criteria Task Force, the Society of Cardiovascular Computed Tomography, the American College of Radiology, the American Heart Association, the American Society of Echocardiography, the American Society of Nuclear Cardiology, the North American Society for Cardiovascular Imaging, the Society for Cardiovascular Angiography and Interventions, and the Society for Cardiovascular Magnetic Resonance. J Am Coll Cardiol. 2011;56:1864–94.
58. Feuchtner GM, Stolzmann P, Dichtl W, et al. Multislice computed tomography in infective endocarditis. Comparison with transesophageal echocardiography and intraoperative findings. J Am Coll Cardiol. 2009;53:436–44.

# Imaging Modality-Independent Anatomy of the Left Heart

**6**

Pascal Thériault-Lauzier and Nicolò Piazza

## 6.1 Introduction

Since its beginnings, fluoroscopy has been and remains the main imaging modality used during percutaneous coronary interventions. However, with the development of structural heart interventions, several additional imaging modalities are required to achieve optimal clinical results. Indeed, echocardiography and computed tomography (CT) are used today for pre-procedural planning, intra-procedural guidance, and post-procedural follow-up of transcatheter structural interventions [1, 2]. In the case of transcatheter valve replacement, interventional cardiologists rely on echocardiography and computed tomography for patient selection, device sizing, and delivery [3, 4]. Herein, we describe an imaging modality-independent terminology to describe the orientation of tomographic data for the specific purpose of left-sided transcatheter cardiac procedures [5–7]. This terminology is intended to be applied to fluoroscopy, CT, echocardiography, and magnetic resonance imaging, thus facilitating the translation between modalities.

## 6.2 Cardiac Imaging Modalities

Introduced in the 1970s, X-ray fluoroscopy is the workhorse of interventional cardiology. Its contrast mechanism is X-ray attenuation, i.e., an X-ray beam decreases in intensity depending on the density and atomic number of the substance it traverses [8]. High-density materials such as calcium, metal, or iodinated contrast agent attenuate the beam more than soft tissue, blood, or water. The simplicity of

P. Thériault-Lauzier • N. Piazza, M.D., Ph.D. (✉)
Interventional Cardiology Department, McGill University Health Center, Glen Hospital/
Royal Victoria Hospital, 1001 Boulevard Décarie, Montréal, QC, Canada, H4A 3J1
e-mail: nicolopiazza@mac.com

© Springer International Publishing AG 2018
C. Tamburino et al. (eds.), *Percutaneous Treatment of Left Side Cardiac Valves*,
https://doi.org/10.1007/978-3-319-59620-4_6

125

this technique constitutes its strength. It provides a high spatial and temporal resolution, at over 30 frames per second. A disadvantage of fluoroscopy is that it relies on carcinogenic ionizing radiation, as well as nephrotoxic iodinated contrast agent. Furthermore, X-ray attenuation offers very limited contrast between different soft tissue structures. Fluoroscopy is not a tomographic imaging method; several viewing angles are required to understand the three-dimensional relationship of anatomical and implanted structures. Viewing angles are described by a cranial (CRA)–caudal (CAU) angulation and a right anterior oblique (RAO)–left anterior oblique (LAO) angulation. In the context of structural heart interventions, fluoroscopy is used for the deployment of devices.

Computed tomography also relies on X-ray attenuation but uses a reconstruction algorithm to generate tomographic images. The information of a given slice is decoupled from that of other slices, thus generating a three-dimensional dataset [8]. In modern multislice computed tomography scanners, the spatial resolution is nearly isotropic, meaning that is almost equal within a slice and across slices. This allows for high-quality multiplanar reconstruction (MPR) and volume rendering techniques to be performed. The high spatial and temporal resolution of ECG-gated multislice CT angiography makes this modality the standard of care for device sizing and procedural planning of transcatheter aortic valve replacement devices. However, CT shares the same disadvantages as fluoroscopy as it also involves ionizing radiation and iodinated contrast agents.

Echocardiography is a widely available imaging modality that uses ultrasound tissue echogenicity as a contrast mechanism [8]. It provides both anatomical and functional information about blood flow and tissue motion. It offers high spatial and temporal resolution but only provides a limited anatomical field of view within a given image. The quality of images depends on the operator experience and skill and on the presence of acoustic windows. It is a crucial modality for the diagnosis and staging of structural heart disease. It is also used for intra-procedural device functional assessment. For valvular interventions, echocardiography is used to assess the presence of residual regurgitation or stenosis after the insertion of a device.

Magnetic resonance (MR) imaging relies on principles of certain atomic nuclei to absorb and then emit radio wave when placed in a strong magnetic field. Depending on the radio wave pulse sequence used, any of several contrast mechanisms can be used to generate tomographic images [8]. MR is particularly interesting since it does not rely on ionizing radiation or on iodinated contrast. In the context of structural heart interventions, MR imaging can be indicated in patients for whom iodinated contrast is contraindicated due to an allergic reaction or due to acute or chronic renal failure. MR is also capable of quantifying blood flow volumes and peak velocities and may therefore be indicated to evaluate the severity of valvular heart disease in patients with poor ultrasound acoustic windows. Post-implantation MR is limited by the presence of susceptibility artifacts caused by the metallic components of various devices.

## 6.3   Heart Anatomy Based on a Unified Terminology

While fluoroscopy, CT, echocardiography, and MR are all fundamentally different, they are used to image the same cardiac structures. Interventional cardiologists rely mostly on pattern recognition rather than three-dimensional anatomical understanding to perform transcatheter procedures. Noninvasive imagers on the other hand have developed a separate terminology to describe the orientation of tomographic images [9–12]. The reliance on multiple imaging modalities each with its own orientation system often results in a disconnect between each modality obfuscating the fact that the same anatomical information is being imaged.

We suggest that describing valve anatomy based on chambers of the heart may facilitate the translation of anatomical information between modalities. This system would enable members of the Heart Team to use the same language to describe common features independently of imaging modality. The concept of heart chamber anatomy originates from echocardiography but can readily be applied to fluoroscopy, CT, or MR.

Because of the fixed coordinate system defined during a CT, MR, or fluoroscopy exam, these modalities are ideal to describe anatomical structures in their attitudinal position [5, 13, 14]. This system assumes that the patient is facing the observer. Structures lying closer to the head are superior, those lying closer the feet are inferior. Structures closer to the observer are anterior, while those that are further are called posterior. Finally, structures at the left of the observer are called right; those on the right of the observer are called left. This system is self-evident for CT, MR, and fluoroscopy, but it is not in the case of echocardiography. Indeed, this observation is particularly significant when considering left ventricle echocardiographic segments. The "anterior" segment lies opposite to the "inferior" segment, which contradicts the fact that two directions are separated by 90° in the attitudinal orientation.

From the standpoint of fluoroscopic c-arm angulations, one can describe specific angulations for each heart chamber view [5–7]. The two-chamber view is best appreciated in a shallow craniocaudal angulation at approximately RAO 30°. This is the typical angulation where a left ventriculogram can be acquired. The three-chamber view can be achieved in a steep RAO caudal angulation or in a steep LAO cranial angulation in some patients. The four-chamber view is located in a steep cranial angulation at approximately LAO 30°. Finally, a short-axis view can be appreciated in a moderate LAO-caudal angulation. Angulations of these views are summarized in Fig. 6.1, which also illustrates the concept of *optimal projection curve* [1, 5–7, 15–23]. In this case, the optimal projection curve of the mitral annulus is shown. Any fluoroscopic view lying on the optimal projection curve corresponds to a perpendicular view of the mitral annulus. Note that this concept can be generalized to any planar structure. The orientation of the two-, three-, and four-chamber view relative to the mitral and aortic valves is demonstrated in Fig. 6.2. We note the four-chamber view at 45° between the two- and three-chamber views, the latter two being mutually 90° apart.

In the next sections, the anatomical features best appreciated in each view are described.

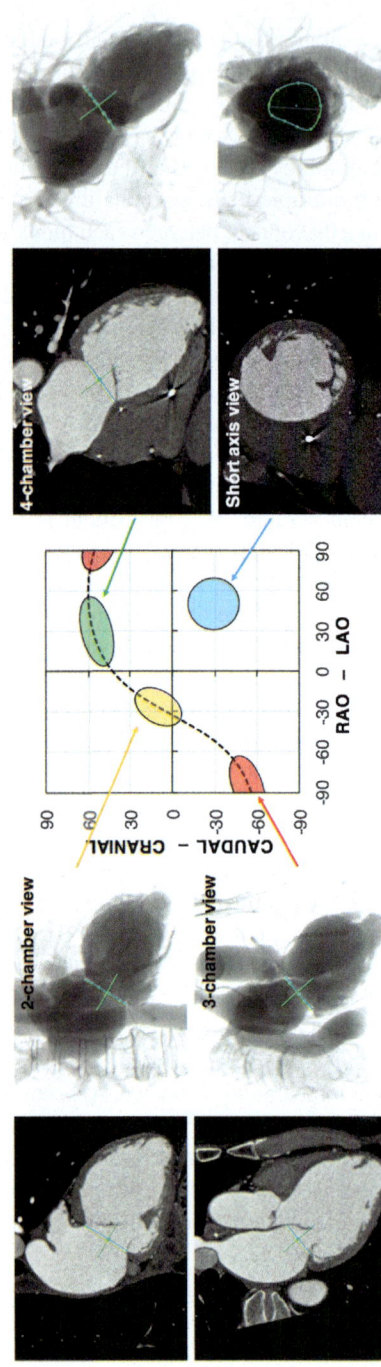

**Fig. 6.1** Fluoroscopic angulations corresponding to standardized views. The optimal projection curve of the mitral annulus is plotted as a *dotted line*. The region of fluoroscopic angulations corresponding to each of the four views is indicated by *arrows*. For each standardized view, a CT slice is shown on the *left*, and a volume-rendered fluoroscopic view is shown on the *right*, both of which are in the same orientation

**Fig. 6.2** Short-axis view
of the heart at the level of
the mitral annulus.
Overlaid on the image are
the orientations of the
two-, three-, and four-
chamber views of the heart

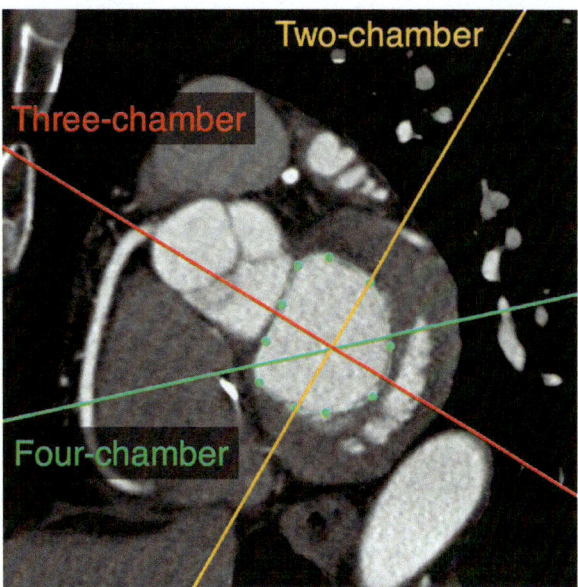

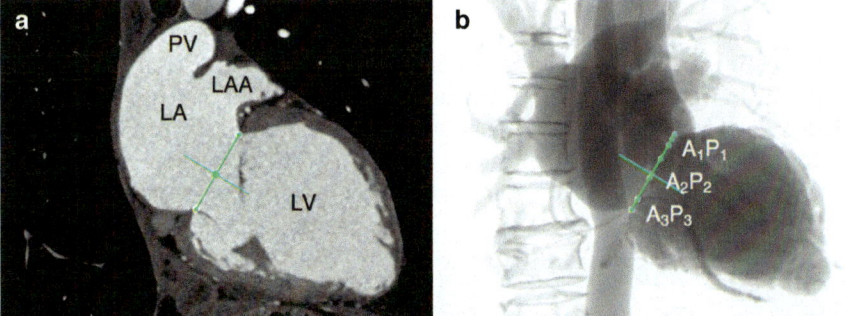

**Fig. 6.3** Two-chamber view. (**a**) Shows a CT slice demonstrating the left atrium (LA) and left ventricle (LV). The left atrial appendage (LAA) is maximally separated from the left superior pulmonary vein (PV). (**b**) Shows a volume-rendered fluoroscopic image demonstrating the overlap of the mitral valve scallops A1 with P1, A2 with P2, and A3 with P3. Note the order of the mitral valve scallops, 1 being superior and lateral and 3 being inferior and posterior. The mitral valve annulus is overlaid in *green*

## 6.4   Three-Chamber View

The three-chamber view (Fig. 6.3) maximally separates the aortic valve from the mitral valve. The minimum diameter of both the aortic and mitral valves is typically visualized in this view. It follows that measurement of each valve dimension in this view can lead to significant underestimation of the average diameter of the valve. In the three-chamber view, the left coronary cusp and non-coronary cusp of the aortic valve are overlapping along the aorto-mitral curtain. Furthermore, the anterior and posterior leaflets of the mitral valve are maximally separated but the subsegments of each leaflet are overlapping.

A three-chamber view can be generated during transthoracic echocardiography using a parasternal long-axis view or an apical view. During transesophageal echocardiography, a mid-esophageal long axis at 120°–140° or a transgastric long axis at 100°–130° can be used.

From an interventional perspective, the three-chamber view is the best view to direct a transapical guidewire from the left ventricle into the left atrium or the ascending aorta. The crossing of the mitral valve can be particularly challenging because of the funnel-like architecture of the left ventricular outflow tract (LVOT), which naturally guides the catheter toward the aortic valve. The LVOT can be avoided by directing the guidewire in the posterior and inferior direction. The three-chamber view is also ideal to direct catheters toward the anterior or posterior leaflet of the mitral valve. For atrial transseptal puncture, the atrial septum is viewed en face with the needle pointing toward the observer. This view can be used to minimize the risk of aortic root perforation during transseptal puncture.

## 6.5    Two-Chamber View

The two-chamber view (Fig. 6.4) has the aortic valve overlapping the mitral valve on fluoroscopy. The maximum diameter of both the aortic and mitral valves is appreciated in this configuration. The anterior and posterior leaflets of the mitral valve are overlapping, thus maximally separating the three scallops of each leaflet; according to Carpentier's classification, A1, A2, and A3 are separated but overlap with P1, P2, and P3. The scallops are ordered from 1 in the left and superior aspect

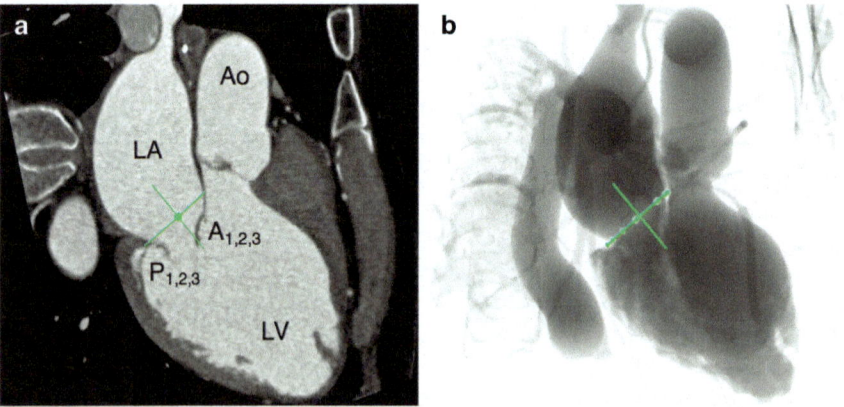

**Fig. 6.4** Three-chamber view. (**a**) Shows a CT slice demonstrating the left atrium (LA), left ventricle (LV), and ascending aorta (Ao). The left atrial appendage (LAA) is maximally separated from the left superior pulmonary vein (PV). Note the separation of the anterior and posterior mitral valve leaflets and overlap of the mitral valve scallops of each leaflet. (**b**) Shows a volume-rendered fluoroscopic image. The mitral valve annulus is overlaid in *green*

to 3 in the inferior and right aspect relative to the mitral valve. The left atrial append-age is appreciated superior to the mitral valve and partially overlaps the ascending aorta. The two papillary muscle bundles are maximally separated in this view.

During transthoracic echocardiography, the two-chamber view can be generated from the apical window. On transesophageal echocardiography, this view is appreciated in mid-esophageal 60°–90° or in transgastric long axis 90°.

From a historical perspective, it is interesting to note that prior to the advent of pre-procedural CT, echocardiography and fluoroscopy were used for TAVR device sizing. Interestingly, an aortogram recorded in a nearly AP orientation was used to measure the diameter of the aortic annulus. This procedure often resulted in the selection of a larger transcatheter device compared to that suggested by echocardiography in a three-chamber view. In the interventional context, the two-chamber view is important to direct catheters toward a mitral valve scallop but cannot differentiate between the anterior or posterior scallops. This is an important point for those performing mitral valve interventions that require the interaction with a specific segment of the valve. The two-chamber view is also important for the left atrial appendage closure since is demonstrates the ostium of the appendage perpendicularly and maximally separated from the left superior pulmonary vein. This allows catheters to be directed toward the appendage thus avoiding the pulmonary vein.

## 6.6    Four-Chamber View

The four-chamber view (Fig. 6.5) shows the left and right ventricles, as well as the left and right atria maximally separated. The interatrial and interventricular septa are perpendicular to the orientation of the screen. The aortic valve overlaps the anterior-inferior aspect of the mitral valve. The commissure of the mitral valve is appreciated in an oblique orientation where different leaflets and scallops are difficult to differentiate.

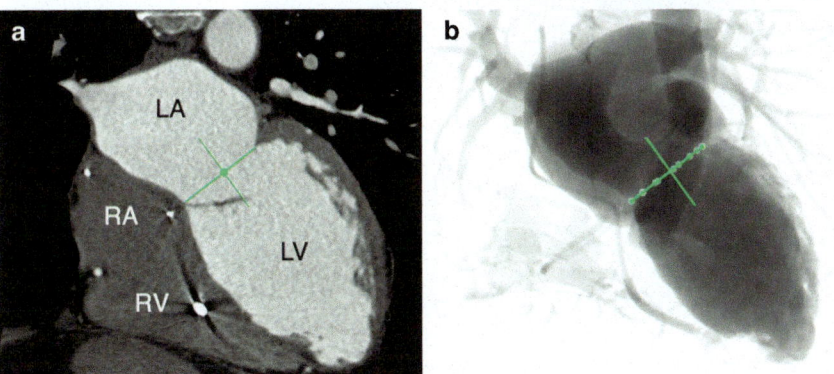

**Fig. 6.5** Four-chamber view. (**a**) Shows a CT slice demonstrating the left atrium (LA), left ventricle (LV), right atrium (RA), and right ventricle (RV). (**b**) Shows a volume-rendered fluoroscopic image. The mitral valve annulus is overlaid in *green*

The four-chamber view can be achieved with transthoracic echocardiography using the apical window. During transesophageal echocardiography, a four-chamber view can be appreciated in a mid-esophageal 10°–20° view. Note the tomographic imaging modalities can achieve a five-chamber view in nearly the same orientation as a four-chamber view by translating the imaging in the anterior and superior direction, which provides visualization of the aortic root, the fifth chamber.

From the interventional perspective, the four-chamber view is interesting to visualize atrial and ventricular septal defects. A catheter can thus be directed toward the defect as is done during transcatheter closure. During transseptal puncture, this view can be used to appreciate the needle perpendicularly as it crosses the atrial septum. However, it does not allow to differentiate the septum from the aortic root as those structures are nearly overlapped in this view.

## 6.7    Short-Axis View

The short-axis view (Fig. 6.6) of the heart shows the mitral valve and left ventricular outflow tract en face. Both the major and minor diameters of the mitral valve can be appreciated. The leaflets of the mitral valves as well as each of the leaflet scallops are maximally separated. This view is also perpendicular to the interatrial and interventricular septum. The aortic root lies anterior and superior to the mitral valve. The ostium of the left atrial appendage is appreciated perpendicularly and overlaps the left superior pulmonary vein in this orientation. The two bundles of papillary muscles are located opposite the left ventricular outflow tract, which is severely foreshortened in this view.

The short-axis view can be achieved using the parasternal or subcostal acoustic windows during transthoracic echocardiography. During transesophageal echocardiography, the short-axis view is obtained from a transgastric 0° configuration.

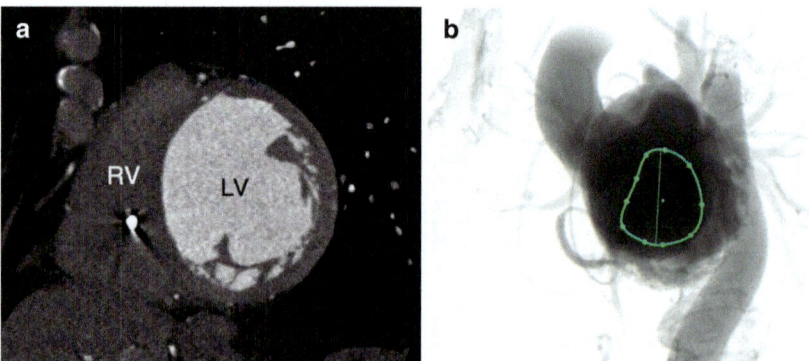

**Fig. 6.6** Short-axis view. (**a**) Shows a CT slice demonstrating the left ventricle (LV) and right ventricle (RV). Interestingly, the two papillary muscle bundles are in a superior–inferior configuration relative to each other. (**b**) Shows a volume-rendered fluoroscopic image. The mitral valve annulus is overlaid in *green*. Note that the left ventricular outflow tract is severely foreshortened in this view and that it lies superior, right, and anterior relative to the two papillary muscle bundles

**Table 6.1** Summary of anatomical structures in different views

| Three-chamber view | Two-chamber view | Four-chamber view | Short-axis view |
|---|---|---|---|
| • Minor axis of the mitral annulus | • Major axis of the mitral valve annulus | • Oblique axis of mitral valve | • Major and minor axes of the mitral valve annulus |
| • Minor axis of the aortic annulus | • Major axis of the aortic annulus | • Oblique axis of aortic valve | • Major and minor axes of the aortic valve annulus |
| • Separation of the anterior and posterior mitral valve leaflets | • Overlap of the anterior and posterior mitral valve leaflets | • Overlap of anterior and posterior mitral valve leaflets | • Separation of the anterior and posterior mitral valve leaflets |
| • Overlap of anterior mitral leaflets scallops (A1, A2, A3) | • Separation of anterior mitral leaflets scallops (A1, A2, A3) | • Overlap of anterior mitral leaflets scallops (A1, A2, A3) | • Separation of the anterior mitral leaflets scallops |
| • Overlap of posterior mitral leaflets scallops (P1, P2, P3) | • Separation of posterior mitral leaflets scallops (P1, P2, P3) | • Overlap of posterior mitral leaflets scallops (P1, P2, P3) | • Separation of the posterior mitral leaflets scallops |
| • Separation of the aortic valve from the mitral valve | • Overlap of the aortic valve and the mitral valve | • Overlap of mitral and aortic valves | • Separation of the aortic and mitral valves |
| • Aortic and mitral valve annulus in plane (along both optimal projection curves) | • Separation of papillary muscles | • Perpendicular view of the atrial and ventricular septa | • Left ventricular outflow tract is severely foreshortened |
| • Overlap of papillary muscles | • Atrial septum nearly in plane | | • Left atrial appendage overlap with left superior pulmonary vein |
| • En face view of the left atrial appendage ostium | • Left atrial appendage separated from left superior pulmonary vein | | |
| • En face view of the atrial septum | | | |

The short-axis view can be used to define the angulation of the left ventricular axis and the direction of the mitral valve during transapical puncture. For transseptal puncture, this view shows the needle perpendicularly. In the context of transcatheter aortic valve replacement or transcatheter mitral valve replacement, this view should not be used during deployment of the device as it provides no information on the depth of implantation in the aortic root or within the mitral annulus (Table 6.1).

## Conclusion

In this chapter, we described standard imaging modality-independent view based on echocardiographic views of the heart. We described the relevance of these views for structural heart interventions. Using a common language between members of the Heart Team should facilitate translation of the wealth of information obtained from noninvasive imaging to the interventional cardiologist.

# References

1. Kurra V, Kapadia SR, Tuzcu EM, et al. Pre-procedural imaging of aortic root orientation and dimensions: comparison between X-ray angiographic planar imaging and 3-dimensional multidetector row computed tomography. JACC Cardiovasc Interv. 2010;3:105–13.
2. Leipsic J, Gurvitch R, Labounty TM, et al. Multidetector computed tomography in transcatheter aortic valve implantation. JACC Cardiovasc Imaging. 2011;4:416–29.
3. Achenbach S, Delgado V, Hausleiter J, Schoenhagen P, Min JK, Leipsic JA. SCCT expert consensus document on computed tomography imaging before transcatheter aortic valve implantation (TAVI)/transcatheter aortic valve replacement (TAVR). J Cardiovasc Comput Tomogr. 2012;6:366–80.
4. Holmes DR Jr, Mack MJ, Kaul S, et al. 2012 ACCF/AATS/SCAI/STS expert consensus document on transcatheter aortic valve replacement. J Am Coll Cardiol. 2012;59:1200–54.
5. Theriault-Lauzier P, Andalib A, Martucci G, et al. Fluoroscopic anatomy of left-sided heart structures for transcatheter interventions: insight from multislice computed tomography. JACC Cardiovasc Interv. 2014;7:947–57.
6. Spaziano M, Theriault-Lauzier P, Meti N, et al. Optimal fluoroscopic viewing angles of left-sided heart structures in patients with aortic stenosis and mitral regurgitation based on multislice computed tomography. J Cardiovasc Comput Tomogr. 2016;10:162–72.
7. Piazza N, Mylotte D, Theriault LP. Fluoroscopic "heart chamber" anatomy—the case for imaging modality-independent terminology. EuroIntervention. 2016;12:Y9–Y15.
8. Bushberg JT. The essential physics of medical imaging. 3rd ed. Philadelphia: Wolters Kluwer Health/Lippincott Williams & Wilkins; 2012.
9. Lang RM, Badano LP, Mor-Avi V, et al. Recommendations for cardiac chamber quantification by echocardiography in adults: an update from the American Society of Echocardiography and the European Association of Cardiovascular Imaging. Eur Heart J Cardiovasc Imaging. 2015;16:233–70.
10. Hahn RT, Abraham T, Adams MS, et al. Guidelines for performing a comprehensive transesophageal echocardiographic examination: recommendations from the American Society of Echocardiography and the Society of Cardiovascular Anesthesiologists. J Am Soc Echocardiogr. 2013;26:921–64.
11. Wharton G, Steeds R, Allen J, et al. A minimum dataset for a standard adult transthoracic echocardiogram: a guideline protocol from the British Society of Echocardiography. Echo Res Pract. 2015;2:G9–G24.
12. Picard MH, Adams D, Bierig SM, et al. American Society of Echocardiography recommendations for quality echocardiography laboratory operations. J Am Soc Echocardiogr. 2011;24:1–10.
13. Anderson RH. Clinical anatomy of the aortic root. Heart. 2000;84:670–3.
14. Piazza N, de Jaegere P, Schultz C, Becker AE, Serruys PW, Anderson RH. Anatomy of the aortic valvar complex and its implications for transcatheter implantation of the aortic valve. Circ Cardiovasc Interv. 2008;1:74–81.
15. Arnold M, Achenbach S, Pfeiffer I, et al. A method to determine suitable fluoroscopic projections for transcatheter aortic valve implantation by computed tomography. J Cardiovasc Comput Tomogr. 2012;6:422–8.
16. Binder RK, Leipsic J, Wood D, et al. Prediction of optimal deployment projection for transcatheter aortic valve replacement: angiographic 3-dimensional reconstruction of the aortic root versus multidetector computed tomography. Circ Cardiovasc Interv. 2012;5:247–52.
17. Cockburn J, Trivedi U, de Belder A, Hildick-Smith D. Optimal projection for transcatheter aortic valve implantation determined from the reference projection angles. Catheter Cardiovasc Interv. 2012;80:973–7.
18. Dvir D, Kornowski R. Percutaneous aortic valve implantation using novel imaging guidance. Catheter Cardiovasc Interv. 2010;76:450–4.

19. Piazza N. Obtaining the correct depth of implant using the FluoroCT Double S curve. London: PCR London Valves; 2015.
20. Piazza N. Facilitating TAVR with supra-annular sizing and double S-curve. Chicago: TVT; 2016.
21. Poon KK, Crowhurst J, James C, et al. Impact of optimising fluoroscopic implant angles on paravalvular regurgitation in transcatheter aortic valve replacements—utility of three-dimensional rotational angiography. EuroIntervention. 2012;8:538–45.
22. Samim M, Stella PR, Agostoni P, et al. Automated 3D analysis of pre-procedural MDCT to predict annulus plane angulation and C-arm positioning: benefit on procedural outcome in patients referred for TAVR. JACC Cardiovasc Imaging. 2013;6:238–48.
23. Tzikas A, Schultz C, Van Mieghem NM, de Jaegere PP, Serruys PW. Optimal projection estimation for transcatheter aortic valve implantation based on contrast-aortography: validation of a Prototype Software. Catheter Cardiovasc Interv. 2010;76:602–7.

# Transcatheter Repair of Mitral Regurgitation: Abbott Vascular MitraClip

**7**

Carmelo Grasso, Maria Elena Di Salvo, Salvatore Scandura, and Sergio Buccheri

Edge-to-edge repair has been used as a surgical technique in open-chest, arrested heart surgery for the treatment of mitral regurgitation (MR) since the early 1990s. With this technique, a portion of the anterior leaflet is sutured to the corresponding portion of the posterior leaflet, creating a point of permanent approximation of the two leaflets and resulting in a double orifice. Mitral valve repair with the MitraClip™ system (Abbott Vascular, Santa Clara, CA, USA) consists of applying a clip at the site of mitral regurgitation, thereby faithfully reproducing the edge-to-edge surgical technique described by Alfieri. In this case the device is applied by means of a catheter introduced through the right common femoral vein under transesophageal echocardiography (TEE) monitoring and general anesthesia.

Leaflet repair using the MitraClip system is one of the most extensively investigated procedures in the field of percutaneous intervention on the mitral valve. To date, more than 35,000 patients have been treated worldwide. In select patients, a high level of safety and efficacy has been consistently identified for this procedure [1, 2].

C. Grasso, M.D. (✉)
Cardiology Division, Structural Heart Disease, Coronary and Peripheral Intervention Laboratory,
Ferrarotto Hospital, Catania, Italy
e-mail: melfat@tiscali.it

M.E. Di Salvo • S. Scandura
Ferrarotto Hospital, University of Catania, Catania, Italy

S. Buccheri
Department of General Surgery and Medical-Surgical Specialties, University of Catania,
Catania, Italy

© Springer International Publishing AG 2018
C. Tamburino et al. (eds.), *Percutaneous Treatment of Left Side Cardiac Valves*,
https://doi.org/10.1007/978-3-319-59620-4_7

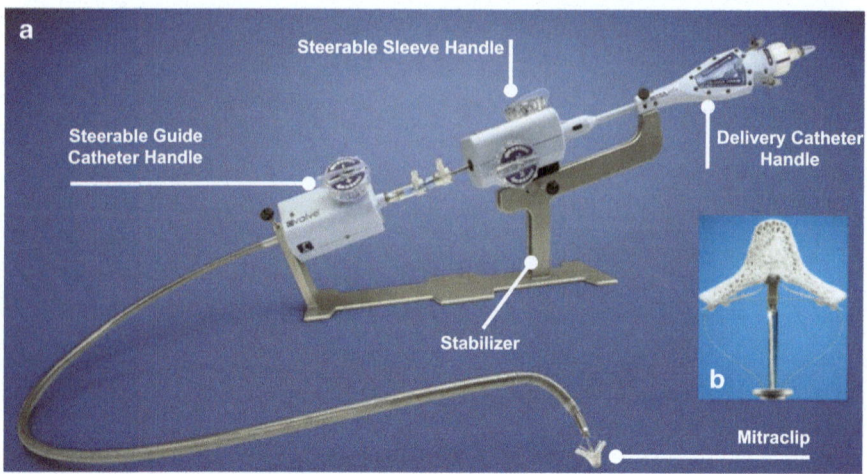

**Fig. 7.1** The MitraClip system. *Panel A* shows the triaxial system. *Panel B* shows the MitraClip device

## 7.1　Description of the Device

The MitraClip system is a catheter-based device designed to perform an edge-to-edge reconstruction of the insufficient mitral valve while the heart is beating and used as an alternative to the conventional surgical approach. The MitraClip system uses a triaxial catheter system (Fig. 7.1) and consists of two different parts, namely, the steerable guide catheter (SGC) and the clip delivery system (CDS). The CDS consists of three major components: the delivery catheter handle, the steerable sleeve handle, and the MitraClip device. The SGC is 24 Fr proximally and 22 Fr distally and is delivered with an echogenic tapered dilator. The dilator allows the introduction of the SGC into the femoral vein and the left atrium (through the interatrial septum) (Fig. 7.2). A knob on the proximal end of the guide catheter allows deflection of the distal tip. Once positioned through the SGC, the CDS is used to advance the MitraClip and allows for different spatial maneuvers to obtain proper positioning of the device between the mitral valve leaflets. The CDS has the MitraClip attached to its distal end and uses two knobs that allow medial-to-lateral and anterior-to-posterior steering (Fig. 7.3). The MitraClip device is a cobalt/chromium implantable device with two arms, covered with polyester fabric and preassembled to the tip of the disposable delivery catheter. On the inner portion of the clip, there are two movable "grippers" adjacent to each arm to secure the leaflets as they are "captured" during closure of the arms. The clip has a locking mechanism to maintain closure. Opening, closing, locking, and detaching the clip are all controlled by the delivery catheter handle mechanisms, which are firmly lodged on a sterilized metal external support, named "stabilizer," placed outside the patient.

　　Three principal components of the CDS allow MitraClip closing/opening and locking/unlocking maneuvers, namely, the arm positioner, the lock lever, and the

**Fig. 7.2** The steerable guide catheter with tapered dilator

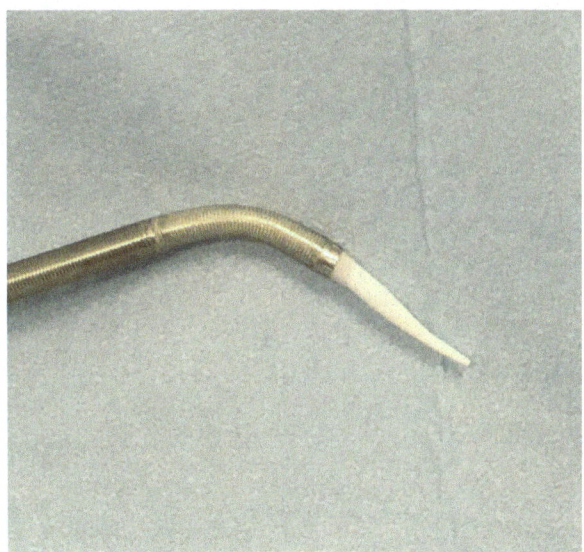

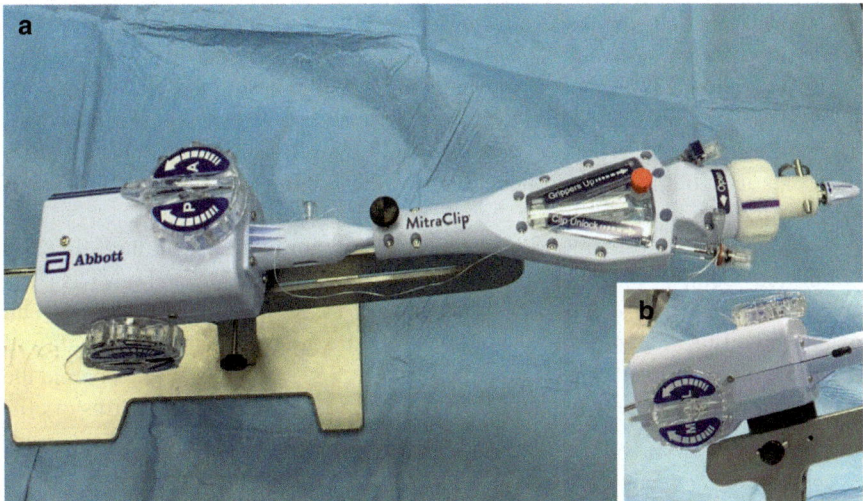

**Fig. 7.3** The clip delivery system. *Panel A* shows the A/P knob and the Smart Handle. *Panel B* shows the M/L knob

gripper lever. The arm positioner is a control knob that enables opening or closing of the clip arms when rotating along specific directions of rotation. The gripper lever raises (in upright position) and lowers (if fully advanced in the catheter handle) grippers through the gripper line. The lock lever unlocks the mechanism that allows opening of the clip arms (upright position) or closing (when fully advanced in the catheter handle). Table 7.1 summarizes the principal maneuvers performed with the CDS during the procedure to obtain desired clip arm angles. Briefly,

**Table 7.1** Principal maneuvers during implant

| Desired arms position | Maneuvers |
|---|---|
| Clip arms opening | Rotate the lock lever outward and fully retract the lever until the mark on the lever is exposed |
| | Turn the arm positioner counterclockwise until desired clip arms angle is reached |
| | Lock the clip by fully advancing the lock lever |
| Clip arms closure | Fully advance lock lever |
| | Turn the arm positioner clockwise |
| Inverting clip arms | Unlock the clip by fully retracting the lock lever |
| | Turn the arm positioner counterclockwise until clip arms are inverted |
| | Lock the clip |
| Final arm angle | Turn the arm positioner in the open direction with lock lever fully advanced |
| | Clip arms should remain in a stable position and a slight delivery catheter shaft deflection should be observed |

opening of the clip arms happens when rotating the arm positioner toward the opening direction with the lock lever upright (unlock position), while rotating the arm positioner toward the opening direction with the lock lever fully advanced induces a slight delivery catheter shaft deflection named "arm angle."

Additional control mechanisms on the system (A/P, M/L, and +/− knobs) allow for tip deflection and fine spatial movements of the clip during the procedure.

Finally, the stabilizer and the silicon pad are useful accessories for the procedure. The stabilizer is used to support and stabilize the SGC and CDS, while the silicon pad helps to avoid accidental movements of the stabilizer-SGC-CDS and further supports the entire system during the procedure.

New technical developments have been recently introduced with the MitraClip NT device. Compared with prior versions of the system, the MitraClip NT is characterized by material and geometrical changes to enhance device steering and maneuverability. A significant change involves the geometry and functionality of the grippers. Changes in gripper material (from elgiloy to nitinol) have increased the gripper drop angle (from 85° to >120°), facilitating leaflet capture in terms of efficiency and durability of grasping (Fig. 7.4).

## 7.2 Patient Selection

A multidisciplinary team, comprising a cardiologist, a cardiac surgeon, and an anesthesiologist, is essential for the proper selection of candidates for MitraClip implantation.

This is generally done in four steps:

- Confirmation of severity of MR
- Assessment of symptoms
- Analysis of surgical risk, life expectancy, and quality of life
- Assessment of procedure feasibility and evaluation of any contraindications for percutaneous treatment

**MitraClip**                                    **MitraClip NT**

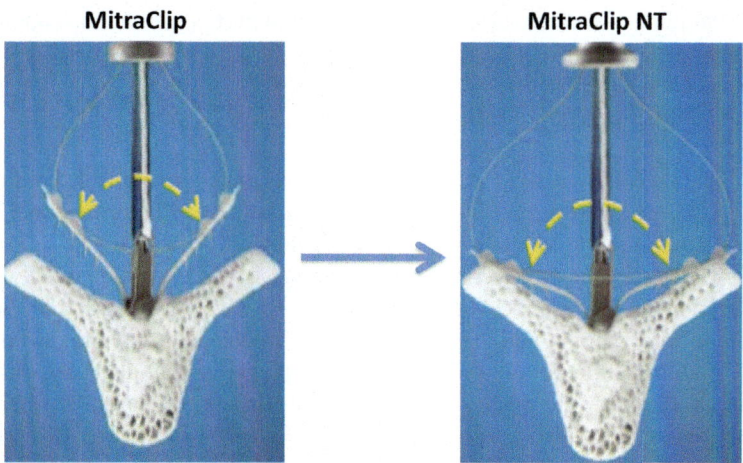

**Fig. 7.4**  Changes in grasping angle with MitraClip NT

Here we will focus our attention mainly on the clinical and anatomical indications and contraindications for percutaneous valve repair with the MitraClip system.

Possible candidates for this procedure are MR patients who meet the criteria of the current guidelines, [3] namely, symptomatic patients with moderate-to-severe (3+) or severe (4+) MR, left ventricular ejection fraction (LVEF) > 30%, left ventricular end-diastolic diameter (LVESD) ≤ 40 mm, or asymptomatic patients with one or more of the following: LVEF between 25 and 60%, LVESD ≥ 45 mm, new-onset atrial fibrillation, and pulmonary hypertension defined as sPAP > 50 mmHg at rest or >60 mmHg on effort. In addition to meeting guideline criteria, patients should be high-risk candidates for mitral valve surgery, including cardiopulmonary bypass. High risk should be established on a consensus between a local independent cardiologist and a cardiac surgeon that conventional surgery would be associated with excessive morbidity and mortality. Criteria of high risk include EuroSCORE II >8%, STS score mortality >4%, combined STS score > 10%, or other risk characteristics not included in the aforementioned scores:

- Hostile chest/chest wall deformities/prior mediastinal irradiation due to neoplasms/mediastinitis
- Frailty (geriatric status scale; ADL/IADL score)
- Liver cirrhosis (Child Pugh A-B/hyperbilirubinemia)
- Morbid obesity (BMI > 40 Kg/m$^2$), severe cachexia (<18 Kg/m$^2$)
- Severe respiratory deficit (VEMS/FCV < 70%, VEMS < 60%)
- Chronic kidney failure (VGF < 90)/dialysis
- Left ventricular failure (EF < 30%)
- Right ventricular failure (TAPSE 14)
- Pulmonary hypertension (sPAP > 55 mmHg)
- Prior endocarditis on electrocatheters
- Chronic degenerative disease of the CNS

- Autoimmune diseases or other diseases requiring prolonged immunosuppressive and cortisone therapy
- Advanced age (>80 years)
- Prior cardiac surgery procedure)

Pre-interventional patient screening includes transthoracic echocardiogram (TTE), TEE, chest x-ray, and invasive cardiac evaluation with coronary angiography, left ventriculography, and right catheterization.

Therefore, together with accurate patient clinical assessment based mainly on the identification of high surgical risk usually due to advanced age and associated comorbidities, it is important to assess some anatomical and morphological parameters, which may rule out not only MitraClip implantation but also prejudice success and duration of the result over time [4]. According to data in the literature, percutaneous mitral valve repair using the MitraClip system requires that patients undergo specific TTE and TEE assessment [4, 5] to identify the anatomical and functional state of the mitral valve, the pathogenesis of the regurgitation, and select patients for whom percutaneous mitral valve repair can achieve an optimal result.

## 7.3 Anatomic and Functional Evaluation of the Mitral Valve

Specific criteria for the selection of candidates for MitraClip implantation are needed to ensure optimal procedural results and increase patient safety. The currently adopted criteria to assess the anatomical suitability for the procedure derive mainly from the EVEREST trial echocardiographic inclusion criteria. The procedure cannot be performed in the presence of a rheumatic valve; therefore, the criteria for exclusion are fibrotic, calcified, or retracted leaflets and severe calcification of the subvalvular apparatus or annulus. In addition, careful assessment of the subvalvular apparatus is needed because the presence of chordal tissue in excess or abnormal chordate implantation, especially in the raphe zone, may negatively influence the clip stability and increase risk of iatrogenic lesions. This assessment should be made solely by TEE in intercommissural view (Fig. 7.5), and, if necessary, the zoom should also be used to avoid amplifying the error. TEE is also needed to exclude any endocarditic processes, including preexisting ones, with splitting of the leaflet or a part of it. Special attention must be paid to the middle scallops (A2–P2), as they are the ideal implantation sites. After careful anatomical assessment of the mitral valve apparatus, functional assessment of the valve has to be jointly made. The anatomical and flow area value should be >4.0 cm$^2$ without any significant transvalvular gradient (Fig. 7.6) [6]. Both degenerative and functional etiologies can be treated if anatomical criteria are met. Therefore, echocardiography is absolutely necessary to assess the tethering and annular deformation indices in functional MR [7]. As regards MitraClip implantation more specifically, if there is tethering, the following exclusion criteria are considered: a coaptation depth $\geq 11$ mm and a coaptation length $< 2$ mm (Fig. 7.7). In the case of degenerative MR, the parameters to be measured are flail gap and flail width [5, 8], with flail being a leaflet with a free

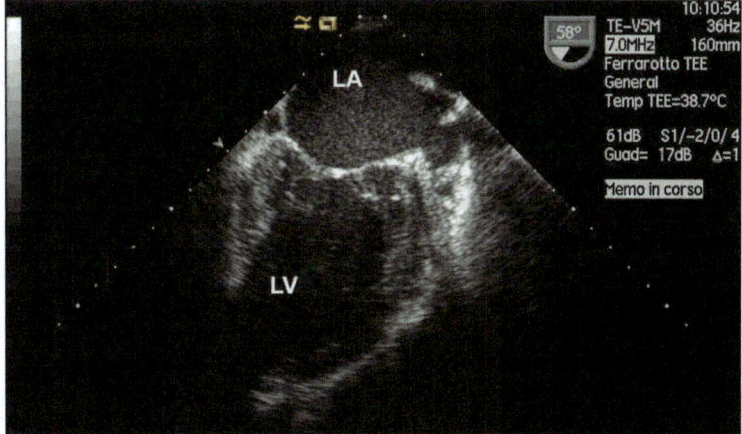

**Fig. 7.5** Transesophageal intercommissural view (~60°). *LA* left atrium, *LV* left ventricle

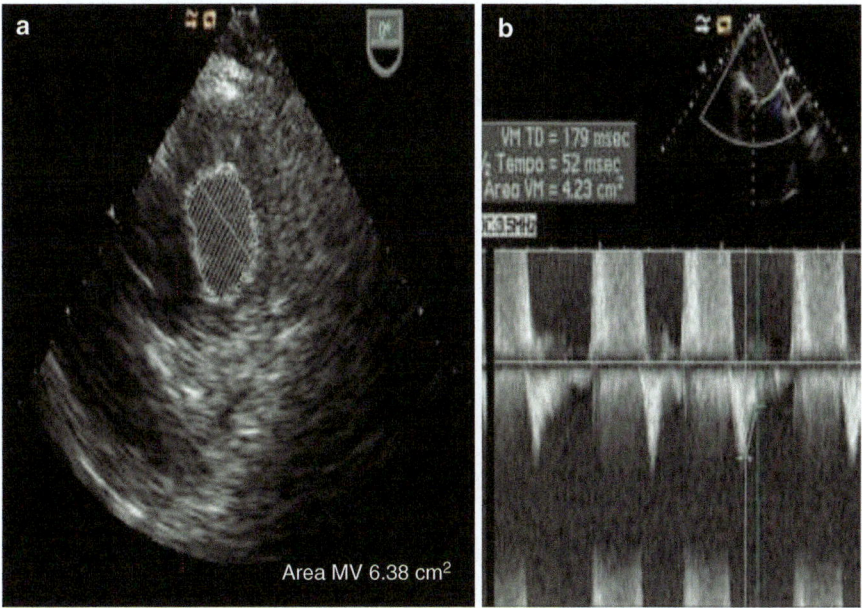

**Fig. 7.6** Transesophageal echocardiography shows a planimetric mitral valve area measured in transgastric view (~0°) (*Panel A*) and with PHT method (*Panel B*)

tip, which passes the opposite leaflet during systole; flail gap, the maximum distance between the edge of the floating leaflet on the ventricular side and the tip of the opposite leaflet on the atrial side (measurement obtained by TEE in four-chamber view ~0°, intercommissural view ~60°, or outflow section at ~120°); and flail width, the width of the floating segment measured along the coaptation line in

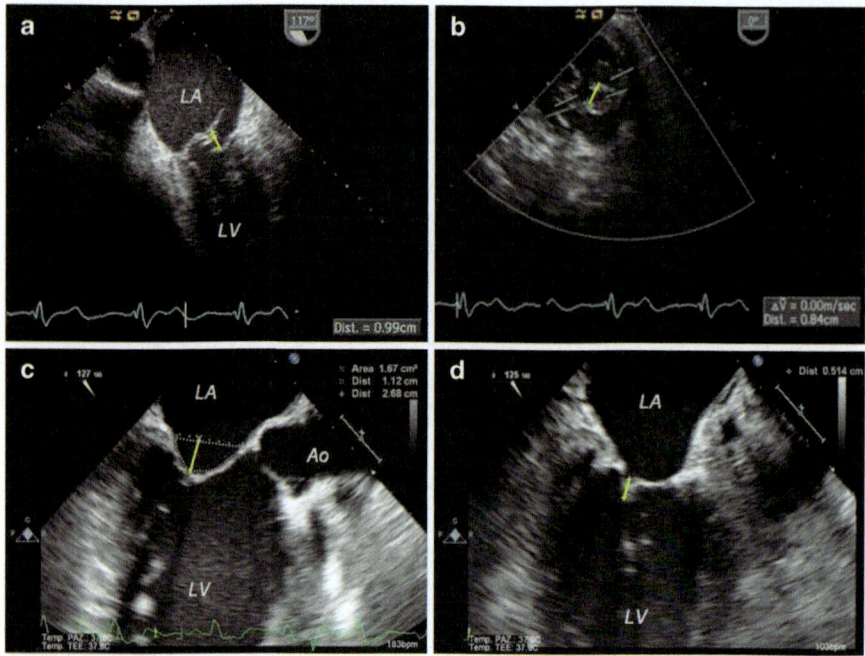

**Fig. 7.7** Anatomical echocardiographic criteria evaluated during patient selection: *Panel A*, flail gap (<10 mm), assessed in long-axis view (four chambers or five chambers), where the larger gap is visible; *Panel B*, flail width (<15 mm), assessed in short-axis view, where the lesion is wider; *Panel C*, coaptation depth (<11 mm); and *Panel D* coaptation length (≥2 mm), both assessed in four-chamber or left ventricular outflow tract view. *LA* left atrium, *LV* left ventricle, *Ao* aorta

the short axis. The anatomical and morphological criteria for proper patient selection are a flail gap < 10 mm and flail width < 15 mm (Fig. 7.7). In addition to the anatomical eligibility criteria illustrated above, echocardiography also allows for the search of additional anatomical contraindications. The exclusion criteria are:

- Intracardial masses and/or thrombotic formations in the heart cavity (Fig. 7.8, Panel A and B)
- Prior mitral valve surgery (valvuloplasty or implantation of biological device) (Fig. 7.8, Panel C)
- Prior implantation of interatrial occlusive device (Fig. 7.8, Panel D)
- Anatomical variants like lipomatosis of the septum, aneurysmal atrial septum, or hypoplasia or surgical closing of the left superior pulmonary vein

The abovementioned should not be considered as absolute contraindications for the procedure, but the operator should be aware of them to decide the transseptal strategy or, as in the case of the pulmonary vein variants, to plan a different route for catheters. Ectasia of the ascending aorta, aortic bulb, or sinuses of Valsalva must be carefully evaluated since all of these conditions can complicate the transseptal

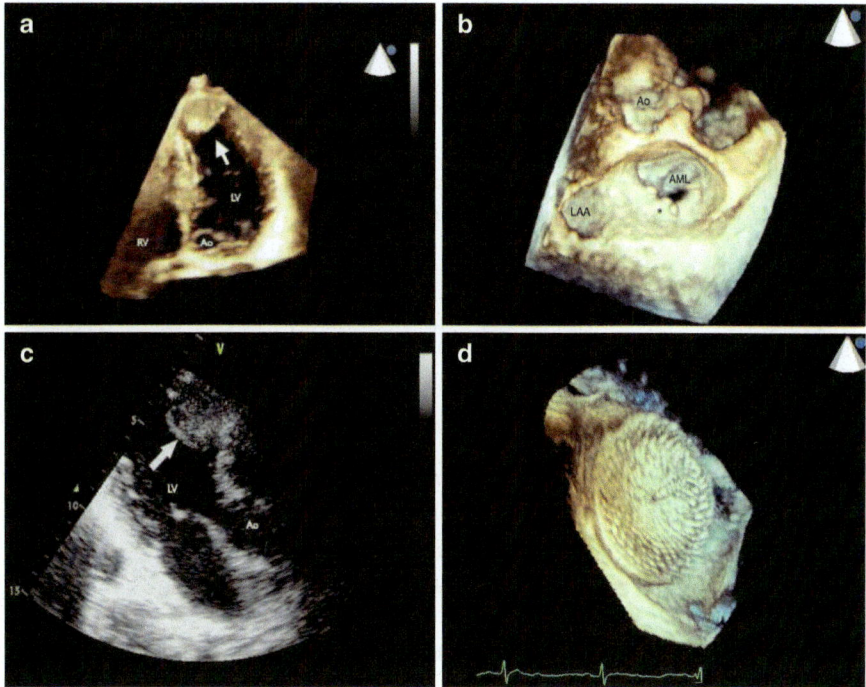

**Fig. 7.8** *Panels A and B*, apical and septal thrombotic formation (*arrow*) in the left ventricle assessed by 3D and 2D transthoracic echocardiography; *Panel C*, 3D echocardiographic atrial view of the mitral valve with a posterior annuloplasty surgical device (*asterisk*); and *Panel D*, 3D transesophageal echocardiogram. Presence of occlusive device in the interatrial septum. *Ao* aorta, *LV* left ventricle, *RV* right ventricle, *AML* anterior mitral leaflet, *LAA* left atrial appendage

puncture and, therefore, should be carefully signaled to the operator. TEE should be used to assess the course of the ascending aorta.

Recently, efficacy and safety of MitraClip implantation has been demonstrated in patients not fulfilling EVEREST anatomic criteria. Attizzani et al. [9] found that 12-month outcomes in this group of patients, characterized by LVESD ≥ 55 mm and LVEF < 25%, are comparable to those of patients selected on the basis of EVEREST anatomic criteria. Along this line, Adamo et al. [10] found that pre-procedural inotropic administration could be useful to improve leaflet coaptation length in dilated ventricles with extreme forms of tethering.

With the increasing experience of operators in managing the device in difficult anatomies, the EVEREST criteria for the selection of patients are obsolete. Today, the most extreme anatomies are treated in high-volume centers by expert operators, after a case-by-case clinical and anatomic selection of patients for MitraClip implantation (Table 7.2). The only concerns regard rheumatic and stenotic valves. Technical advances introduced with the new-generation device (MitraClip NT) will likely help new operators to shorten their learning curve and broaden the kinds of patients and anatomies treated even in start-up or intermediate centers.

**Table 7.2** Suitability by echo criteria and center experience

| Optimal | Limited suitability | Inappropriate |
|---|---|---|
| Pathology in segment 2 | Pathology in segment 1 or 3 | Leaflet perforation or cleft |
| No calcification | – Slight calcification outside the grasping area<br>– Ring calcification<br>– Annuloplasty with ring | Severe calcification |
| Valve area >4 cm$^2$ | Valve area >3 cm$^2$ and good leaflet mobility | Mitral stenosis (<3cm$^2$, gradient >5 mmHg) |
| Length of the posterior leaflet >10 mm | Length of the posterior leaflet 7–10 mm | Length of the posterior leaflet <7 mm |
| Coaptation depth <11 mm | Coaptation depth >11 mm | |
| Normal thickness and mobility of the leaflets | Restriction (Carpentier IIIB) | Rheumatic thickening and restriction (Carpentier IIIA) |
| MR with prolapse<br>– Flail size <15 mm<br>– Flail gap <10 mm | Flail size >15 mm only with large mitral annulus and option for more than 1 clip | Barlow's disease |
| ***Start-up centers*** | ***Intermediate centers*** | ***High-volume centers*** |

## 7.4 Procedure and Technical Aspects

Before the procedure, all patients are administered a single dose of broad-spectrum antibiotic IV (intravenous) for prophylactic purposes. If a patient is on oral anticoagulant therapy, this must be lowered for 3 days before the procedure to obtain an international normalized ratio ≤ 1.7 and replaced with heparin. If low molecular weight heparin is administered, it must be suspended, ideally, 12 h before the procedure, while unfractionated heparin should be stopped at least 4 h before surgery.

The procedure is performed in the cardiac catheterization laboratory under echocardiography and fluoroscopic guidance, with the patient usually under general anesthesia. Emergency surgical backup should be available for each procedure, because in case of complications during the procedure, it may be necessary to convert to an open surgical procedure. During the procedure, invasive arterial pressure is monitored through the radial or the femoral artery, and a central venous catheter is placed in the right internal jugular or subclavian vein. The right femoral vein is cannulated with a 12 Fr introducer sheath, and a baseline right heart catheterization is performed. In order to evaluate the acute hemodynamic effects of the MitraClip device, intracardiac pressure and flow measurements are taken at baseline and 10 min after device deployment (Table 7.3). Baseline activated clotting time (ACT) has to be determined following venous access for the endovascular procedure. ACT and heparin administration should be recorded throughout the procedure, and a final ACT level should be documented before leaving the catheterization laboratory.

The procedure can be divided into five steps: (1) transseptal puncture and SGC insertion, (2) straddling and steering of the clip, (3) alignment with the mitral valve and commissure line, (4) grasping of the leaflets, and (5) final evaluation.

**Table 7.3** Catheterization measurements obtained before clip implantation and ≥10 min after clip deployment

| Measurements |
|---|
| PCWP or left atrial pressure (*a* wave/*v* wave/mean pressure) with simultaneous left ventricular pressure |
| Pulmonary artery pressure (systolic/diastolic/mean pressure) |
| Right atrial pressure |
| Left ventricular peak systolic and end-diastolic pressure |
| Systemic arterial pressure (systolic/diastolic/mean pressure) |
| Cardiac output |

*PCWP* pulmonary capillary wedge pressure

1. *Transseptal puncture and SGC insertion*

   After the right catheterization is performed, an 8 Fr Mullins sheath is introduced over a 0.35 guidewire, and a transseptal puncture is performed using a Brockenbrough needle under TEE guidance. Many operators use a radiofrequency (RF) system in case of difficult puncture or to improve precision. This is a critical point of the procedure, because the puncture has to be located in the posterosuperior part of the fossa ovalis in order to obtain enough space in the left atrium (LA) for a safe and optimal orientation of the steerable distal part of the CDS. In this phase, the height of the transseptal puncture from the valve plane is very important as well, because if the puncture is too low, there is not enough space to move freely inside the LA, while if it is too high, it is not possible for the CDS to reach the coaptation zone. An optimal distance is about 35–45 mm from the valve plane depending on the type of disease (DMR vs. FMR). The location of the lesion is important because to reach a medial lesion, the puncture should be higher, and in the case of a lateral lesion, a lower puncture should be performed. Once the LA is entered with the 8 Fr sheath, the left pulmonary vein is cannulated directly with the Mullins sheath or with a 6 Fr multipurpose catheter. After angiography (Fig. 7.9, Panel A) of the pulmonary vein, a 260 cm Amplatz Super Stiff guidewire is left in place. Following transseptal crossing, 100 IU/kg of UFH or alternative anticoagulation therapy is administered, according to standard hospital practice, maintaining an ACT of >250 s throughout the procedure. The 24 Fr guiding catheter is then introduced into the LA (Fig. 7.9, Panel B), and the dilator is carefully and slowly retrieved to avoid the formation of vacuum air bubbles.

2. *Straddling and steering of the clip*

   This step can be carried out using only fluoroscopy in most cases. If the atrium is large enough, the easiest and fastest maneuver is to complete the straddling (aligning the two markers on the CDS shaft with the marker on the tip of the SGC) pointing with the clip to the pulmonary vein (Fig. 7.9, Panel C) to have more room and steering (bending the delivery system, since the clip is toward the mitral valve) by going simultaneously posterior with the SGC and medial with the medial/lateral (M/L) knob. An excessive use of the M-knob should be avoided to create less tension in the system.

3. *Alignment with the mitral valve and commissure line*

The delivery system is then advanced in the LA, and the distal steerable part is manipulated in the atrium to obtain a perpendicular and central position with respect to the mitral valve leaflets coaptation line. Under echocardiography and fluoroscopic guidance, the clip is steered until axially aligned and centered over the origin of the regurgitant jet. The correct trajectory of the clip and the perpendicularity of the two arms with respect to the mitral leaflet coaptation line are checked using TEE standard views (see echocardiographic guidance). Once the system has been aligned, the clip with opened arms is advanced into the left ventricle (Fig. 7.9, Panel D).

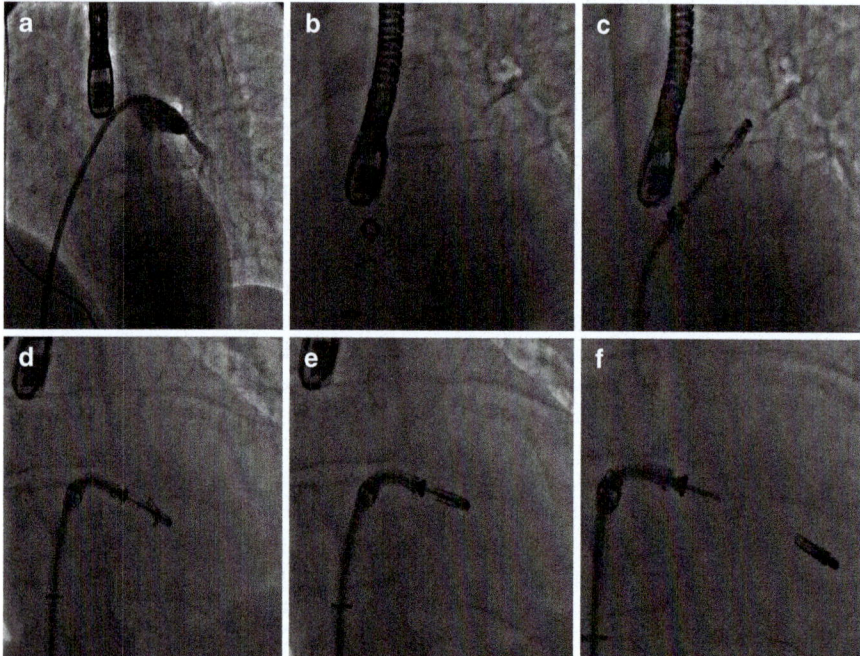

**Fig. 7.9** Once the left atrium (LA) is entered with the 8 Fr sheath, the left pulmonary vein (PV) is cannulated, and a stiff guidewire is left in place after angiography of the vein (*Panel A*). The 24 Fr steerable guide catheter (SGC) is then introduced in the LA, and the dilator is carefully and slowly retrieved to avoid vacuum air bubbles (*Panel B*). The clip delivery system (CDS) is then advanced in the LA (*Panel C*), and the distal steerable part is manipulated in the atrium to obtain a perpendicular and central position with respect to the mitral valve leaflets coaptation line. Once the system has been aligned, the clip, with opened arms, is advanced into the left ventricle (*Panel D*), and under transesophageal guidance the arms grasp the leaflets. When a double orifice has been created and the echocardiography confirms regurgitation reduction and optimal and stable grasp of both leaflets, the clip arms are closed (*Panel E*), locked, and detached and the SGC and CDS are withdrawn (*Panel F*)

4. *Grasping of the leaflets*

This step is performed under TEE guidance (use of X-plane is advised). The clip with the arms opened is gently retracted toward the atrium trying to accommodate both leaflets. The grippers are then dropped, and the arms closed to grasp the leaflets (Fig. 7.9, Panel E). The technique of grasping is different when dealing with FMR or DMR, and even the number of clips needed should vary.

5. *Final evaluation*

When a double orifice has been created, and the echocardiography confirms reduction of regurgitation and optimal and stable grasp of both leaflets (see echocardiographic guidance), the clip arms are completely closed and locked, and the clip is detached (Fig. 7.9, Panel F), following the procedural steps provided by the company regarding the locker line and the gripper line retrieval. The delivery system is then straightened slightly and withdrawn, paying attention to avoid damage of the left atrial wall. Finally, the guiding catheter is pulled away. If the position is judged suboptimal by TEE evaluation, the clip can be reopened and repositioned; if the clip must be withdrawn into the LA, the arms may be inverted in the ventricle, providing a smooth profile for retraction to prevent entangling the *chordae tendineae*. When necessary, for example, in the case of degenerative MR or ruptured *chordae tendineae* with wide prolapse, a second clip can be implanted, usually very close to the first implanted clip (Fig. 7.10). While the implantation of a second clip is predictable when a flail is present, the need for a second clip in other scenarios is evaluated on a case-by-case basis. Right cardiac catheterization is finally performed to record the post-procedural pressure and the final results (Fig. 7.11) (Table 7.3). The guiding catheter is removed, ACT control is done, heparin reversal with protamine sulfate is started, and venous femoral access is closed using a "figure-of-eight" superficial stitch (Fig. 7.12).

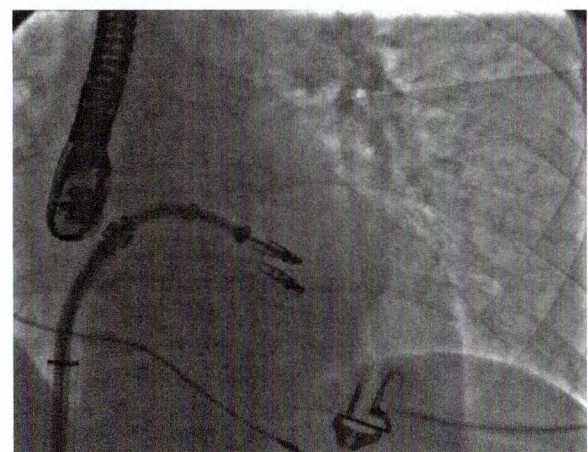

**Fig. 7.10** In select cases, a second clip can be implanted, usually very closely to the first implanted one

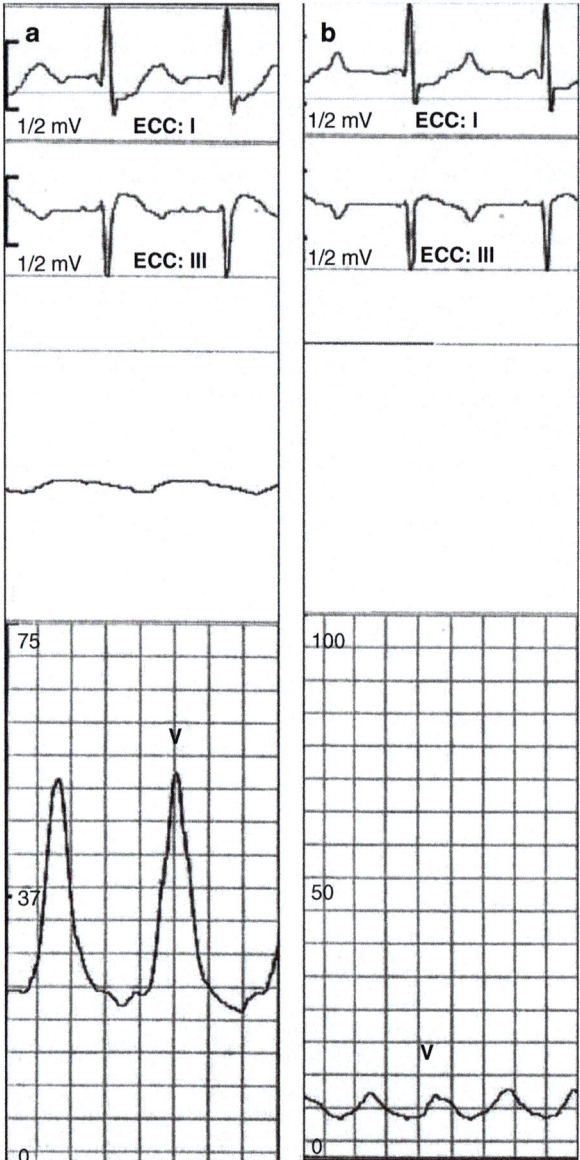

**Fig. 7.11** Pulmonary wedge pressure recorded in basal condition shows a high *v* wave (*Panel A*) secondary to severe mitral regurgitation. After clip implantation, the *v* wave is reduced (*Panel B*). The parallel *a* wave reduction indicates diminished end-diastolic pressure

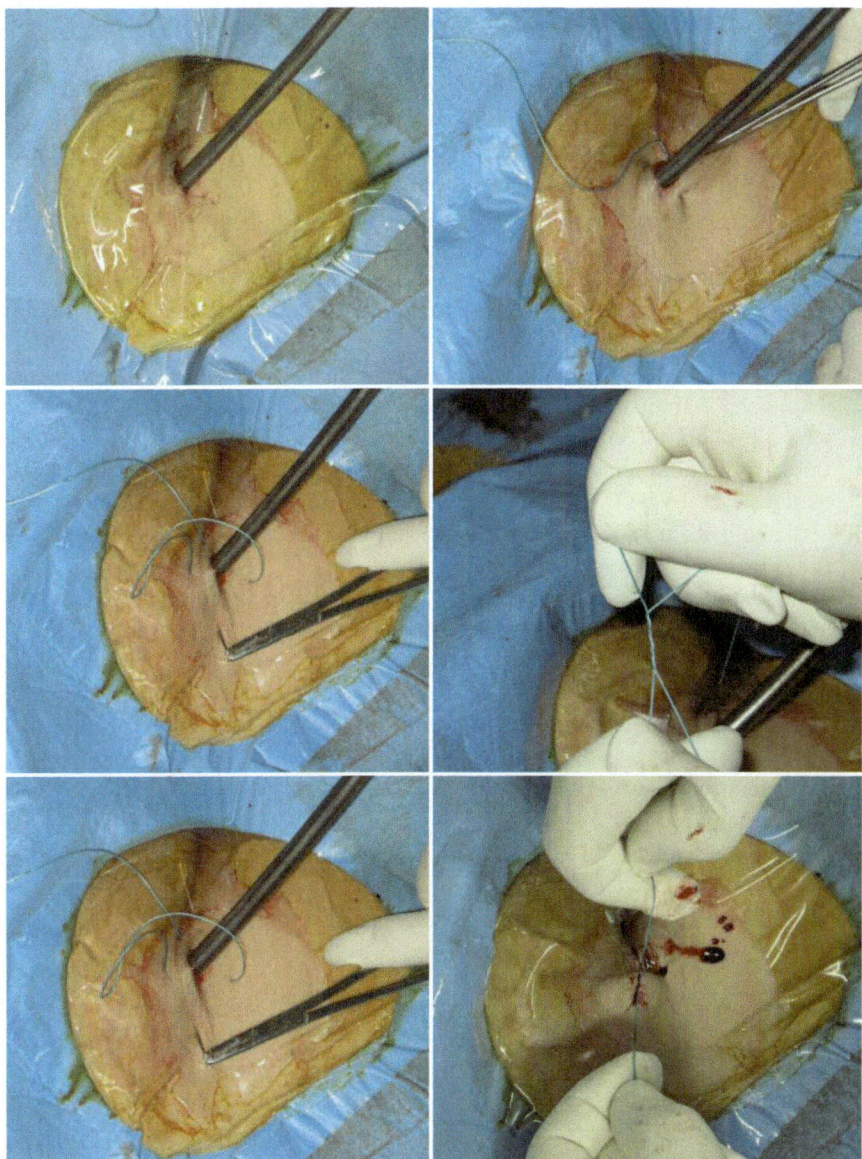

**Fig. 7.12** Venous femoral access closing with a "figure-of-eight" superficial stitch

## 7.5     Intraprocedural Echocardiography Monitoring

TEE during the procedure provides guidance for the operator and makes it possible to obtain information on the morphofunctional characteristics of the mitral valve, assess the degree of regurgitation and biventricular function, as well as the immediate result, and to exclude any complications.

Four views are mainly used during the procedure and are defined as "key views":

- Mid-esophageal view (~0°–90°) for the study of the interatrial septum and to follow the catheters during the transseptal approach and movements in the left atrium (Fig. 7.13).
- Two-chamber intercommissural view (~60°) showing the anterolateral and posteromedial commissure and part of the mitral valve scallops (P3-A2-P1). This view allows for the midlateral (ML) orientation of the system.
- Low-axis mid-esophageal view (~120°–150°), also defined as left ventricular outflow tract (LVOT) view. This view shows the P2-A2 scallops in addition to the aortic bulb and part of the ascending aorta. This view allows for the anteroposterior orientation of the system.
- Transgastric short-axis view (~0°–30°), which shows the mitral valve in the short axis. This view is essential in guiding the clip perpendicularly to the coaptation line.

The procedure can be illustrated in five basic steps:

1. Performance of transseptal puncture
2. Axial orientation of the system
3. Grasping of leaflets
4. Post-grasping assessment
5. Clip release

### 7.5.1    Step 1: Transseptal Puncture

In this procedure the transseptal puncture is a crucial moment. The puncture site has to be "precise" since fluoroscopic guidance does not provide robust guidance. A puncture of the septum in the posterior and superior position is required at about 4 cm above the mitral annular plane (Fig. 7.14) to allow for subsequent optimal maneuverability of the system. TEE monitoring of the puncture requires a short-axis view on the base (0°–30°) with the aorta at the center of the view as the anterior reference point for the interatrial septum. This view allows the interventional cardiologist to orient the catheter anteroposteriorly over the interatrial septum. Superoinferior orientation is obtained with the bicaval view (about 90°), which displays the atrial outlet of the superior vena cava (upper point of reference) and inferior vena cava (lower point of reference). Ideally, the transseptal puncture should be made through the posterior-mid aspect of the fossa in a posterior and superior

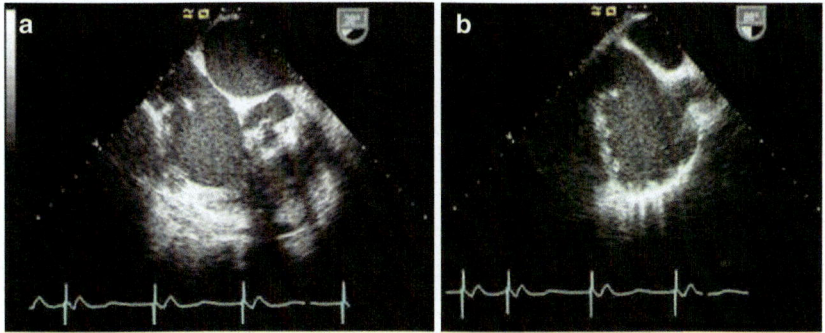

**Fig. 7.13** Trans-esophageal echocardiogram at ~40° (**a**) and ~90° (**b**) for the study of the inter-atrial septum, with respect to the aorta, superior and inferior vena cava

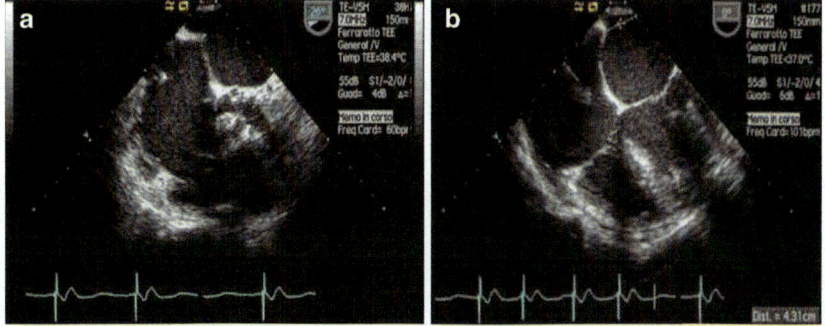

**Fig. 7.14** Trans-esophageal echocardiography guidance during the transeptal puncture, showing the catheter positioned at ~4 cm from the mitral valve (panel a). The measurement has to be performed in four-chamber view (0°, panel b)

direction. As previously reported, the distance between the site of the puncture and the annulus plane is also important in order to move the catheter freely inside the LA and reach the leaflets. The catheter is visualized in all the views to accurately find the point where it is wedged inside the septum (Fig. 7.14), causing what is known as the "tenting effect," and to follow the needle until it passes the septum and enters the LA. After transseptal puncture, TEE guides the catheters into the LA and the placement of the guiding catheter in the upper left pulmonary vein. A radiopaque and echogenic ring identifies the tip of the guiding catheter (Fig. 7.15). The clip is advanced through this guidewire. Ideally, the tip of the catheter should be positioned in the upper short-axis view to avoid contact with the lateral and posterior walls of the LA. The "X-plane" modality view of the 3D echocardiography provides, at the same time, an ultrasound view perpendicular to the reference view, allowing concomitant visualization of the interatrial septum in the short-axis and bicaval views (Fig. 7.16), thereby helping the operator in guiding the Brockenbrough needle over the interatrial septum in order to make the puncture in the correct position.

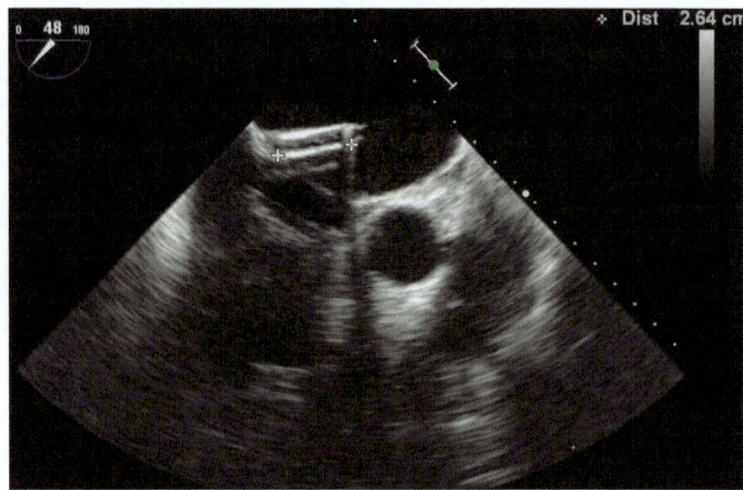

**Fig. 7.15** Trans-esophageal echocardiographic view showing the tip of the SGC in left atrium. The optimal distance from the interatrial septum is about 2 cm

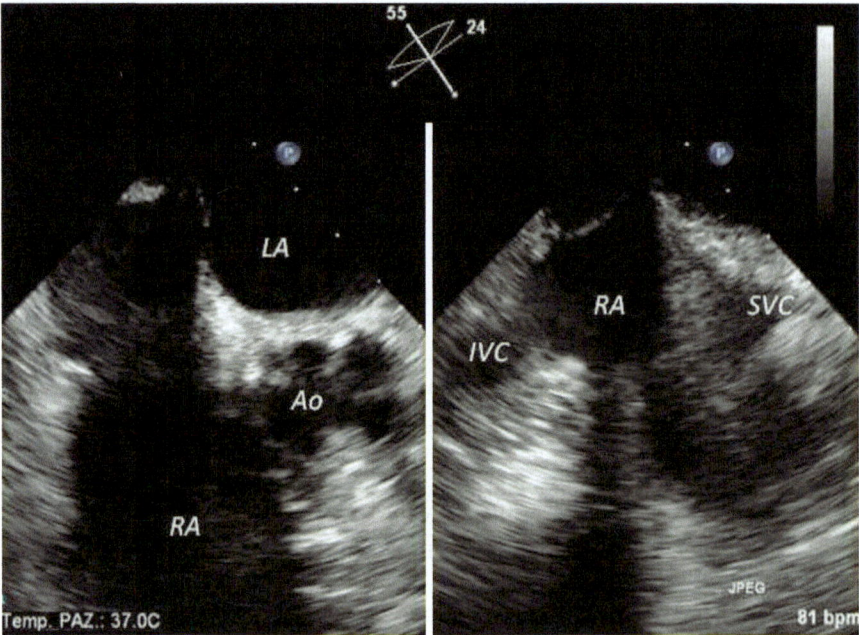

**Fig. 7.16** X-plane orthogonal visualization of the interatrial septum in short-axis and bicaval view. *LA* left atrium, *RA* right atrium, *Ao* aorta, *SVC* superior vena cava, *IVC* inferior vena cava

## 7.5.2   Step 2: Axial Orientation of the System

Once transseptal puncture is made, the following step is the axial alignment of the clip perpendicular to the mitral valve annular plane and parallel to the antegrade flow direction. The course of the system must be carefully followed by TEE to ensure proper passage into the left ventricle and proper clip placement (Table 7.4). The clip is generally oriented with small and fine movements. Two useful views have been already described:

- LVOT long-axis view, allowing anterior-to-posterior clip orientation
- Intercommissural view, allowing medial-to-lateral clip orientation

Generally, clip alignment perpendicular to the coaptation line is made in the transgastric short-axis view. This view is also used for further movements in either the anteroposterior or latero-medial direction. Real-time 3D (RT 3D) examination of the mitral valve could further facilitate optimal alignment of the system by using a zoomed en face view of the valve (Fig. 7.17). The ideal prerelease positioning of

**Table 7.4** Transesophageal echocardiographic projections during the procedure used for correct orientation of the MitraClip system

| Projection | Degrees | View | Alignment |
|---|---|---|---|
| Two chambers (IC) | ~60° | Anterolateral commissure, Posteriormedial commissure, Scallops P3-A2-P1 | Mediolateral |
| Mid-esophageal long axis (LVOT) | ~120°–150° | Scallops A2-P2, aortic bulb and part of ascending aorta | Anteroposterior |
| Transgastric short axis | ~0°–30° | Mitral valve short axis | Perpendicularity to coaptation line; mediolateral |

**Abbreviations**: *IC* inter-commissural, *LVOT* left ventricle outflow tract

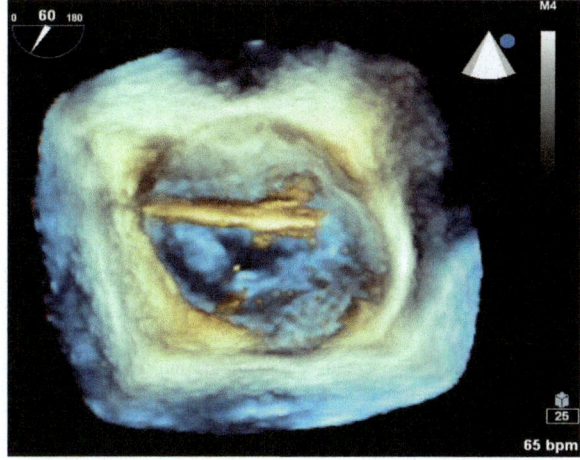

**Fig. 7.17** 3D echocardiography to guide optimal positioning of the clip with respect to the mitral valve

the clip delivery system is just above the regurgitant orifice showing maximal PISA effect ("split the jet"). System orientation should then be checked during system advancement in the left ventricle since rotation can occur in this step. Again, an RT 3D view from the ventricular aspect of the mitral valve can be used to maintain the system perpendicular to the coaptation line.

### 7.5.3 Step 3: Grasping of Leaflets

Once the device is satisfactorily oriented, both leaflets should be anchored, usually in the long-axis LVOT and intercommissural views (120° and 60°–70°, respectively) to better visualize the two leaflets. Special attention must be paid to proper insertion of the leaflets inside the clip to prevent embolism or device detachment. If grasping is inadequate, the clip can be released and repositioned. TEE is used not only to guide anchorage but also to check grasping in the various views (Fig. 7.18). RT 3D TEE can be useful for anatomic assessment of grasping, thereby confirming the correct insertion of the leaflets inside the closed clip, by means of the most common 3D views, namely, atrial and ventricular views (see Fig. 2.86) or various sections that can be obtained on multiple planes (see Fig. 2.87).

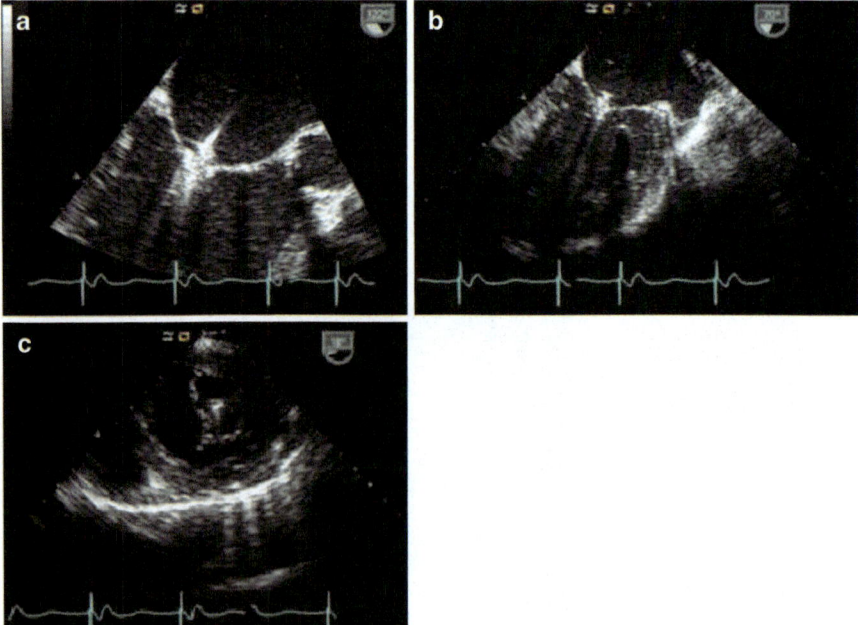

**Fig. 7.18** Trans-esophageal echocardiographic evaluation of the leaflets grasping in long-axis view (**a**), intercommissural two-chamber view (**b**) and trans-gastric short-axis view (**c**)

### 7.5.4   Step 4: Post-grasping Assessment

After checking the anchoring of both leaflets, residual MR and transmitral diastolic gradient must be assessed using continuous-wave Doppler before releasing the clip. Double-orifice insertion should be checked in both the intercommissural and short-axis views. If the result is not satisfactory, the leaflets are released and the clip is repositioned. An adequate grasp of both mitral leaflets does not ensure an acceptable reduction in the degree of mitral regurgitation. Suboptimal MR reduction can derive from a non-perpendicular placement of the clip in relation to the jet's origin or capture of the chordae or margin of the leaflets by clip arms. Therefore, careful assessment of residual MR is made before releasing the clip. If results are suboptimal even after adequate clip deployment, a second clip can be implanted. Because, with the clip in situ, the regurgitant jet can become highly eccentric, it is absolutely mandatory that the Nyquist limits and color gain are identical to the initial assessments if there is no residual, as these factors may affect jet size.

### 7.5.5   Step 5: Clip Release

After adequate reduction in the degree of regurgitation, the clip is released, and the system and guidewire are withdrawn. The data obtained from echocardiography are compared with the hemodynamic and angiographic data. TEE is also useful in assessing procedural complications such as pericardial effusion, intracardiac thrombus formation, and the entity of residual interatrial shunt after transseptal puncture (Fig. 7.19). RT 3D TEE allows for the observation of the results from both the atrium and ventricle, documenting any sign of eccentricity of the dual orifices

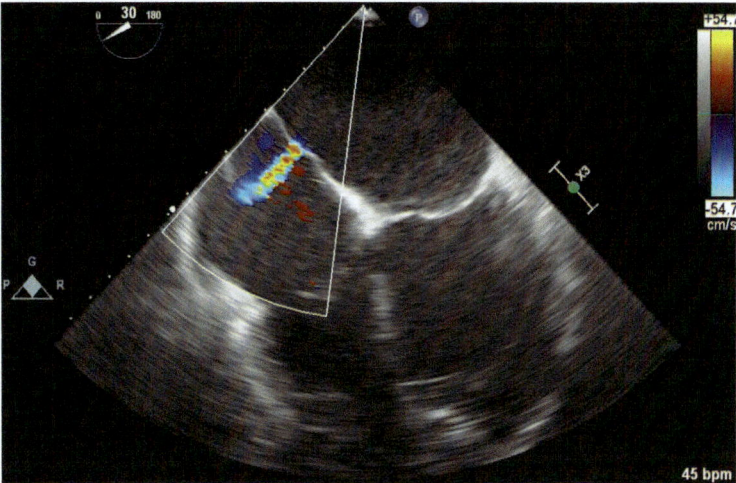

**Fig. 7.19**  Residual inter-atrial shunt after SGC removal

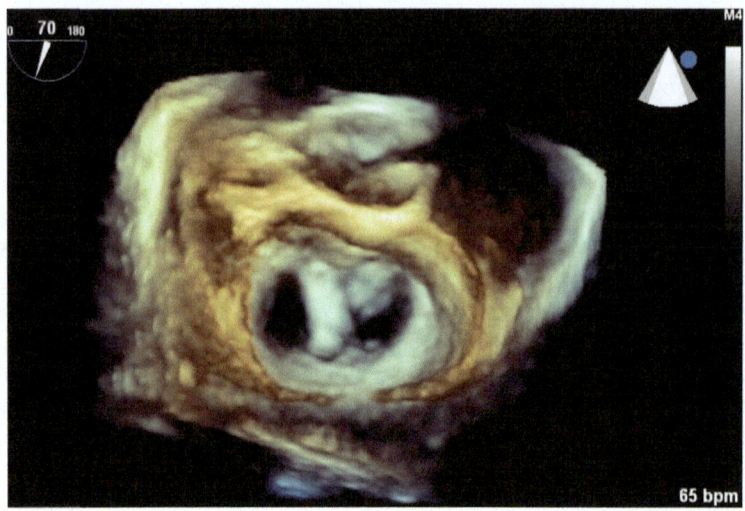

**Fig. 7.20** 3D-real time atrial view of the double orifice mitral valve after clip deployment

created by the device (Fig. 7.20). Moreover, 3D color displays also provide good definition of the site(s) of any residual regurgitation [11].

The use of 3D echocardiography during the MitraClip procedure is associated with shorter procedural time, leading to a reduction in the exposure to fluoroscopy. Biner et al. [12] have reported that procedural guidance based on combined 2D and 3D imaging was associated with a shorter time for first clip deployment and a reduction in procedural time by 28% or 40 min ($p = 0.035$).

## References

1. Wan B, Rahnavardi M, Tian DH, Phan K, Munkholm-Larsen S, Bannon PG, Yan TD. A meta-analysis of MitraClip system versus surgery for treatment of severe mitral regurgitation. Ann Cardiothorac Surg. 2013;2(6):683–92. doi:10.3978/j.issn.2225-319X.2013.11.02.
2. D'ascenzo F, Moretti C, Marra WG, Montefusco A, Omede P, Taha S, Castagno D, Gaemperli O, Taramasso M, Frea S, Pidello S, Rudolph V, Franzen O, Braun D, Giannini C, Ince H, Perl L, Zoccai G, Marra S, D'Amico M, Maisano F, Rinaldi M, Gaita F. Meta-analysis of the usefulness of Mitraclip in patients with functional mitral regurgitation. Am J Cardiol. 2015;116(2):325–31. doi:10.1016/j.amjcard.2015.04.025.
3. Joint Task Force on the Management of Valvular Heart Disease of the European Society of Cardiology (ESC), European Association for Cardio-Thoracic Surgery (EACTS), Vahanian A, Alfieri O, Andreotti F, Antunes MJ, Barón-Esquivias G, Baumgartner H, Borger MA, Carrel TP, De Bonis M, Evangelista A, Falk V, Iung B, Lancellotti P, Pierard L, Price S, Schäfers HJ, Schuler G, Stepinska J, Swedberg K, Takkenberg J, Von Oppell UO, Windecker S, Zamorano JL, Zembala M. Guidelines on the management of valvular heart disease (version 2012). Eur Heart J. 2012;33(19):2451–96. doi:10.1093/eurheartj/ehs109.
4. Feldman T, Wasserman HS, Herrmann HC, et al. Percutaneous mitral valve repair using the edge-to-edge technique: six-month results of the EVEREST phase I clinical trial. J Am Coll Cardiol. 2006;46:2134–40.

5. Silvestry FE, Rodriguez LL, Herrmann HC, et al. Echocardiographic guidance and assessment of percutaneous repair for mitral regurgitation with the Evalve MitraClip: lessons learned from EVEREST I. J Am Soc Echocardiogr. 2007;20:1131–40.
6. Herrmann HC, Kar S, Siegal R, et al. Effect of percutaneous mitral repair with the MitraClip device on mitral valve area and gradient. EuroIntervention. 2009;4:437–42.
7. De Bonis M, Lapenna E, La Canna G, et al. Mitral valve repair for functional mitral regurgitation in end-stage dilated cardiomyopathy. Circulation. 2005;112:402–8.
8. Wunderlich NC, Siegel RJ. Peri-interventional echo assessment for the MitraClip procedure. Eur Heart J Cardiovasc Imaging. 2013;14(10):935–49. doi:10.1093/ehjci/jet060.
9. Attizzani GF, Ohno Y, Capodanno D, Cannata S, Dipasqua F, Immé S, Mangiafico S, Barbanti M, Ministeri M, Cageggi A, Pistritto AM, Giaquinta S, Farruggio S, Chiarandà M, Ronsivalle G, Schnell A, Scandura S, Tamburino C, Capranzano P, Grasso C. Extended use of percutaneous edge-to-edge mitral valve repair beyond EVEREST (Endovascular Valve Edge-to-Edge Repair) criteria: 30-day and 12-month clinical and echocardiographic outcomes from the GRASP (Getting Reduction of Mitral Insufficiency by Percutaneous Clip Implantation) registry. JACC Cardiovasc Interv. 2015;8(1 Pt A):74–82. doi:10.1016/j.jcin.2014.07.024.
10. Adamo M, Chiari E, Curello S, Maiandi C, Chizzola G, Fiorina C, Frontini M, Cuminetti G, Pezzotti E, Rovetta R, Lombardi CM, Manzato A, Metra M, Ettori F. Mitraclip therapy in patients with functional mitral regurgitation and missing leaflet coaptation: is it still an exclusion criterion? Eur J Heart Fail. 2016;18(10):1278–86. doi:10.1002/ejhf.520.
11. Zamorano JL, Badano LP, Bruce C, et al. EAE/ASE recommendations for the use of echocardiography in new transcatheter interventions for valvular heart disease. J Am Soc Echocardiogr. 2011;24:937–65.
12. Biner S, Perk G, Saibal K, et al. Utility of combined two-dimensional and three-dimensional transesophageal imaging for catheter-based mitral valve clip repair of mitral regurgitation. J Am Soc Echocardiogr. 2011;24:611–7.

# Transcatheter Repair of Mitral Regurgitation: Edwards Cardioband

# 8

Carmelo Grasso, Sebastiano Immè, Sarah Mangiafico, and Giuseppe Ronsivalle

## 8.1 Description of the Device

The Cardioband is a device designed to perform direct percutaneous transfemoral annuloplasty by means of a half ring implanted on the posterior annulus, with beating heart, and under fluoroscopic and transesophageal echocardiography (TEE) guidance. The device is fixed in situ thanks to a series of helical anchors and is equipped with a system that allows adjustment of the degree of annular reduction to achieve a good result in terms of residual mitral regurgitation, without creating stenosis.

The procedure is associated with a much lower risk of mortality compared with surgical annuloplasty and is therefore reserved for patients who are not candidates for cardiac surgery due to the high risk of intra- and postoperative mortality.

The Cardioband can be employed to correct functional mitral regurgitation secondary to dilation of the left ventricular cavity and subsequent anatomical distortion of the entire valvular apparatus constituting the mitral valve.

## 8.2 Components of the Device

The Cardioband system consists of a half ring (implant) and three main accessories:

C. Grasso, M.D. (✉)
Cardiology Division, Structural Heart Disease, Coronary and Peripheral Intervention Laboratory, Ferrarotto Hospital, Catania, Italy
e-mail: melfat@tiscali.it

S. Immè • S. Mangiafico • G. Ronsivalle

Division of Cardiology, Ferrarotto Hospital, University of Catania, Italy

© Springer International Publishing AG 2018
C. Tamburino et al. (eds.), *Percutaneous Treatment of Left Side Cardiac Valves*,
https://doi.org/10.1007/978-3-319-59620-4_8

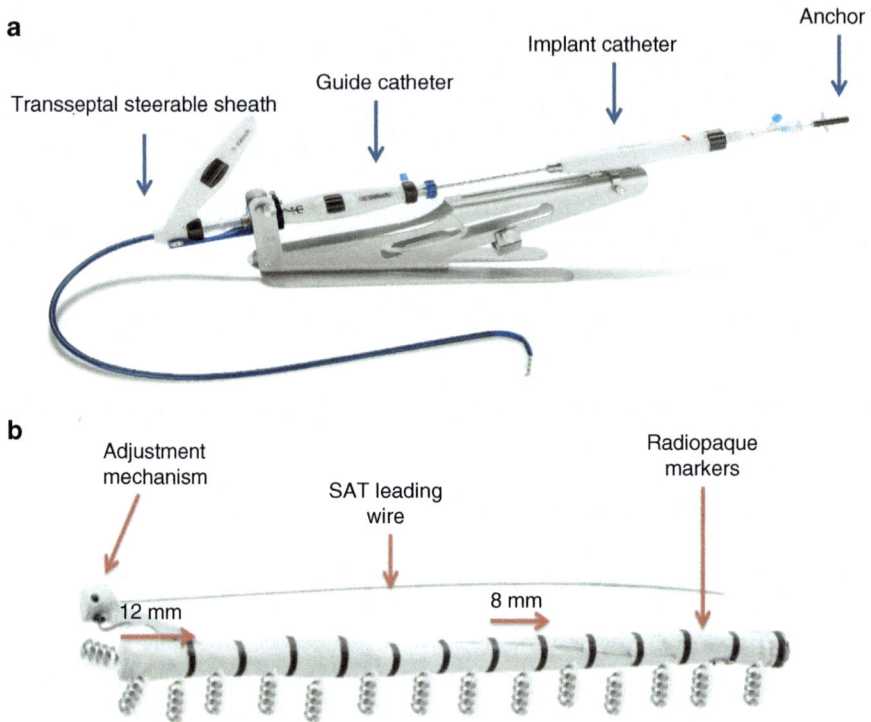

**Fig. 8.1** (**a**) Cardioband delivery system, implant delivery system (IDS), and transseptal steerable sheath (TSS). (**b**) The implant, the spool, and implantable metal anchors

1. *The implant* is a polyester sleeve with radiopaque markers spaced 8 mm apart. The sleeve, available in six lengths, is mounted on the delivery system, and the anchor is deployed from the internal part. Inside the sleeve, there is a metal alloy contraction wire connected to an adjusting spool that allows shortening the implant at the end of the procedure to reduce the anteroposterior distance of the mitral annulus.

   The final implant size is adjusted to the patient's needs under TEE guidance, and the maneuver can be completely reversed.

2. *TF delivery system*: The Cardioband delivery system (CDS) consists of the implant delivery system (IDS) and a 25 Fr transseptal steerable sheath (TSS) that is able to change its curvature by means of a knob, as well as the position and height of the implant by means of clockwise and counterclockwise movements of the handle. The IDS is composed of the steerable guide catheter (GC) that allows, with the aid of a knob, the further adjustment of the position and angle. This varies with the implantation site and the implant catheter (IC), with the Cardioband implant mounted on its distal end (Fig. 8.1), which thanks to another knob at the end allows the advancement of the implant and, hence, the deployment of the anchors.

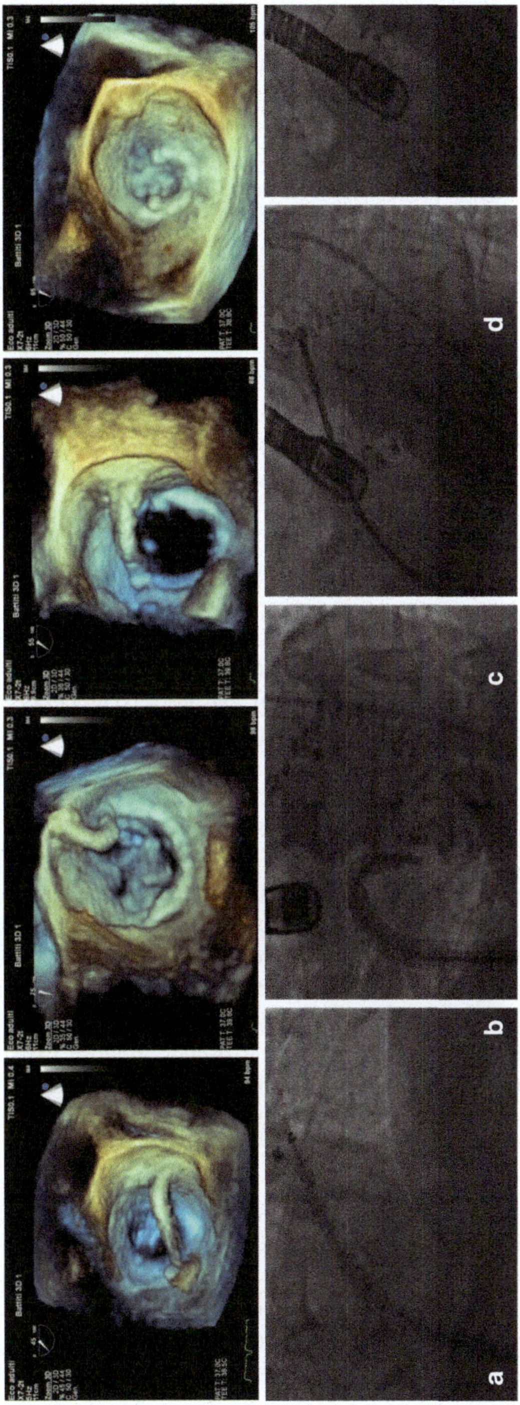

**Fig. 8.2** Three-dimensional echocardiography (surgical view) and corresponding fluoroscopic view: (**a**) placement of the first screw in the anterolateral commissure, (**b**) placement of the last screw in the posteromedial commissure (hooking phase), (**c**) implant completed before cinching, (**d**) Cardioband after final cinching

3. *Implantable metal anchors and anchor delivery shafts*: Stainless implantable anchors, 6 mm in length, are used to fasten the Cardioband implant to the annulus (Fig. 8.1). Between 12 and 17 anchors are implanted using the delivery shaft. The anchors are fully repositionable and retrievable until deployed. The anchors are screwed inside the fabric by means of a torque limiter that adapts to the delivery shaft and limits the maximum torsion torque applicable to the single anchor, thus highlighting any excess torque resulting from incorrect positioning.
4. *Size adjustment tool (SAT)*: The distal tip of the SAT is connected by means of a guide wire to the implant, and at the end of the procedure, it is slid on the guidewire until it engages with the spool, which acts as an actuator for shortening the implant.

## 8.3    Patient Selection

Patients are evaluated by a heart team, composed of an interventional cardiologist, an echocardiographic cardiologist, a cardiac surgeon, and a cardiac anesthesiologist in order to always choose the repair technique best suited to each individual patient.

Percutaneous repair can be considered if the patient has a contraindication for surgical repair of valve disease due to a high risk of mortality or intra- and postop complications.

Transthoracic echocardiography (TTE), TEE, and cardiac computed tomography with contrast agent are always done and sent to the core lab to assess the technical feasibility of the procedure. The Cardioband can correct moderate-to-severe or severe functional mitral regurgitation resulting from a primitive pathology of the left ventricle, which has led over time to a progressive dilation, with an increase in the diameters and volumes of the ventricular chamber.

Cardioband implantation can be carried out in forms of both ischemic (prior acute myocardial infarction) and nonischemic functional mitral regurgitation.

Patients must be symptomatic, in NYHA functional classes II–IV, and/or present with clinical evidence of heart failure despite optimal medical therapy. If the patient can benefit from cardiac resynchronization therapy (CRT), this procedure must be performed before the repair of the mitral valve.

Patients with a complex or mixed etiology of mitral regurgitation must be excluded. Any ruptures of the *chordae tendineae*, pseudoprolapse, extreme tethering (coaptation depth, tethering height > 11 mm), overdilated left ventricle (left ventricular end-diastolic diameter < 70 mm, sphericity index < 0.7), or presence of aneurysms of the ventricular walls are all contraindications for treatment with Cardioband.

Patients with severe right heart failure due to right ventricular dysfunction and/or severe tricuspid regurgitation must also be excluded.

The possible exclusion criteria include anatomical criteria that cannot be neglected. The course of the circumflex artery must always be evaluated for proximity to the insertion point of the first anchor of the Cardioband.

Another anatomical exclusion criterion is the presence of calcification of the annulus or of the valve leaflets, which may hinder implantation and is thoroughly evaluated by TTE, TEE, and cardiac CT, which are always performed during screening.

Clinical and instrumental exclusion criteria (absolute contraindication) are presence of active bacterial endocarditis, major organic lesions with retraction of the chordae or congenital defects with alteration of valve tissue, inability to perform TEE, patients allergic to nickel, patients allergic or intolerant to treatment with anticoagulants or antiplatelet agents, and patients with severe reaction to contrast agent who cannot be properly pretreated.

Other clinical and instrumental criteria that represent important contraindications (relative contraindications), evaluated from time to time in the individual patients, are prior coronary or carotid artery percutaneous revascularization in the previous 30 days or revascularization or carotid endarterectomy in the 3 months prior to implant, past stroke, or transient ischemic attack within the previous 6 months, with evidence of significant carotid artery stenosis (>70%, at color Doppler ultrasonography of the SAT), kidney failure treated with dialysis, history of bleeding or blood clotting disorders, and severe pulmonary hypertension (sPAP > 70 mmHg).

## 8.4 Procedure

The procedure is performed under general anesthesia and fluoroscopic and 2D and 3D TEE guidance. A simulation of the entire procedure is carried out at the core lab using the cardiac CT of the patient to identify the correct points and angles for the deployment of the anchors. Implantation starts from the anterolateral commissure and ends at the posteromedial commissure after fastening the anchors spaced at a distance of 8 mm along the entire posterior annulus.

Femoral vein access is obtained. Following echo-guided transseptal puncture, systemic heparinization is performed to achieve an activated clotting time between 250 and 300 s.

The TSS is then placed in the left atrium. The IDS is then advanced through the TSS and guided so that the tip of the IC is placed above the anterolateral commissure. This maneuver can be facilitated by using an Iron Man guidewire in the left ventricle through the anterolateral commissure. Once the ideal location for the delivery of the first anchor is identified under fluoroscopy (LAO and RAO predetermined by CT) and 2D and 3D TEE, it is screwed and released after checking proper anchoring with push-and-pull testing under fluoroscopy. The first three anchors are implanted in the first 12 mm to give greater stability and pulling strength to the implant. The next anchors are spaced apart every 8 mm.

The sequence for positioning and delivering each anchor is the following:

1. Navigation under ultrasound guidance using the 3D en face reconstruction (surgical view) and fluoroscopic guidance in LAO-CAU view

2. Check of the entry angle and proximity to the hinge point by 2D ultrasound with X-plane
3. Insertion of the anchor under fluoroscopic guidance in RAO-CRA view
4. Push-and-pull test to check secure deployment of the anchor under 2D ultrasound
5. Release of the anchor and passage to the next deployment site

It is very important to carefully check the positioning of the first anchor because a good result of the implant depends on its correct positioning.

Once the last anchor is positioned, the implant is released from the IDS, which is then removed.

The SAT is then inserted through the TSS, over the implant guidewire, until its distal end reaches the adjustment spool of the implant. After SAT connection, the implant is contracted by clockwise rotation of the adjustment roller. This maneuver is carried out progressively, reaching the various degrees of shortening at intervals of 5 min to allow the cardiac tissue to adapt and to avoid excessive tension.

The degree of residual regurgitation, size of the annulus, and transmitral gradient are measured at each step. When the appropriate size of the system is reached, the SAT detaches from the adjusting spool, leaving the implant with the degree of contraction obtained (Fig. 8.2).

## 8.5    Echocardiographic Guidance

As already mentioned, patients who can potentially benefit from treatment with Cardioband are those with functional mitral regurgitation. This form is secondary to left ventricular dilation and systolic dysfunction, in which the individual components of the valve (papillary muscles, *chordae tendineae*, valve leaflets) are anatomically healthy, and essentially the left ventricular disease is the real cause of the valve defect.

A distinction can be made between two categories of patients with functional mitral regurgitation, i.e., ischemic and nonischemic functional mitral regurgitation, both of which are eligible for repair with Cardioband.

In the ischemic form, in which the valve failure is linked to an alteration of the limited regional kinetics (often inferior and/or posterior), left ventricular dysfunction will be mild or moderate in severity, and there will be a displacement of the posteromedial papillary muscle, tethering of the posterior leaflet (associated or not with pseudoprolapse), and often eccentric regurgitant jet. These patients do not appear to be the ideal candidates for this type of percutaneous repair.

In ischemic functional mitral regurgitation with significant left ventricular dysfunction, instead, it is often possible to observe remodeling of the ventricular cavity into a spherical shape and subsequent downward and outward displacement of both the anterolateral and posteromedial papillary muscles, with traction on the *chordae tendineae* and the leaflets, thus making the coaptation point lower inside left ventricle. In extreme cases, even a coaptation gap will be observed.

Along with the displacement of the papillary muscles, there is often the dilation of the annulus, which often involves an increase in the septolateral or anteroposterior diameter, thus making the annulus to develop a circular shape (loss of annular contraction).

The gradual expansion of the annulus leads to a loss of the typical saddle shape, and this will result in further stress on the valve leaflets. To quantify annular dilation, the anteroposterior or septolateral diameter (SL) and the intercommissural diameter (CC) need to be measured by echocardiography. Since the annulus tends to develop a spherical shape, the measurements will tend to be similar in advanced forms.

Potentially, these patients can be the ideal candidates for percutaneous repair by Cardioband.

A substantially superimposable mechanism is present in the case of nonischemic functional mitral regurgitation, often defined as idiopathic, in which the displacement of the papillary muscles, annular dilation, and intraventricular pressure are decisive in the onset of regurgitation, as in advanced ischemic forms.

In the echocardiographic assessment of patients, careful attention needs to be paid to the assessment of the left ventricle by acquiring the following measurements under transthoracic echocardiography:

– End-diastolic diameter (EDD) and end-systolic diameter (ESD) in parasternal long axis view in M-mode and 2D (always acquire a parasternal short axis view to assess regional and annulus kinetics)
– Left ventricular end-systolic and end-diastolic volume in apical four-chamber and apical two-chamber view
– Left ventricular sphericity index, also in apical four-chamber view

Optimal evaluation of the annulus certainly requires measuring (TTE) the septo-lateral diameter in the apical three-chamber view and the intercommissural diameter in the apical two-chamber view in systole and diastole.

A morphological characteristic of functional mitral regurgitation is certainly tenting of the valve leaflets, which tend to have a lower coaptation point inside the left ventricle.

There are several parameters to assess and estimate tenting, some of which are absolutely indispensable:

– Coaptation depth, i.e., the vertical distance between the ideal coaptation plane of the leaflets at the level of the annulus and the actual coaptation point
– Coaptation length or residual coaptation surface
– Tenting area, which measures the tent area by tracing the area between the line of the ideal coaptation point at the level of the annulus and the actual coaptation point

Evaluation of the extent of regurgitation is certainly the most important aspect in both TTE and TEE.

We should always keep in mind that there is no absolutely reliable method for the estimation of mitral regurgitation (quantitative, semiquantitative, invasive, and non-invasive methods), that there are continuous variations in the extent depending on hemodynamic conditions, and that the extent of regurgitation calls for a clinical instrumental counterpart to make an accurate assessment.

However, many methods are described in the literature for the evaluation of mitral valve regurgitation, and there are studies in progress on many others.

We will describe some that we have selected for potential accuracy, reproducibility, ease of acquisition, and immediate use.

We start by evaluating the morphology of the valve, with particular attention to the leaflets and to the possible presence of calcifications of the annulus that could make the implantation of Cardioband cumbersome.

Semiquantitative methods include color Doppler, which allows us to estimate the area of the regurgitant jet in the left atrium.

We can thus identify:

- *The convergence zone*, i.e., the zone immediately before the valve where the flow converges and accelerates before entering the regurgitation orifice.
  - Using the proximal isovelocity surface area (PISA) method and imagining it as a hemisphere, we can calculate the amount of flow passing through this surface. Therefore, this gives us an estimate of the effective regurgitant orifice area (EROA).
  - With the advent of three-dimensional (3D) echocardiography, it is possible to directly measure the effective regurgitant orifice area without having to resort to PISA.
- *Vena contracta (VC)*, i.e., the area in which the regurgitant jet reaches its smallest dimensions immediately after the regurgitation orifice. The use of the VC as a parameter for assessing the extent of regurgitation is based on the principle that the width of the jet is correlated with the size of the anatomical orifice.
  - It is necessary to carry out the measurement perpendicular to the commissural line and, hence, in parasternal or apical long axis view, and in transesophageal long axis view. Since the measurement is just of a few millimeters, a zoom with a good degree of resolution is needed.
- *Turbulence zone* in the post-orifice left atrium: this evaluation allows the estimation of the regurgitation fraction (compared with the size of the left atrium) and the regurgitant volume. The 3D color echocardiography allows the visualization of the regurgitant jet, and the direct measurement is more accurate than the diameter of the regurgitation orifice.

Other methods that can be used to complete a thorough examination to estimate mitral regurgitation include:

- The intensity of the continuous-wave Doppler signal.
- The pattern of the pulmonary venous flow obtained by pulsed Doppler, which will give two peak velocities, systolic and diastolic, and a small reverse wave, which is the expression of atrial contraction. The increase in pressure in the left atrium due to severe mitral regurgitation determines a reduction in systolic velocity.
- The E-wave velocity (quick filling) of the transmitral flow is a simple and reproducible parameter. It is the expression of the pressures in the left atrium; in the absence of mitral stenosis, the finding of an $E/A$ ratio > 1.5 and an E-wave velocity > 2 m/s are qualitative indices of hemodynamically significant regurgitation.
- The estimate of the dimensions of the left atrium and of sPAP is an indirect parameter for the evaluation of the degree of severity of mitral regurgitation.

3D echocardiography is certainly the method of choice for the evaluation of many valve diseases. It provides optimal evaluation of valve leaflets and of the annulus and subvalvular apparatus. Moreover, 3D visualization of TEE surely represents an indispensable part for guiding the interventional procedure of Cardioband.

# Transcatheter Repair of Mitral Regurgitation: Kardia Carillon

**9**

Sebastiano Immè, Antonio Popolo Rubbio, Stefano Cannata, and Salvatore Scandura

## 9.1    Description of the Device

The CARILLON™ Mitral Contour System™ Model XE2 (Cardiac Dimension® Inc., Kirkland, WA, USA) is a device designed for indirect percutaneous mitral valve (MV) annuloplasty through the coronary sinus (CS). It received the CE mark in August 2011 for use in [1, 2].

The device consists of a proprietary implant, designed for permanent implantation in the CS to reshape the mitral annulus (MA), and a catheter-based delivery system, which consists of a delivery catheter and the so-called handle assembly [3].

The implant features a wire-shaping ribbon (connector), positioned between two interwoven anchors to form a figure-of-eight or semi-helical shape. The shaping ribbon, made of nickel and titanium, is designed to be deployed, tensioned, and fastened inside the CS (Fig. 9.1). The characteristic arc shape of the ribbon allows orientation of the implant to facilitate release in the CS. Indirect annuloplasty exploits the strategic anatomical position of the CS [1, 4], which runs parallel to the posterolateral MA, thus embracing about two thirds of the circumference of the annulus. The CS is separated from the MA by nonfibrous myocardial tissue. Its shortening, therefore, allows creation of a tension that is exerted on the posterior part of the peri-annular tissue, thus causing an anterior deflection of the posterior MA, with consequent reduction of the area of the MA.

The ends of the implant comprise the distal and proximal crimp tube, where the respective anchors in nitinol are located (Fig. 9.2). The distal anchor, which is smaller,

S. Immè, MD, PhD (✉)
Centro Cuore Morgagni, Pedara, Catania, Italy
e-mail: sebastiano.imme@alice.it

A.P. Rubbio • S. Cannata • S. Scandura
Cardiac-Thoracic-Vascular Department, Ferrarotto Hospital,
University of Catania, Catania, Italy

© Springer International Publishing AG 2018
C. Tamburino et al. (eds.), *Percutaneous Treatment of Left Side Cardiac Valves*,
https://doi.org/10.1007/978-3-319-59620-4_9

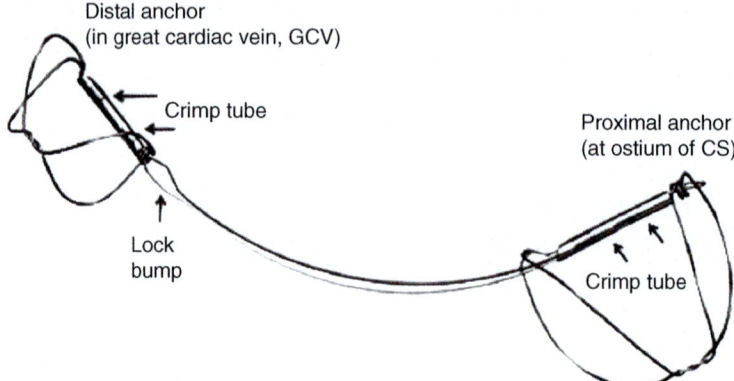

Distal anchor
(in great cardiac vein, GCV)

Crimp tube

Proximal anchor
(at ostium of CS)

Lock
bump

Crimp tube

**Fig. 9.1** CARILLON™. Depiction of the implant

**Fig. 9.2** Anchor
architecture
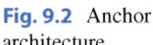

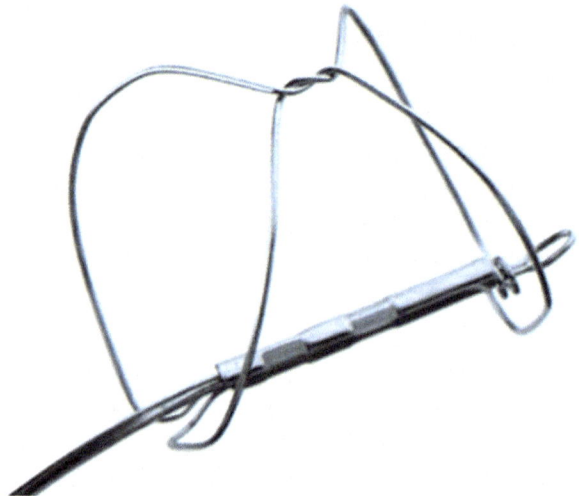

is positioned in the great cardiac vein (GCV), while the proximal anchor, which is larger, is positioned in the proximal CS, contiguous to the anterior commissure of the MV. As regards anatomical variability between individuals, there are up to 37 different combinations of implant sizes that take into account the length of the ribbon (60, 70, 80 mm) and various diameters for the proximal anchor (12–20 mm) and distal anchor (7–14 mm) [5]. To determine the most appropriate measure, a thorough pre-procedure study phase is needed; it takes into account the geometry of the CS, as well as its length and diameter and its anatomic relationships with the coronary arteries.

The delivery catheter (Fig. 9.3) is a custom catheter composed of a metal braid reinforced polymer sheath with a Luer Y-connector. At the distal end, the catheter curves and features a radiopaque tip. The catheter has an actual length of 70 cm, with an outer diameter of 9 Fr (3.0 mm) and an inner diameter of 7.5 Fr (2.5 mm), and is able to accommodate a 0.035″ guidewire or a flexible diagnostic catheter with an outer diameter of 7 Fr.

The second element of the delivery system is the handle assembly (Fig. 9.4), composed of the cartridge, the sheath-pusher assembly, and the handle. In its packaging, the

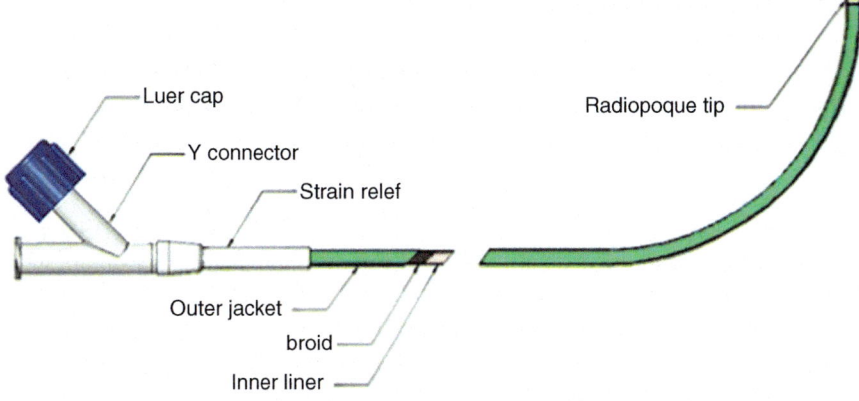

**Fig. 9.3** Delivery catheter, composed of a lateral port that can be used to inject contrast medium, and a straight port for advancement and removal of a measuring device and for implant introduction

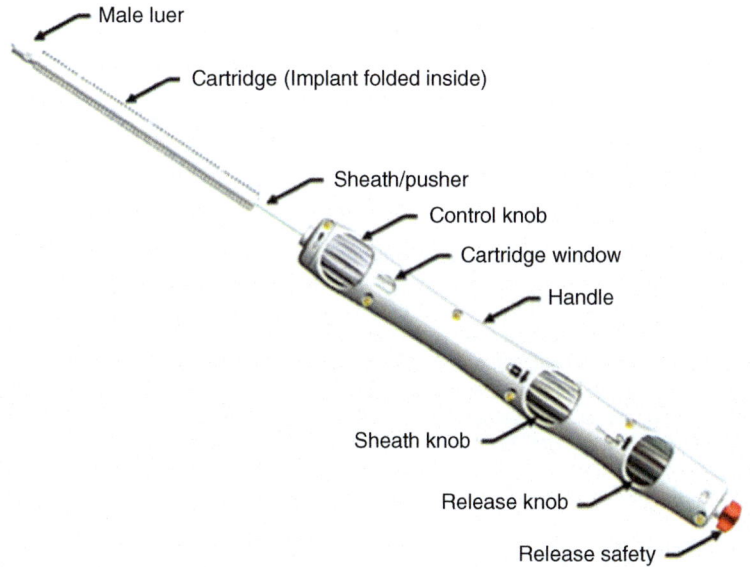

**Fig. 9.4** Handle assembly

implant, folded in unlocked position, is loaded into the cartridge. The male Luer, which represents the distal portion of the cartridge, is connected to the straight port of the proximal end of the delivery catheter. The sheath-pusher assembly is composed of a pusher, lock wire, tether wire, and a polymeric sheath for locking the proximal anchor. It allows the placement, deployment, and decoupling of the implant from the handle assembly.

The handle will also consist of rotating knobs that allow the operator to maneuver the deployment, locking, decoupling, and removal of the implant, thus providing a safe release mechanism.

All system components are for single use only.

## 9.2    Patient Selection

Today, a number of MV percutaneous repair techniques are available for interventional cardiologists. Obviously, the most suitable percutaneous treatment options vary from patient to patient. Therefore, the Heart Team plays a crucial role in the case-by-case assessment and in correctly determining the procedure indication and surgical risk.

The target population for percutaneous treatment with the CARILLON™ system includes patients with dilated cardiomyopathy and symptomatic heart failure who, despite optimal medical therapy, continue to be in NYHA class III/IV, suffering from moderate-to-severe functional (ischemic or nonischemic) mitral regurgitation (MR).

Apart from the manufacturer's indications, the main inclusion and exclusion criteria for this procedure are the result of real-life clinical practice and of pilot studies on the device, such as the AMADEUS (CARILLON Mitral Annuloplasty Device European Union Study), a prospective multicenter singlearm feasibility study, which was one of the first to assess the safety and efficacy of the CARILLON™ system in patients with functional MR [6], followed by the TITAN trial (The Transcatheter Implantation of the CARILLON Mitral Annuloplasty Device), a prospective, nonrandomized study that evaluated the second generation of the device [7].

These criteria for inclusion and exclusion are listed in Table 9.1.

**Table 9.1**  Major inclusion and exclusion criteria

| |
|---|
| *Inclusion criteria* |
| Age over 18 years |
| Ischemic or nonischemic dilated cardiomyopathy with systolic HF |
| Moderate-to-severe or severe chronic FMR, symptomatic in NYHA class III-IV, or asymptomatic, but with LVEF ≤40%, LVEDD ≥55 mm |
| Patients at high surgical risk, including patients with CABG or prior heart surgery |
| Functional capacity estimated at 6-min walking test, with distance comprised at least between 150 and 450 m |
| Insufficient optimal medical therapy (β-blocker plus ACE inhibitors or sartans, with stable dose for at least 1 month and an adjustable dose of diuretic for at least 3 months) |
| *Exclusion criteria* |
| Evidence of a history of myocardial infarction or CABG or unstable angina in the previous 3 months |
| PCI in the previous 30 days |
| Mild or moderate FMR, in symptomatic patient in NYHA class II or in non-optimized pharmacological treatment |
| DMR |
| Need for heart surgery within 1 year for other reason or need for emergency heart surgery |
| Pacing involving the CS (e.g., in the case of CRT) or other catheters or devices inside the CS |
| Pathologies of the mitral valve of organic and degenerative nature, e.g., rheumatic valve, myxomatous valve, structural abnormalities of leaflets, severe calcification of the mitral annulus, or prior surgical annuloplasty by prosthetic ring or valve replacement |
| Allergy to nickel, titanium, or nickel/titanium (NITINOL) as a relative contraindication |
| Contraindications to TEE |

*HF* heart failure, *FMR* functional mitral regurgitation, *NYHA* New York Heart Association, *LVEF* left ventricular ejection fraction, *LVEDD* left ventricular end-diastolic diameter, *CABG* coronary artery bypass graft, *PCI* percutaneous coronary intervention, *DMR* degenerative mitral regurgitation, *CS* coronary sinus, *CRT* cardiac resynchronization therapy, *TEE* transesophageal echocardiography

## 9.3     Procedural and Technical Aspects

The procedure is carried out in the cath lab under guidance with fluoroscopy and transesophageal echocardiography (TEE). It can be performed either under deep sedation or general anesthesia. General anesthesia is generally preferred considering the discomfort that TEE can cause in patients during a procedure, the length of which, according to the data reported in the literature, is about 40 min on average and varies depending on the experience of the operator and the learning curve.

The procedure requires several clinicians: an interventional cardiologist, an echocardiographic cardiologist, an anesthesiologist, a nurse, and a cath lab technician. The cath lab should have emergency surgical back-up in case of complications requiring a change from a percutaneous to open-chest procedure.

Patient preparation involves a first phase for the assessment of blood tests, including standard exams such as a complete blood count and renal function and blood coagulation tests. In patients with history of chronic kidney disease or high levels of creatinine, it may be necessary to deliver liquids IV in the run-up to the procedure in order to avoid contrast-induced nephropathy. The CARILLON™ implantation procedure does not, in itself, require the administration of a significant amount of contrast medium, but it can be used during the angiographic assessment of the CS or adjacent coronary arteries. Therefore, good hydration or the use of other means to protect against contrast-induced nephropathy may be necessary. Cases of contrast-induced nephropathy after the implantation of the CARILLON™ have been documented [6, 7]. Any vitamin K antagonist oral anticoagulants must be discontinued approximately 3 days prior to the procedure and replaced with low-molecular-weight heparin to achieve an international normalized ratio (INR) of <1.7 or, better, of <1.5. In patients under treatment with new oral anticoagulants, it is necessary to suspend anticoagulant treatment 24–48 h before the procedure, depending on the molecule and on the renal function of the patient. For prophylactic purposes, all patients also receive a single IV dose of broad-spectrum antibiotic with a long half-life. In view of the procedure, a preliminary anesthesia consult should be carried out in addition to a chest X-ray as basic imaging to identify any contraindications to patient intubation.

Once in the cath lab, the patient receives deep sedation or general anesthesia. In the latter case, the patient is intubated and vital signs are monitored. During the procedure, constant measurement of systemic blood pressure and of oxygen saturation and ECG monitoring are carried out. If necessary, intra-procedure inotropes, such as dobutamine, dopamine, or adrenaline, can be administered depending on the hemodynamics of the patient and on the evaluation of the anesthesiologist. The patient is heparinized, and activated clotting time (ACT) is monitored at set intervals to maintain an ACT of >200 s. Through ACT monitoring every 30 min, it is possible to decide whether to administer heparin again during the procedure to ensure adequate patient anticoagulation.

The CARILLON™ system is implanted according to standard catheterization techniques. Unlike other MV percutaneous repair techniques like the MitraClip system or direct annuloplasty, there is no need to puncture the interatrial septum. The procedure provides for the preparation of the right internal jugular venous access to cannulate the CS and of an arterial access for invasive monitoring of blood pressure, as well as for assessments by coronary angiography at the start of the procedure and just before the release of the device, given the contiguity of the CS with the coronary arteries. A diagonal or ramus branch can be found between the CS and MA in 16% of patients [4]. The relationship between the CS and the left circumflex artery (LCA), which runs between the CS and the MA, is more significant, accounting for a percentage ranging between 64 and 80% of cases [8–10]. In the latter case, the LCA could be compressed frequently due to extrinsic compression [11]. In addition, the obtuse marginal branches originating from the LCA may be potentially involved [12]. For the same reason, the CARILLON™ should not be released at a site where the compression of the CS on a coronary artery can compromise the integrity of a previously implanted stent.

The first step of the procedure consists in a coronary angiography to assess a possible coronary disease, the anatomy, and the coronary flow at baseline, and especially of the LCA, and to locate the CS ostium during the venous injection of the contrast medium.

The second step is the cannulation of the CS. The puncture of the right internal jugular vein is made by standard technique with a 9 Fr introducer, which is capable of lodging a 6 or 7 Fr multipurpose diagnostic catheter and a 0.035″ (0.89 mm) hydrophilic guidewire. The angled catheter, together with the delivery catheter, is advanced along the guidewire toward the CS. The shape of the angled catheter allows the cannulation of the anterior interventricular branch of the GCV, which is the anatomical landmark for insertion in the CS. Once the CS is cannulated, the guidewire, together with the delivery catheter, is advanced up to the distal portion of the vein. Under fluoroscopy it can be observed that the delivery catheter is correctly positioned at the distal end of the CS. The guidewire and angled catheter are then removed, and the delivery catheter is carefully de-aired. A catheter with radiopaque marker (e.g., a 5 Fr) is then advanced through the delivery catheter to its end. Another coronary angiogram is done, this time by moving the image intensifier to an oblique right anterior view with caudal angulation. The specific reason for this step is to analyze the contiguity relationship between the LCA and GCV which will be marked by the delivery catheter and the radiopaque marker. The anatomical assessment of the venous structures is then completed by venography of the GCV/CS system. The image intensifier will then be moved to an oblique left anterior projection with caudal angulation, and another coronary angiogram of the left coronary artery is done, followed by venography.

The marker catheter, besides being a point of reference, will be used as a calibration system to assess the length and diameter of the venous system and the appropriate site for the anchoring of the implant in the CS. This step also includes an assessment of any torsion in the venous system, of any individual anatomical variants, and of the presence of satellite branches, as well as the relationship with the LCA. If the vein that can be used for implantation is not long enough, the marker catheter is then removed, and the guidewire and angled catheter are reinserted to make the delivery catheter advance further to the anterior interventricular vein to make sure that there is sufficient space for the release of the implant.

Once the anatomical assessments are completed, it is necessary to choose the size of the most appropriate implant. In order to generate a tension of at least 3 cm (preferably 4–5 cm), a vein length of at least 9 cm (preferably 11 cm) is needed, using a device with connector at least 60 mm long. In case of longer veins, you will need to opt for a device length of 80 mm, which is the maximum allowed. Once you have assessed the appropriate device measures, the marker catheter can be removed.

The next step is the introduction of the device and the release of the distal anchor in the distal part of the GCV. When positioning the distal anchor, pull the delivery system slightly to allow a passive expansion of the nitinol meshes [6] and then advance the delivery catheter to allow reaching the maximum diameter of the anchors (Fig. 9.5).

Once the distal anchor is positioned in the CS with the control knob and after checking by coronary angiography that the distal release does not compromise the arterial flow of the LCA, the device is pulled gradually by hand to generate an adequate tension to indirectly create a fold in the tissue around the annulus and hence reduce the coaptation gap between the two valve leaflets. The ultimate result is a reduction in MR. TEE at this stage will allow assessment of the degree of MR

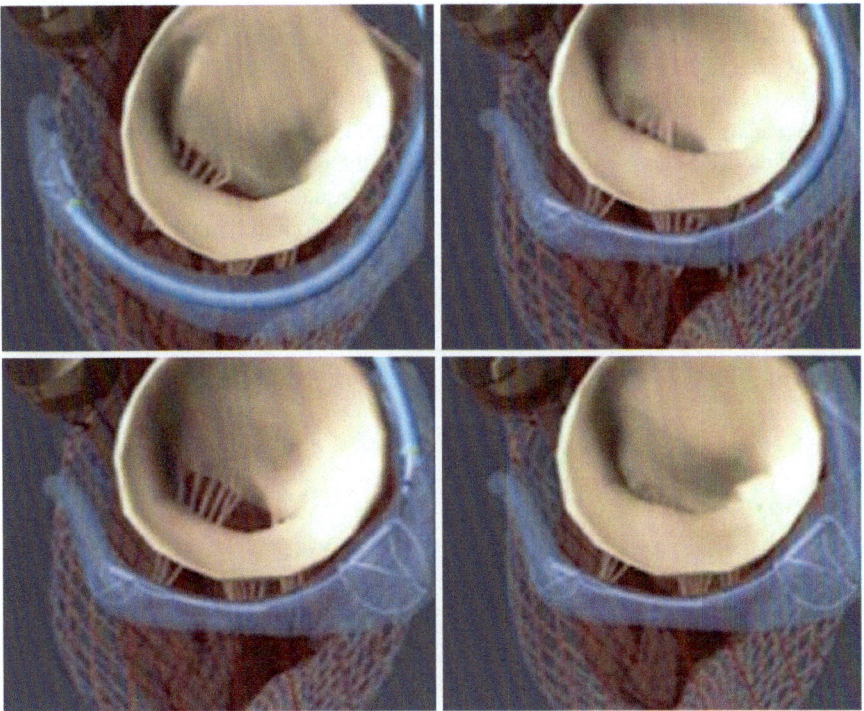

**Fig. 9.5** The different steps of the procedure, with the advancement of the distal and proximal anchor and mesh opening

reduction. Once the procedure is completed, another assessment by coronary angiography may be needed to reevaluate any extrinsic compressions on the arterial system that could compromise the technical success of the procedure. A venogram will determine whether the venous system has been damaged. If technical success has been achieved, also place the proximal anchor and check the final result in terms of residual MR by TEE [13–15].

After positioning the CARILLON™, any other potential procedure can be carried out, including edge-to-edge percutaneous repair [16]. It has also been demonstrated that in patients in need of cardiac resynchronization therapy devices following implantation, the CARILLON™ system leaves enough space to implant another catheter in the CS [17, 18] but no earlier than 3–6 months after the procedure to ensure complete encapsulation of the implant. The system also does not prevent any conversion of the procedure to a conventional surgical approach (Fig. 9.6).

Intra- and post-procedure complications [6, 7, 13, 19] can include cases of perforation or dissection of the CS, which in some cases may have a self-limiting course or lead to pericardial effusion requiring pericardiocentesis. Data in the literature shows that these complications related to the cannulation of the CS are also correlated with the learning curve, as demonstrated by those observed in early cardiac resynchronization studies, which similarly required an approach with CS cannulation [20]. The first generation of the device showed cases of slippage of the distal anchor, which prevented the final release of the implant, but this issue was solved by modifying the shape of the anchors which are now twisted at the apex to increase rigidity. One of the other complications can be the reduced strength of the metal, which can result in failure of the device. In this case as well, reengineering of the device, as shown in the TITAN study [7], has led to a reduction in the number of cases of device failure, with an improvement in the general outcome. Other possible events of device failure can be related to an inadequate MR reduction or compression of the coronary arteries. In the event of arterial compression or inadequate MR reduction, or of inappropriate placement of the device inside the CS, the CARILLON™ system can be retrieved through a specific capture system and safely repositioned [21] (Fig. 9.7). The position of the implant can thus be modified, or, if

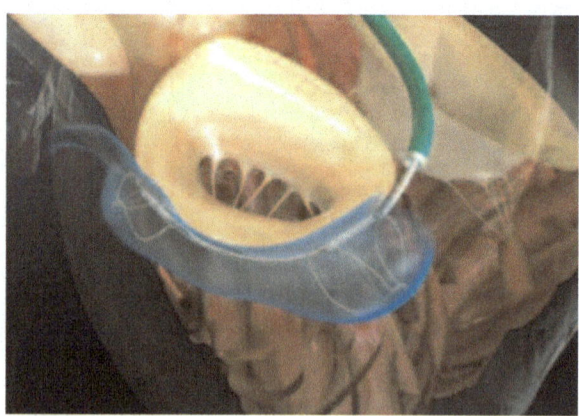

**Fig. 9.6** Final placement of the CARILLON™ device in the coronary sinus

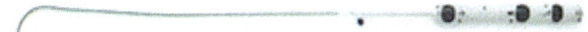

**Fig. 9.7** Recapture system attached to the handle assembly allows recompression and optimization of final position in the coronary sinus or recapture of the device prior to decoupling from the handle assembly

necessary, the implant attached to the handle assembly can be removed and the procedure abandoned. Particular attention must be paid to this stage, since the implant can no longer be retrieved once it is decoupled from the handle assembly. This is undoubtedly an advantage of the CARILLON™ system compared with other devices for indirect annuloplasty. The first generation of the device, in fact, had problems in the anchoring process [6], but this drawback was promptly solved by following generations of the device. In addition, it should be borne in mind that the components of the CARILLON™ system are for single use. Therefore, if an additional implant attempt is planned, the procedure must be repeated entirely, with a new implant and a new delivery system.

Once the procedure is completed, the patient is awakened and extubated. While still in the cath lab, particular attention at this stage will be paid to the onset of alterations in pressure and/or cardiac rhythm, desaturation, and bleeding.

The patient is then transferred and monitored in the cardiac ICU for close monitoring of vital signs and laboratory tests. The post-procedure management of the patient includes the assessment of the onset of fever, hemodynamic or cardiac rhythm alterations, desaturation, and fluid balance alterations or late bleedings linked to major or minor vascular complications at the access site, which may or may not require concentrated red blood cell transfusions. The laboratory tests requiring special attention are therefore the CBC, hemoglobin, BUN, creatinine, and electrolytes, as well as myocardium-specific enzymes, and especially creatine kinase MB. Considering that patients receiving this procedure are patients with functional MR and a history of systolic heart failure, NT-proBNP should be monitored as a laboratory indicator of decompensation. Before discharge, we recommend assessing technical success by follow-up transthoracic echocardiogram to identify any residual MR or to rule out the presence of pericardial effusion.

## 9.4 Echocardiographic Assessment

Intra-procedure TEE represents a key element of the procedure, since the MV and its components cannot be viewable with X-rays by fluoroscopy alone [22]. 3D reconstruction of the TEE also allows us to better determine the anatomical features of the MA [23], the saddle or hyperbolic paraboloid shape of which cannot be assessed by 2D imaging alone, because it tends to greatly simplify the anatomy of the MA, presenting it as a planar ring [24, 25]. TEE provides vital information in guiding the procedure and will be used to evaluate the degree of intra- and post-procedure MR until completion of the procedure. In light of this, a unified protocol for image acquisition is needed [26]. A multiplanar probe must be used; in addition to standard 2D assessment, 3D assessment with full-volume, real-time, and zoom 3D imaging is also needed. The anatomy of the MA is best viewed using 3D full volume and 3D zoom formats.

Echocardiographic monitoring is started after inducing general anesthesia. The assessment of the MV before implant provides for standard assessments, including a mid-esophageal view at 0°–180° to have an initial assessment of the left atrium and left atrial appendage and to view the outflow of the pulmonary veins, and then follows the assessment of the mitral leaflets to rule out any degeneration of the MV, such as the presence of major calcifications that may compromise the effectiveness of the device in indirectly reducing the MA [8, 9]. It should be borne in mind that these assessments, both by transthoracic echocardiography and TEE, in compliance with the guidelines of the American Society of Echocardiography [27], are part of the pre-procedure assessment phase, but at this phase they are used as further confirmation. The projections at 0°, 30°, 60°, 90°, and 120° are used to assess the surface area of the left atrium, the dimensions of the MA, and the MR jet area. Projections at 30° and 120° are used to assess the vena contracta, the effective regurgitant orifice, and regurgitant volume, while flow and the diameter of the left ventricle outflow tract can be viewed at 0° and 120°.

To view the CS, the probe must be run through the distal esophagus. During the procedure, this view allows you to display the proximal anchor of the device. In addition to monitoring proper implantation, TEE also identifies any complications related, for example, to the acute formation of thrombi, perforation of the CS with cardiac tamponade, or excessive tension on the MV generating mitral stenosis.

At the end of the procedure, if there are no complications and residual MR, the device is permanently released and the procedure is concluded.

## References

1. Maniu CV, Patel JB, Reuter DG, et al. Acute and chronic reduction of functional mitral regurgitation in experimental heart failure by percutaneous mitral annuloplasty. J Am Coll Cardiol. 2004;44:1652–61.
2. Kaye DM, Byrne M, Alferness C, et al. Feasibility and short-term efficacy of percutaneous mitral annular reduction for the therapy of heart failure-induced mitral regurgitation. Circulation. 2003;108:1795–7.
3. Cardiac Dimensions Inc. Submission File Cardiac Dimensions.
4. Lansac E, Di Centa I, Al Attar N, et al. Percutaneous mitral annuloplasty through the coronary sinus: an anatomic point of view. J Thorac Cardiovasc Surg. 2008;135:376–81.
5. Cardiac Dimensions Inc. CARILLON® Mitral Contour System® Instructions for Use.
6. Schofer J, Siminiak T, Haude M, et al. Valvular heart disease. Percutaneous mitral annuloplasty for functional mitral regurgitation. Results of the CARILLON mitral annuloplasty device European Union Study. Circulation. 2009;120:326–33.
7. Siminiak T, Wu JC, Haude M, et al. Treatment of functional mitral regurgitation by percutaneous annuloplasty: results of the TITAN Trial. Eur J Heart Fail. 2012;14:931–8.
8. Chiam PTL, Ruiz CE. Percutaneous transcatheter mitral valve repair. JACC Cardiovasc Interv. 2011;4:1–13.
9. Tops LF, Van De Veire NR, Schuijf JD, et al. Noninvasive evaluation of coronary sinus anatomy and its relation to the mitral valve annulus: implications for percutaneous mitral annuloplasty. Circulation. 2007;115:1426–32.

10. Choure AJ, Garcia MJ, Hesse B, et al. In vivo analysis of the anatomical relationship of coronary sinus to mitral annulus and left circumflex coronary artery using cardiac multidetector computed tomography: implications for percutaneous coronary sinus mitral annuloplasty. J Am Coll Cardiol. 2006;48:1938–45.
11. Goldberg SL, Van Bibber R, Schofer J, et al. The frequency of coronary artery compression and management using a removable mitral annuloplasty device in the coronary sinus. J Am Coll Cardiol. 2008;51:28.
12. Van Mieghem NM, Piazza N, Anderson RH, et al. Anatomy of the mitral valvular complex and its implications for transcatheter interventions for mitral regurgitation. J Am Coll Cardiol. 2010;56:617–26.
13. Feldman T, Cilingiroglu M. Percutaneous leaflet repair and annuloplasty for mitral regurgitation. J Am Coll Cardiol. 2011;57:529–37.
14. Siminiak T, Firek L, Jerzykowska O, et al. Percutaneous valve repair for mitral regurgitation using the Carillon™ Mitral Contour System™. Description of the method and case report. Kardiol Pol. 2007;65:272–8.
15. Goldberg SL, Lipiecki J, Sievert H, et al. The Carillon Mitral Contour transcatheter indirect mitral valve annuloplasty system. EuroIntervention. 2015;11:W64–6.
16. Grasso C, Attizzani GF, Ohno Y, et al. Catheter-based edge-to-edge mitral valve repair after percutaneous mitral valve annuloplasty failure. JACC Cardiovasc Interv. 2014;7:e85–6.
17. Hoppe UC, Brandt MC, Degen H, et al. Percutaneous mitral annuloplasty device leaves free access to cardiac veins for resynchronization therapy. Catheter Cardiovasc Interv. 2009;74:506–11.
18. Siminiak T, Jerzykowska O, Kalmucki P, et al. Cardiac resynchronization therapy after percutaneous trans-coronary-venous mitral annuloplasty. Kardiol Pol. 2013;71:1293–4.
19. Feldman T, Ali O. Transcatheter mitral valve interventions: current status and future perspective. EuroIntervention. 2012;8:Q53–9.
20. Angel RL, Abraham WT, Curtis AB, et al. Safety of transvenous cardiac resynchronization system implantation in patients with chronic heart failure: combined results of over 2,000 patients from a multicenter study program. J Am Coll Cardiol. 2005;46:2348–56.
21. Klein N, Pfeiffer D, Goldberg S, et al. Mitral annuloplasty device implantation for non-surgical treatment of mitral regurgitation: clinical experience after the approval studies. J Invasive Cardiol. 2016;28:115–20.
22. Jerzykowska O, Kałmucki P, Wołoszyn M, et al. Echocardiographic evaluation of percutaneous valve repair in patients with mitral regurgitation using the CARILLON system. Kardiol Pol. 2010;68:57–63.
23. Kalyanasundaram A, Qureshi A, Nassef L, et al. Functional anatomy of normal mitral valve-left ventricular complex by real-time three-dimensional echocardiography. J Heart Valve Dis. 2010;19:28–34.
24. Levine RA, Handschumacher MD, Sanfilippo AJ, et al. Three-dimensional echocardiographic reconstruction of the mitral valve, with implications for the diagnosis of mitral valve prolapse. Circulation. 1989;80:589–98.
25. Kwan J, Qin J, Popovic Z, et al. Geometric changes of mitral annulus assessed by real-time 3-dimensional echocardiography: becoming enlarged and less nonplanar in the anteroposterior direction during systole in proportion to global left ventricular systolic function. J Am Soc Echocardiogr. 2004;17:1179–84.
26. Lancellotti P, Moura L, Pierard L, et al. European Association of Echocardiography recommendations for the assessment of valvular regurgitation. Part 2: mitral and tricuspid regurgitation (native valve disease). Eur J Echocardiogr. 2010;11:307–32.
27. Zoghbi WA, Enriquez-Sarano M, Foster E, et al. Recommendations for evaluation of the severity of native valvular regurgitation with two-dimensional and Doppler echocardiography. J Am Soc Echocardiogr. 2003;16:777–802.

# Transcatheter Repair of Mitral Regurgitation: Other Devices and Novel Concepts

# 10

Ted Feldman, Mayra Guerrero, Michael H. Salinger, and Justin P. Levisay

## 10.1 Introduction

For many years percutaneous mitral repair was synonymous with the MitraClip device, since no other repair therapies were available. Over the past 2 years, three additional repair technologies have received EC approval. These four devices, MitraClip, Cardiac Dimensions Carillon, Valtech Cardioband, and Mitralign, are described in the preceding chapters. Numerous other repair devices and concepts have been described. The great challenges for mitral regurgitation (MR) repair devices are reflected in the fact that many novel device approaches for MR treatment have already fallen by the wayside. A variety of new device approaches are in the early stages of development. The typical sequence of development includes bench and preclinical animal testing, first in human intraoperative testing and finally percutaneous delivery for clinical use. The many other devices in the development pathway are in the earliest stages at the time of this writing. Many have been used only in preclinical or surgical applications.

The usual classification for percutaneous mitral repair devices includes leaflet repair, direct and indirect annuloplasty, chamber remodeling, and neochordal implantation. This classification includes some overlap. For example, some of the annuloplasty devices are implanted into the ventricular side of the mitral valve annulus and subannular myocardium and, therefore, may also contribute to some degree of chamber remodeling.

T. Feldman, MD, FESC, FACC, MSCAI (✉)
Cardiology Division, Evanston Hospital,
Walgreen Building 3rd Floor, 2650 Ridge Ave, Evanston, IL 60201, USA

NorthShore University HealthSystem, Evanston, IL, USA
e-mail: tfeldman@tfeldman.org

M. Guerrero, M.D., F.A.C.C., F.S.C.A.I. • M.H. Salinger, M.D., F.A.C.C., F.S.C.A.I.
J.P. Levisay, M.D., F.A.C.C., F.S.C.A.I.
NorthShore University HealthSystem, Evanston, IL, USA

© Springer International Publishing AG 2018
C. Tamburino et al. (eds.), *Percutaneous Treatment of Left Side Cardiac Valves*,
https://doi.org/10.1007/978-3-319-59620-4_10

In addition to the complexity of creating MR repair devices that can be implanted percutaneously and also reduce MR, the appropriate patient population must be defined. Devices and approaches that may be suitable for degenerative MR may or may not also be used for functional MR. While the MitraClip device was initially intended for degenerative MR, we have found its largest application in functional MR. Neochordal implantation will clearly be used for degenerative MR. Functional MR poses a special problem since no prior surgical therapies have demonstrated important survival benefit in this population, and even the clinical impact of surgical repair for functional MR remains unclear.

This review will describe many of the devices in this area of development, some at only the concept stages, others with open surgical approaches, and some with early human transapical or percutaneous experience.

## 10.2 Leaflet Repair

The first mitral repair device with significant use in patients is the MitraClip, based on the Alfieri edge-to-edge or double-orifice surgical repair. Surgical leaflet repair has historically been used for degenerative MR, but the widespread use of MitraClip for functional MR makes it possible to consider leaflet repair devices more broadly. One leaflet approach that used a suture to create an edge-to-edge repair, the Edwards Mobius (Edwards Lifesciences, Irvine, CA) leaflet repair system, was used in a small number of patients before the effort was discontinued [1].

*Cardica Mitral Repair*: Edge-to-edge repair, Cardica Inc. (Redwood City, CA), sells automated stapling or anastomosis systems [2]. They have developed a concept for edge-to-edge mitral repair using a staple-like implant delivered with a transseptal catheter system (Fig. 10.1). The guide catheter has mechanisms for centering and stabilizing the delivery system. The guide catheter includes a clip channel, at least one hook channel, and at least one sling channel and a clip applier, which is movable within the clip channel. The hook and sling channels are alternately positioned and evenly spaced around the perimeter of the guide catheter. The clip or staple has at least three tines and is used to approximate or fasten the anterior and posterior mitral leaflets.

*Cardiosolutions MitraSpacer*: The MitraSpacer (West Bridgewater, MA) is a hydraulically inflated balloon that is anchored in the left ventricular apex and positioned in the regurgitant mitral orifice [3]. The device fills the space of the regurgitant orifice or malcoapting segments (Fig. 10.2). The balloon is about the size of a small chili pepper. The balloon is connected to a port just below the patient's skin and can be inflated or deflated over time depending on the patient's condition. A compassionate use first in human surgical implant was successfully performed in March 2015 at King's College Hospital in London, and the results were presented at the EuroPCRLondon Valves meeting in 2015. This patient developed recurrence of MR and underwent successful addition of 2.5 mL fluid to the balloon injected through the subcutaneous port, resulting in improvement of MR.

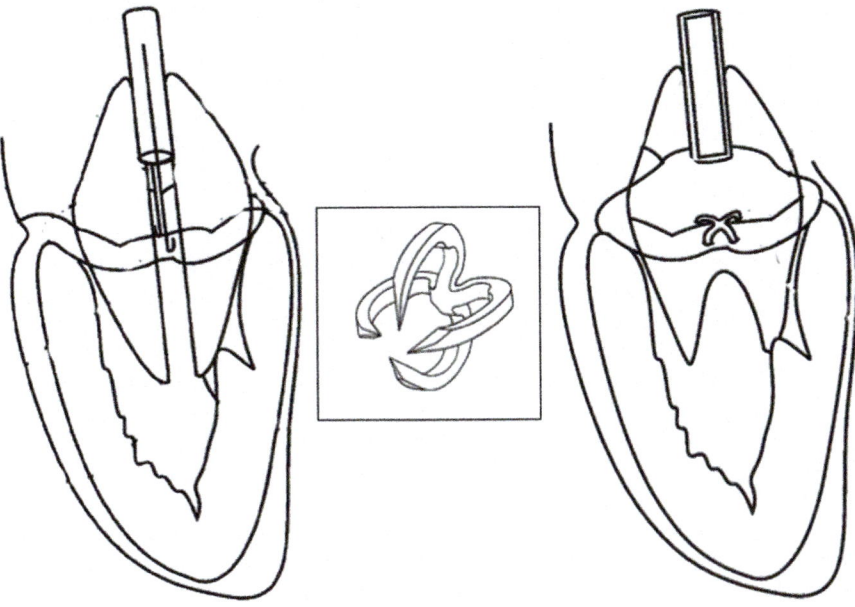

**Fig. 10.1** Cardiac edge-to-edge mitral repair using a staple-like implant delivered with a transseptal catheter system. Drawing from US Patent 8,888,794, filed July 26, 2013

**Fig. 10.2** Cardiosolutions MitraSpacer is a hydraulic balloon that is anchored in the left ventricular apex and positioned in the regurgitant mitral orifice. The balloon, the volume of which is adjustable, fills the space of the regurgitant orifice or malcoapting segment

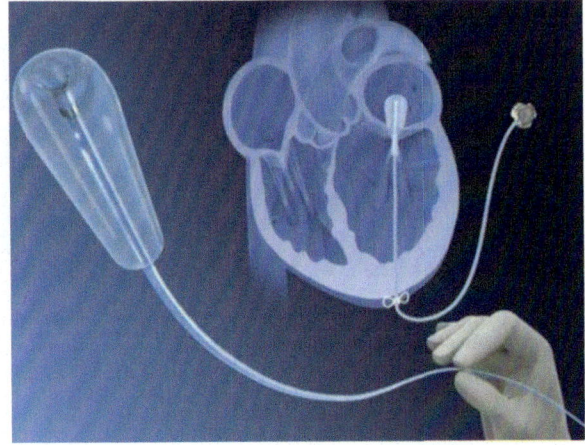

*Middle Peak Medical*: The Middle Peak (Palo Alto, California) device is an implant that functions as a posterior mitral leaflet replacement (Figs. 10.3 and 10.4). This neo-leaflet is made of dual layer ePTFE. The device is implanted directly over the existing posterior leaflet. It provides a new surface onto which the anterior leaflet can coapt. This serves several functions, including annuloplasty, by diminishing the annular area, a direct leaflet repair, and chordal support. It is intended for either

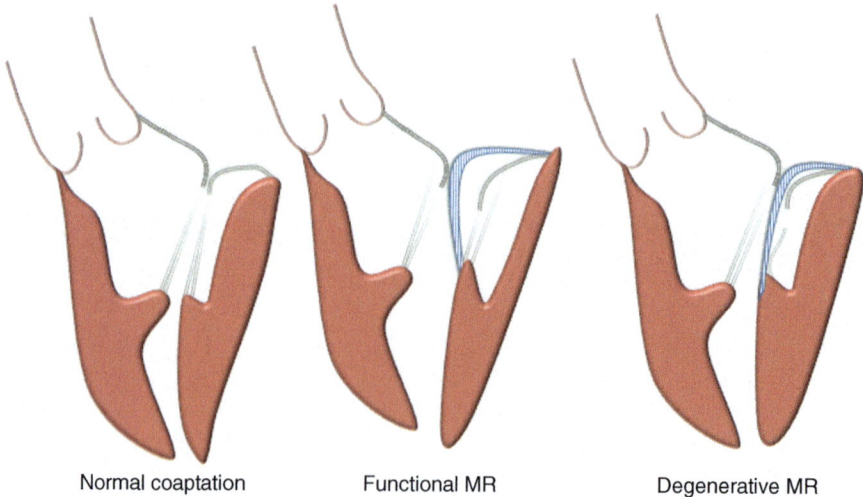

Normal coaptation          Functional MR          Degenerative MR

**Fig. 10.3** The Middle Peak device is an implant that functions as a posterior mitral leaflet replacement. It provides a new surface onto which the anterior leaflet can coapt

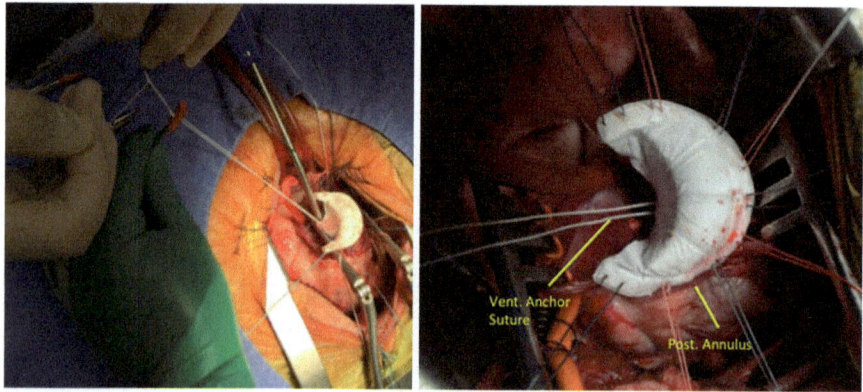

**Fig. 10.4** Intraoperative photos of Middle Peak device implantation. The Middle Peak device is implanted directly over the existing posterior leaflet. This provides several functions, including annuloplasty by diminishing the annular area, a direct leaflet repair, and chordal support. This neo-leaflet is made of dual layer ePTFE

surgical or transseptal delivery. Surgical implants have been performed in humans, and the transcatheter option is under development.

*MitraFlex*: The TransCardiac Therapeutics MitraFlex (Atlanta, GA) artificial chords and leaflet plication device are designed for a direct thorascopic approach through the apex of a beating heart [4]. MitraFlex fulfills several functions, including stabilizing and centering the leaflets, automating the capture and connection of the approximate midpoint of the leaflets, implanting artificial chordae tendineae, and reducing the annulus. Figure 10.5 shows a patent drawing. There are no published reports on the use of this system.

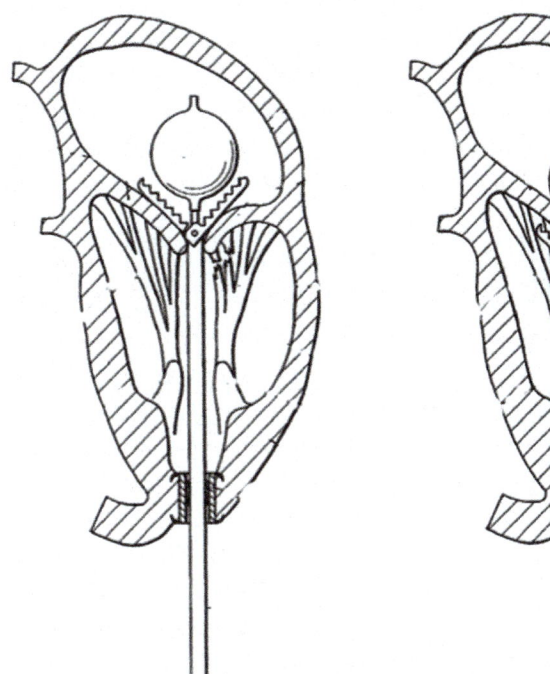

**Fig. 10.5** The TransCardiac Therapeutics MitraFlex artificial chords and leaflet plication device fulfills several functions, including stabilizing and centering the leaflets, automating the capture and connection of the approximate midpoint of the leaflets, implanting artificial chordae tendineae, and reducing the annulus

## 10.3  Indirect Annuloplasty

The only indirect annuloplasty device with EC approval and clinical use is the Cardiac Dimensions Carillon coronary sinus implant. Two indirect annuloplasty systems have previously failed, due to device fracture or coronary sinus erosion. The Edwards Monarc device (Edwards Lifesciences, Irvine, CA) used a springlike contraction band anchored with self-expanding stents at either end. The connection between the band and the stents fractured in several cases. The Viacor PTMA system (Viacor, Inc., Wilmington, MA) used nitinol rods to compress the posterior mitral annuls from within the coronary sinus, and device fractures resulted in coronary sinus perforation.

*Arto-MVRx*: The Arto System, by MVRx, Inc. (Belmont, California), is a permanent implantable device comprised of two anchors, deployed in the lateral wall of the left atrium and the atrial septum, respectively [5]. This was previously known as the PS3 system. A bridge between the two anchors provides a means for reduction of the minor axis of the mitral valve (Fig. 10.6). The procedure is performed under general anesthesia and fluoroscopic and transesophageal echocardiographic guidance. Using magnetically linked catheters and routine catheter exchanges, a coronary sinus

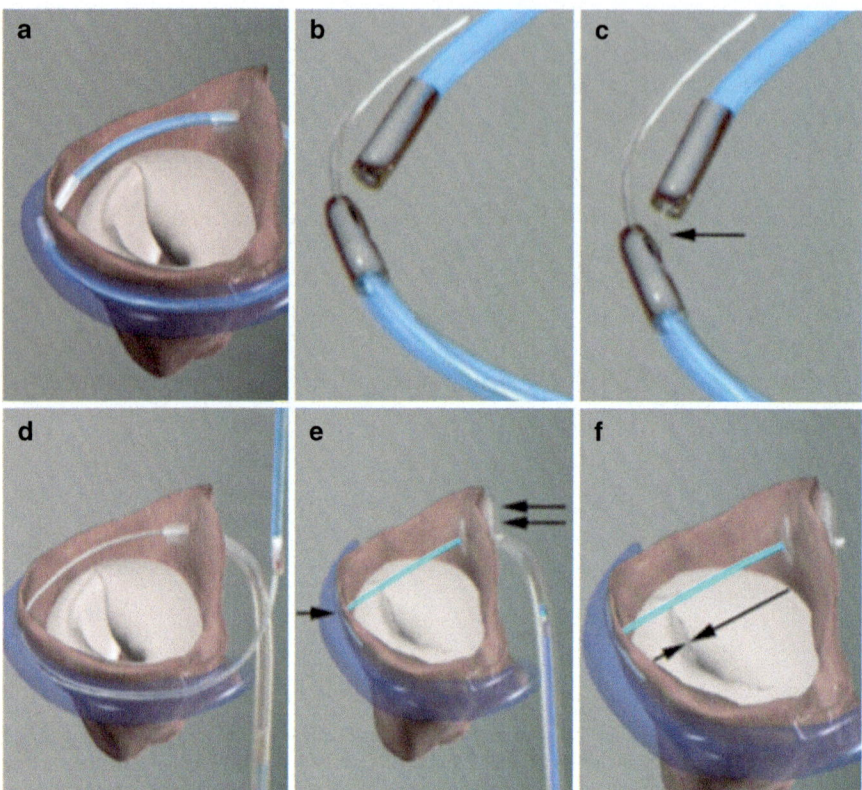

**Fig. 10.6** The Arto System implantation procedure. (**a**) Great cardiac vein (GCV) and left atrial (LA) MagneCaths in position and magnetically linked behind the P2 segment of the posterior mitral leaflet. (**b**) Close-up of magnetically linked LA and GCV MagneCaths. Each magnetic catheter has a specific shape and lumen to direct and receive the crossing wire. (**c**) The crossing wire (*arrow*) is pushed from the GCV into the LA MagneCath. The MagneCaths are aligned to direct the wire safely from the GCV to the LA through the atrial wall. (**d**) After using an exchange catheter, the loop guidewire in place across left atrium. This guidewire directs the placement of the GCV anchor (T-bar) and septal anchor. (**e**) The MVRx System in place before tensioning. T-Bar, *single arrow*; septal anchor, *double arrow*. (**f**) Tensioning of the bridge results in precise shortening of the mitral annulus anteroposterior diameter (*arrows*) and elimination of FMR; once the final position is attained, the suture is cut and secured with a suture lock

anchor (T-bar) is placed and connected by an adjustable length suture to the atrial septal anchor. The suture is tensioned to indirectly decrease the anteroposterior (AP) diameter of the mitral annulus, which results in reduction of MR. Since the implant is atrial, there is no hemodynamic instability or ventricular arrhythmias. Device efficacy is seen immediately at the time of implantation. The Arto system is adjusted with tensioning or relaxing the suture prior to lock and release of the device. The system is recapturable and retrievable during the deployment.

Clinical data from 11 patients implanted with the Arto system has been published in the MitrAl ValvE Repair Clinical Trial (MAVERIC Trial, clinicaltrials.gov identifier NCT02302872) [6]. All patients were deemed to be at high surgical risk by the heart team and were symptomatic, with most in NYHA Class III or IV. There were no procedural safety events and two clinical events within the 30-day follow-up period. One patient underwent uncomplicated surgical drainage of pericardial effusion without recurrence, and one patient had asymptomatic dislocation of the coronary sinus T-bar and underwent successful elective surgical MV replacement. At 6 months, MR grade, LV volumes, mitral annular dimensions, and functional status all improved. Pre-procedure FMR was grade 3–4+ in 90% and at 6 months was grade 1–2+ in 80%. EROA by PISA at baseline was 30.3 ± 11.1, decreasing at 6 months to 13.7 ± 8.6 mm². Regurgitant volumes decreased from 45.4 ± 15.0 to 19.9 ± 11.6 mL. LVESVi decreased from 77.5 ± 24.3 to 68.2 ± 28.2 mL/m² and LVEDVi 118.7 ± 28.6 to 104.9 ± 30.2 mL/m² at 6 months. Mitral annular anteroposterior diameter decreased from 45.0 ± 3.3 to 38.9 ± 2.7 mm. Functional status was NYHA Class III or IV in 81.8% and Class I/II in 18.2% at baseline, improving at 6 months to 50% Class III and 50% Class I/II. Enrollment of up to 20 additional patients at three sites (Riga, Latvia, Massy, France and London, United Kingdom) is underway in Phase II of the MAVERIC trial.

## 10.4    Direct Annuloplasty

There are two EC-approved percutaneous direct annuloplasty devices, the Valtech Cardioband (Valtech Cardio, Or Yehuda, Israel) and the Mitralign system (Mitralign, Inc., Tewksbury, MA). The Cardioband most closely resembles a surgical annuloplasty, while the Mitralign system uses pledgets to plicate the mitral annulus, similar to some established surgical suture annuloplasty procedures [7, 8]. Indirect annuloplasty has the potential to be simpler than direct annuloplasty, but direct approaches have the advantage of closer approximation of established surgical annuloplasty. Several other novel annuloplasty devices have been employed preclinically, used with surgical implants, or are in early human use.

*Cerclage annuloplasty*: This is a creative method for mitral annuloplasty. A wire loop is created encompassing the coronary sinus, basal myocardium, and right atrial chamber (Fig. 10.7) [9]. Annular tension is introduced through a "cerclage" suture that traverses the coronary sinus and basal septal myocardium and is secured within the right atrium. Circumferential tension is intended to reduce annular dilation and enhance mitral leaflet coaptation by introducing radial force uniformly, independent of the rotational orientation of the commissures. For cerclage, 9Fr introducer sheaths are placed percutaneously into the right jugular and femoral veins and 6Fr introducer sheaths into a femoral artery. A guidewire loop is created around the mitral annulus and LV outflow tract and then exchanged for a suture. The guidewire traverses the coronary sinus and the proximal great cardiac vein into the first septal perforator vein toward the basal interventricular septum. It is then directed across a short segment of myocardium to reenter a right heart chamber where it is snared and exchanged for a suture and tension fixation device. To conduct cerclage, a transjugular balloon-tipped guiding catheter is introduced into the

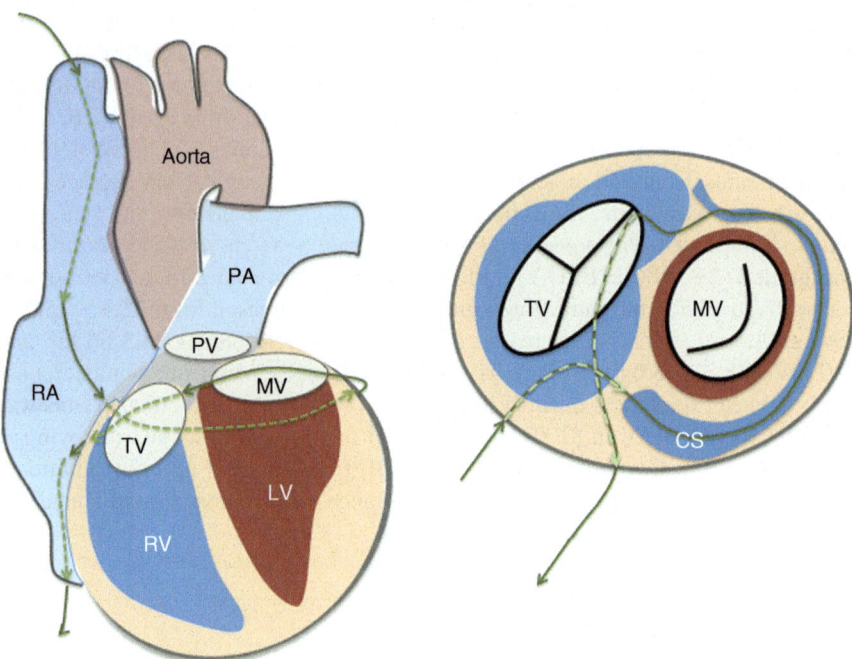

**Fig. 10.7** Cerclage annuloplasty. A guidewire is placed via the coronary sinus and then into a coronary vein. It is passed through the septal myocardium into the right ventricular outflow tract or right atrium to encircle the mitral annulus. *CS* coronary sinus, *LV* left ventricle, *MV* mitral valve, *PA* pulmonary artery, *PV* pulmonic valve, *RA* right atrium, *RV* right ventricle, *TV* tricuspid valve

coronary sinus, the occlusion balloon inflated, and a retrograde coronary contrast venogram opacifies the great cardiac vein and septal perforator veins. A stiff 0.014″ guidewire is steered into the first basal septal perforator vein. Once a right heart chamber is entered, the guidewire is snared and replaced with a braided nonabsorbable tension suture.

A unique feature of the cerclage procedure incorporates the use of circumflex coronary artery protection. The coronary sinus frequently crosses over the circumflex or one of its branches. The cerclage procedure utilizes a relatively rigid spacer device, shaped somewhat like a piece of elbow macaroni. This spacer protects the coronary from compression by the cerclage loop.

A single-center feasibility study is being conducted in Korea (ClinicalTrials.gov identifier NCT02471664). Inclusion criteria include NYHA Class III–IV with symptomatic severe functional MR despite optimal medical treatment. Optimal medical therapy includes an ACE inhibitor or angiotensin receptor blocker, β-blocker, and aldosterone antagonists for at least 3 months unless the patient is contraindicated or intolerant. Key exclusion criteria include LV ejection fraction lower than 25%, anomalies of the coronary sinus, or preexisting coronary sinus devices such as implantable cardioverter defibrillator or pacemaker, or 2:1 or higher grade AV block. Several patients have been treated successfully.

*Micardia Encor adjustable surgical annuloplasty ring*: This is currently a surgical annuloplasty ring with a percutaneous adjustment mechanism (R&D Surgical Ltd, UK) [10]. The concept is that late postoperative adjustment of the ring could be an advantage. The ring is deformable, nickel–titanium based. It is heated for 45 s, which induces a change of geometry to a preformed reduced anterior–posterior diameter.

In a clinical trial of 94 patients, a smaller ring size was implanted in patients with ischemic mitral regurgitation to "downsize" the mitral annulus [11]. A permanent lead was attached to the ring in the P2/P3 region. It was routed through the atrial wall to a subcutaneous pocket. If an adjustment was required, the lead was accessed by a small incision and connected to a generator. The ring adjusted its form during the activation procedure to a preformed shape with a reduced anterior–posterior diameter. The median age was 71 (range 64–75) years with EuroSCORE II 6.7 ± 6.3. Two-thirds were male, 48% had ischemic MR, 37% had dilated cardiomyopathy, and 15% degenerative disease. Operative mortality was 1%, and the 1-year survival was 93%. Ring adjustment was attempted in 12 patients at a mean interval of 9 ± 6 months after surgery. In three of these attempts, a technical failure occurred. In one patient, mitral regurgitation was reduced two grades, in two patients mitral regurgitation was reduced one grade, and in six patients mitral regurgitation did not change significantly. The mean grade of mitral regurgitation changed from 2.9 ± 0.9 to 2.1 ± 0.7 ($P = 0.02$). Five patients were reoperated after 11 ± 9 months (ring dehiscence, 2; failed adjustment, 3). Based on this early experience, the authors concluded that an adjustable ring may provide an additional option for recurrent MR. A percutaneous version, enCorTC, is under development.

*Millipede*: This is an annuloplasty ring that is anchored to the mitral (or tricuspid) annulus using screws and is then mechanically cinched to reduce the mitral annular circumference (Fig. 10.8). It is a complete ring (Millipede, LLC, Ann Arbor, MI) [12]. The cinching or adjustment is done in real time with echo guidance to optimize the reduction of MR. Several patients have had operative implants. A catheter system for percutaneous delivery is under development. An international trial, Annular Reshaping of the Mitral Valve for MR Using the Millipede IRIS System,

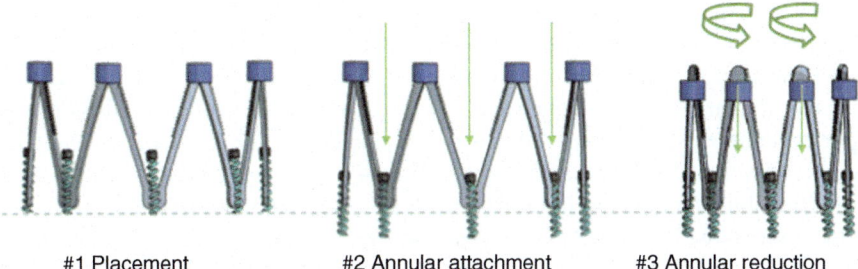

#1 Placement          #2 Annular attachment          #3 Annular reduction

**Fig. 10.8** Millipede annuloplasty ring is a complete ring that is anchored in the mitral or tricuspid annulus using screws and is then mechanically cinched to reduce the mitral annular circumference. The cinching or adjustment is done in real time with echo guidance to optimize the reduction of MR

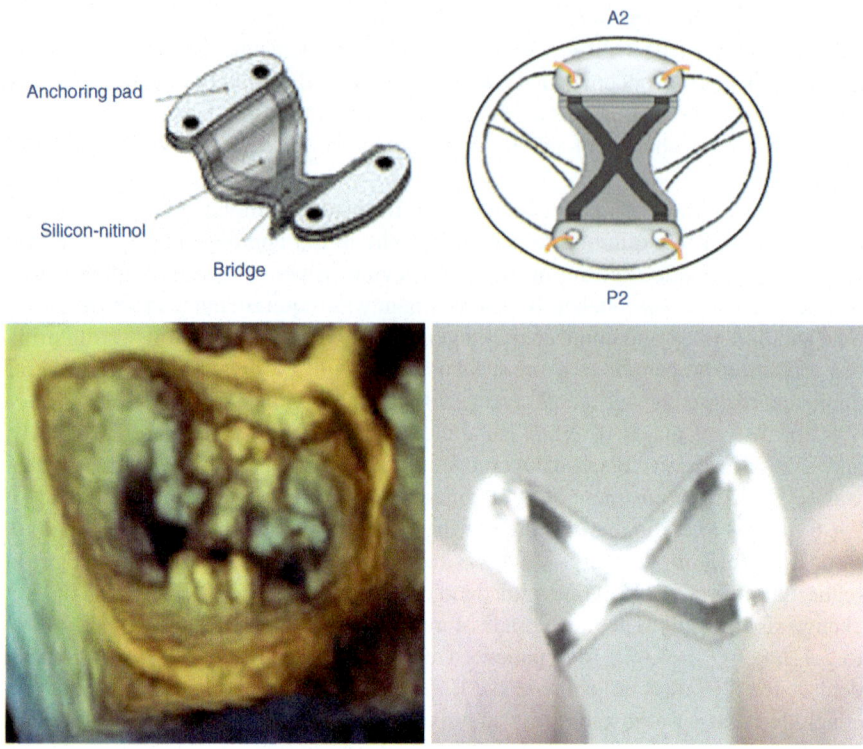

**Fig. 10.9** Mitral bridge is a novel surgical annular repair device that is sutured from the septal to the lateral annulus. It is placed between A2 and P2 at annular level with standard sutures

for symptomatic severe MR (effective regurgitant orifice (ERO) $\geq 0.2$ cm$^2$ for secondary MR, ERO $\geq 0.4$ cm$^2$, for primary MR) is registered with ClinicalTrials.gov Identifier NCT02607527 anticipating enrollment of approximately ten patients beginning March 2016.

*Mitral bridge*: This is a novel surgical annular repair device. Rather than encircling the mitral annulus with a ring, a nitinol bridge is sutured from the septal to the lateral annulus (Fig. 10.9). It is placed between A2 and P2 at annular level with standard sutures. It is available in five sizes from 22 to 30 mm. Thirty-four patients have been treated in an EC-approved trial. Three-quarters had Type I MR with annular dilatation, and one-quarter had Type III-b ischemic MR. Chronic AF was present in 88%. All 34 successful implants resulted in a decrease of MR to <1+. One patient developed a paravalvular leak and required reoperation at 7 months post implantation, and one developed a paravalvular leak and required catheter closure after 18 months. The device is unique in that it reduces and stabilizes the anteroposterior annular dimension without the use of annular trigone-to-trigone anchoring. It has been hypothesized that part of the mechanism of action for MitraClip is anteroposterior annular stabilization by the tissue bridge that develops after edge-to-edge repair [13].

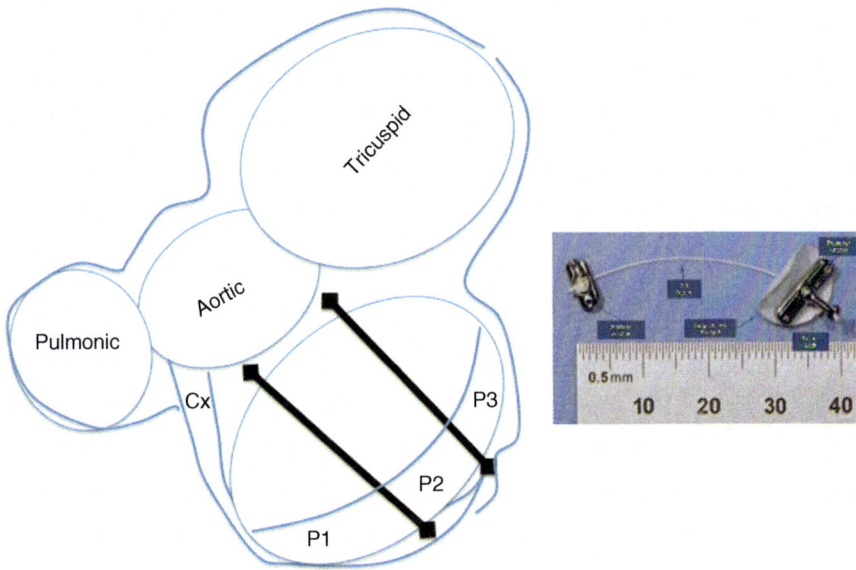

**Fig. 10.10** Transapical segmental reduction annuloplasty (TASRA) is based on the experimental concept of septal–lateral annular cinching. A suture is placed from mid-anterior annulus to the posterior LV wall to accomplish annular cinching

*MitraSpan TASRA*: The TASRA technique (Belmont, MA), Transapical Segmental Reduction Annuloplasty, is based on the experimental concept of septal–lateral annular cinching (SLAC). The SLAC concept was first described in adult sheep with acute ischemic MR produced by circumflex occlusion. A suture is placed from the mid-anterior annulus to the posterior LV wall (Fig. 10.10). This resulted in an anteroposterior reduction of 22% [14]. Subsequent studies found MR elimination in a chronic ischemic sheep model, with preservation of both leaflet mobility and the normal saddle shape of the mitral annulus [15, 16]. The feasibility of suture implants is generally established by the precedents of the components of the procedure, including neochordal implants, the Myocor device [17], and suture annuloplasty. There is some evidence of trigone anchoring as the most secure.

The device system is transapical and low profile (12 F or 9 + 5 F). It allows for a direct approach to the critical locations for device implantation using short tools. Tissue crossing uses a 0.018″ wire. There are pledgeted anchors on the LV side and by the trigones. The procedure is TEE-guided, with pre-procedure planning with multi-slice CT.

The safety of implants and biocompatibility of the polyester suture and stainless steel anchors have been demonstrated in preclinical studies of 60 acute and chronic porcine implants with up to 12 weeks pathology and in 18 consecutive chronic animal implants out to 30 days. In these preclinical studies, efficacy to reduce annular diameter by 20–40% was confirmed.

A human feasibility study of the MitraSpan device (SPARE-MR) has been initiated outside the USA. The major inclusion criteria include moderate–severe, symptomatic, secondary MR with LVEF 20–50%. An IDE early feasibility study has been approved by the FDA. The long-term goal is to develop nearly percutaneous LV access with a procedure that could include both a subvalvular/papillary displacement component and an annular correction.

*QuantumCor*: The QuantumCor (QuantumCor, Inc., Lake Forest, CA) system uses a radiofrequency system to shrink collagen, resulting in remodeling of the annulus. The RF energy is administered with electrodes that are delivered transseptally. In preclinical work described in 2008, the device was evaluated in 16 animals [18]. Acutely, all responded appropriately with a mean septal–lateral reduction of 21.7%. Seven animals survived for 4–180 days, in which the mean septal–lateral reduction was 26.5%, with some expectation that additional remodeling might occur as the collagen matrix heals.

*Valcare AMEND*: Valcare (Herzliya Pituach, Israel) has developed a minimally invasive D-shaped ring technology, the AMEND device, which emulates a surgical closed, semirigid D-shaped annuloplasty ring (Fig. 10.11) [20]. The system is

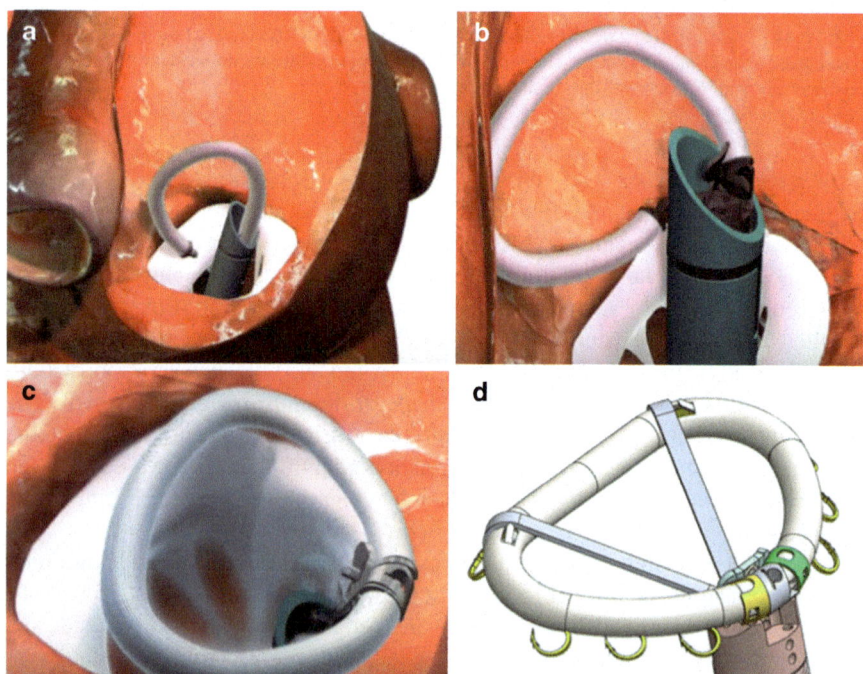

**Fig. 10.11** The Valcare AMEND device emulates a closed surgical semirigid D-shaped annuloplasty ring. (**a**) The system is delivered via apical LV access into the mitral annulus in a linear configuration through a catheter to the target site. (**b**) As it is advanced, it changes geometry above the annulus using a series of remotely activated mechanisms [19]. (**c**) The result is a complete D-shaped ring. (**d**) A series of 12 anchors in four zones that are independently deployed attach the ring to the annulus

delivered via apical LV access into the mitral annulus. The implant is delivered under fluoroscopic and echo guidance in a linear configuration through a catheter to the target site, and as it is advanced from the guide catheter system, it changes geometry above the annulus using a series of remotely activated mechanisms. The result is a complete D-shaped ring. A series of 12 anchors in four zones that are independently deployed attach the ring into the annulus. The posterior anchors are placed first and then pulled toward the anterior side to reduce the anteroposterior dimension, thus reducing the septal–lateral dimension and mitral circumference. This technology creates an opportunity to use it as a platform for mitral valve replacement, possibly using valve prosthesis proven in aortic position. The system has been tested in preclinical models.

## 10.5    Chamber and Annular Remodeling

It has been recognized for many years that direct surgical annuloplasty is effective at reducing MR severity in functional MR but that recurrence rates are as high as almost 60% in the first 2 years after annuloplasty [21] and that annuloplasty has no direct effect on LV function, which is at the root of functional MR. Only one device has ever shown a survival advantage compared to annuloplasty for functional MR in a randomized trial, the Myocor Coapsys system (Myocor, Maple Grove, MN). This device remodeled both the mitral annulus and the LV, but unfortunately the manufacturer lost funding and went out of business in 2008. Other devices have effects on both annular and LV remodeling.

*Guided Delivery Systems*: The Accucinch System (Guided Delivery Systems, Santa Clara, CA) implants multiple anchors in the mitral basal annular myocardium. A tether connects the anchors, and tension of the catheter diminishes the mitral annular circumference (Fig. 10.12). This approach results in both diminution of the annular circumference and, at the same time, stabilization or remodeling of the basal LV myocardium. The concept is thus a combination of LV remodeling and annuloplasty.

The Guided Delivery Systems Accucinch device places a delivery system below the posterior mitral leaflet on the ventricular side, through which between 10 and 20 nitinol anchors are delivered. Thus, the base of the LV is remodeled at the same time as the annulus. These anchors are tethered by a drawstring, which is tensioned to reduce the mitral annulus. An incomplete ring approach has some precedents in surgery. Surgical annular plication without placement of an annular ring has shown some efficacy in reducing MR.

Several patients have been treated over the last few years as the system has evolved, but there is no published experience. A Feasibility Study Using the Accucinch System in the Left Ventricular Reshaping of the Mitral Apparatus to Reduce Functional Mitral Regurgitation and Improve Left Ventricular Function Trial (LV RECOVER, ClinicalTrials.gov identifier NCT02153892) has been designed. The inclusion criteria include patients with severe symptomatic functional MR of $\geq$3+ secondary to LV or annular remodeling, as measured in

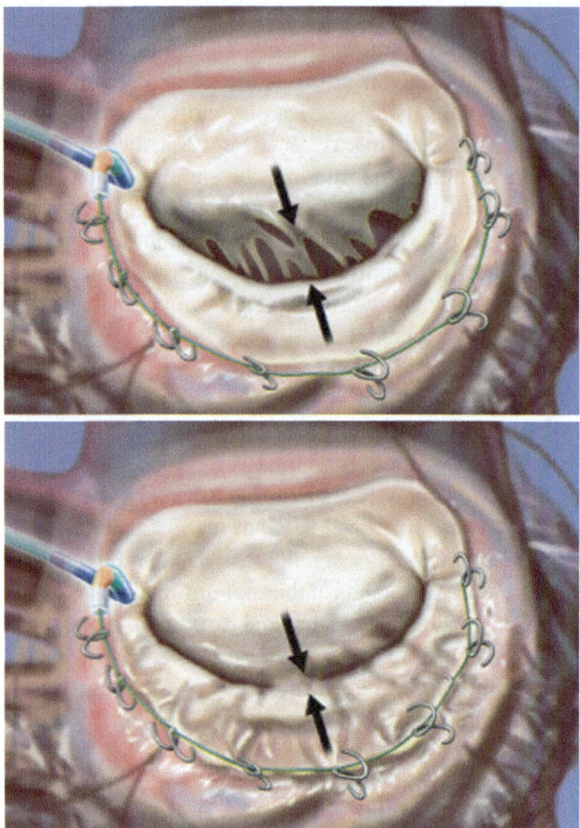

**Fig. 10.12** The Guided Delivery Systems Accucinch device is delivered through retrograde cath-eterization of the LV (**a**). The *arrows* highlight the separation of the leaflet edges, which define the regurgitant orifice. Anchors are placed in the posterior mitral annulus and connected with a "draw-string" to cinch the annular circumference. When the cord is tightened, the basilar myocardium and annulus draw the mitral leaflets together to decrease the regurgitant orifice (**b**); artwork by Craig Skaggs. From Feldman T, Young A. Percutaneous approaches to valve repair for mitral regurgitation. J Am Coll Cardiol. 2014;63: 2057–68

accordance with the current ASE guidelines and suitable for treatment in accordance with the current AHA/ACC guidelines with LVEF ≥20% and ≤40%, stable cardiac medical regimen for heart failure for at least 1 month, and stable NYHA Classification (Class III and above) for at least 1 month. A second study, Percutaneous Left Ventricular Reshaping to Reduce Functional Mitral Regurgitation and Improve LV Function (LVRESTORESA), is also listed on the ClinicalTrials.gov web site (identifier NCT01899573). This second investigation is being conducted in Medellin, Colombia. When updated to December 1, 2015, there were ten patients enrolled in the two trials. A third study, Safety and Performance of the Accucinch System NCT02624960, apparently planned in

Germany and the UK, is a single-arm, multicenter, open-label controlled study that will assess the safety and performance of the Accucinch System to induce left ventricular reverse remodeling and reduce the severity of functional mitral regurgitation in symptomatic adult patients with mitral regurgitation and left ventricular remodeling due to dilated cardiomyopathy (ischemic or nonischemic etiology) and who are at high operative risk. Enrollment has not been reported and targeted completion is set for 2019.

*Mardil extracardiac annuloplasty*: BACE (Basal Annuloplasty of the Cardia Externally, Mardil, Inc. Minneapolis, MN) is a tension band with inflatable silicone chambers that is wrapped around a section of the heart and is thus an extra-cardiac device (Fig. 10.13). BACE does not require open-heart surgery. The company is developing a tool to implant the BACE device through a small incision, as a minimally invasive procedure. After the device is sutured to the heart, the chambers are filled with saline via tubing connected to subcutaneous ports. The saline applies pressure at the basal LV to approximate the mitral leaflets. The saline levels can be adjusted during or after the procedure to provide the appropriate pressure needed to minimize functional MR. The pilot clinical study enrolled 11 patients at medical centers in India and showed clinical efficacy and no device-related safety concerns. Results in five patients have been published [22]. All five patients were male, NYHA Class III, with LVEF of 20–40%. Epicardial application and adjustment of the BACE device was performed on a beating heart with effective reduction in FMR to grade <1. All five patients also had three bypass grafts. Reduction in MR was sustained for at least 6 months, and there were no unanticipated or device-related

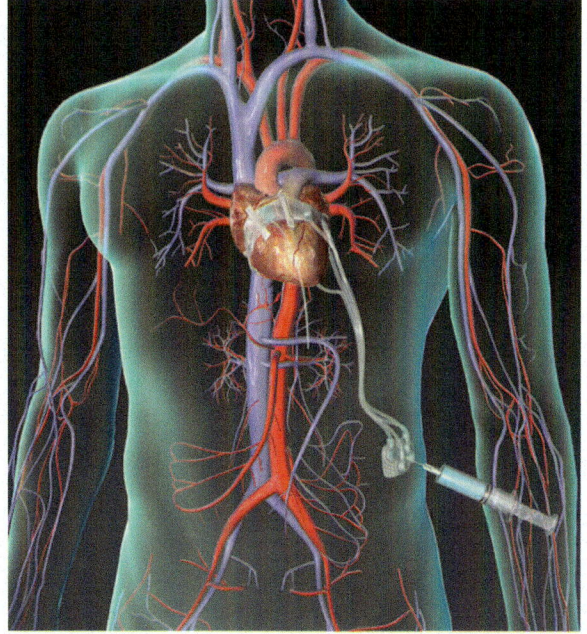

**Fig. 10.13** BACE (Basal Annuloplasty of the Cardia Externally) is a tension band with inflatable silicone chambers that is wrapped around a section of the heart and is thus an extra-cardiac device. After the device is sutured to the heart, the chambers are filled with saline via tubing connected to subcutaneous ports. The saline applies pressure at the basal LV to approximate the mitral leaflets. The saline levels can be adjusted during or after the procedure to provide the appropriate pressure needed to minimize functional MR

adverse events. The system is being further studied in a 14-patient trial, the Evaluation of the Minimally Invasive VenTouch System in the Treatment of Functional MR (ClinicalTrials.gov Identifier NCT02671799), with centers recruiting in France and Malaysia and additional centers planned in Canada, the Czech Republic, and the Netherlands. There is also progress in a CE Mark study with 30 implants performed worldwide out of a total enrollment of 50.

## 10.6   Chordal Repair

The use of artificial chordae tendineae is an established repair method for degenerative MR. Methods for implanting neo-chordae via transapical beating-heart approaches have been developed and commercialized, and percutaneous approaches are under development.

*Harpoon*: This is another transapical system for placement of ePTFE neochords. The system uses echo guidance for real-time titration of the chordal length (Fig. 10.14). The delivery system is 6F. The chords have a preformed ePTFE knot that is formed on the atrial surface of the leaflet, which securely anchors the suture. The anchoring is equivalent to that accomplished with surgical chord placement. Normal chords have a pull-out force of 0.1–0.3 N. Conventional surgical chords have a pull-out force of 8.34 ± 3.29 N, while for Harpoon chords the pull-out force measured 8.58 ± 3.34 N, tested in 11 hearts during bench testing.

An early feasibility study was done in ten patients, in 2015, in Warsaw [23]. The population was at low risk, with normal LVEF, a mean age of 66 years, and a mean STS risk of 1.26%. Preoperative MR grade by core laboratory was severe in all patients. There was 100% procedural success. A mean of 3.6 chords per patient was placed. The introducer time was 36 min, and skin-to-skin time was 107 min. At 30-day follow-up echo, the MR grade was none or trace in most and moderate in two of the seven who had reached that time point. There was no perioperative mortality, stroke, or blood transfusion. There were two reoperations for delayed tamponade on postoperative days 5 and 13 and one late reoperation for recurrent MR on postoperative day 72.

*MISTRAL*: The MISTRAL Chordal repair (Mitralix Ltd, Jerusalem) uses a transseptally delivered 3D nitinol spiral-shaped atraumatic wire implant for grasping the chordae tendineae from both mitral valve leaflets in order to bring them closer together (Fig. 10.15). When the spiral is rotated, the chordae become closer, the gap between the leaflets is decreased, and coaptation is significantly improved. The system relies on a 12F off-the-shelf guide catheter (Agilis, St. Jude Medical, St. Paul, MN). The delivery system is 7.5F. By transseptal percutaneous approach, the 12F guiding catheter is delivered into the left atrium and steered towards the mitral valve, and the applicator catheter end is advanced into the left ventricle. The MISTRAL ventricular spiral is released, and by echo guidance, the spiral is turned to capture anterior and posterior leaflet chordae. The spiral is turned back and forth, and the regurgitant jet is measured by echo until the desired outcome is achieved. The applicator catheter is then drawn back to the atrium, and the atrial spiral is released. Some implants have been done in an acute porcine model, and one

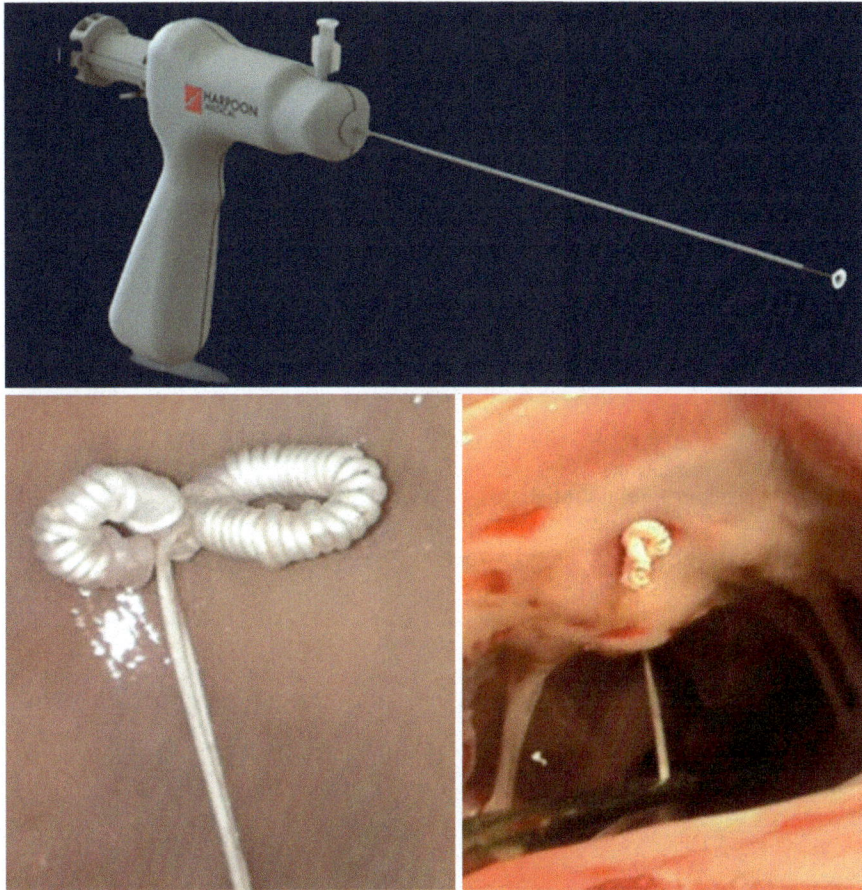

**Fig. 10.14** Harpoon is another transapical system for placement of ePTFE neochords. The delivery system is 6F. The chords have a preformed ePTFE knot that is formed on the atrial surface of the leaflet, which securely anchors the suture. The anchoring is equivalent to that accomplished with surgical chord placement. The system uses echo guidance for real-time titration of the chordal length

procedure was done, in January 2016, in a patient with tricuspid valve regurgitation, under compassionate use.

*Mitralis*: Mitralis (Norwell, MA) has described a system for degenerative mitral regurgitation with a leaflet restraint, still in the concept stage (Fig. 10.16). This system uses an annular anchor and extensions anchored in the LV and so is not distinctly either an annuloplasty or a chordal device. An annuloplasty device is placed along the mitral annulus, and an anchor is then embedded into tissue in the left ventricle. A restraining matrix is extended between the annuloplasty member and the LV anchor such that the restraining matrix is draped over a leaflet of the mitral valve. Adjustment of the restraining matrix is performed to correct one or more prolapsing segments of the leaflet.

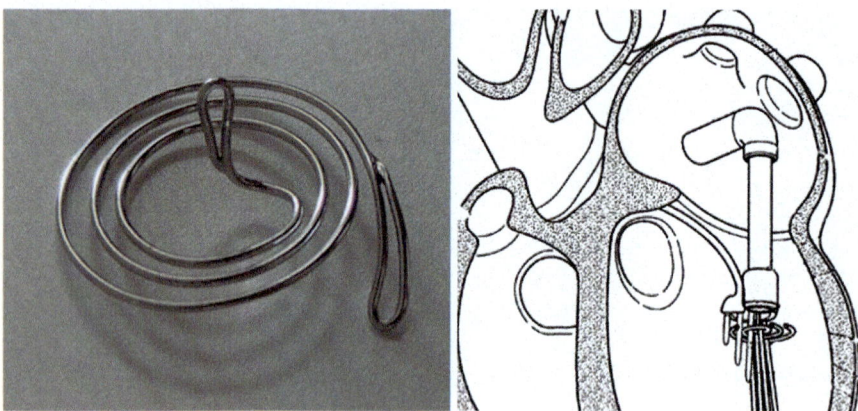

**Fig. 10.15** The MISTRAL chordal repair uses a transseptally delivered 3D nitinol spiral-shaped wire implant for grasping the chordae tendineae from both mitral valve leaflets in order to bring them closer together. When the spiral is rotated, the chordae become closer, the gap between the leaflets is decreased, and coaptation is significantly improved

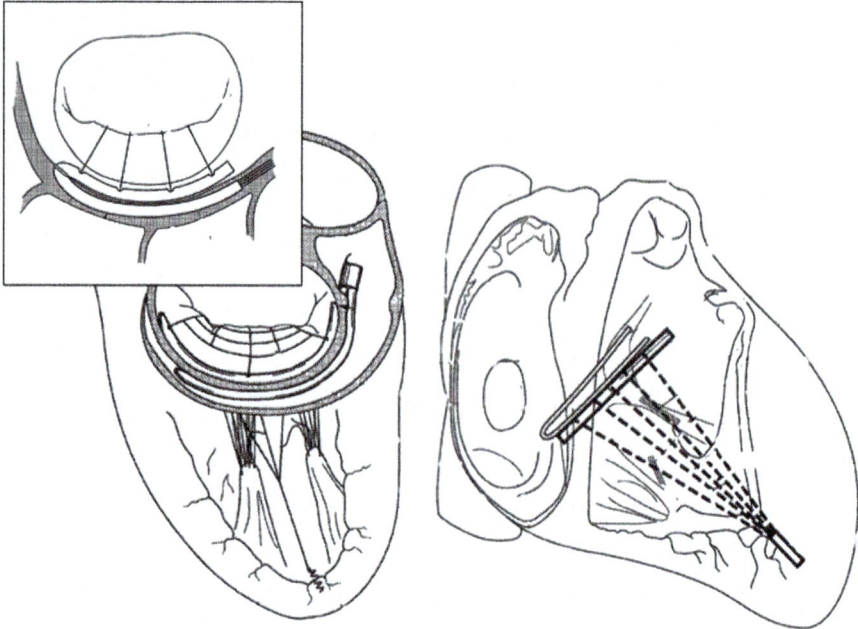

**Fig. 10.16** Mitralis has described a system for degenerative MR, still in the concept stage. This system uses an annular anchor and extensions anchored in the LV, so it is not distinctly either an annuloplasty or a chordal device. An annuloplasty device is placed along the mitral annulus, and an anchor is then embedded into tissue in the left ventricle. A restraining matrix is extended between the annuloplasty member and the LV anchor such that the restraining matrix is draped over a leaflet of the mitral valve. Adjusting the restraining matrix is done to correct one or more prolapsing segments of the leaflet

*NeoChord*: The transapical off-pump mitral valve intervention with neochord implantation (TOP-MINI) is performed using the NeoChord DS1000 system (NeoChord, Inc., Eden Prairie, MN) under 2D and 3D transesophageal echocardiography guidance for both implantation and tension adjustment of the neochordae [24, 25]. The Transapical Artificial Chordae Tendineae (TACT) trial showed that the procedure is feasible and reproducible, with low rate of complications [26]. A recent registry confirmed the acute safety of the procedure, with improved clinical outcomes compared with previous published reports [27]. Further outcomes have been reported at 3 months [28]. Forty-nine patients with severe symptomatic degenerative MR were treated. Median age was 72 years (IQR 58–78) and median Euroscore-I was 3.26% (IQR 0.88–8.15); 89.8% presented with posterior leaflet prolapse, 8.2% with anterior prolapsed, and 2% with bileaflet prolapse. Acute procedure success, defined as successful placement of at least three neochords with residual MR less than 2+, was achieved in all patients. In-hospital mortality was 2%. At 30 days, major adverse events included one AMI (2%) successfully treated percutaneously and one case of sepsis (2%), with no stroke or bleeding events. At 3 months, overall survival was 98%. MR was absent in 33.4%, grade 1+ in 31.2%, and grade 2+ in 25%; 10.4% developed recurrent severe MR due to anterior native chord rupture. Four of these were successfully reoperated. At 3 months follow-up, freedom from reoperation was 91.7 ± 4%.

*Valtech V-Chordal*: Degenerative MR frequently (84%) involves ruptured or elongated chordae. Conventional surgical procedures involve creation of neochordae using Gore-tex suture anchored in the papillary muscle and are technically challenging. Estimation of proper length is made on a flaccid heart. Improper chordal length contributes to residual MR. The V Chordal Adjustable Artificial Chordae System (Or Yehuda, Israel) proposes accurate and reliable fixation to the head of the papillary muscle using beating-heart procedures. Fine-tuning of the leaflet coaptation length and depth is possible with millimeter resolution, and off-pump adjustment of chordal length is done under physiological loading conditions. In animal models there is an excellent tissue ingrowth. Surgical feasibility has been shown in six patients in a European study. Four patients completed 1 year of follow-up. The accumulated implant time was about 10 years, with one death, which was not device-related, 3 months post procedure.

A conceptual transfemoral V Chordal procedure has several steps. Reaching the papillary muscle is accomplished by placing a wire through the mitral valve, inserting a chordae-capturing device over it, and advancing the capturing device to the papillary muscle. Anchoring to the papillary muscle is done using the chordae-capturing device for advancement of an anchor to the papillary muscle. The capturing device is removed, leaving the anchor in place. A guide wire exits from the anchor. Grasping of the leaflets is accomplished by advancing a grasping device over the wire that extends from the anchor. The clip is positioned at the location of the prolapse. The clip is attached to the leaflet, connecting the adjustment element to the anchor. Length adjustment is made with an adjustment tool over the wire to minimize MR, with further adjustment as needed before detaching the system and leaving the implant in place. Each of the component steps is based on existing capabilities from other device developments.

### Conclusions

There are a remarkable number and spectrum of devices under development for percutaneous mitral repair. The slow development of catheter mitral replacement systems and the growing positive international experience with the EC- and US-approved repair devices suggest there will be a role for percutaneous mitral repair for at least the near future, if not indefinitely.

## References

1. Webb JG, Maisano F, Vahanian A, Mundt B, Naqvi TZ, Bonan R, Zarbatany D, Buchbinder M. Percutaneous suture edge-to-edge repair of the mitral valve. EuroIntervention. 2009;5(1):86–9.
2. http://www.cardica.com/contact-us.php. Accessed 28 Apr 2016.
3. http://www.cardiosolutionsinc.com/mitra-spacer.html. Accessed 28 Apr 2016.
4. http://www.transcardiac.com/products/. Accessed 28 Apr 2016.
5. Rogers JH, Macoviak JA, Rahdert DA, Takeda PA, Palacios IF, Low RI. Percutaneous septal sinus shortening: a novel procedure for the treatment of functional mitral regurgitation. Circulation. 2006;113:2329–34.
6. Rogers JH, Thomas M, Morice MC, Narbute I, Zabunova M, Hovasse T, Poupineau M, Rudzitis A, Kamzola G, Zvaigzne L, Greene S, Erglis A. Treatment of heart failure with associated functional mitral regurgitation using the ARTO system: initial results of the first-in-human mitral valve repair clinical trial (MAVERIC). JACC Cardiovasc Interv. 2015;8(8):1095–104. doi:10.1016/j.jcin.2015.04.012. Epub 24 June 2015.
7. Barlow CW, Ali ZA, Lim E, Barlow JB, Wells FC. Modified technique for mitral repair without ring annuloplasty. Ann Thorac Surg. 2003;75:298–300.
8. Nagy ZL, Peterffy A. Mitral annuloplasty with a suture technique. Eur J Cardiothorac Surg. 2000;18:739–41.
9. Kim JH, Kocaturk O, Ozturk C, Faranesh AZ, Sonmez M, Sampath S, Saikus CE, Kim AH, Raman VK, Derbyshire JA, Schenke WH, Wright VJ, Berry C, McVeigh ER, Lederman RJ. Mitral cerclage annuloplasty, a novel transcatheter treatment for secondary mitral valve regurgitation: initial results in swine. J Am Coll Cardiol. 2009;54(7):638–51. doi:10.1016/j.jacc.2009.03.071.
10. http://www.rdsurgical.com/MiCardiaEnCorSQ.htm. Accessed 28 Apr 2016.
11. Andreasa M, Dollb N, Livesey S, Castella M, Kocher A, Casselman F, Voth V, Bannister C, Palacios JFE, Pereda D, Laufer G, Czesla M. Safety and feasibility of a novel adjustable mitral annuloplasty ring: a multicentre European experience. Eur J Cardiothorac Surg. 2015;1–6. doi:10.1093/ejcts/ezv015.
12. Smith TW, Bolling SF, Rogers JH. Next-generation percutaneous mitral and tricuspid valve repair approaches. Cardiac Interventions Today August/September 2009.
13. Feldman T, Kar S, Elmariah S, Smart SC, Trento A, Siegel RJ, Apruzzese P, Fail P, Rinaldi MJ, Smalling RW, Hermiller JB, Heimansohn D, Gray WA, Grayburn PA, Mack MJ, Lim DS, Ailawadi G, Herrmann HC, Acker MA, Silvestry FE, Foster E, Wang A, Glower DD, Mauri L, for the EVEREST II Investigators. Randomized comparison of percutaneous repair and surgery for mitral regurgitation 5-year results of EVEREST II (endovascular valve edge-to-edge repair study). J Am Coll Cardiol. 2015;66:2844–54.
14. Timek TA, Lai DT, Tibayan F, Liang D, Daughters GT, Dagum P, Ingels NB Jr, Miller DC. Septal-lateral annular cinching abolishes acute ischemic mitral regurgitation. J Thorac Cardiovasc Surg. 2002;123(5):881–8.
15. Tibayan FA, Rodriguez F, Langer F, Zasio MK, Bailey L, Liang D, Daughters GT, Ingels NB Jr, Miller DC. Does septal-lateral annular cinching work for chronic ischemic mitral regurgitation? J Thorac Cardiovasc Surg. 2004;127(3):654–63.

16. Timek TA, Lai DT, Liang D, Tibayan F, Langer F, Rodriguez F, Daughters GT, Ingels NB Jr, Miller DC. Effects of paracommissural septal-lateral annular cinching on acute ischemic mitral regurgitation. Circulation. 2004;110(11 Suppl 1):II79–84.
17. Grossi EA, Patel N, Woo YJ, Goldberg JD, Schwartz CF, Subramanian V, Feldman T, Bourge R, Baumgartner N, Genco C, Goldman S, Zenati M, Wolfe JA, Mishra YK, Trehan N, Mittal S, Shang S, Mortier TJ, Schweich CJ. Outcomes of the RESTOR-MV trial (Randomized evaluation of a surgical treatment for off-pump repair of the mitral valve). J Am Coll Cardiol. 2010;56:1984–93.
18. Goel R, Witzel T, Dickens D, Takeda PA, Heuser RR. The QuantumCor device for treating mitral regurgitation: an animal study. Catheter Cardiovasc Interv. 2009;74(1):43–8. doi:10.1002/ccd.21.
19. https://www.youtube.com/watch?v=tQY-BJZpKKw. Accessed 20 May 2016.
20. http://www.valcaremedical.com/. Accessed 20 May 2016.
21. Goldstein D, Moskowitz AJ, Gelijns AC, Ailawadi G, Parides MK, Perrault LP, Hung JW, Voisine P, Dagenais F, Gillinov AM, Thourani V, Argenziano M, Gammie JS, Mack M, Demers P, Atluri P, Rose EA, O'Sullivan K, Williams DL, Bagiella E, Michler RE, Weisel RD, Miller MA, Geller NL, Taddei-Peters WC, Smith PK, Moquete E, Overbey JR, Kron IL, O'Gara PT, Acker MA, CTSN. Two-year outcomes of surgical treatment of severe ischemic mitral regurgitation. N Engl J Med. 2016;374(4):344–53.
22. Raman J, Jagannathan R, Chandrashekar P, Sugeng L. Can we repair the mitral valve from outside the heart? A novel extra-cardiac approach to functional mitral regurgitation. Heart Lung Circ. 2011;20:157–62.
23. Gammie JS, Bartus K, Kolsut P, Gackowski A, D'Ambra MN, Hung JW, Sadowski J, Kapelak B, Kusmierczyk M, Bilewska A, Szymanski P, Ghoreishi M. Harpoon mitral valve repair: design and update. Presented at TCT 2015.
24. Seeburger J, Borger MA, Tschernich H, Leontjev S, Holzhey D, Noack T, Ender J, Mohr FW. Transapical beating heart mitral valve repair. Circ Cardiovasc Interv. 2010;3(6):611–2.
25. Colli A, Manzan E, Fabio FZ, Sarais C, Pittarello D, Speziali G, Gerosa G. TEE-guided transapical beating-heart neochord implantation in mitral regurgitation. JACC Cardiovasc Imaging. 2014;7(3):322–3. doi:10.1016/j.jcmg.2014.01.003.
26. Seeburger J, Rinaldi M, Nielsen SL, Salizzoni S, Lange R, Schoenburg M, Alfieri O, Borger MA, Mohr FW, Aidietis A. Off-pump transapical implantation of artificial neo-chordae to correct mitral regurgitation: the TACT Trial (Transapical Artificial Chordae Tendineae) proof of concept. J Am Coll Cardiol. 2014;63(9):914–9.
27. Colli A, Manzan E, Rucinskas K, Janusauskas V, Zucchetta F, Zakarkaitė D, Aidietis A, Gerosa G. Acute safety and efficacy of the NeoChord procedure. Interact Cardiovasc Thorac Surg. 2015;20(5):575–80; discussion 580–1.
28. Colli A, Manzan E, Zucchetta F, Bizzotto E, Besola L, Bagozzi L, Bellu R, Sarais C, Pittarello D, Gerosa G. Transapical off-pump mitral valve repair with Neochord implantation: early clinical results. Int J Cardiol. 2016;204:23–8.

# Transcatheter Mitral Valve Implantation

**11**

Adrian Attinger-Toller, Anson Cheung, and John G. Webb

## 11.1 Introduction

Mitral regurgitation (MR) is the most common cardiac valve pathology in Western countries. The estimated prevalence of moderate and severe MR in the USA is 2–2.5 million [1], and its presence may contribute to an impaired prognosis [2–7]. Furthermore, MR is the second most frequent valve disease requiring surgery in Europe [8]. In degenerative MR, surgical treatment by reconstruction rather than replacement is well established based on excellent long-term outcomes and effective reduction of MR [9]. For functional MR, however, isolated mitral valve (MV) surgery is less well established due to less favorable surgical results and the lack of evidence for the benefit of surgery over medical therapy [10].

Though surgery remains the gold standard treatment for significant MR, many patients, regardless of MR etiology, are declined surgery due to their high operative risk [11]. The Euro Heart Survey revealed that up to 50% of patients hospitalized with symptomatic severe MR are not referred for MV surgery, mainly because of advanced age, comorbidities, and left ventricular (LV) dysfunction [8]. The desire for less invasive approaches has led to the development of a variety of percutaneous approaches for treating MR. This chapter aims to introduce five transcatheter MV implantation (TMVI) devices, which are the only MV valves currently being used in human trials.

A. Attinger-Toller • A. Cheung • J.G. Webb (✉)
Center for Heart Valve Innovation, St Paul's Hospital, Vancouver, BC, Canada
e-mail: webb@providencehealth.bc.ca

© Springer International Publishing AG 2018
C. Tamburino et al. (eds.), *Percutaneous Treatment of Left Side Cardiac Valves*,
https://doi.org/10.1007/978-3-319-59620-4_11

### 11.1.1 Transcatheter MV Repair

Several percutaneous transcatheter MV repair technologies have recently emerged as possible alternatives to open heart surgery for high-risk patients. The MitraClip™ system was one of the first transcatheter devices to be commercialized and is now widely available [12–14]. Other transcatheter devices using the concepts of annuloplasty, chordal implantation, and LV remodeling are undergoing evaluation [15–17].

### 11.1.2 Transcatheter MV Implantation

Like transcatheter aortic valve replacement, transcatheter mitral valve implantation (TMVI) may have the potential to become an alternative to surgery in high-risk patients with severe MR. In contrast to repair, TMVI has the potential to reduce MR to a similar extent as that achieved with surgery, with the potential for reducing invasiveness and procedural risk. Importantly, TMVI may offer wider applicability across patients and disease variations compared with repair.

The first experimental off-pump TMVI via the left atrium was reported in 2005 [17], and the first-in-human percutaneous TMVI was performed in June, 2012, with the CardiAQ valve system. Since then, several medical device companies have been competing to bring suitable transcatheter valves to the market.

## 11.2 Challenges for TMVI Devices

Device design faces a variety of challenges in targeting the most complex of the heart's four valves. In contrast to the aortic valve, the MV has a larger and noncircular saddle-shaped annulus and a complex subvalvular apparatus. Due to the close anatomical relationship between the MV and the left ventricular outflow tract (LVOT), implantation of a prosthetic MV has the potential for LVOT obstruction. These attributes, together with the absence of calcification in MR, and high mitral transvalvular systolic gradients, have made development of a transcatheter MV device more difficult. Table 11.1 lists anatomical, hemodynamical, and technical challenges of TMVI devices.

## 11.3 Patient Selection

There remains a great deal to learn about which patients may benefit from TMVI. As with other valve procedures, patient selection is determined by anatomical and clinical criteria. Discussion of patients by a heart team and detailed imaging are imperative for patient selection and preprocedural planning. Because the technique is still evolving, only patients who pose a high risk for surgery due to comorbidities have been treated. Anatomical selection criteria are discussed below.

**Table 11.1**  Challenges of TMVI devices

| | |
|---|---|
| Valve position | Truly percutaneous, transfemoral access to MV challenging |
| | – Multidimensional, highly curved catheter course |
| | Possible access routes: transapical, transseptal, transatrial |
| Valve anatomy | – Asymmetrical saddle-shaped mitral annulus |
| | – Complex subvalvular apparatus composed of leaflets, annulus, chordae tendineae, and papillary muscles |
| | – Mandatory to preserve LV geometry |
| | – Irregular geometry of the mitral leaflets |
| | – No stable calcified structure for anchoring in most cases[a] |
| Dynamic environment | Dynamic changes in mitral annular geometry (shape/size) during the cardiac cycle: |
| | – Overall reduction of annular area up to 30% |
| | – Reduction of annular circumference up to 15% |
| | High dislodgment forces: |
| | – Displacement or migration of device during continuous cyclic movements of the annulus and LV base |
| | – High transvalvular gradients |
| Device requirements | – Balanced radial stiffness: |
| |     To resist dynamic environment and avoid frame fracture |
| |     At the same time: no perforation of adjacent structures due to device stiffness |
| | – Durable valve materials to withstand the loads generated |
| | – No LVOT obstruction, occlusion of circumflex coronary artery, compression of coronary sinus, or disruption of major conduction system |
| | – Large delivery systems due to large annular size |
| Hemodynamic performance | PVL should be minimized: |
| | – Regurgitation poorly tolerated in the mitral position as a result of the higher pressure gradient across the valve |
| | – PVL may result in hemolysis. |
| Other issues | – Thrombogenicity in the setting of a dilated LA and atrial fibrillation |
| | – Possibility of reoperation or TMVI-in-TMVI still unclear |

Adapted from Ole De Backer et al. Circ Cardiovasc Interv. 2014 Jun;7(3):400–9
*LA* left atrium, *LV* left ventricle, *LVOT* left ventricular outflow tract, *MV* mitral valve, *PVL* paravalvular leak, *TMVI* transcatheter mitral valve implantation
[a]In some patients with MV stenosis, it is possible to anchor the device in the severely calcified mitral annulus

## 11.4  Preprocedural Imaging

Preprocedural imaging is pivotal for determining patient eligibility and device sizing. Transthoracic echocardiography (TTE) remains the first imaging technique for diagnosing and quantifying MV pathology. However, preprocedural three-dimensional (3D) transesophageal echocardiography (TEE) improves morphological and functional MV evaluation. Multislice computed tomography (CT) with its high spatial resolution and 3D data may be the modality of choice for morphological and geometrical evaluation of the MV and surrounding structures. Though less often used in clinical practice, cardiac magnetic resonance permits accurate assessment of anatomy and function of the MV and can be helpful in some cases [18].

### 11.4.1 Determining TMVI Feasibility and Preprocedural Planning

Given the variability of anchoring mechanisms and dimensions, relevant anatomy for determining TMVI feasibility depends on which device is being used. For all TMVI devices, proper sizing of the mitral annulus (MA), as well as a detailed characterization of the landing zone and adjacent structures, is required. Due to dynamic variability, dimensions should be assessed at multiple phases throughout the cardiac cycle. Calcification of cardiac structures needs to be assessed in detail, because excessive mitral annular, valvular, or subvalvular calcification can interfere with proper seating and fixation of the bioprosthetic valve. Finally, assessment of LV size is important, because small LV cavities with hyperdynamic function may not allow room for the TMVI frame [19].

#### 11.4.1.1 Mitral Annulus

The annulus is defined by the junction of the left atrium, left ventricle, and mitral leaflets, resulting in a 3D saddle-shaped configuration with anterior and posterior peaks. The posterior annulus is formed by a well-defined, distinct fibrous structure consisting of the junction of the left atrium, the left ventricle, and insertion of the posterior mitral leaflet. Due to the continuous transition of the anterior mitral leaflet into the intervalvular fibrosa (aortomitral "curtain" or "continuity"), the anterior annulus is more difficult to define. Though the annulus can be visualized by echocardiography and CT, two-dimensional (2D) measurements incompletely describe the complex 3D geometry, and yielded values are strongly dependent on their exact orientation. 3D annular segmentation on echocardiography and CT overcomes these measurement limitations, permitting assessment of area, perimeter, and other measurements. Simplified, the so-called method of "least squares planes" provides 2D measurements from the 3D contour by projecting the 3D contour onto a 2D plane and thus provides valuable information needed to choose a prosthetic valve size [19]. This method also permits definition of an axis that is oriented perpendicularly to the 2D plane while transecting the centroid (Figs. 11.1 and 11.2) [19].

#### 11.4.1.2 Mitral Leaflets, Chords, and Papillary Muscles

Leaflet anatomy, length, thickness, and calcification can be important for device anchoring. An adequate gap between the papillary muscle and the mitral leaflet may be necessary for devices that anchor behind the leaflets. Insertion of a papillary muscle directly into a leaflet can interfere with device anchoring [19]. In some cases, specific chordal anatomies can interfere with positioning and fixation.

#### 11.4.1.3 Annular Calcification

Mitral annular calcification (MAC) is a common degenerative process of the fibrous annulus and is associated with advancing age and end-stage renal disease. MAC is

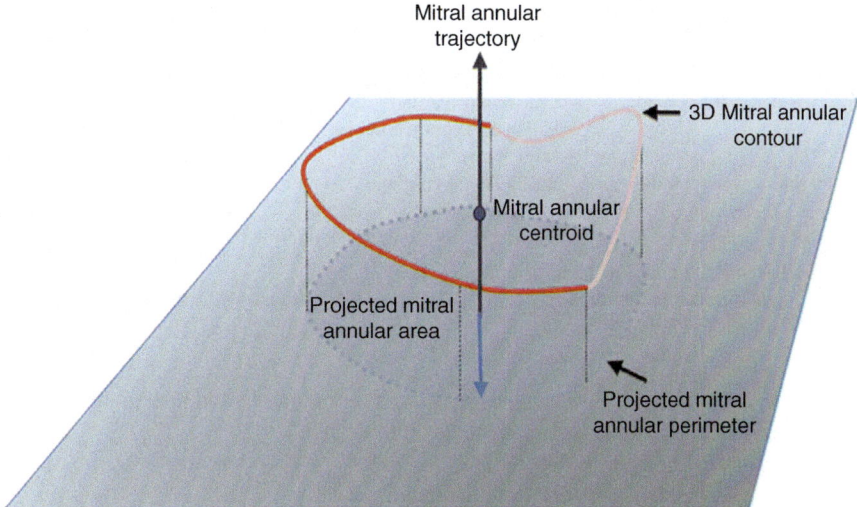

**Fig. 11.1** Projection of 3D mitral annulus onto a 2D plane. The 2D mitral annular area is assessed using the method of least squares, similar to projecting the contour onto a plane. Orientation of the plane and annular trajectory are obtained by the least squares plane calculation. The actual 2D annular plane has the identical orientation as the projection but transects through the geometrical centroid

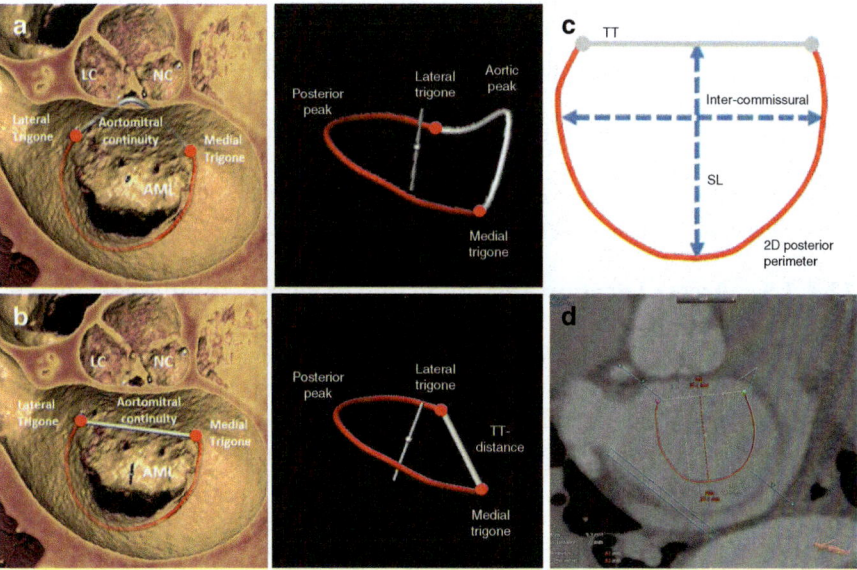

**Fig. 11.2** 3D mitral annular segmentation on CT. Annular segmentation is performed by generating a cubic spline interpolation of manually placed seeding points along the 3D annular contour. This segmentation results in a saddle-shaped mitral annular contour with an anterior/aortic peak and nadirs at the fibrous trigones (**a**). The contour is truncated at a virtual line connecting both trigones, excluding the aortic peak, resulting in a D-shape contour (**b**). Important measurements are the projected area septal-to-lateral (SL) and intercommissural distances; the latter is oriented perpendicularly to SL while transecting through the centroid (**c** and **d**)

**Table 11.2** Risk factors for LVOT obstruction

| | |
|---|---|
| Aortomitral angulation | Angle between the MA trajectory[a] and the LVOT long axis: <br> – Low risk if parallel <br> – High risk if perpendicular |
| LV size | Small LV cavity |
| Interventricular septum | – Basal, septal bulging <br> – Basal hypertrophy (>15 mm) |
| Device-related factors | Extension of device protrusion into the LV and device flaring |

*LVOT* left ventricular outflow tract, *MA* mitral annulus

[a]Axis that is oriented perpendicularly to the 2D plane while transecting the geometrical center of the MA

present in approximately 6% of the general older population and presents a concern for patients undergoing surgery, as well as TMVI [19].

#### 11.4.1.4   Predicting LVOT Obstruction

TMVI devices consist of circumferentially covered stent frames, which can significantly protrude into the LV cavity or displace the anterior mitral leaflet, and potentially encroach upon the LVOT. Because of this protrusion, a "neo-LVOT" is created by the device, the anterior mitral leaflet, and the interventricular septum. Predisposing factors for LVOT obstruction include anatomical- and device-related factors. LVOT anatomy is influenced mainly by the configuration of the interventricular septum, LV size, and the aortomitral angulation. Furthermore, extensive device protrusion into the left ventricle and device flaring can lead to LVOT obstruction (Table 11.2).

Though limited, virtual CT TMVI simulation can predict neo-LVOT geometry by embedding a cylindrical or device-specific contour into the CT dataset (Fig. 11.3). However, to date there are no established cutoff values for minimal neo-LVOT area that indicate an increased risk of LVOT obstruction [19].

#### 11.4.1.5   Access Location and Prediction of Fluoroscopic Angulation

Post-processing of CT data allows identification of the ideal LV access point, which is commonly located laterally or anteriorly to the true apex. To facilitate coaxial device deployment, coplanar fluoroscopic projections are used during TMVI. Mitral annular plane segmentation on CT can provide these projection angulations for intraprocedural fluoroscopy.

## 11.5   Transcatheter Mitral Valve Implantation

Currently, all devices are deployed transapically (Table 11.3). The CardiAQ TMVI system is unique at this time in also being compatible with transseptal implantation. Procedures are performed under general anesthesia, with hemodynamic monitoring in an operating room.

**Fig. 11.3** Prediction of neo-LVOT dimensions. End-systolic CT datasets of a patient with prior bioprosthetic valve replacement. Three-chamber (**a**) and LVOT short-axis (**b**) views showing a simulated cylindrical device (23 mm), oriented perpendicularly to the annular plane

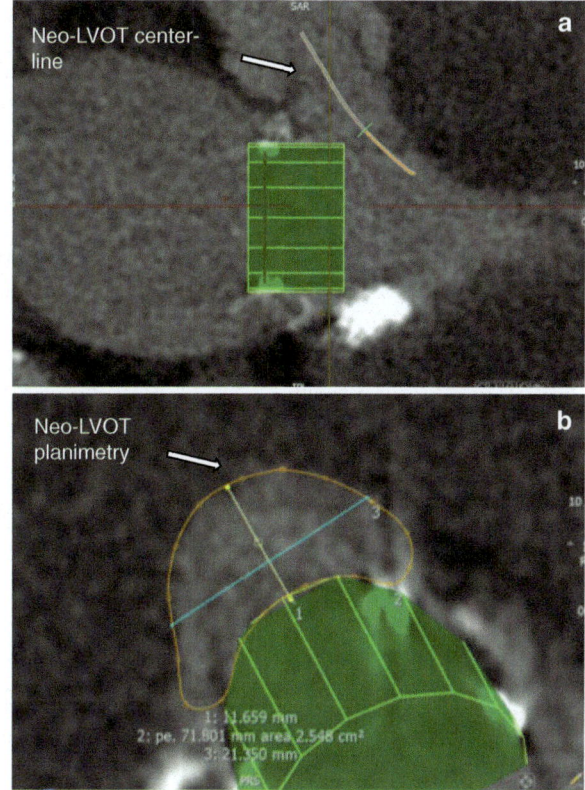

Generally, in transapical procedures, the ventricular apex is approached through a left lateral thoracotomy, and the apex is punctured lateral to the ventricular apex. A soft J-tip guidewire is advanced through the left ventricle and, retrograde, through the mitral valve into the left atrium. The transcatheter valve delivery catheter is typically advanced over the wire into position. Coaxial positioning can be achieved by direct manipulation of the apical delivery system and evaluated by 2D and 3D TEE.

In transfemoral procedures, percutaneous access is obtained in a femoral vein, and a transseptal puncture is made. Typically, the puncture site is high or midway up on the posterior aspect of the interatrial septum to facilitate crossing the mitral valve. An exchange length guidewire is advanced through the mitral valve and into the left ventricle. If necessary, the guidewire can be passed out of the LVOT into the aorta or even snared and exteriorized from a femoral artery, forming a venoarterial loop. Subsequently, the delivery catheter is advanced across the septum into the left ventricle. Coaxial alignment of the valve can be achieved by active flexion of the delivery catheter or alternatively by advancing or retracting either the delivery system or the wire.

For both antegrade and retrograde approaches, it is very important to ensure that the ventricular wire does not pass under chords that might be damaged or interfere

**Table 11.3** Overview of TMVI devices

| Device | CardiAQ TMVI system | Tiara transcatheter heart valve | FORTIS transcatheter mitral valve | Tendyne TMVI system | Intrepid transcatheter mitral valve |
|---|---|---|---|---|---|
| Manufacturer | Edwards Lifesciences Inc. | Neovasc Inc. | Edwards Lifesciences Inc. | Abbott Inc. | Medtronic Inc. |
| Human implants | + | + | + | + | + |
| Access | TA/TS | TA | TA | TA | TA |
| Nitinol frame | + | + | + | + | + |
| Pericardial leaflet tissue type | Bovine | Bovine | Bovine | Porcine | Bovine |
| Trileaflet valve | + | + | + | + | + |
| Symmetric leaflets | + | − | + | + | + |
| Implant shape | Circular | D-shaped | Circular | D-shaped | Circular |
| Seal | Pericardial | Synthetic | Synthetic | Synthetic | Synthetic |
| Fixation: | | | | | |
| Atrial flange | + | + | + | + | + |
| Apical tether | − | − | − | + | − |
| Barbs/tines | + | − | − | − | + |
| Clips/tabs/paddles | + | + | + | − | − |
| Radial force | − | − | − | − | − |
| Requires normal PML | − | − | + | − | − |
| Requires posterior ridge | − | + | − | − | − |
| Requires normal AML | − | − | + | − | − |
| Recapture/retrieval | − | − | − | Retrievable | Retrievable |
| Suitable for | | | | | |
| Functional MR | + | + | + | + | + |
| Degenerative MR | ± | + | − | + | + |
| Sheath size | 36 Fr | 32 Fr | 42 Fr | 32 Fr | 35 Fr |

*AML* anterior mitral leaflet, *MR* mitral regurgitation, *PML* posterior mitral leaflet, *TA* transapical, *TS* transseptal, *TMVI* transcatheter mitral valve implantation

with delivery catheter passage or device fixation. A J-tip guidewire is less likely to pass under a chord than a straight wire. A typical maneuver is to pass an inflated balloon over the wire and verify that this passes freely through the left ventricle to the valve.

## 11.5.1 Intraprocedural Imaging

Intraprocedural imaging is done with TEE and fluoroscopy. By compressing the left ventricle with a finger epicardially or epicardial ultrasound, the location of the ventricular puncture can be confirmed. To determine the correct placement of the guidewire across the MA, and to position the guidewire in the roof of the LA, continuous imaging is performed using fluoroscopy and TEE. The delivery system is

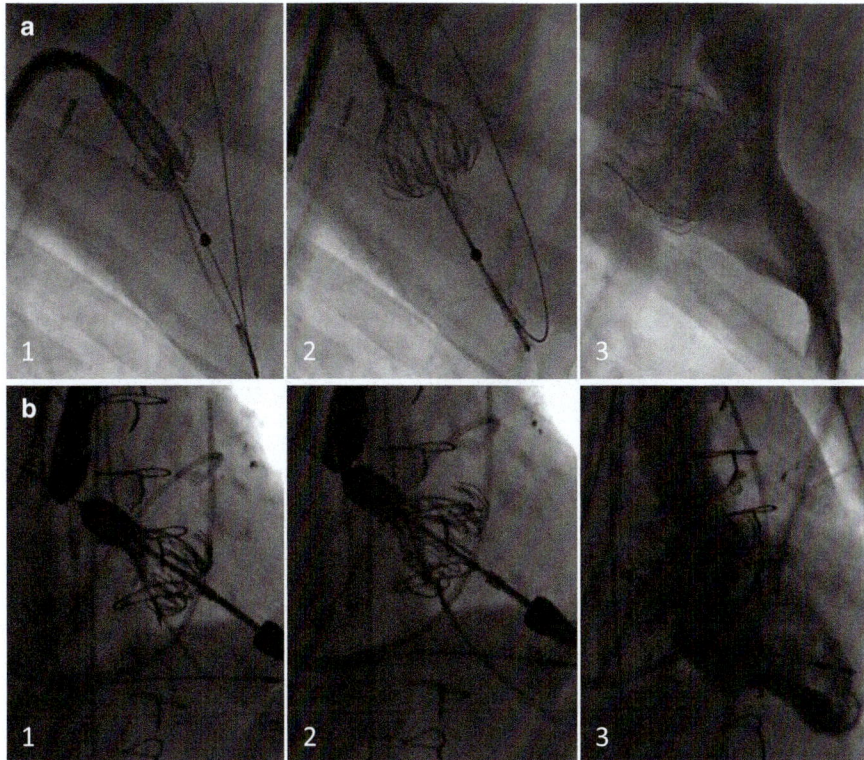

**Fig. 11.4** Deployment sequence of a CardiAQ valve under fluoroscopic guidance. Transseptal (**a**) and transapical approach (**b**): (*1*) leaflet capture; (*2*) valve expansion; (*3*) valve release

introduced, and the device is deployed under both fluoroscopic and TEE guidance (Fig. 11.4), thus confirming free passage from the apex to the left atrium and ensuring alignment of the flat portion of D-shaped devices or specific anchoring mechanism with the mitral apparatus. Immediately following deployment, 2D and 3D imaging confirm appropriate seating, stability, radial orientation, relationship to the captured leaflets, and prosthetic valve function (Fig. 11.5).

Follow-up imaging is done most conveniently by TTE to assess valve function (MV orifice area; central or paravalvular mitral regurgitation) [19].

## 11.6 Transcatheter MV Systems

To date, the following five transcatheter MV systems have been implanted in humans:

- CardiAQ TMVI System (Edwards Lifesciences Inc., USA)
- Tiara transcatheter valve (Neovasc Inc., Canada)

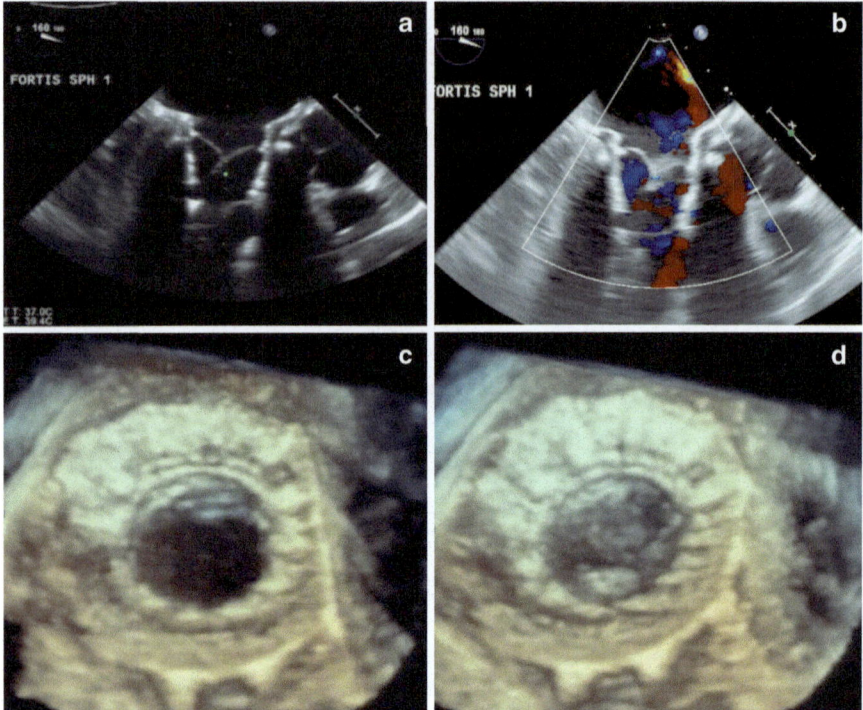

**Fig. 11.5** Echocardiographic images after deployment of a FORTIS valve. (**a** and **b**) Evaluation after TMVI showing an accurate and stable position of the bioprosthetic valve and only trace para-valvular regurgitation. (**c** and **d**) Three-dimensional images showing the bioprosthesis during dias-tole and systole

- – FORTIS transcatheter mitral valve (Edwards Lifesciences, USA)
- – Tendyne TMVI System (Abbott Inc., USA)
- – Intrepid transcatheter mitral valve (Medtronic Inc., USA).

Each of these systems offers innovative design solutions to overcome the chal-lenging anatomy of the MV complex. All current devices incorporate a self-expandable nitinol frame, three pericardial leaflets, and a synthetic fabric or pericardial seal (Fig. 11.6). Table 11.3 provides an overview of their specific characteristics.

## 11.6.1 CardiAQ TMVI System

### 11.6.1.1 Device
The CardiAQ bioprosthesis (Edwards Lifesciences Inc., USA) consists of a self-expanding nitinol frame, which carries three leaflets of bovine pericardial tissue (Fig. 11.7). The device does not rely on radial force for fixation to the annulus.

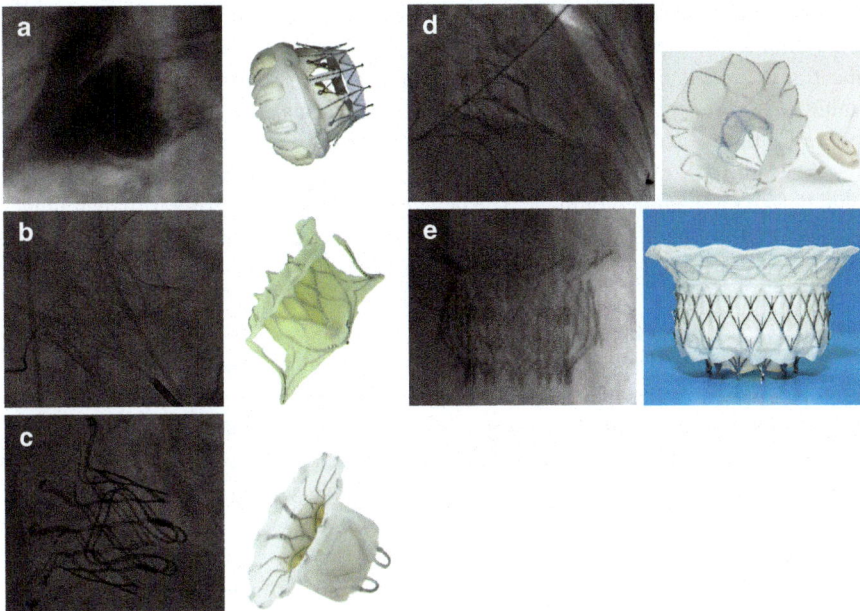

**Fig. 11.6** Overview of the five transcatheter mitral valve systems that have been implanted in humans. (**a**) CardiAQ valve. (**b**) Tiara valve. (**c**) FORTIS. (**d**) Tendyne valve. (**e**) Intrepid valve

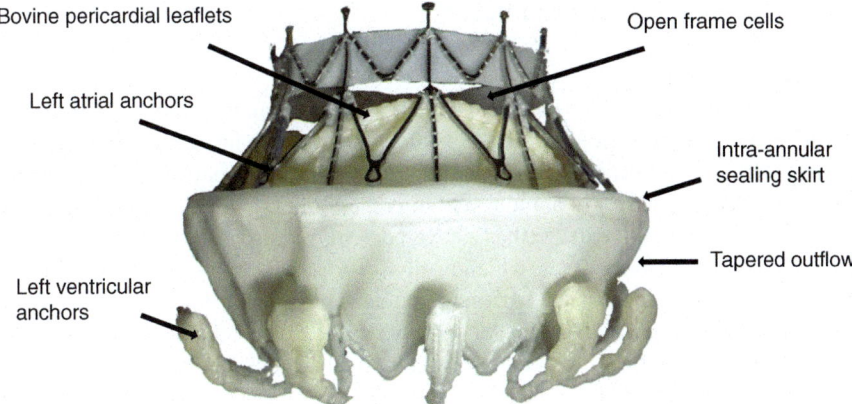

**Fig. 11.7** CardiAQ valve. The valve consists of a self-expanding nitinol frame that carries three leaflets of bovine pericardial tissue. The anchoring mechanism of the CardiAQ valve preserves chords and utilizes native leaflets to secure the position. Also, load distribution among annulus, leaflets, and chords is promoted. The valve is designed to promote physiological flow and eliminate mitral regurgitation. The supra-annular position and the tapered outflow of the device minimize the risk of LVOT obstruction. The intra-annular sealing skirt is designed to minimize paravalvular leak. The frame cells of the inflow section are open to ensure atrial flow

Sealing and anchoring are achieved by two sets of opposing anchors which grasp the mitral leaflets from the left atrial and LV side. Additionally, foreshortening of the frame creates a clamping action that anchors the valve above and below the annulus, preserving the chordae and papillary apparatus. The frame is covered by a polyester fabric seal to reduce paraprosthetic leaks. To ensure accurate placement, the different steps of valve deployment are controllable, and the valve is repositionable before the final deployment. The device can either be inserted truly percutaneously through the femoral vein using a transseptal access to the left atrium (antegrade) or transapically (retrograde) [20].

### 11.6.1.2    Clinical Experience

In June, 2012, the first-in-human TMVI was done in Copenhagen, Denmark in a high-risk patient with severe, symptomatic MR. Despite successful antegrade transseptal implantation of the first-generation, porcine pericardial CardiAQ valve, with stable position and hemodynamics, the patient died 3 days post-procedure of multiorgan failure. The second-generation CardiAQ valve was first implanted in 2014, using a transapical delivery system [21]. Subsequently 14 patients were treated under compassionate use protocols (Table 11.4). Two procedural deaths were reported (TVT Chicago 2016), one due to entrapment in the mechanical aortic valve and one as a result of malpositioning due to sub-leaflet calcification. Currently, patients are being enrolled in a US early feasibility study and a CE Mark trial, utilizing both transapical and transseptal accesses.

## 11.6.2    Tiara Transcatheter Valve

### 11.6.2.1    Device

The Tiara valve (Neovasc Inc., Canada) is a self-expanding bioprosthesis with cross-linked bovine pericardial tissue leaflets mounted inside a metal alloy frame (Fig. 11.8). The atrial portion of the valve is anatomically shaped to fit the asymmetric and D-shaped mitral annulus and to prevent impingement of the LVOT. The ventricular portion of the device has a covered skirt to prevent paravalvular leakage, as well as three anchoring tabs, which firmly secure the Tiara valve onto the fibrous trigones and the posterior shelf of the annulus. These features prevent retrograde dislodgement during systole. The Tiara valve can be resheathable, repositionable, and retrievable until the final step of ventricular deployment. The device is implanted

Table 11.4  Clinical outcome after TMVI

| Device | CardiAQ TMVI system | Tiara transcatheter heart valve | FORTIS transcatheter mitral valve | Tendyne TMVI system | Intrepid transcatheter mitral valve |
|---|---|---|---|---|---|
| Patients treated (*n*) | 14 | 17 | 13 | 37 | 17 |
| Procedural success | 9/11 (82%) | 14 (82%) | 10/13 (77%) | 26/28 (93%) | 15 (88%) |
| Early mortality | 6/12 (50%) | 3 (18%) | 5/13 (39%) | 1/23 (4%) | 4 (24%) |

Adapted from Gregg W. Stone, TVT Chicago 2016

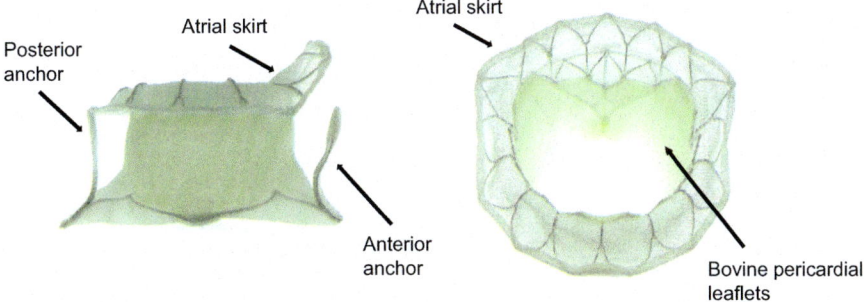

**Fig. 11.8** Tiara valve. The anatomical D-shape of the valve, the atrial skirt that engages the atrial aspect of the mitral annulus, one posterior and two anterior anchors as well as the saddle-shaped valve are clearly seen

transapically using a 32 French (F) delivery catheter for the 35 mm and a 36 F catheter for the 40 mm device.

The Tiara valve can be used for both functional and degenerative mitral regurgitation. Relative anatomical exclusions include very large annular dimensions and severe mitral and subvalvular calcification [22].

### 11.6.2.2  Clinical Experience

The first two cases of human Tiara valve implantation were in 2014, in Vancouver, Canada. Both patients had severe ischemic cardiomyopathies with poor LV functions, severe functional MR, and prohibitive comorbidities. Device implantation was successful, with good results. Repeat TTEs at 4 weeks showed normal valve function with no relevant paravalvular leak, normal transmitral gradients, and no LVOT obstruction. The first patient, however, had persistent symptoms related to congestive heart failure and chronic renal failure leading to death 69 days postprocedure. The second patient remained well at 2.5 years, with a significant clinical improvement [22]. At TVT Chicago 2016, implantation of the Tiara valve system was reported in 17 high-risk patients (Table 11.4). In 14 patients, Tiara was successfully implanted as intended, resulting in a stable and well-anchored prosthetic valve, without paravalvular leakage. There were no procedural deaths, though three patients required conversion to surgical valve replacement due to valve malposition. Two patients with preprocedural severe MR and low EF (20%) are alive and well 2 years post implant, with no recurrent MR or PVL and well-functioning Tiara on TTE follow-up.

### 11.6.3  FORTIS Transcatheter Mitral Valve

### 11.6.3.1  Device

The Edwards FORTIS valve is made of a self-expanding nitinol stent with three bovine pericardial leaflets (Fig. 11.9). The valve consists of a cylindrical central valve

**Fig. 11.9** FORTIS valve. Two flexible arms respect the aortomitral anatomy and prevent aortic sinus impingement; the adaptable flange flexes to D-shape in patient anatomy as needed; the circular valve with symmetric leaflets minimizes leaflet closing stress under high ventricular pressures; the cylindrical frame ensures optimal laminar flow, and wide paddles capture the native leaflets for secure anchoring

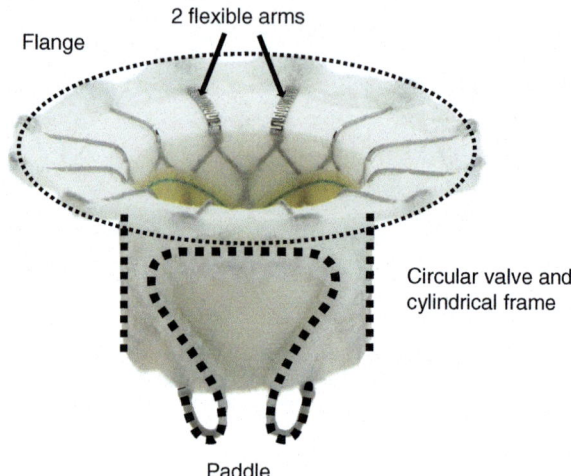

body, two paddles, and an atrial flange. The central valve harbors the three leaflets. The outside of the stent is cloth covered to prevent mitral leaflet injury and provide a platform for tissue ingrowth after implantation. The paddles are located in the outflow of the central valve body. The paddles anchor the FORTIS device by capturing the mitral leaflets in such a way that the native leaflets are secured between the valve body and the paddles. The atrial flange is positioned at the inflow portion of the valve body and is made of multiple nitinol struts covered with cloth. Two of the struts are more flexible than the rest to prevent interference with the aortic valve function. The atrial flange rests on the base of the left atrium and allows tissue endothelialization.

The FORTIS valve is loaded into a 42 F transapical delivery system. The delivery system allows stepwise release of the valve as well as recapturability and repositionability to a certain point during deployment (Fig. 11.10). Multiple radiopaque markers on the delivery system facilitate positioning and deployment of the device under fluoroscopy and echocardiography [23].

### 11.6.3.2    Clinical Experience

In February 2014, the first patient was treated with the FORTIS valve. So far, there are reports of 20 high-risk patients who underwent implantation of the FORTIS valve. From the ongoing feasibility trial protocol in the USA, results for 13 of these patients are available [23]. Implantation of the device was successful in ten patients (Table 11.4). Two patients had to be converted to surgery due to malposition of the device and chordal entanglement of the balloon before device implantation. One patient had partial migration of the device 4 days after the procedure because of incomplete posterior leaflet capture. Valve thrombosis was documented in isolated cases, leading to recommendations for more aggressive anticoagulation. The longest survival of the patients treated with the FORTIS valve was in Vancouver, Canada, and was 2 years. Recently the Edwards FORTIS and the CardiAQ valve programs have been merged.

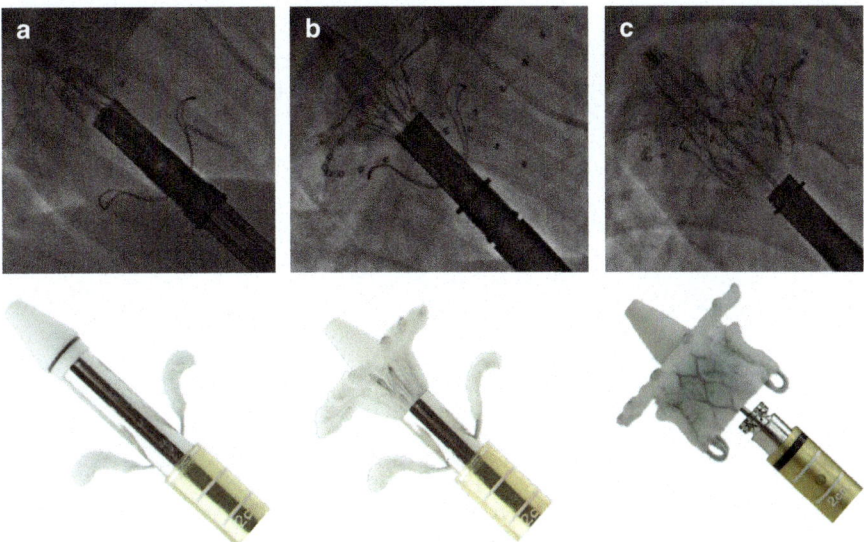

**Fig. 11.10** Deployment sequence of a FORTIS valve. (**a**) Leaflet capture; (**b**) flange release; (**c**) valve release

### 11.6.4 Tendyne TMVI System Device

#### 11.6.4.1 Device

The Tendyne valve (Abbott Inc., USA) is a trileaflet porcine, pericardial valve (Fig. 11.11). The device consists of an atrial flange, a ventricular body made of two self-expanding nitinol stents that house the valve leaflets, and a ventricular fixation system composed of a tether attached to the stent. The atrial flange offers atrial sealing and anchoring. The inner stent is one size and circular to maintain a consistent, large, effective orifice area ($>3.0$ cm$^2$); the outer stent is D-shaped, which helps seat the valve. The prosthetic valve is delivered transapically through a 32 F sheath and is secured via a tether (neochordae) near the LV apex using a pad that sits on the epicardium. The device is designed to be fully retrievable, and can be repositioned, even after full deployment [24].

#### 11.6.4.2 Clinical Experience

Initial experience with the Tendyne valve was with patients undergoing planned surgical MV replacement in Asuncion, Paraguay (2013). Two patients received a Tendyne implant and were monitored for 2 h post implant prior to planned removal and conventional surgical MV repair. After the valve implantation, good valve function was documented, with no coronary artery restriction, LVOT obstruction, or systolic anterior motion of the MV in either patient [24]. Following this, the bioprosthetic device has been implanted in 37 patients (32 EFS implants, 5 compassionate use implants) worldwide (Table 11.4). Outcomes of 23 patients were shown at TVT 2016 in Chicago. At 30 days, one patient died of sepsis. Function of the

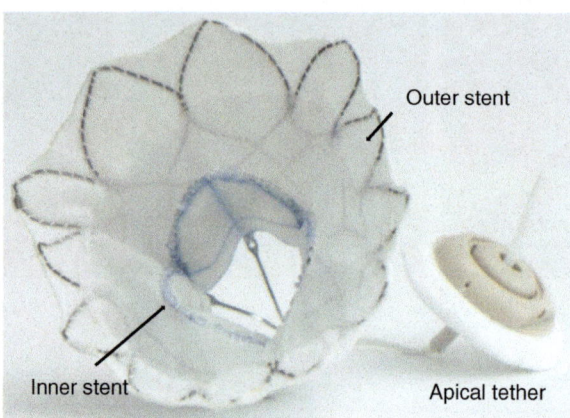

**Fig. 11.11** Tendyne valve. Adapted from Neal Moat, TVT Chicago 2016. The valve consists of an atrial flange, a ventricular body made of two self-expanding nitinol frames (inner stent circular; outer stent D-shaped) that house the porcine pericardial valve leaflets and a ventricular fixation system composed of tethering strings attached to the stent. The Tendyne valve has a large valve size matrix with multiple outer frame sizes, whereas there is only one size for the inner stent ensuring a large effective orifice area

Tendyne valve was reported to be good, with only mild MR in 4 patients and no MR in 15 patients.

### 11.6.5 Intrepid Transcatheter Mitral Valve

#### 11.6.5.1 Device
The Intrepid (Medtronic Inc., USA) valve is a trileaflet pericardial valve sewn onto a self-expanding nitinol frame (Fig. 11.12). The bioprosthetic valve features a large inflow atrial portion that is responsible for sealing and a short outflow ventricular portion to avoid LVOT obstruction. The bioprosthesis does not rely on outward radial forces for anchoring. Instead, it uses the native mitral apparatus for axial fixation. Attached to the outflow section of the frame, the device has support arms that function to capture the anterior and posterior MV leaflets and engage the submitral apparatus. Leaflet capture also minimizes the risk of systolic anterior motion. The valve is designed to be fully retrievable, and it is possible to refold and withdraw the valve via a catheter in case a bailout procedure is needed. Similar to a minimally invasive MV repair, the current device is delivered transatrially to avoid further damage to the LV wall. A transseptal delivery system is under development [25].

#### 11.6.5.2 Clinical Experience
At TVT Chicago, outcomes of 17 patients were presented. Successful implantation of the Intrepid valve has been reported in 15 patients, with an early mortality of 24% (Table 11.4).

Outer stent

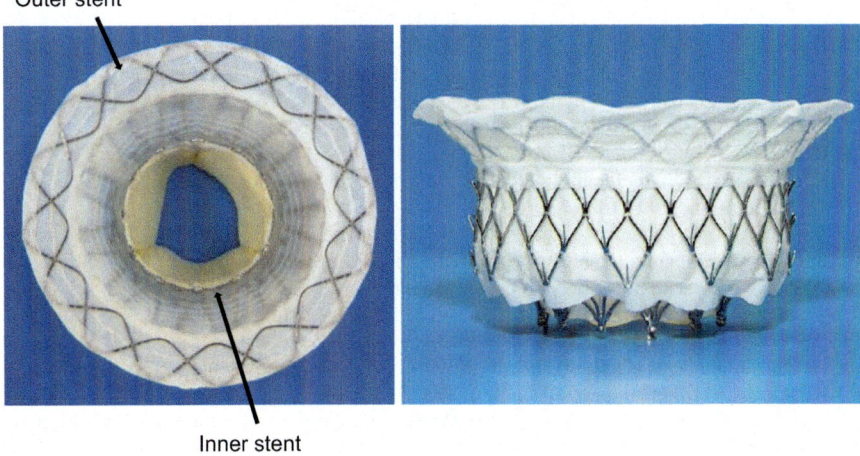

Inner stent

**Fig. 11.12** Intrepid valve. The twelve valve is a trileaflet bovine pericardial valve consisting of a self-expanding inner and an outer stent. For fixation the valve uses the mitral apparatus (axial fixation)

**Conclusion**

Due to the large number of high-risk patients with significant mitral valve disease, transcatheter options will be of increasing importance. TMVI offers great potential to expand treatment options for these patients. However, multiple technical challenges still have to be overcome before TMVI for native mitral valve disease becomes an option in daily practice.

# References

1. Nkomo VT, Gardin JM, Skelton TN, Gottdiener JS, Scott CG, Enriquez-Sarano M. Burden of valvular heart diseases: a population-based study. Lancet. 2006;368:1005–11.
2. Grigioni F, Enriquez-Sarano M, Zehr KJ, Bailey KR, Tajik AJ. Ischemic mitral regurgitation: long-term outcome and prognostic implications with quantitative Doppler assessment. Circulation. 2001;103:1759–64.
3. Bursi F, Enriquez-Sarano M, Nkomo VT, et al. Heart failure and death after myocardial infarction in the community: the emerging role of mitral regurgitation. Circulation. 2005;111:295–301.
4. Lamas GA, Mitchell GF, Flaker GC, et al. Clinical significance of mitral regurgitation after acute myocardial infarction. Survival and ventricular enlargement investigators. Circulation. 1997;96:827–33.
5. Trichon BH, Felker GM, Shaw LK, Cabell CH, O'Connor CM. Relation of frequency and severity of mitral regurgitation to survival among patients with left ventricular systolic dysfunction and heart failure. Am J Cardiol. 2003;91:538–43.
6. Ling LH, Enriquez-Sarano M, Seward JB, et al. Clinical outcome of mitral regurgitation due to flail leaflet. N Engl J Med. 1996;335:1417–23.
7. Avierinos J-FF, Gersh BJ, Melton LJ, et al. Natural history of asymptomatic mitral valve prolapse in the community. Circulation. 2002;106:1355–61.

8. Iung B, Baron G, Butchart EG, et al. A prospective survey of patients with valvular heart disease in Europe: the euro heart survey on Valvular heart disease. Eur Heart J. 2003;24:1231–43.
9. Vahanian A, Alfieri O, Andreotti F, et al. Guidelines on the Management of Valvular Heart Disease (version 2012). The joint task force on the management of Valvular heart disease of the European Society of Cardiology (ESC) and the European Association for Cardio-Thoracic Surgery (EACTS). Giornale Italiano di Cardiologia (2006). 2013;14:167–214.
10. Gillinov AM, Wierup PN, Blackstone EH, Bishay ES, Cosgrove DM, White J, Lytle BW, PM MC. Is repair preferable to replace-ment for ischemic mitral regurgitation? J Thorac Cardiovasc Surg. 2001;122:1125–41.
11. Mirabel M, Iung B, Baron G, et al. What are the characteristics of patients with severe, symptomatic, mitral regurgitation who are denied surgery? Eur Heart J. 2007;28:1358–65.
12. Alfieri O, Maisano F, De Bonis M, et al. The double-orifice technique in mitral valve repair: a simple solution for complex problems. J Thorac Cardiovasc Surg. 2001;122:674–81.
13. Feldman T, Kar S, Rinaldi M, et al. Percutaneous mitral repair with the MitraClip system: safety and midterm durability in the initial EVEREST (endovascular valve edge-to-edge REpair study) cohort. J Am Coll Cardiol. 2009;54:686–94.
14. Tamburino C, Ussia GP, Maisano F, et al. Percutaneous mitral valve repair with the MitraClip system: acute results from a real world setting. Eur Heart J. 2010;31:1382–9.
15. Chiam PT, Ruiz CE. Percutaneous transcatheter mitral valve repair: a classification of the technology. JACC Cardiovasc Interv. 2011;4:1–13.
16. Cubeddu RJ, Palacios IF. Percutaneous techniques for mitral valve disease. Cardiol Clin. 2010;28:139–53.
17. Seeburger J, Rinaldi M, Nielsen SL, Salizzoni S, Lange R, Schoenburg M, Alfieri O, Borger MA, Mohr FW, Aidietis A. Off-pump transapical implantation of artificial neochordae to correct mitral regurgitation: the TACT trial (Transapical artificial chordae Tendinae) proof of concept. J Am Coll Cardiol. 2014;63:914–9.
18. Debonnaire P, Palmen M, Marsan NA, Delgado V. Contemporary imaging of normal mitral valve anatomy and function. Curr Opin Cardiol. 2012 Sep;27(5):455–64.
19. Blanke P, Naoum C, Webb J, Dvir D, Hahn RT, Grayburn P, Moss RR, Reisman M, Piazza N, Leipsic J. Multimodality imaging in the context of transcatheter mitral valve replacement: establishing consensus among modalities and disciplines. JACC Cardiovasc Imaging. 2015;8(10):1191–208.
20. Ussia GP, Quadri A, Cammalleri V, De Vico P, Muscoli S, Marchei M, Ruvolo G, Sondergaard L, Romeo F. Percutaneous transfemoral-transseptal implantation of a second-generation CardiAQ™ mitral valve bioprosthesis: first procedure description and 30-day follow-up. EuroIntervention. 2016;11(10):1126–51.
21. Sondergaard L, Brooks M, Ihlemann N, Jonsson A, Holme S, Tang M, Terp K, Quadri A. Transcatheter mitral valve implantation via transapical approach: an early experience. Eur J Cardiothorac Surg. 2015;48(6):873–7.
22. Verheye S, Cheung A, Leon M, Banai S. The Tiara transcatheter mitral valve implantation system. EuroIntervention. 2015;11(Suppl W):W71–2.
23. Bapat V, Lim ZY, Boix R, Pirone F. The Edwards Fortis transcatheter mitral valve implantation system. EuroIntervention. 2015;11(Suppl W):W73–5.
24. Perpetua EM, Reisman M. The Tendyne transcatheter mitral valve implantation system. EuroIntervention. 2015;11(Suppl W):W78–9.
25. Piazza N, Treede H, Moat N, Sorajja P, Popma J, Grube E, Bolling S, Adams D. The Medtronic transcatheter mitral valve implantation system. EuroIntervention. 2015;11(Suppl W):W80–1.

# Transcatheter Therapy for Mitral Regurgitation: A Review of the Literature

# 12

Sergio Buccheri and Davide Capodanno

Growing evidence in the literature testifies to the clinical safety and efficacy of the percutaneous treatment of mitral regurgitation (MR) [1, 2]. The available data are mainly from multicenter registries or from case studies collected prospectively in individual centers. Data from randomized trials is rather limited [3]. Among the different techniques available for interventional treatment of the mitral valve, percutaneous repair with the MitraClip System (Abbott Vascular, Santa Clara, CA) has definitely been the most studied technique, and the one with the most data currently available, though the feasibility and safety data for other percutaneous techniques (Cardioband, Mitralign, Carillon, transcatheter implantable mitral valve) have recently been published [4, 5].

## 12.1 The EVEREST Studies: From the Initial Stage to the Randomized Study

The first data on the efficacy and safety of the MitraClip System were reported by EVEREST (Endovascular Valve Edge-to-Edge Repair Study) I and pre-randomization EVEREST II "start-up experience" studies [6, 7]. These studies were designed as prospective multicenter studies to evaluate the safety and initial feasibility of percutaneous MR repair with the MitraClip System. The EVEREST studies enrolled a total of 107 patients, of whom 62% were over the age of 65, and 21% had functional MR. The mean left ventricular ejection fraction (EF) in the population was 62%. The acute success of the procedure, defined as a reduction of the degree

S. Buccheri
Ferrarotto Hospital, University of Catania, Via Citelli 6, 95124 Catania, Italy

D. Capodanno (✉)
Department of General Surgery and Medical-Surgical Specialties, University of Catania, Catania, Italy

Ferrarotto Hospital, University of Catania, Via Citelli 6, 95124 Catania, Italy
e-mail: dcapodanno@gmail.com

© Springer International Publishing AG 2018
C. Tamburino et al. (eds.), *Percutaneous Treatment of Left Side Cardiac Valves*,
https://doi.org/10.1007/978-3-319-59620-4_12

of MR $\leq$ 2+, was obtained in 74% of patients, and 64% of the enrolled patients were discharged with an MR $\leq$ 1+. The procedure was ineffective in 11 patients, of whom 8 for inability to reduce MR and 3 due to complications during transseptal puncture. There were no cases of intraoperative death. In the group of treated patients, there was no case of device embolization, while a partial clip detachment from a single leaflet was reported in ten (9%) patients. At 30 days of follow-up, ten patients (9%) had experienced a major adverse event, including a non-procedural death in a patient who had not received MitraClip. Analysis of the follow-up showed that freedom from death at 3 years was 90%, while freedom from surgery was 76%. The primary efficacy end point (composite of freedom from MR > 2+, cardiac surgery for valve dysfunction and death) was reached in 66% of cases at 1 year, in 65% at 2 years, and in 63% at 3 years. Superimposable results in the acute and in the medium term were also reported in patients with functional MR. In a period of 3.2 years, however, 32 patients (30%) needed subsequent surgery to treat recurrent MR. An analysis of 65 patients also showed a significant improvement in the functional class and symptoms reported by the patients after MitraClip implantation (92% in NYHA functional class I–II at 12 months). In aggregate, EVEREST showed that the MitraClip System is safe and feasible, with a good percentage of success in patients considered at high surgical risk. These studies have laid the foundations, and supported the design, of the randomized EVEREST study (EVEREST II) [3].

The EVEREST II trial randomized a total of 279 patients suffering from MR for treatment with MitraClip or surgery and had a ratio of 2:1, respectively. All the enrolled patients had MR $\geq$ 3+ and were eligible for both types of treatment. A total of 73% of the patients in the MitraClip group had degenerative MR. The safety end point set for the study was defined as the composite of death, myocardial infarction, stroke, reoperation, transfusions, and renal failure, while the primary composite end point for efficacy was freedom from death and from surgery for MR repair/replacement and improvement of MR by a grade.

The EVEREST trial has provided several results of great interest. In the intention-to-treat analysis, the efficacy end point was reached in 55% of patients treated with MitraClip compared with 78% of patients treated with surgery ($p = 0.007$), while the rate of major adverse events was significantly higher in the surgical group as a result of the higher number of postoperative transfusions needed. The specific analysis concerning the improvement in the grade of MR showed that 41 patients, i.e., about a quarter of the population assigned to treatment with MitraClip, were discharged with residual MR grades of 3+/4+, and, among them, 28 patients required subsequent surgical treatment. All patients treated surgically were discharged with a residual grade of MR of <2+. Treatment with MitraClip reached the non-inferiority margin, compared with surgery, for the primary efficacy end point. In the follow-up at 2 years, there were no significant differences in mortality between the two groups. Echocardiographic evaluations showed that both treatments accounted for significant reductions in end-diastolic and end-systolic volumes and an increase in left ventricular EF at 12 months. Surgical treatment, however, resulted in a greater reduction of the end-diastolic volume and a greater increase in EF, compared with treatment with MitraClip

($p = 0.004$ and $p = 0.005$, respectively). A significant improvement in the quality of life in both groups was found, with a transient decrease in the quality of life at 30 days in patients treated surgically. In the exploratory analysis of subgroups of the study, the benefits of surgery were attenuated in patients aged 70 years and over, with an EF of <60%, and with functional MR.

The long-term results of the EVEREST trial [8] showed a substantial stability of the results in 210 patients analyzed at 5 years of follow-up. Interestingly, though treatment with MitraClip had led to a greater need for reoperation due to early recurrence of MR, between 6 months and 5 years, the efficacy in reducing the degree of MR was maintained in both groups. In addition, there appeared to be no differences in mortality in the long-term follow-up.

## 12.2   Data from the Real World: An Analysis of Registries

The data derived from the EVEREST randomized trial highlighted the feasibility and procedural safety of percutaneous repair with MitraClip, thus encouraging a broader use of the device. Numerous experiences published in the literature [9–12] have reported data on procedural success and on the clinical impact of MitraClip implantation in non-select patients. Interesting evidence confirming the efficacy of the device has also been found in the real world.

Two large US registries, EVEREST II HRR (Endovascular Valve Edge-to-Edge REpair STudy High-Risk registry) and REALISM, have provided the first results after MitraClip implantation in the real world [9]. The enrolled patients were elderly (mean age $76 \pm 11$ years), and in 70% of cases had severe functional MR. The combined analysis of the two registries, for a total of 351 patients, of whom 327 with follow-up available at 12 months, found a procedural success (MR $\leq$ 2+) in 86% of cases. In the follow-up, 84% patients maintained the procedural results in terms of improvement in the grade of MR. Compared with the pre-procedural clinical conditions, a significant reduction was found in the percentage of patients in NYHA class III–IV, as was an improvement in the quality of life. The annualized rate of heart failure hospitalizations was significantly reduced (from 0.79% to 0.41%). The estimated survival rate at 12 months, using the Kaplan-Meier method, was 77.2%.

ACCESS-EU (a two-phase observational study of the MitraClip System in Europe), a large European multicenter registry, substantially confirmed the results of previous experiences [10]. A total of 567 patients treated with MitraClip in 14 European centers were enrolled in the registry. The enrolled patients were elderly, at high surgical risk (mean logistic EuroSCORE of 23.0%), and with an EF $\leq$ 40% in 52.7% of cases. At 1 year, the mean survival and the rate of patients with MR $\leq$ 2+ were 81.8% and 78.9%, respectively. A total of 36 patients required re-surgery at 12 months.

Similarly, the European Sentinel Registry reported the procedural data and clinical outcomes of 628 patients treated with MitraClip in 25 European centers (8 countries) [11]. In this case, as well, the treated patients were elderly, at high surgical risk (logistic EuroSCORE of 20.4%), and 72% of cases were affected with functional

MR. The acute procedural success rate was 95.2%. Intrahospital mortality was low (2.9%), while mortality in the follow-up at 1 year was 15.3%.

One of the largest currently available body of cases is the Transcatheter Mitral Valve Interventions (TRAMI) multicenter registry [12]. The TRAMI registry analyzed the data of 828 patients treated with MitraClip in Germany. In this registry, too, the patients enrolled in the analysis were elderly and at high surgical risk (mean age of 76 years and with mean logistic EuroSCORE of 20.0%). In the follow-up at 12 months, a significant improvement was recorded in the quality of life (10 points on the EuroQuol visual analogue scale) and in the NYHA functional class (63.3% of patients in NYHA functional class I compared with 11% at the baseline evaluation). The mortality rate at 1 year in this large cohort was 20.3%. Interestingly, among the independent predictors of mortality, the highest risk (hazard ratio [HR] 4.36, $p < 0.0001$) was associated with procedural failure, defined as residual severe MR, conversion to open heart surgery, or procedural failure of the operator.

The prognostic impact of acute procedural success was confirmed by the Italian multicenter registry GRASP-IT (Getting Reduction of mitrAl inSufficiency by Percutaneous clip implantation in ITaly) [13]. The GRASP-IT registry analyzed the clinical outcomes in 304 patients enrolled in four centers in Italy. The patients suffered from functional MR in 79% of cases, and 63% of patients were in NYHA functional class III–IV. Acute procedural success was determined in 92% of patients. In the GRASP-IT registry, mortality at 30 days and 1 year was 3.4% and 10.8%, respectively. The independent predictors of mortality in this group of patients were procedural success (HR 0.18, 95% confidence interval [CI] 0.06–0.51), functional/ischemic etiology (HR 2.12, 95% CI 1.15-3.91), and clinical presentation in NYHA functional class IV (HR 3.38, 95% CI 1.71–6.66).

Sorajja et al. [14] recently reported the short-term clinical outcome (30 days) in patients who received a MitraClip implant in the post-approval commercial experience with the device in the United States (Society of Thoracic Surgeons/American College of Cardiology Transcatheter Valve Therapy Registry). The 563 patients included in the analysis were at high surgical risk (mean STS score for the estimated mortality rate of 7.9%) and had degenerative MR in 90.8% of cases. This registry also recorded high percentages of acute procedural success (93%), with low intrahospital and 30-day mortality (2.3% and 5.8%, respectively).

Finally, there are other national and multinational registries, with smaller patient populations (the Mitra-Swiss and Asia-Pacific registries) [15, 16]. The safety and efficacy outcomes of the MitraClip System have been confirmed in these smaller cohorts, as well. Table 12.1 summarizes the main clinical characteristics, the procedural success, and survival in the various registries hitherto analyzed.

## 12.3 Meta-analyses in the Literature

Meta-analyses represent the highest level of evidence in the literature because they condense the results of individual studies with appropriate statistical techniques and, thus, make it possible to analyze larger samples and to investigate the presence and sources of heterogeneity among the published studies.

**Table 12.1** Main clinical characteristics, procedural success and mortality in different registers

| Register | Number of patients | Age | Logistic Euro SCORE°/STS score* | Functional MR | Procedural success | Mortality at 30 days | Mortality at 1 year |
|---|---|---|---|---|---|---|---|
| EVEREST HRR and REALISM (aggregated data) [9] | 351 | 76 ± 11 | 11.3 ± 7.7%* | 70.1% | 86% | 4.8% | 22.8% |
| ACCESS-EU [10] | 567 | 74 ± 10 | 23.0 ± 18.3° | 77.1% | 90% | 3.4% | 17.3%, |
| SENTINEL [11] | 628 | 74 ± 10 | 20.4 ± 16.7% | 72% | 95.4% | NR | 15.3% |
| TRAMI [12] | 749 | 76 (71–81) | 20 (12–31)/6.0 (4–11) | 71.3% | 97% | 4.5% | 20.3% |
| GRASP-IT [13] | 304 | 72 ± 10 | 6 (3–11)[a] | 79% | 91.7% | 2.6% | 12.5% |
| STS/TVT Commercial experience [16] | 564 | 83 (74–87) | 7.9 (4.7–12.2)* | 9.2% | 93.1% | 5.8% | NR |
| Mitra-Swiss [14] | 100 | 72 ± 12 | 16.9% | 62% | 85% | NR | 15.4% |
| MARS [15] | 142 | 71 ± 12 | 16.8 ± 14.6/7.4 ± 8.1 | 53.5% | 93% | 5.6% | NR |

*NR* not reported

[a]Risk estimate by EuroSCORE II

°EuroSCORE

*STS score

Vakil et al. [17] analyzed the safety and efficacy data of the device reported in 16 studies (total of 2980 patients). The mean estimated procedural success was 91.4%, with intra-procedural and 30-day mortality of 0.1% and 4.2%, respectively. Adverse procedural events were infrequent and often related to the need for transfusions.

Wan et al. [18], instead, conducted a meta-analysis of studies, showing the comparative results of the treatment of MR with the MitraClip device or surgery. Though this analysis was limited by the small number of studies included ($n = 4355$ patients in the MitraClip group and 288 in the surgical group), no significant differences in mortality were found between the different modes of treatment at 30 days (1.7% vs. 3.5%; OR, 0.66; 95% CI: 0.17–2.52; $p = 0.54$) and at 12 months (7.4% vs. 7.3%; OR, 1.18; 95% CI: 0.56–2.48; $p = 0.66$) despite a higher mean EuroSCORE in patients treated with MitraClip. The presence of residual post-procedural MR of >2 was significantly more frequent in the MitraClip group (17.2% vs. 0.4%; OR, 20.72; 95% CI: 4.91–87.44; $p < 0.0001$). The rate of neurological adverse events was similar between the two groups (0.85% vs. 1.74%; OR, 0.58; 95% CI: 0.15–2.23; $p = 0.43$).

Finally, D'Ascenzo et al. [19] reported the main clinical outcomes in functional MR patients treated with MitraClip. The analysis included a total of nine studies (875 patients). At a mean follow-up of 9 months, the mortality "pooled across studies" was 15% (78 events), and 11% of patients showed residual moderate-to-severe MR. In addition, 78% of patients were in NYHA class I/II at follow-up, and this data was associated with a significant improvement in the distance covered during the 6-min walking test (average increase of 100 m compared with the baseline value).

## 12.4    MitraClip: Future Research Areas

The US guidelines recommend treatment with MitraClip in inoperable patients, with primitive etiology, and with reasonable life expectancy (evidence class IIb, level B) [20]. The European guidelines consider the MitraClip therapy option in functional MR; however, they stress the absence of randomized data with supporting data solely from registries [21]. Along this line, the principal research effort is aimed at supporting the use of MitraClip in patients with functional MR (whether ischemic or nonischemic). The design of future randomized studies is shown in Table 12.2. The recent publication of international standardized criteria (MVARC criteria) for the evaluation and the "reporting" of the main safety and clinical efficacy outcomes in patients treated with MitraClip will allow a clearer interpretation of the results from these studies [22, 23]. The MVARC criteria will also be useful for conducting aggregated analyses at study level to increase the statistical power and to assess the consistency of the results in larger samples. The timeline of the main studies (published and expected) is shown in Fig. 12.1.

**Table 12.2** Main characteristics of future randomized studies

| Trial | Inclusion criteria | Target patients number | Control arm | Follow-up | Primary end point | Expected completion date |
|---|---|---|---|---|---|---|
| COAPT | Symptomatic functional MR (≥3+) due to cardiomyopathy of either ischemic or nonischemic etiology; LVEF ≥20% and ≤50% | 555 | Patients managed nonsurgically based on standard hospital clinical practice | 12 and 24 months (safety and efficacy endpoints, respectively) | *Safety:* Composite of Single Leaflet Device Attachment, device embolizations, endocarditis requiring surgery, mitral stenosis requiring surgery, LVAD implant, heart transplant, and any device-related complications requiring surgery. *Efficacy:* Recurrent heart failure (HF) hospitalizations | July 2018 (primary outcome measures) |
| MATTERHORN | Patients with moderate-to-severe mitral regurgitation (MR) of functional pathology and reduced left ventricular function (LVEF ≥20% and ≤45%) considered to be at high surgical risk | 210 | Reconstructive mitral valve surgery | 12 months | Composite of death, rehospitalization for heart failure, reintervention (repeat operation or repeat intervention), assist device implantation, and stroke (whatever is first) | December 2017 |
| MITRA-FR | Severe secondary mitral regurgitation with LVEF between 15 and 40%, NYHA functional class ≥2; Minimum of 1 hospitalization for heart failure within 12 months | 288 | Optimal medical therapy | 12 months (24 months for cost-effectiveness analysis) | Composite of all-cause mortality and unplanned hospitalizations for heart failure | October 2017 |

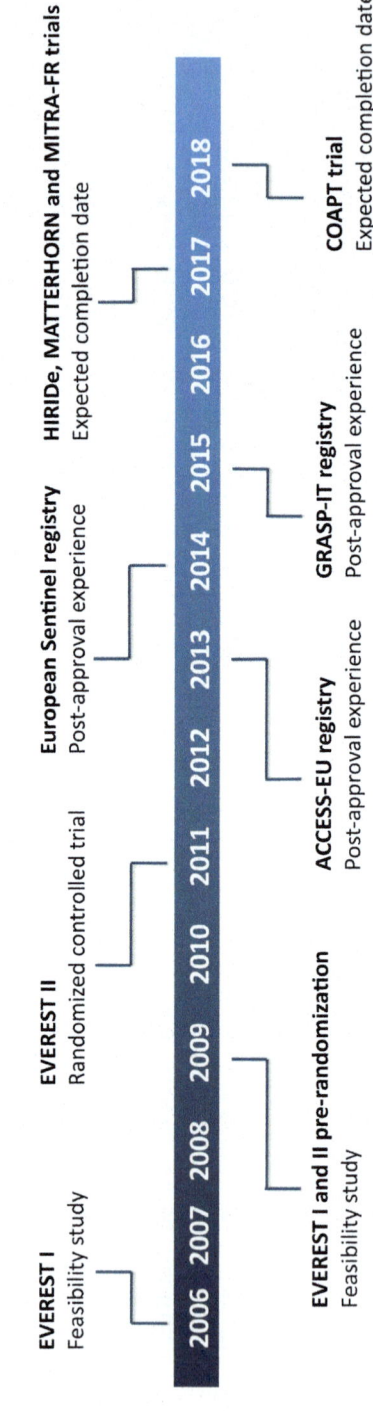

**Fig. 12.1** Timeline of principal studies investigating the MitraClip repair system

## 12.5    Percutaneous Annuloplasty: Additional Targets in Interventional Treatment of the Mitral Valve

The main limit in the percutaneous treatment of MR has been the absence of alternative strategies for repairing the leaflets. In fact, the duration of valve repair becomes questionable in the absence of additional repair strategies for other anatomical components of the mitral apparatus (e.g., the mitral annulus). Along this line, different techniques have been developed, and are currently available to perform mitral valve percutaneous annuloplasty. The first device to obtain the CE mark (2011) was the "CARILLON" indirect annuloplasty system.

The initial data on the feasibility of implantation were obtained with AMADEUS (CARILLON Mitral Annuloplasty Device European Union Study) (Table 12.3) [24]. In this study, implantation success and the acute reduction of MR were obtained in 30 of 48 patients (62.5%) with severe functional MR. The rate of major adverse events at 30 days was 13%. In the follow-up at 6 months, the implantation of the device resulted in a significant improvement in quality of life and the distance covered during the 6-min walking test. The TITAN study [25] later confirmed the initial results obtained with the implantation of the device and compared the clinical results with those of a cohort of non-implanted patients. After 12 months, 36 patients who were implanted with the device had a reduction in the grade of MR, with an improvement of at least one NYHA class in 80% of patients ($p < 0.001$). The rate of major adverse events at 30 days was 1.9%. In both studies, one of the main limitations of implantation of the device was the course and the potential risk of compressing the circumflex artery. In addition, fracturing of the nitinol structure of the device often occurred. In order to overcome this limit, the TITAN II study [26] evaluated the safety and procedural efficacy of a modified version of the device. The study was carried out in 36 patients and substantially confirmed the previous results and clinical outcomes. There were no fractures of the device. The randomized study entitled REDUCE FMR (CARILLON Mitral Contour System for Reducing Functional Mitral Regurgitation, NCT02325830) is currently recruiting patients. It will assess the efficacy of the Carillon implant in patients with severe functional MR compared with patients treated with medical therapy.

The first feasibility results for devices suitable for direct percutaneous annuloplasty (Cardioband and Mitralign) were recently obtained by Maisano et al. [4], who reported encouraging data on the use of the Cardioband. Implantation feasibility in 31 patients was 100%, resulting in a significant reduction of the septolateral dimensions of the left ventricle (from $36.8 \pm 4.8$ to $29 \pm 5.5$ mm after the procedure, $p < 0.01$). None of the patients experienced severe MR after implantation, and in the follow-up at 30 days, 88% of the patients showed a grade of residual MR $\leq$2+. There were no cases of procedural death. A similar procedural safety profile, though with a lesser degree of implantation feasibility, was found with the Mitralign device [5]. In fact, implantation was effective in 50 of 74 candidates for implantation, with no cases of intra-procedural death. However, there were four cases of cardiac tamponade. The follow-up echocardiographic analysis at 6 months

**Table 12.3** Main characteristics and clinical results of studies on percutaneous annuloplasty

| Study | Device | Patients | Age (years) | Ejection fraction (%) | Implant success | Follow-up (months) | Mortality | Principal findings |
|---|---|---|---|---|---|---|---|---|
| TITAN | Carillon | 53 | 62 ± 13 | 28 ± 8 | 68% | 24 | 22.6% | Reduction in LV systolic and diastolic volumes, significant improvement in 6MWD |
| TITAN II | Carillon | 36 | 71 ± 9 | 34 ± 10 | 83% | 12 | 19.4% | Reduction in FMR and improvements in functional class and 6-min walk tests |
| AMADEUS | Carillon | 48 | 64.4 | 29.6 | 62.5% | 6 | 2.2% (30 days) | Significant improvement in 6MWT distance and quality of life |
| Maisano et al. | Cardioband | 31 | 72 ± 7 | 34 ± 11 | 100% | 1 | 6.5% (in-hospital) | Significant reduction in the septolateral dimension in all but two patients, MR ≤ 2 in 85% of patients at 1 month |
| Nickenig et al. | Mitralign | 71 | 68 ± 11 | 34 ± 8 | 70.4% | 6 | 12.2% | Evidence of reverse LV remodeling, significant reduction of the anterior-posterior and septal-lateral dimensions, improvement in NYHA class and 6MWD |

showed an average 1.3 reduction in the grade of MR, with significant valvular remodeling (reduction of the septolateral and anteroposterior diameter, reduction of the tenting area, and increase in the coaptation length) and ventricular remodeling (reduction of the ventricular end-diastolic diameters and volumes). There was also a reduction in the percentage of patients in NYHA functional class III/IV at follow-up.

## 12.6 Transcatheter Implantable Mitral Valve: A Glimpse into the Future

The first clinical experiences with implants in humans of devices for MR transcatheter implantation have recently been reported. Various devices will make their clinical debut in the near future, including Tendyne (Abbott Vascular, Santa Clara, California), CardiAQ (Edwards Lifesciences, Irvine, California), Tiara (Neovasc, Richmond, British Columbia, Canada), Twelve (Medtronic, Minneapolis, Minnesota), NaviGate (NaviGate Cardiac Structures, Lake Forest, California), HighLife (HighLife Inc., Paris, France), and the MValve (MValve Technologies, San Diego, California) [27–29]. Future fields of research concerning patient selection, technical and procedural optimization, and the study of post-implant clinical outcomes will probably be among the most important and active areas of research in structural interventional cardiology.

## References

1. Wan B, Rahnavardi M, Tian DH, Phan K, Munkholm-Larsen S, Bannon PG, Yan TD. A meta-analysis of MitraClip system versus surgery for treatment of severe mitral regurgitation. Ann Cardiothorac Surg. 2013;2(6):683–92. doi:10.3978/j.issn.2225-319X.2013.11.02.
2. D'ascenzo F, Moretti C, Marra WG, Montefusco A, Omede P, Taha S, Castagno D, Gaemperli O, Taramasso M, Frea S, Pidello S, Rudolph V, Franzen O, Braun D, Giannini C, Ince H, Perl L, Zoccai G, Marra S, D'Amico M, Maisano F, Rinaldi M, Gaita F. Meta-analysis of the usefulness of Mitraclip in patients with functional mitral regurgitation. Am J Cardiol. 2015;116(2):325–31. doi:10.1016/j.amjcard.2015.04.025.
3. Feldman T, Foster E, Glower DD, Kar S, Rinaldi MJ, Fail PS, Smalling RW, Siegel R, Rose GA, Engeron E, Loghin C, Trento A, Skipper ER, Fudge T, Letsou GV, Massaro JM, Mauri L, EVEREST II Investigators. Percutaneous repair or surgery for mitral regurgitation. N Engl J Med. 2011;364(15):1395–406. doi:10.1056/NEJMoa1009355.
4. Maisano F, Taramasso M, Nickenig G, Hammerstingl C, Vahanian A, Messika-Zeitoun D, Baldus S, Huntgeburth M, Alfieri O, Colombo A, La Canna G, Agricola E, Zuber M, Tanner FC, Topilsky Y, Kreidel F, Kuck KH. Cardioband, a transcatheter surgical-like direct mitral valve annuloplasty system: early results of the feasibility trial. Eur Heart J. 2016;37(10):817–25. doi:10.1093/eurheartj/ehv603.
5. Nickenig G, Schueler R, Dager A, Martinez Clark P, Abizaid A, Siminiak T, Buszman P, Demkow M, Ebner A, Asch FM, Hammerstingl C. Treatment of chronic functional mitral valve regurgitation with a percutaneous annuloplasty system. J Am Coll Cardiol. 2016;67(25):2927–36. doi:10.1016/j.jacc.2016.03.591.
6. Feldman T, Wasserman HS, Herrmann HC, Block P, Gray W, Hamilton A, Zunamon A, Homma S, Di Tullio MR, Kraybill K, Merlino J, Martin R, Rodriguez L, Stewart WJ, Whitlow P, Wiegers SE, Silvestry FE, Foster E, Feldman T. Percutaneous mitral valve repair using the

edge-to-edge technique six-month results of the EVEREST phase I clinical trial. J Am Coll Cardiol. 2006;46:2134–40.

7. Feldman T, Kar S, Rinaldi M, Fail P, Hermiller J, Smalling R, Whitlow PL, Gray W, Low R, Herrmann HC, Lim S, Foster E, Glower D, EVEREST Investigators. Percutaneous mitral repair with the MitraClip system: safety and midterm durability in the initial EVEREST (endovascular valve edge-to-edge REpair study) cohort. J Am Coll Cardiol. 2009;54:686–94.

8. Feldman T, Kar S, Elmariah S, Smart SC, Trento A, Siegel RJ, Apruzzese P, Fail P, Rinaldi MJ, Smalling RW, Hermiller JB, Heimansohn D, Gray WA, Grayburn PA, Mack MJ, Lim DS, Ailawadi G, Herrmann HC, Acker MA, Silvestry FE, Foster E, Wang A, Glower DD, Mauri L, EVEREST II Investigators. Randomized comparison of percutaneous repair and surgery for mitral regurgitation: 5-year results of EVEREST II. J Am Coll Cardiol. 2015;66(25):2844–54. doi:10.1016/j.jacc.2015.10.018.+.

9. Glower DD, Kar S, Trento A, Lim DS, Bajwa T, Quesada R, Whitlow PL, Rinaldi MJ, Grayburn P, Mack MJ, Mauri L, McCarthy PM, Feldman T. Percutaneous mitral valve repair for mitral regurgitation in high-risk patients: results of the EVEREST II study. J Am Coll Cardiol. 2014;64(2):172–81. doi:10.1016/j.jacc.2013.12.062.

10. Maisano F, Franzen O, Baldus S, Schäfer U, Hausleiter J, Butter C, Ussia GP, Sievert H, Richardt G, Widder JD, Moccetti T, Schillinger W. Percutaneous mitral valve interventions in the real world: early and 1-year results from the ACCESS-EU, a prospective, multicenter, nonrandomized post-approval study of the MitraClip therapy in Europe. J Am Coll Cardiol. 2013;62(12):1052–61. doi:10.1016/j.jacc.2013.02.094.

11. Nickenig G, Estevez-Loureiro R, Franzen O, Tamburino C, Vanderheyden M, Lüscher TF, Moat N, Price S, Dall'Ara G, Winter R, Corti R, Grasso C, Snow TM, Jeger R, Blankenberg S, Settergren M, Tiroch K, Balzer J, Petronio AS, Büttner HJ, Ettori F, Sievert H, Fiorino MG, Claeys M, Ussia GP, Baumgartner H, Scandura S, Alamgir F, Keshavarzi F, Colombo A, Maisano F, Ebelt H, Aruta P, Lubos E, Plicht B, Schueler R, Pighi M, Di Mario C, Transcatheter Valve Treatment Sentinel Registry Investigators of the EURObservational Research Programme of the European Society of Cardiology. Percutaneous mitral valve edge-to-edge repair: in-hospital results and 1-year follow-up of 628 patients of the 2011-2012 pilot European sentinel registry. J Am Coll Cardiol. 2014;64(9):875–84. doi:10.1016/j.jacc.2014.06.1166.

12. Puls M, Lubos E, Boekstegers P, von Bardeleben RS, Ouarrak T, Butter C, Zuern CS, Bekeredjian R, Sievert H, Nickenig G, Eggebrecht H, Senges J, Schillinger W. One-year outcomes and predictors of mortality after MitraClip therapy in contemporary clinical practice: results from the German transcatheter mitral valve interventions registry. Eur Heart J. 2016;37(8):703–12. doi:10.1093/eurheartj/ehv627.

13. Capodanno D, Adamo M, Barbanti M, Giannini C, Laudisa ML, Cannata S, Curello S, Immè S, Maffeo D, Bedogni F, Petronio AS, Ettori F, Tamburino C, Grasso C, GRASP-IT Investigators. Predictors of clinical outcomes after edge-to-edge percutaneous mitral valve repair. Am Heart J. 2015;170(1):187–95. doi:10.1016/j.ahj.2015.04.010.

14. Sorajja P, Mack M, Vemulapalli S, Holmes DR Jr, Stebbins A, Kar S, Lim DS, Thourani V, McCarthy P, Kapadia S, Grayburn P, Pedersen WA, Ailawadi G. Initial experience with commercial transcatheter mitral valve repair in the United States. J Am Coll Cardiol. 2016;67(10):1129–40. doi:10.1016/j.jacc.2015.12.054.

15. Sürder D, Pedrazzini G, Gaemperli O, Biaggi P, Felix C, Rufibach K, der Maur CA, Jeger R, Buser P, Kaufmann BA, Moccetti M, Hürlimann D, Bühler I, Bettex D, Scherman J, Pasotti E, Faletra FF, Zuber M, Moccetti T, Lüscher TF, Erne P, Grünenfelder J, Corti R. Predictors for efficacy of percutaneous mitral valve repair using the MitraClip system: the results of the MitraSwiss registry. Heart. 2013;99(14):1034–40. doi:10.1136/heartjnl-2012-303105.

16. Yeo KK, Yap J, Yamen E, Muda N, Tay E, Walters DL, Santoso T, Liu X, Jansz P, Yip J, Zambahari R, Passage J, Koh TH, Wang J, Scalia G, Kuntjoro I, Soesanto AM, Muller D. Percutaneous mitral valve repair with the MitraClip: early results from the MitraClip Asia-Pacific registry (MARS). EuroIntervention. 2014;10(5):620–5. doi:10.4244/EIJV10I5A107.

17. Vakil K, Roukoz H, Sarraf M, Krishnan B, Reisman M, Levy WC, Adabag S. Safety and efficacy of the MitraClip® system for severe mitral regurgitation: a systematic review. Catheter Cardiovasc Interv. 2014;84(1):129–36. doi:10.1002/ccd.25347.
18. Wan B, Rahnavardi M, Tian DH, Phan K, Munkholm-Larsen S, Bannon PG, Yan TD. A meta-analysis of MitraClip system versus surgery for treatment of severe mitral regurgitation. Ann Cardiothorac Surg. 2013;2(6):683–92. doi:10.3978/j.issn.2225-319X.2013.11.02.
19. D'ascenzo F, Moretti C, Marra WG, Montefusco A, Omede P, Taha S, Castagno D, Gaemperli O, Taramasso M, Frea S, Pidello S, Rudolph V, Franzen O, Braun D, Giannini C, Ince H, Perl L, Zoccai G, Marra S, D'Amico M, Maisano F, Rinaldi M, Gaita F. Meta-analysis of the usefulness of Mitraclip in patients with functional mitral regurgitation. Am J Cardiol. 2015;116(2):325–31. doi:10.1016/j.amjcard.2015.04.025.
20. Nishimura RA, Otto CM, Bonow RO, Carabello BA, Erwin JP III, Guyton RA, O'Gara PT, Ruiz CE, Skubas NJ, Sorajja P, Sundt TM III, Thomas JD, American College of Cardiology/American Heart Association Task Force on Practice Guidelines. 2014 AHA/ACC guideline for the management of patients with valvular heart disease: executive summary: a report of the American College of Cardiology/American Heart Association task force on practice guidelines. J Am Coll Cardiol. 2014;63(22):2438–88. doi:10.1016/j.jacc.2014.02.537.
21. Ponikowski P, Voors AA, Anker SD, Bueno H, Cleland JG, Coats AJ, Falk V, González-Juanatey JR, Harjola VP, Jankowska EA, Jessup M, Linde C, Nihoyannopoulos P, Parissis JT, Pieske B, Riley JP, Rosano GM, Ruilope LM, Ruschitzka F, Rutten FH, van der Meer P, Authors/Task Force Members; Document Reviewers. 2016 ESC guidelines for the diagnosis and treatment of acute and chronic heart failure: the task force for the diagnosis and treatment of acute and chronic heart failure of the European Society of Cardiology (ESC). Developed with the special contribution of the heart failure association (HFA) of the ESC. Eur J Heart Fail. 2016;18(8):891–975. doi:10.1002/ejhf.592. [Epub ahead of print]
22. Stone GW, Vahanian AS, Adams DH, Abraham WT, Borer JS, Bax JJ, Schofer J, Cutlip DE, Krucoff MW, Blackstone EH, Généreux P, Mack MJ, Siegel RJ, Grayburn PA, Enriquez-Sarano M, Lancellotti P, Filippatos G, Kappetein AP, Mitral Valve Academic Research Consortium (MVARC). Clinical trial design principles and endpoint definitions for transcatheter mitral valve repair and replacement: part 1: clinical trial design principles: a consensus document from the mitral valve academic research consortium. J Am Coll Cardiol. 2015;66(3):278–307. doi:10.1016/j.jacc.2015.05.046.
23. Stone GW, Adams DH, Abraham WT, Kappetein AP, Généreux P, Vranckx P, Mehran R, Kuck KH, Leon MB, Piazza N, Head SJ, Filippatos G, Vahanian AS, Mitral Valve Academic Research Consortium (MVARC). Clinical trial design principles and endpoint definitions for transcatheter mitral valve repair and replacement: part 2: endpoint definitions: a consensus document from the mitral valve academic research consortium. J Am Coll Cardiol. 2015;66(3):308–21. doi:10.1016/j.jacc.2015.05.049.
24. Schofer J, Siminiak T, Haude M, Herrman JP, Vainer J, Wu JC, Levy WC, Mauri L, Feldman T, Kwong RY, Kaye DM, Duffy SJ, Tübler T, Degen H, Brandt MC, Van Bibber R, Goldberg S, Reuter DG, Hoppe UC. Percutaneous mitral annuloplasty for functional mitral regurgitation: results of the CARILLON mitral Annuloplasty device European Union study. Circulation. 2009;120(4):326–33. doi:10.1161/CIRCULATIONAHA.109.849885.
25. Siminiak T, Wu JC, Haude M, Hoppe UC, Sadowski J, Lipiecki J, Fajadet J, Shah AM, Feldman T, Kaye DM, Goldberg SL, Levy WC, Solomon SD, Reuter DG. Treatment of functional mitral regurgitation by percutaneous annuloplasty: results of the TITAN trial. Eur J Heart Fail. 2012;14(8):931–8. doi:10.1093/eurjhf/hfs076.
26. Lipiecki J, Siminiak T, Sievert H, Müller-Ehmsen J, Degen H, Wu JC, Schandrin C, Kalmucki P, Hofmann I, Reuter D, Goldberg SL, Haude M; for the TITAN II Investigators. Coronary sinus-based percutaneous annuloplasty as treatment for functional mitral regurgitation: the TITAN II trial. Open Heart. 2016;3. doi:10.1136/openhrt-2016-000411.
27. Cheung A, Webb J, Verheye S, Moss R, Boone R, Leipsic J, Ree R, Banai S. Short-term results of transapical transcatheter mitral valve implantation for mitral regurgitation. J Am Coll Cardiol. 2014;64(17):1814–9. doi:10.1016/j.jacc.2014.06.1208.

28. Søndergaard L, De Backer O, Franzen OW, Holme SJ, Ihlemann N, Vejlstrup NG, Hansen PB, Quadri A. First-in-human case of transfemoral CardiAQ mitral valve implantation. Circ Cardiovasc Interv. 2015;8(7):e002135. doi:10.1161/CIRCINTERVENTIONS.115.002135.
29. Perpetua EM, Reisman M. The Tendyne transcatheter mitral valve implantation system. EuroIntervention. 2015;11 Suppl W:W78–9. doi:10.4244/EIJV11SWA23.

# Part II

# Aortic Valve Disease

# Anatomy of the Aortic Valve

# 13

Francesca Indorato, Silvio Gianluca Cosentino,
and Giovanni Bartoloni

The earliest documented interest in the anatomy of the aortic valvar complex stems from the Renaissance, with the description and drawings by Leonardo da Vinci (1513). Today, the need for accurate knowledge of the aortic valvar complex is imperative, especially for percutaneous therapies of the aortic valve.

The substantial changes in size and shape of the valve cusps and leaflets that occur during the cardiac cycle are facilitated by a highly complex internal microarchitecture. The layered structure of the aortic valve is formed by a dense collagenous layer close to the outflow surface, which provides the primary strength component, a central core of loose connective tissue, and an elastin layer below the inflow surface [1].

The aortic valve should be considered within the wider context of its anatomical and functional unit, namely, the aortic root. The latter is the connection between the left ventricle and the ascending aorta, and is located on the right, posteriorly to the subpulmonary infundibulum; its posterior margin is wedged between the mitral valve orifice and the muscular portion of the interventricular septum. The aortic root goes from the basal plane where the aortic valve leaflets enter the left ventricle to the peripheral point where they enter the sinotubular junction (Fig. 13.1) [2]. About two-thirds of the circumference of the lower part of the aortic root are connected to the muscular portion of the interventricular septum.

F. Indorato (✉)
Postgraduate School of Legal Medicine, University of Catania, Catania, Italy
e-mail: fra.indorato@gmail.com

S.G. Cosentino
Bachelor of Science, University of Catania, Catania, Italy
e-mail: silvio.cosentino@gmail.com

G. Bartoloni
Professor of Anatomic Pathology - Postgraduate School of Cardiology,
University of Catania, Catania, Italy
e-mail: gbartolo@unict.it

© Springer International Publishing AG 2018
C. Tamburino et al. (eds.), *Percutaneous Treatment of Left Side Cardiac Valves*,
https://doi.org/10.1007/978-3-319-59620-4_13

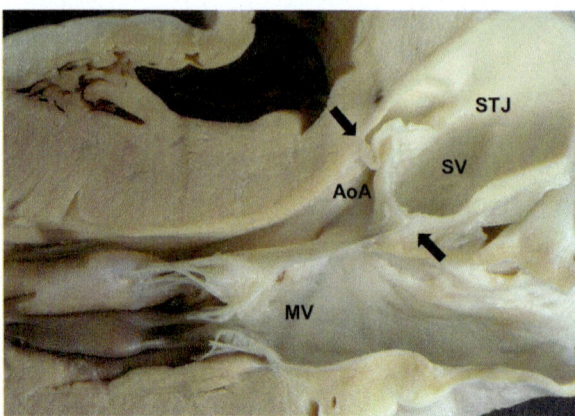

**Fig. 13.1** Long axis showing the aortic root between the aortic annulus (*AoA*) and the sinotubular junction (*STJ*). *SV* sinus of Valsalva, *black arrows* margins of aortic annulus, *MV* mitral valve

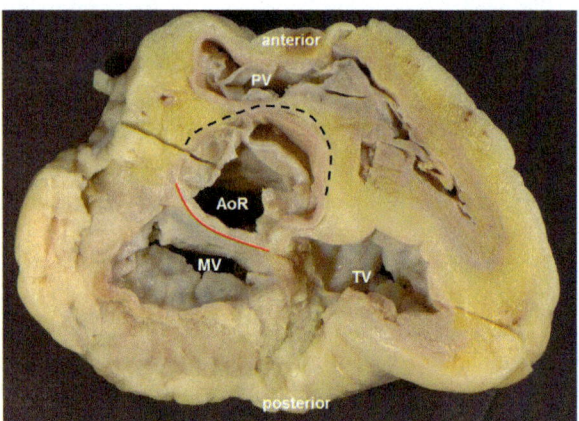

**Fig. 13.2** Short-axis view of the cardiac basis: about two-thirds of the circumference of the lower part of the aortic root are connected to the muscular portion of the interventricular septum (*black dotted line*). The remaining one-third is in continuity with the anterior aortic leaflet (*red line*). *AoR* aortic root, *MV* mitral valve, *PV* pulmonary valve, *TV* tricuspid valve

The remaining one-third is in continuity with the aortic leaflet of the mitral valve (Fig. 13.2). Its components include the annulus, valve leaflets, commissures, sinuses of Valsalva, sinotubular junction, and interleaflet triangles.

## 13.1    The Annulus

The aortic root contains at least three circular rings and one crown-like ring [3]. The valvular leaflets are attached throughout the length of the root. The three-dimensional arrangement of the leaflets takes the form of a three-pointed crown, with the hinges from the supporting ventricular structures forming the crown-like ring. The base of the crown is a virtual ring, commonly known as the "annulus," formed by the plane joining the basal points where the leaflets enter the left ventricle. The crown's upper part is a true ring, called the sinotubular junction, forming the point where the aortic root opens into the ascending aorta. The semilunar lines of attachment cross another true ring, the anatomic ventriculo-aortic junction. Though there have been generic descriptions of the annulus, in the aortic valve it can be said that the annulus takes on the cylindrical shape of the aortic root, in which the valve leaflets are supported by a crown-shaped structure [2].

The diameter of the aortic annulus in a normal adult usually ranges between 21 and 24 mm [4].

## 13.2  The Leaflets

The aortic valve is normally tricuspid. The valve's proper functioning depends on the correct relationship between the leaflets inside the aortic root. The leaflets consist of a core of fibrous tissue inside an endothelial sheath on both the arterial and ventricular side. The locus where they originate from the supporting ventricular structures gives way to the fibroelastic walls of the aortic valvar sinuses and marks off the anatomic ventriculo-aortic junction.

Each leaflet is composed of an attachment, body, coaptation surface, and lunule with the nodules of Arantii. The nodules of Arantii are located halfway on the free margin of the coaptation surface. On both sides of this nodule, there is a thin portion called a "lunule"; it consists of a margin, which is thin at its free end and continues into the coaptation area where the three leaflets meet and allow for complete valve closing. The lunules are attached to the wall of the aortic root in the area of the commissures. The main part of each leaflet is called "body." As specified above, the attachment is the area where the leaflet joins the aortic root [5]. Considering the size of the leaflets, it can be said that the non-coronary leaflet tends to be larger, followed by the left coronary leaflet, and the right coronary leaflet, though these differences are not significant (Fig. 13.3) [4, 6, 7].

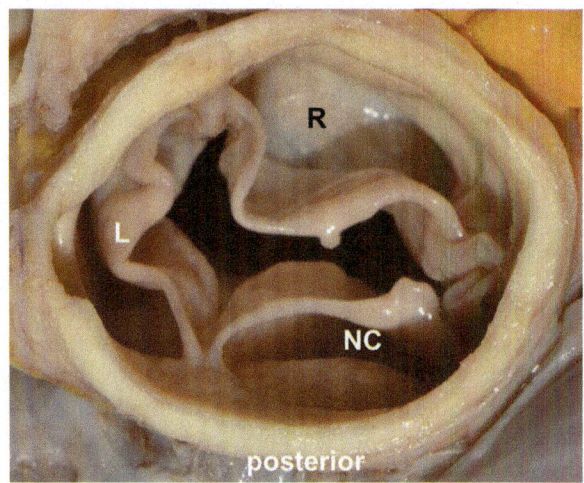

**Fig. 13.3** Aortic view showing the left (*L*), right (*R*), and non-coronary (*NC*) cusps

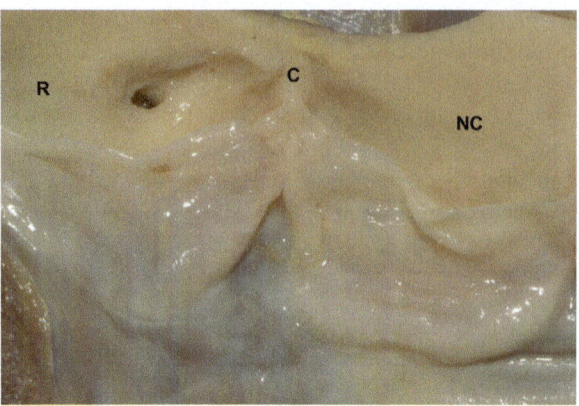

**Fig. 13.4** The commissure between the right (*R*) and non-coronary (*NC*) leaflets

## 13.3 The Commissures

The top of the crown-shaped structure in the area where the lunules of two leaflets are attached to the aortic wall at the sinotubular junctions is called the commissure (Fig. 13.4).

There are three commissures. The commissure between the right and left leaflets is located anteriorly, more or less in front of the matching commissure of the pulmonary valve. The one between the right and non-coronary leaflets is located anteriorly to the right, and the one between the left and non-coronary leaflets is usually located on the posterior face of the aortic root. The commissures have a fibrous structure and support the valvular leaflets located above the three triangular areas called interleaflet triangles.

## 13.4 The Interleaflet Triangles

As a result of the semilunar attachment of the aortic valvular leaflets, there are three triangular extensions of the left ventricular outflow tract that reach to the level of the sinotubular junction [8]. These triangles are formed not of ventricular myocardium but of the thinned fibrous walls of the aorta between the expanded sinuses of Valsalva.

The triangle between the right and left sinuses is located in front of the pulmonary valve. The triangle between the right and non-coronary sinuses is located in front of the right atrium and is proximally in continuity with the membranous septum. This is the area where the conduction system is closely linked to the aortic root. This has major implications, allowing for the introduction of alterations in conduction following percutaneous aortic valve replacement. The bundle of His is an anterior extension of the atrioventricular node. It penetrates through the central fibrous portion just below the lower margin of the membranous ventricular septum at the ridge of the muscular ventricular septum right below this triangle, which is closely interconnected with the septal leaflet of the tricuspid valve.

Finally, the triangle between the left and non-coronary sinuses is inferiorly in direct continuity with the aortic or anterior leaflet of the mitral valve. These triangles separate and mark off the three sinuses in a normal valve (Fig. 13.5) [3, 9].

## 13.5   The Sinuses of Valsalva

The sinuses of Valsalva are defined as expanses separating the ventricle and aorta (Figs. 13.1 and 13.6).

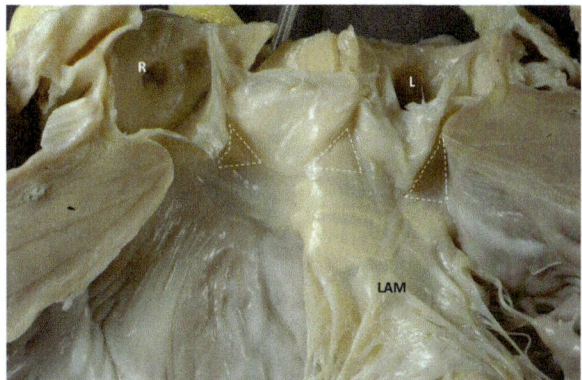

**Fig. 13.5**   Interleaf triangles. *L* left coronary ostium, *LAM* anterior mitral leaflet, *R* right coronary ostium

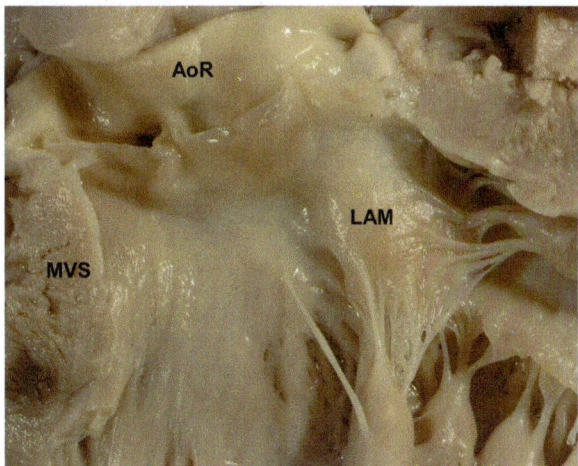

**Fig. 13.6**   Gross view of the left ventricular outlet: the posterior sinus of Valsalva wedged between the orifice of the anterior mitral leaflet (LAM) and the muscular ventricular septum (MVS). *AoR* aortic root

They border superiorly or distally with the sinotubular junction, and inferiorly or proximally with the valvar leaflet attachments. Each sinus takes its name from the coronary cusp it originates from (right, left, or non-coronary) [10] (Fig. 13.3).

The coronary orifices normally originate from the two anterior right and left sinuses of Valsalva, usually right below the sinotubular junction. Their origin may vary from patient to patient. The distance from the annular plane can vary greatly, and there are some congenital anatomic variants, which are very often associated with the bicuspid aortic valve [11]. Knowledge of the precise position of the coronary, ostia, and accurate measurement of the distance from the annulus is of the utmost importance during the screening of patients undergoing percutaneous aortic valve replacement. If this distance is too small, there is a risk of coronary occlusion by the aortic leaflets displaced by the device.

## 13.6    The Sinotubular Junction

The sinotubular junction marks the transition from the aortic root to the ascending aorta, and also the upper part of the attachment of each valve leaflet (Fig. 13.1). The mean diameter of the sinotubular junction ranges between 22 and 26 mm [4]. Dilation of the aortic root at this point has been associated with the onset of aortic failure.

## References

1. Schoen FJ. Evolving concepts of cardiac valve dynamics: the continuum of development, functional structure, pathobiology, and tissue engineering. Circulation. 2008;118:1864–80.
2. Hokken RB, Bartelings MM, Bogers AJ, Gittenberger-de Groot AC. Morphology of the pulmonary and aortic roots with regard to the pulmonary autograft procedure. J Thorac Cardiovasc Surg. 1997;113:453–61.
3. Anderson RH. Clinical anatomy of the aortic root. Heart. 2000;84:670–3.
4. Silver MA, Roberts WC. Detailed anatomy of the normally functioning aortic valve in hearts of normal and increased weight. Am J Cardiol. 1985;55:454–61.
5. Misfeld M, Sievers H. Heart valve macro- and microstructure. Philos Trans R Soc Lond Ser B Biol Sci. 2007;362:1421–36.
6. Vollebergh FE, Becker AE. Minor congenital variations of cusp size in tricuspid aortic valves. Possible link with isolated aortic stenosis. Br Heart J. 1977;39:1006–11.
7. Kunzelman KS, Grande KJ, David TE, et al. Aortic root and valve relationships. Impact on surgical repair. J Thorac Cardiovasc Surg. 1994;107:162–70.
8. Sutton JP III, Ho SY, Anderson RH. The forgotten interleaflet triangles: a review of the surgical anatomy of the aortic valve. Ann Thorac Surg. 1995;59:419–27.
9. Piazza N, de Jaegere P, Schultz C, et al. Anatomy of the aortic valvar complex and its implications for transcatheter implantation of the aortic valve. Circ Cardiovasc Interv. 2008;1:74–81.
10. Mihaljevic T, Sayeed MR, Stamou SC, Paul C. Pathophysiology of aortic valve disease. In: Cohn LH, editor. Cardiac surgery in the adult. New York: Mc Graw-Hill; 2008.
11. Roberts WC. The congenitally bicuspid aortic valve. A study of 85 autopsy cases. Am J Cardiol. 1970;26:72–83.

# Aortic Stenosis: Epidemiology and Pathogenesis

**14**

Simona Gulino, Alessio Di Landro, and Antonino Indelicato

Aortic (valve) stenosis (AS) is an obstruction to blood ejection from the left ventricle (LV) due to a fixed or dynamic stenosis located in the aortic valve, either over (supravalvular) or below it (subvalvular) [1]. AS is the most frequent form and accounts for the majority of congenital forms and for all of the acquired forms. AS is also the most frequent valvular heart disease in Western countries. In the Cardiovascular Health Study (5201 men and women over the age of 65), 26% of study participants had a thickening of the valve or calcification without significant obstruction, with a slight predominance of the disorder noted in men; 2% of all patients had frank AS [2]. Prevalence of aortic sclerosis increases with age: 20% in patients aged 65–75, 35% in those aged 75–85, and 48% in patients older than 85, while frank AS for the same age groups was 1–3%, 2–4%, and 4%, respectively. The most common cause is degenerative calcific valvular disease, with an incidence of 2–7% in the population over the age of 65 [3]. The mechanism by which a tricuspid aortic valve becomes stenotic is judged to be similar to that of atherosclerosis, as the initial plaque of AS is like that in coronary artery disease [4]. Risk factors commonly associated with coronary artery disease—including age, male gender, hyperlipidemia, evidence of active inflammation—seem to play a role in the development of AS, and both diseases are often present in the same individual [5–7]. Though debated, the use of statins is thought to slow the early progression of AS, while it is ineffective in the late course of the disease [8–11]. The initial and further evolution of AS usually occurs in the sixth, seventh, and eighth decades of life. The characteristic morphological appearance of the calcific AS consists in the presence of fibrous and calcific tissue on thickened cusps, preventing valve opening during outflow (Fig. 14.1). Calcific AS is determined mainly by solid calcium deposits in the valve cusps rather than fusion of the commissures, and calcification starts in the fibrous part of the valve. The stratified microscopic structure is usually preserved.

S. Gulino (✉) • A. Di Landro • A. Indelicato
Division of Cardiology-Ferrarotto Hospital, University of Catania, Catania, Italia
e-mail: si.gulino@gmail.com

© Springer International Publishing AG 2018
C. Tamburino et al. (eds.), *Percutaneous Treatment of Left Side Cardiac Valves*,
https://doi.org/10.1007/978-3-319-59620-4_14

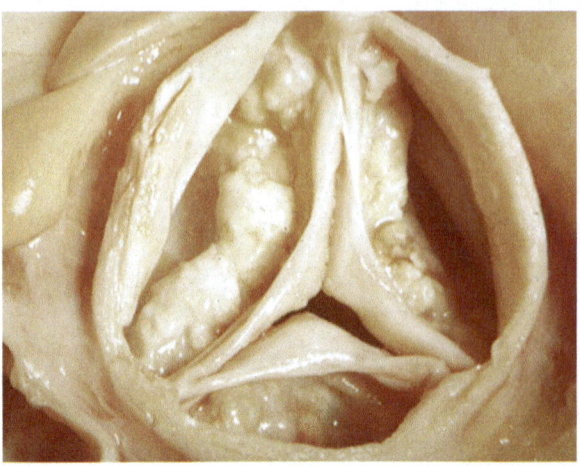

**Fig. 14.1** Calcific aortic stenosis. Calcium deposits are present on cusps without fusion of commissures

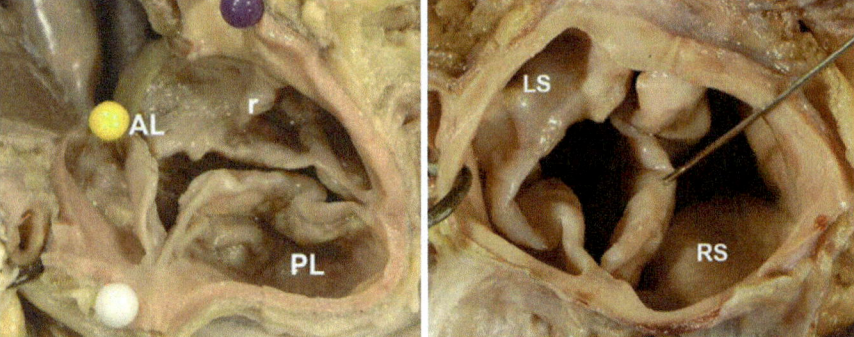

**Fig. 14.2** Bicuspid aortic valve. *AL* anterior leaflet, *LS* left sinus, *PL* posterior leaflet, *r* raphe, *RS* right sinus

The process of calcific aortic valve degeneration is secondary to inflammatory and proliferative changes, with accumulation of lipids, hyperactivity of angiotensin-converting enzymes, and infiltration of macrophages and T lymphocytes [12, 13]. These lesions involve the typical early chronic inflammatory cell infiltrates (macrophages and T lymphocytes) as the first ultrastructural changes, and lipid deposits and fibrotic thickening with collagen and elastin [14, 15].

Between 1 and 2% of children (mostly males) have a bicuspid aortic valve, at times associated with aortic coarctation (Fig. 14.2, Table 14.1). The epidemiological contribution of a bicuspid aortic valve to AS is greater than that of calcific tricuspid aortic valve [16, 17]. The pathogenic process underlying bicuspid AS is similar to that of the tricuspid aortic valve. Nonetheless, the onset of bicuspid AS occurs two decades earlier compared with tricuspid AS. This earlier onset is probably due to the unfavorable hemodynamic conditions of the bicuspid aortic valve. In most cases the cusps have different dimensions, and a median raphe is often present due

**Table 14.1** Sievers bicuspid aortic classification

| | 0 raphe - Type 0 | | 1 raphe - Type 1 | | | 2 raphes - Type 2 |
|---|---|---|---|---|---|---|
| Main category: number of raphes | 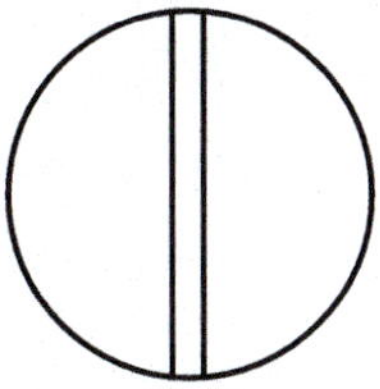 21 (7) | | 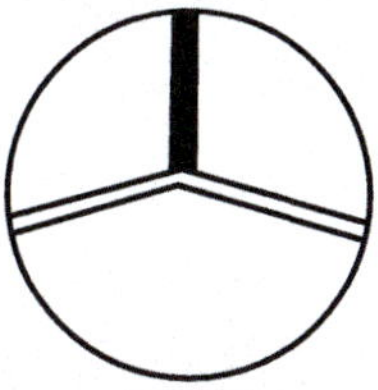 269 (88) | | |  14 (5) |
| 1.subcategory: spatial position of cusps in Type 0 and raphes in Types 1 and 2 | lat 13 (4) 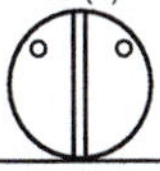 | ap 7 (2) 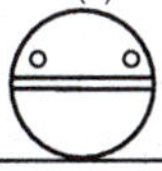 | L-R 216 (71)  | R-N 45 (15) 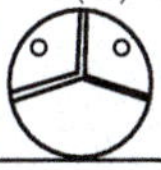 | N-L 45 (15) 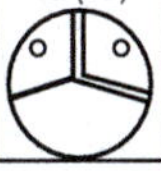 | L-R/R - N 14 (5) 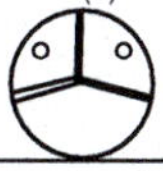 |
| 2. subcategory: | | | | | | |
| VALVULAR FUNCTION I | 6 (2) | 1 (0.3) | 79 (26) | 22 (7) | 3 (1) | 6 (2) |
| VALVULAR FUNCTION S | 7 (2) | 5 (2) | 119 (39) | 15 (5) | 3 (1) | 6 (2) |
| VALVULAR FUNCTION B (I + S) | | 1 (0.3) | 15 (5) | 7 (2) | 2 (1) | 2 (1) |
| VALVULAR FUNCTION No | | | 3 (1) | 1 (0.3) | | |

The main category (types 0, 1, 2) indicates the presence of 0, 1, or 2 raphe. First subcategory defines the cusps spatial disposition (type 0) and different raphe distribution patterns (type 1, 2): type 0 accounts for anteroposterior and latero-lateral patterns; L-R, R-N, and N-L display the relation between the cusps involved in fusion in type 1 and L-R/R-N in type 2 (R = right coronary cusp, L = left coronary cusp, N = noncoronary cusp). The second subcategory indicates aortic valve functional status (I for insufficiency, S for stenosis, B for steno-insufficiency, and No for normal functioning)

to their incomplete splitting. At birth, bicuspid aortic valves are not usually stenotic but are predisposed to gradually becoming so, owing to sclerosis and calcifications of mechanical origin, the processes of which lead to AS. Usually, calcifications develop in the raphe site (Fig. 14.3).

## 14.1 Congenital AS

Most cases of congenital AS are diagnosed and treated in early childhood and adolescence; a first diagnosis in adult age occurs in few cases. Anatomically, congenital AS presents with a unicuspid unicommissural valve, and is never associated with survival in adult age. Less frequently, the disease is attributable to a bicuspid aortic valve [16]. Its natural history is characterized by death during childhood, or symptoms that lead to valve replacement. Sudden death in asymptomatic individuals is common, while angina and heart failure are infrequent [18]. The absence of symptoms related to heart failure is due in part to the compensation mechanisms of the left ventricle, consisting in concentric hypertrophy in response to pressure overload, followed by an increase in the ejection fraction and reduced wall stress [19].

**Fig. 14.3** Stenotic
bicuspid aortic valve

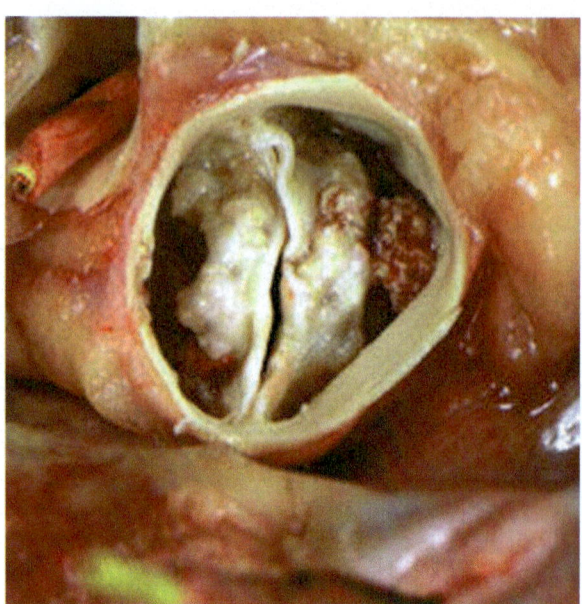

**Fig. 14.4** Rheumatic
aortic valve with
characteristic fusion of
commissures

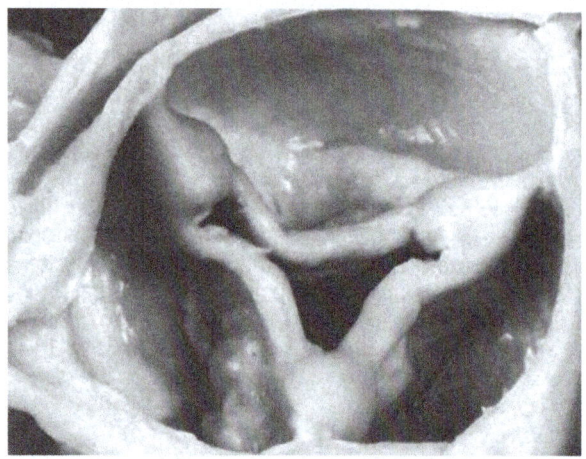

AS of rheumatic origin is the rarest form, though it is the most common cause in developing countries, almost always associated with mitral valve disease such as sequelae of rheumatic fever. It is the result of adhesion and fusion of commissures and cusps, causing retraction and stiffening of their free edges; calcified nodules develop on both surfaces and the orifice is reduced to a small round or triangular opening (Fig. 14.4). Functionally, a rheumatic aortic valve is often insufficient as well as stenotic.

## 14.2   Pathophysiology

The aortic valve area (AVA) in adults is about 3.0 cm$^2$ and varies within a range of 2.5–5 cm$^2$ depending on body surface area. In males, a transvalvular pressure gradient can be measured when the AVA is reduced by at least 50% below normal [20, 21]. Aortic stenosis exerts a resistance to ventricular outflow, and in order to maintain its outflow, the LV develops a higher systolic pressure. Pressure overload leads to concentric hypertrophy of the ventricular walls, namely, the heart's main compensation mechanism to cope with LV outflow obstruction. As a result of hypertrophy, left ventricular diastolic compliance tends to reduce, while end-diastolic pressure rises without necessarily giving rise to ventricular decompensation [22]. Left atrial contraction plays an important role in ensuring adequate filling pressure in the LV. In these patients, the loss of synchronous and vigorous pump function, as in the case of atrial fibrillation or atrioventricular dissociation, can cause rapid functional and clinical deterioration [23]. With a further rise in afterload, the LV adopts additional compensatory mechanisms, such as an increase in preload and myocardial contractility. Both of these expedients maintain normal left ventricular systolic pump function. When the preload reserve limit is reached (afterload mismatch) [24], or myocardial contractility is reduced, left ventricular systolic pump function becomes abnormal. Clinically, manifest heart failure is usually the result of this alteration in pump function. In these cases it is difficult to distinguish whether low left ventricular ejection fraction is secondary to reduced contractility or to an excessive increase in afterload [25]. Left ventricular systolic dysfunction can result from myocardial ischemia, even in the presence of normal epicardial coronary arteries. The increase in myocardial muscle mass due to left ventricular hypertrophy leads to an increase of myocardial oxygen demand, which exceeds oxygen supply. Myocardial ischemia is the result of (1) increased diastolic filling pressure of the left ventricle, which exceeds the coronary perfusion pressure, especially at a subendocardial level; (2) reduced diastolic coronary filling time due to tachycardia (i.e., during exercise); and (3) reduced myocardial capillary density [26–28].

The onset of the typical triad of symptoms of AS (angina, syncope, and heart failure) is a crucial moment in the natural history of the disease [29]. The mortality rate of an individual with symptoms rises to 25% per year (Fig. 14.5).

The narrowing of the aortic orifice by half determines a mild obstruction of cardiac output, thus generating a small pressure gradient across the valve. However, further reductions in valve area progressively produce a greater left ventricular pressure overload. Though still the subject of debate, many researchers consider ventricular hypertrophy to be a compensatory mechanism in response to pressure overload of the left ventricle, and to the increase in the afterload [30–33]. Afterload is generally quantified as wall stress, according to Laplace's law (=pr/2th). The increased pressure (p) is compensated by the increase in wall thickness (th) to keep a normal level of stress on the wall. The normalization of the afterload through the compensation of left ventricular hypertrophy is essential to preserve ejection fraction

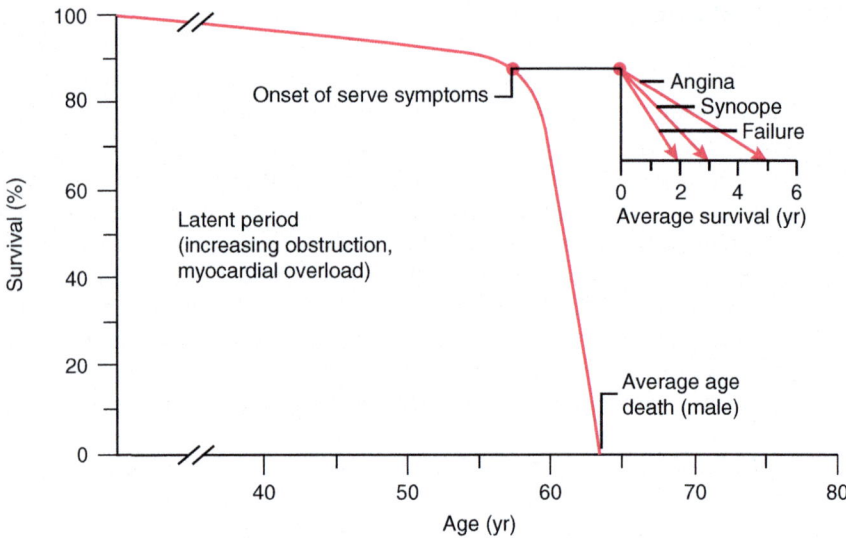

**Fig. 14.5** Ross survival curve in patient with aortic stenosis. The onset of severe symptoms greatly reduces survival after a long asymptomatic period

and stroke volume. However, ventricular hypertrophy also implies a reduced coronary reserve and is associated with diastolic dysfunction and increased mortality [28, 34–39]. One of the causes of reduced coronary reserve is the reduced growth of capillaries in the hypertrophic wall of the left ventricle, and the consequent increase in intercapillary distance. The increased filling pressure needed to stretch the thickened ventricular walls also exerts compression on the endocardium, further reducing the coronary reserve. The onset of angina is, however, correlated with the extent of valve obstruction and with diastolic filling time. The onset of dyspnea is the warning sign of the worst scenario for patients with AS. While concentric hypertrophy increases cardiac output on the one hand, on the other it is associated with diastolic dysfunction. During the active relaxation of the myocardial fibers, intracellular calcium is sequestered again by the sarcoplasmic reticulum and is hence not available for actomyosin contractility. In concentric hypertrophy, this mechanism is delayed and, in turn, delays the passive filling of the left ventricle, thus reducing the time for blood to pass from the atrium to the ventricle. Moreover, the increased wall thickness requires a greater filling pressure to reach an adequate diastolic volume [40]. This increase of the diastolic pressure results in pulmonary edema and dyspnea.

Concentric hypertrophy is not compensatory in all cases. The failure to normalize the excessive afterload results in reduced systolic performance and cardiac output [41]. Finally, the reduced contractility further reduces the ejection fraction [25].

Syncope is one of the most dangerous symptoms in AS. Its mechanisms are not completely known. Usually, syncope develops during physical exercise, when the peripheral resistance forces of the circulatory system are reduced and the increase in cardiac output is, unlike in healthy individuals, insufficient to increase blood pressure due to the reduced stroke volume through the narrow aortic orifice.

A significant reduction in blood pressure is therefore observed during physical activity that leads to syncope [42]. Exercise-induced ischemia can also generate ventricular arrhythmias, which are, in turn, the cause of syncope.

# References

1. Rahimtoola SH. Aortic valve disease. In: Fuster V, Alexander RW, O'Ruourke RA, editors. Hurst's the heart. 11th ed. New York: McGraw Hill; 2004. p. 1987–2000.
2. Supino PG, Borer JS, Preibisz J, Bornstein A. The epidemiology of valvular heart disease: a growing public health problem. Heart Fail Clin. 2006;2:379–93.
3. Vahanian A, Baumgartner H, Bax J, et al. Guidelines on the management of valvular heart disease: the task force on the management of valvular heart disease of the European Society of Cardiology. Eur Heart J. 2007;28:230–68.
4. Otto CM, Kuusisto J, Reichenbach DD, Gown AM, O'Brien KD. Characterization of the early lesion of 'degenerative' valvular aortic stenosis: histological and immunohistochemical studies. Circulation. 1994;90:844–53.
5. Aronow WS, Ahn C, Kronzon I, Goldman ME. Association of coronary risk factors and use of statins with progression of mild valvular aortic stenosis in older persons. Am J Cardiol. 2001;88:693–5.
6. Otto CM, Lind BK, Kitzman DW, Gersh BJ, Siscovick DS. Association of aortic-valve sclerosis with cardiovascular mortality and morbidity in the elderly. N Engl J Med. 1999;341:142–7.
7. Taylor HA Jr, Clark BL, Garrison RJ, et al. Relation of aortic valve sclerosis to risk of coronary heart disease in African-Americans. Am J Cardiol. 2005;95:401–4.
8. Rajamannan NM, Otto CM. Targeted therapy to prevent progression of calcific aortic stenosis. Circulation. 2004;110:1180–2.
9. Novaro GM, Tiong IY, Pearce GL, Lauer MS, Sprecher DL, Griffin BP. Effect of hydroxy-methylglutaryl coenzyme a reductase inhibitors on the progression of calcific aortic stenosis. Circulation. 2001;104:2205–9.
10. Cowell SJ, Newby DE, Prescott RJ, et al. A randomized trial of intensive lipid-lowering therapy in calcific aortic stenosis. N Engl J Med. 2005;352:2389–97.
11. Moura LM, Ramos SF, Zamorano JL, et al. Rosuvastatin affecting aortic valve endothelium to slow the progression of aortic stenosis. J Am Coll Cardiol. 2007;49:554–6.
12. Olsonn M, Thyberg J, Nilsson J. Presence of oxidized low-density lipoproteins in nonrheumatic stenotic aortic valves. Arterioscler Thromb Vasc Biol. 1999;19:1218.
13. O'Brien KD, Shavelle DM, Caulfield MT, et al. Association of ACE with low density lipoprotein in aortic valvular lesions and in human plasma. Circulation. 2002;106:2224–30.
14. Freeman RV, Otto CM. Spectrum of calcific aortic valve disease: pathogenesis, disease progression and treatment strategy. Circulation. 2005;111:3316–26.
15. Olsson N, Delsgaaro CJ, Haegerstrand A, et al. Accumulation of T-lymphocytes and expression of interleukin-2 receptor in non-rheumatic stenotic aortic valves. J Am Coll Cardiol. 1994;23:1162–70.
16. Roberts WC, Ko JM. Frequency by decades of unicuspid, bicuspid, and tricuspid aortic valves in adults having isolated aortic valve replacement for aortic stenosis, with or without associated aortic regurgitation. Circulation. 2005;111:920–5.
17. Aboulhosn J, Child JS. Left ventricular outflow obstruction: subaortic stenosis, bicuspid aortic valve, supravalvular aortic stenosis, and coarctation of the aorta. Circulation. 2006;114:2412–22.
18. Keane JF, Driscoll DJ, Gersony WM, et al. Second natural history study of congenital heart defects: results of treatment of patients with aortic valvular stenosis. Circulation. 1993;87:116–27.
19. Donner R, Carabello BA, Black I, Spann JF. Left ventricular wall stress in compensated aortic stenosis in children. Am J Cardiol. 1983;51:946–51.

20. Bonow RO, Carabello BA, Chatterjee K, et al. ACC/AHA 2006 guidelines for the management of patients with valvular heart disease. J Am Coll Cardiol. 2006;48:1–148.
21. Tobin JR Jr, Rahimtoola SH, Blundell PE, et al. Percentage of left ventricular stroke work loss: a simple hemodynamic concept for estimation of severity in valvular aortic stenosis. Circulation. 1967;35:868–79.
22. Hess OM, Villari B, Krayenbuehl HP. Diastolic dysfunction in aortic stenosis. Circulation. 1993;87:73–6.
23. Braunwald E, Fraham CJ. Studies on the Starling's law of the heart. IV. Observation on hemodynamic functions of the left atrium in man. Circulation. 1961;24:633–42.
24. Ross J Jr. Afterload mismatch and preload reserve: a conceptual framework for the analysis of ventricular function. Prog Cardiovasc Dis. 1976;18:255–64.
25. Huber D, Grimm J, Koch R, et al. Determinants of ejection performance in aortic stenosis. Circulation. 1981;64:126–34.
26. Johnson LL, Sciacca RR, Ellis K, et al. Reduced left ventricular myocardial blood flow per unit mass in aortic stenosis. Circulation. 1978;57:582–90.
27. Marcus ML, Doty DB, Horatzka LF, et al. Decreased coronary reserve. A mechanism for angina pectoris in patients with aortic stenosis and normal coronary arteries. N Engl J Med. 1982;46:1362–6.
28. Gould KL, Carabello BA. Why angina in aortic stenosis with normal coronary arteriograms? Circulation. 2003;107:3121–3.
29. Ross J Jr, Braunwald E. Aortic stenosis. Circulation. 1968;38:61–7.
30. Grossman W, Jones D, McLaurin LP. Wall stress and patterns of hypertrophy in the human left ventricle. J Clin Invest. 1975;53:332–41.
31. Koide M, Nagatsu M, Zile MR, et al. Premorbid determinants of left ventricular dysfunction in a novel model of gradually induced pressure overload in the adult canine. Circulation. 1997;95:1349–51.
32. Rogers JH, Tamirisa P, Kovacs A, et al. RGS4 causes increased mortality and reduced cardiac hypertrophy in response to overload. J Clin Invest. 1999;104:567–76.
33. Hill JA, Karimi M, Kutschke W, et al. Cardiac hypertrophy is not a required compensatory response to short-term pressure overload. Circulation. 2000;101:2863–9.
34. Levy D, Garrison RJ, Savage DD, Kannel WB, Castelli WP. Prognostic implications of echocardiographically determined left ventricular mass in the Framingham heart study. N Engl J Med. 1990;322:1561–6.
35. Gaasch WH, Zile MR, Hoshino PK, Weinberg EO, Rhodes DR, Apstein CS. Tolerance of the hypertrophic heart to ischemia: studies in compensated and failing dog hearts with pressure overload hypertrophy. Circulation. 1990;81:1644–53.
36. Marcus ML, Doty DB, Hiratzka LF, Wright CB, Eastham CL. Decreased coronary reserve: a mechanism for angina pectoris in patients with aortic stenosis and normal coronary arteries. N Engl J Med. 1982;307:1362–6.
37. Breisch EA, White FC, Bloor CM. Myocardial characteristics of pressure overload hypertrophy: a structural and functional study. Lab Investig. 1984;51:333–42.
38. Rajappan K, Rimoldi OE, Camici PG, et al. Functional changes in coronary microcirculation after valve replacement in patients with aortic stenosis. Circulation. 2003;107:3170–5.
39. Zile MR, Brutsaert DL. New concepts in diastolic dysfunction and diastolic heart failure: part II—causal mechanisms and treatment. Circulation. 2002;105:1503–8.
40. Hess OM, Ritter M, Schneider J, Grimm J, Turina M, Krayenbuehl HP. Diastolic stiffness and myocardial structure in aortic valve disease before and after valve replacement. Circulation. 1984;69:855–65.
41. Gunther S, Grossman W. Determinants of ventricular function in pressure-overload hypertrophy in man. Circulation. 1979;59:679–88.
42. Schwartz LS, Goldfischer J, Sprague GJ, Schwartz SP. Syncope and sudden death in aortic stenosis. Am J Cardiol. 1969;23:647–58.

# Aortic Stenosis: Diagnosis

# 15

Ines Monte, Rita Sicuso, and Vera Bottari

## 15.1 Non-Invasive Diagnosis

The diagnosis of aortic stenosis (AS) is reached through clinical and instrumental assessment of patients [1]. The symptomatic forms are characterized by angina, dyspnea, and syncope, but the diagnostic suspicion can be supported by the presence of typical physical signs, such as harsh diamond-shaped systolic murmur, often matched by a more intense fremitus along the right upper sternal margin and irradiated to the neck, *parvus et tardus* pulse, fourth sound, and attenuation or disappearance of the aortic component of the second sound. A complete picture of heart failure can be found where a systolic murmur is often faint or lacking. In asymptomatic forms, physical findings can be the only evidence of aortic valve (AV) disease. With regard to instrumental examinations, standard electrocardiogram (ECG) can highlight signs of left ventricular hypertrophy. However, even in the more severe forms of AS, ECG may not show any alteration.

*Chest X-ray* commonly shows a normal cardiac picture, with dilatation of the proximal ascending aorta (post-stenotic) and valve calcification in the lateral views. The increase in cardiac area and signs of pulmonary edema can be seen in the case of heart failure. When heart failure happens because of an afterload mismatch, the heart volume is generally normal.

The staple examination for noninvasive diagnosis of AS is *transthoracic bidimensional echocardiography (TTE) with Doppler examination (2D Doppler)* [2–4]. This method allows clinicians to:

- Assess the presence, etiology, and severity of valve stenosis
- Quantify the degree of heart function impairment
- Identify associated valve diseases
- Assess valve apparatus anatomy

I. Monte (✉) • V. Bottari • R. Sicuso
General Surgery and Medical-Surgery Specialities, University of Catania, Catania, Italy
e-mail: inemonte@unict.it

© Springer International Publishing AG 2018
C. Tamburino et al. (eds.), *Percutaneous Treatment of Left Side Cardiac Valves*,
https://doi.org/10.1007/978-3-319-59620-4_15

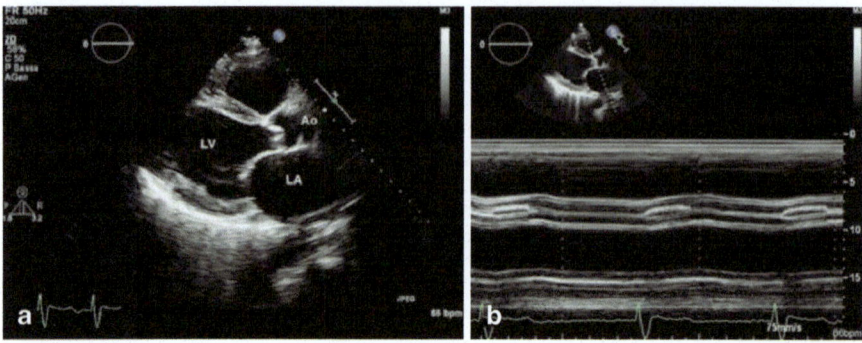

**Fig. 15.1** (**a**) Transthoracic echocardiogram, long-axis view, showing a calcified and stenotic aortic valve. (**b**) M-mode image in parasternal long-axis view: reduced opening of aortic leaflets during systolic phase. *Ao* aorta, *LA left* atrium, *LV left* ventricle

TTE gives very accurate morphological and functional information on the aortic valve, identifying the number of cusps, the thickening pattern, and the motility. It allows for the detection of some anatomical features of the valve apparatus, which can guide the diagnosis, such as the presence of a bicuspid aortic valve, and marked calcifications, which are predictors of rapidly progressing valve disease or commissural fusion, typical of the rheumatic form. Leaflet motility may help to estimate the severity of the valve disease. Severe AS is unlikely if at least a cusp opens well and the other two are stiff, while a calcified and immobile aortic valve is the sign of a severe stenosis (Fig. 15.1).

Doppler assessment allows estimation of the severity of AS by considering the following parameters:

- Peak velocity of the antegrade aortic systolic jet ($V_{max}$)
- Transvalvular maximum ($\Delta P_{max}$) and mean ($\Delta P_{mean}$) gradients
- Valve area by means of the continuity equation (CE-AVA)

The shape of the Doppler velocity curve allows assessment of the severity of AS, as the maximum peak is later and the curve has a rounded shape in the more severe obstructions. In addition, it can be useful in distinguishing fixed from dynamic obstructions, as the latter have a late peak, often with a concave curve at the beginning of the systole.

$V_{max}$ through a narrow aortic valve is measured by continuous wave Doppler (CWD), aligning the ultrasound beam as best as possible with the jet direction through various acoustic windows: apical, suprasternal, right parasternal, and, on rare occasions, subcostal. $V_{max}$ is defined as the highest velocity signal obtained from any acoustic window (Fig. 15.2).

$\Delta P_{max}$ is calculated from $V_{max}$ using the simplified Bernoulli equation as $\Delta P_{max} = 4 V^2_{max}$, while $\Delta P_{mean}$ is calculated by tracing the outer edge of the dark "envelope" of the velocity curve. A function included in most clinical instrument measurement package averages is the instantaneous gradient over the ejection period. The velocity/time integral (VTI) is calculated at the same time.

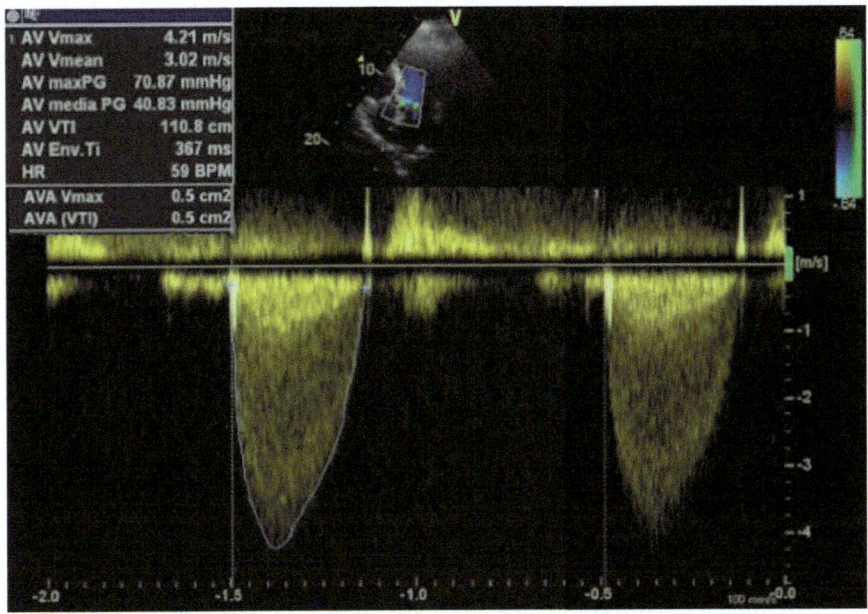

AV Vmax        4.21 m/s
AV Vmean       3.02 m/s
AV maxPG       70.87 mmHg
AV media PG    40.83 mmHg
AV VTI         110.8 cm
AV Env.Ti      367 ms
HR             59 BPM
AVA Vmax       0.5 cm2
AVA (VTI)      0.5 cm2

**Fig. 15.2** Continuous wave (CW) Doppler recordings at the level of a stenotic aortic orifice in five-chamber apical view. Peak velocity (*AV* $V_{max}$) is more than 4 m/s and the mean gradient (*AV media PG*), obtained when tracking the velocity wave, is about 40 mmHg

Of course, an underestimated $V_{max}$ gives a proportionally greater underestimation of the gradients, considering the squared relationship that exists between velocity and pressure gradient. Underestimated Doppler gradients are usually the result of inadequate signal recording or inaccurate alignment of the ultrasound beam, while overestimation can be secondary to a high cardiac output and associated subvalvular stenosis. In the case of high cardiac output, it must be borne in mind that the simplified Bernoulli equation assumes that the proximal velocity ($V_{prox}$) can be ignored, a reasonable assumption if it is <1 m/s. Otherwise, $V_{prox}$ should be included in the Bernoulli equation so that $\Delta P_{max} = 4\ (V^2_{max} - V^2_{prox})$ when calculating maximum gradients, in order to avoid overestimation. It is more problematic to include proximal velocity in mean gradient calculations, and this approach is not clinically used. In this situation, maximum velocity and gradient should be used to grade stenosis severity (a $V_{max}$ of 4.0 m/s corresponds to a $\Delta P_{max}$ of 64 mmHg).

AVA is calculated based on the continuity equation, except that the SV ejected through the LV outflow tract (LVOT) all passes through the stenotic orifice and thus the SV is equal at both sites: $AVA = A_{LVOT}\ x\ VTI_{LVOT}/VTI_{AV}$.

Calculation of CE-AVA requires three measurements: the velocity-time integral of the antegrade aortic systolic jet ($VTI_{AV}$) recorded by CWD; the velocity-time integral of the flow in the LVOT ($VTI_{LVOT}$), recorded by pulsed Doppler (PWD), with the sample volume moved apically 0.5–1.0 cm from the annulus to obtain a laminar flow curve without spectral dispersion (Fig. 15.3); and LVOT diameter for calculation of a circular cross-sectional area (CSA) at this site. LVOT diameter

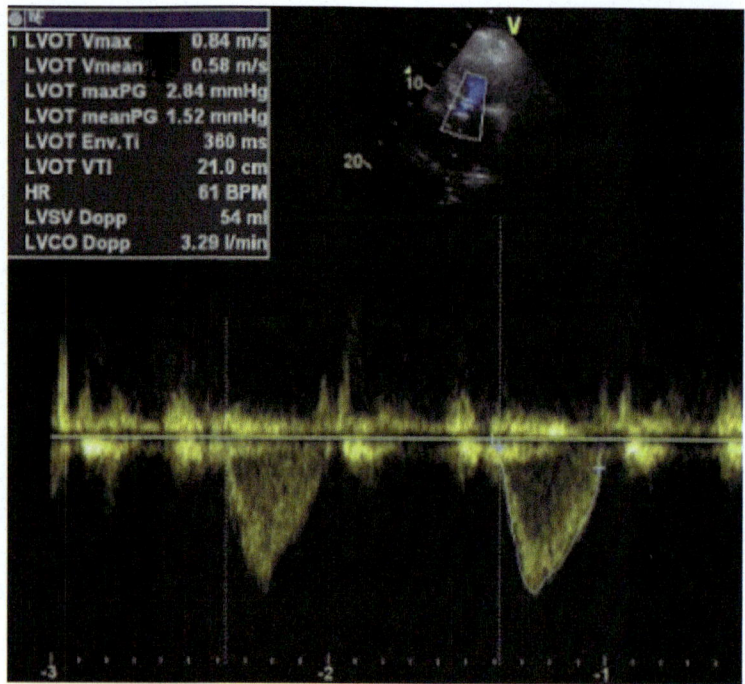

**Fig. 15.3** Pulsed wave (PW) Doppler recording on the left ventricle outflow tract, obtained in five chambers apical view, with sample volume placed about 0.5 cm below the aortic valve

should be calculated on 2D images, using the distance between the inner margin of the septal endocardium and the inner margin of the anterior mitral leaflet during systole in the parasternal long-axis view (Fig. 15.4). This measurement is the main source of errors in calculating the continuity equation (squared relationship). Therefore, when it is not possible to obtain an adequate image at TTE, transesophageal echocardiogram (TEE) is recommended.

The CE measures the effective AVA that is smaller than the anatomic AVA, due to contraction of the flow stream in the orifice. Though the difference between effective and anatomic AVA may account for some of the discrepancies between Doppler and catheterization, there now are ample clinical outcome data validating the use of the continuity equation. The weight of the evidence now supports the concept that effective, not anatomic, AVA is the primary predictor of clinical outcome.

Moreover, it must be borne in mind that the CE is affected by flow changes, with minimal effects in the case of AS and normal LV function, but more evident in the case of low-flow conditions. LV dysfunction can result in decreased cusp opening and a small effective orifice area even though severe stenosis is not present.

There is a simplified CE, using peak velocities instead of mean velocities, considering that the systolic ejection time and morphology of the velocity curves in the LVOT and at the stenotic AV are very similar.

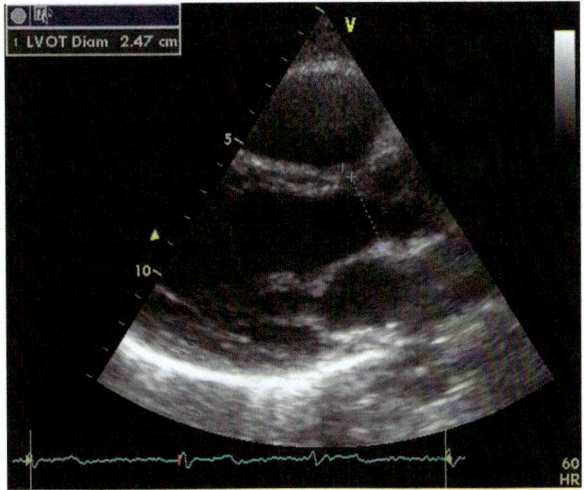

**Fig. 15.4** Measurement of the diameter of the left ventricle outflow tract in parasternal long-axis view, done in midsystole, within 0.5–1.0 cm of the valve orifice

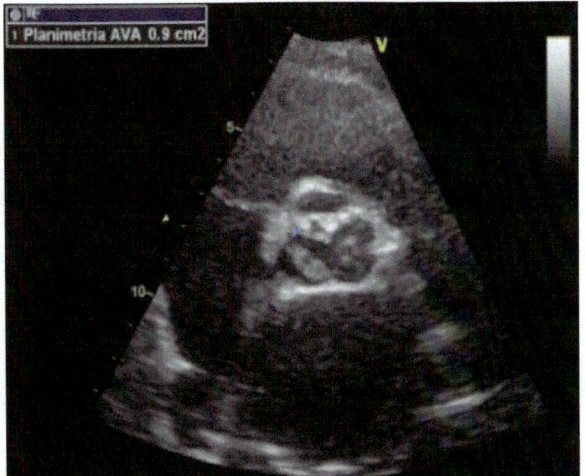

**Fig. 15.5** Planimetry of the aortic orifice, transthoracic echocardiogram, short-axis view

The velocity ratio (VR) has been introduced in order to reduce errors due to the calculated LVOT diameter. It consists of the relationship between PWD velocity in the LVOT and CWD velocity through the AV. In the absence of stenosis, the VR is around one.

Direct planimetry of the AVA is not routinely performed since, especially in the case of an extremely calcified aortic valve, orifice identification is difficult (Fig. 15.5).

In the global assessment of a patient, it is necessary to check for associated valve and/or heart diseases, for both therapeutic and prognostic purposes. Mitral regurgitation (MR) should be carefully assessed. MR can often be overestimated due to high left ventricular pressures secondary to AS. On the other hand, a severe MR, by reducing the transaortic flow, can lead to underestimation of AS. Aortic regurgitation (AR) is present in about 80% of patients with AS, but in most cases, it is either mild or moderate. Severe AR, by causing a high transaortic flow, can lead to overestimation of the $\Delta P_{mean}$ and AS.

The morphological and functional assessment of the left and right chambers (diameters, wall thickness, volumes, ventricular contractile function) provides information on AS severity, left ventricular hypertrophy, and systolic and diastolic function, with obvious prognostic and therapeutic implications (Fig. 15.6). Similar considerations apply to estimation of the pulmonary pressure and the resulting overload affecting the right ventricle (Fig. 15.7).

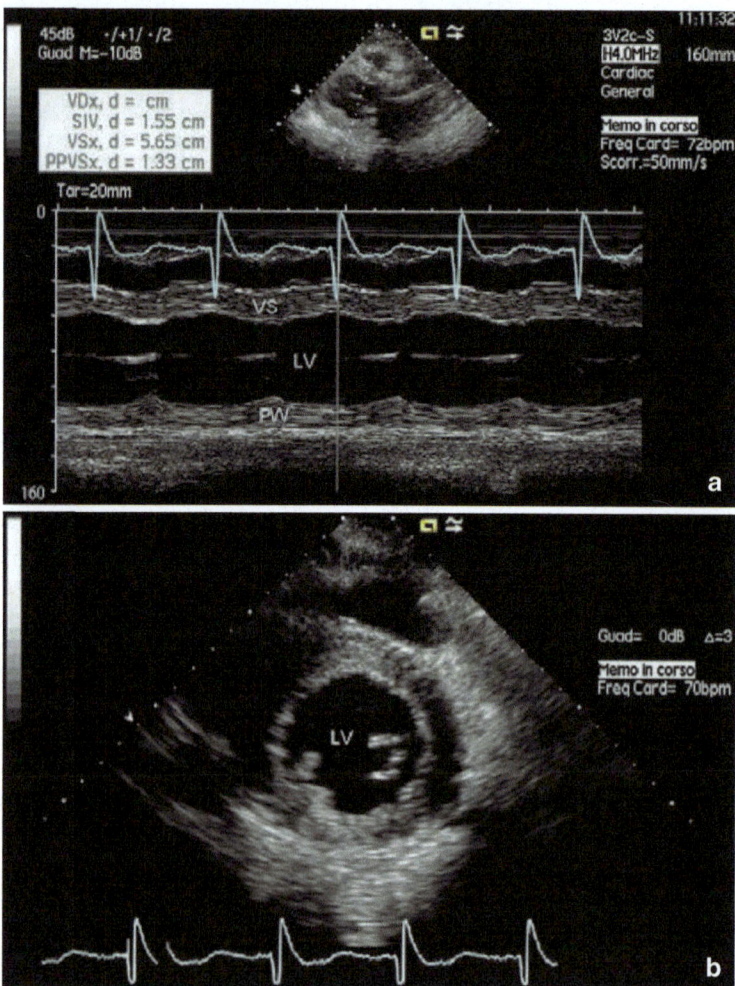

Fig. 15.6 (a) M-mode echocardiogram in a patient with severe aortic stenosis who has developed moderate ventricular hypertrophy. *LV* left ventricle, *PW* posterior wall, *VS* ventricular septum. (b) 2D echocardiogram, short-axis view, showing concentric left ventricular hypertrophy. *LV* left ventricle

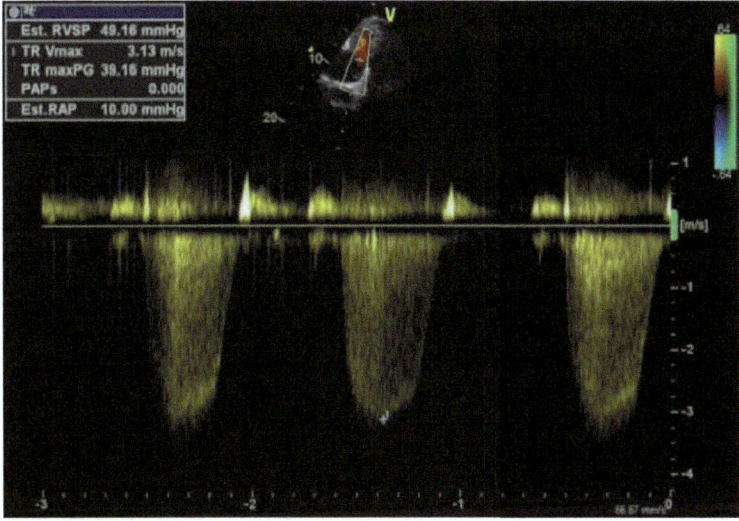

**Fig. 15.7** CW Doppler recording showing the tricuspid regurgitant jet velocity

The 2014 AHA/ACC guidelines for the management of patients with valvular heart disease [5] have provided a classification of the valvular AS stages, defined by valve anatomy, hemodynamics, and patient's symptoms (Table 15.1).

The most recent European Guidelines are consistent with the US Guidelines regarding the hemodynamic definition of severe AS [6].

The most typical form of severe AS is high-gradient AS (HGAS). In this setting, LVEF is generally preserved. However, some patients can present with HGAS and reduced LVEF, though asymptomatic.

Nevertheless, a severe AS may exist in the presence of low gradients and velocities, when the transvalvular flow is reduced (SVI $\leq$ 35 mL/m$^2$). This happens mainly when LVEF is reduced, as in the classical low-flow, low-gradient AS (LFLGAS). There is a subset of patients who present with severe AS and low gradients and velocity, despite a preserved LVEF ($\geq$50%). This subset has been termed as "paradoxical" low-flow, low-gradient AS (PLFLGAS) [6–10].

Clinicians must appreciate that AS is not a simple obstruction but involves a complex pathological interaction among LV, AV, and peripheral circulation.

Distinctive features of PLFLGAS are (Table 15.2):

- Reduced SVI $\leq$ 35 mL/m$^2$ and preserved LVEF $\geq$50%.
- Higher valvuloarterial impedance. Zva = SAP + $\Delta P_{mean}$/SVI (the ratio of the LV systolic pressure to the SVI, where SAP is the systolic arterial pressure measured at the time of echocardiography).
- More pronounced concentric remodeling, mainly due to reduced size of left ventricular cavity.
- Increased intrinsic left ventricular systolic dysfunction.

**Table 15.1** Stages of valvular AS

| Stage | Definition | | Hemodynamics |
|---|---|---|---|
| A | At risk of AS (previous congenital, flogistic or sclerotic anomalies) | | $V_{max}$ <2 m/s |
| B | Progressive AS | | Mild AS $V_{max}$ <2 m/s or $\Delta p_{mean}$ <20 mm Hg Moderate AS $V_{max}$ 3.0–3.9 mm Hg or $\Delta p_{mean}$ 20–39 mm Hg |
| C | Asymptomatic severe AS | C1 Normal LVEF | $V_{max}$ ≥4 m/s or $\Delta p_{mean}$ ≥40 mm Hg AVA ≤1.0 cm$^2$ (or AVAi ≤0.6 cm$^2$/m$^2$) |
| | | C2 Reduced LVEF <50% | Very severe AS $V_{max}$ ≥5 m/s or $\Delta p_{mean}$ ≥60 mm Hg |
| D | Symptomatic severe AS | D1 High-gradient | $V_{max}$ ≥4 m/s or $\Delta p_{mean}$ ≥40 mm Hg AVA ≤1.0 cm$^2$ (or AVAi ≤0.6 cm$^2$/m$^2$) |
| | | D2 Low-flow/low-gradient with reduced LVEF | $V_{max}$ <4 m/s or $\Delta p_{mean}$ <40 mm Hg |
| | | D3 Low-flow/low-gradient with preserved LVEF >50% (Paradoxical) | AVA ≤1.0 cm$^2$ (or AVAi ≤0.6 cm$^2$/m$^2$) Svi <35 mL/m$^2$ |

Adapted from 2014 AHA/ACC Guidelines for the Management of Patients with Valvular Heart Disease [5]

**Table 15.2** "Paradoxical" low flow-low gradient aortic stenosis distinctive features

- Reduced indexed stroke volume ≤35 mL/m$^2$, preserved LVEF ≥50%
- Higher valvuloarterial impedance. Zva = SAP + $\Delta P_{mean}$/SVI
- More pronounced concentric remodelling
- Increased intrinsic left ventricular systolic dysfunction

Thus, a greater afterload characterizes the hemodynamic picture where the valvular stenosis is at least as severe as in normal-flow patients and systemic arterial compliance is markedly lower. The chronic exposure to a high level of afterload eventually exceeds the limit of LV compensatory mechanisms and leads to an intrinsic impairment of myocardial function, as evidenced by lower values of mid-wall fractional shortening (MWFS) and a decrease in cardiac output.

In this context, LVEF turns out to be a quite rough tool and may not be able to detect a low-flow condition. LVEF normally tends to be higher according to the degree of concentric remodeling, so that such patients usually display a hypernormal LVEF (>70%). Thus, an LVEF >50% cannot exclude the presence of intrinsic myocardial dysfunction and shortening.

Moreover, under the same LVEF, the smaller the chamber, the smaller is the produced SV.

The specific role of diastolic dysfunction is probably limited in this setting, since no meaningful differences have been found between NF and PLF patients regarding the presence and the severity of this hemodynamic element.

PLFLGAS can frequently be misdiagnosed and inappropriately treated, even if symptomatic.

However, this subset of AS patients remains challenging. Few studies have concluded that they are likely at an advanced stage of their disease due to a long-standing exposition to it and have a poor prognosis if managed medically, while others have proposed that they may frequently have just moderate stenosis or, in any case, a similar outcome to the one usual for this condition [7, 8, 11–13].

Many reasons could account for these considerable discrepancies. First, calculation errors in determining SV and VA by Doppler echocardiography have to be considered. Moreover, Doppler measurements tend to underestimate flow, resulting in eventual underestimation of VA and erroneous assumption of low-flow conditions. Blood pressure can indirectly affect the assessment of AS severity through concomitant changes in transvalvular flow. The response of these hemodynamic parameters in individual patients is both variable and unpredictable, so AS severity should be assessed in a normotensive state. Most patients in this setting are elderly and female, with a small body size, so the valve area should be indexed to body size because an apparently small valve area may be only moderate AS in this context. Finally, an inconsistency in the definition of severe AS by current guidelines should be considered. While peak velocity cutoffs and mean gradient are usually consistent, the corresponding valve area cutoff is usually closer to $0.8 \text{ cm}^2$. In fact, a cutoff of $1 \text{ cm}^2$, though highly sensitive for severe AS, yields a low specificity for either peak velocity >4 m/s or mean gradient >40 mmHg. The majority of AS patients who are symptomatic have a valve area $< 0.75 \text{ cm}^2$, with many fewer symptomatic patients needing intervention in the $0.75–1 \text{ cm}^2$ cohort. A cutoff valve area for severe AS $\leq 0.8 \text{ cm}^2$ ($0.45 \text{ cm}^2/\text{m}^2$) would appropriately reclassify some patients with "severe" AS into moderate severity, with implications for defining severe AS in low-flow states.

Unfortunately, excluding a pseudo-severe AS in a low-flow setting remains a challenge.

In the presence of LFLGAS, a dobutamine stress test can be conclusive [14, 15]. Infusion of low-dose dobutamine at gradually increasing doses (starting from 5 µg/kg/min with 5 µg/kg/min increases every 3–5 min until a maximum dose of 20 µg/kg/min), by increasing cardiac output, can increase the pressure gradient, leaving the AVA unaltered and so confirming a truly severe AS ($V_{max} \geq 4$ m/s with a VA $\leq 1.0 \text{ cm}^2$ at any point during the test protocol). On the other hand, in the case of an aortic pseudostenosis, where a weak LV is not able to generate sufficient contractile strength to fully open the valve, the increase in cardiac output increases the AVA, with a minimal change in gradient. In cases in which there is no increase in EF or cardiac output (lack of contractile reserve, usually defined as an increase in SV < 20%), this test cannot distinguish between the two conditions. However, this finding is of outmost prognostic importance, as predictive of adverse outcomes and high operating risk. In the evaluation of a PLFLGAS, a low-dose dobutamine test can be administered, but its role in this setting is not well established [6].

Moreover, the pressure recovery (PR) phenomenon may be responsible for Doppler gradients that are substantially higher and a valve area that is substantially lower than those determined invasively. When blood accelerates across a restrictive orifice, pressure energy, proximal to the stenosis, is converted to kinetic energy, whereas, distal to the stenosis, blood decelerates again. Kinetic energy gained during flow acceleration must be converted to another form of energy during flow deceleration. Kinetic energy dissipates into heat due to turbulences and viscous losses in the case of a dilated ascending aorta; instead, kinetic energy is reconverted into potential energy, with a corresponding increase in pressure (so-called PR) in the case of laminar transvalvular flow and a normal caliber of the proximal ascending aorta. However, in most adults with native AS, the magnitude of pressure recovery is small and can be ignored as long as the diameter of the aorta is >30 mm [6, 7].

Careful evaluation of symptoms, measuring of neurohormones, evaluation of valve area, degree of calcification, amount of myocardial scar by transesophageal echocardiography (TEE), multislice computed tomography (MSCT), and/or cardiovascular magnetic resonance (CMR) and catheterization can play an important role in a low-flow condition. Measurement of global longitudinal strain (GLS) by 2D speckle tracking method, at rest and during dobutamine stress, can be helpful in enhancing diagnosis and risk stratification in LFLGAS [16].

The tomographic nature of 2D echo, the inability to view the entire AV valve apparatus (valve, root, and ascending aorta) in order to understand the spatial relationships among its components, and the need for geometrical assumptions about the morphology of the structures of the valve apparatus limit the utility of 2DE for the selection of patients who may benefit from percutaneous/surgical replacement. Dynamic stereoscopic visualization of the aortic valve with *three-dimensional echocardiography (3DE)* improves the diagnostic potential of ultrasound in AV disease [17–20].

Three-dimensional data volumes that contain the aortic valve apparatus can be subsequently split and rotated to obtain a dynamic and anatomically oriented view of the aortic valve, which can be viewed from different perspectives: from the aortic root, the ventricular outflow tract, as well as from any plane, either longitudinal or oblique, as may be needed. Valve visualization from the aortic root perspective is the most favorable to assess its morphology (Fig. 15.8), while the view from the ventricular outflow tract is the most suitable to visualize tumors, vegetations, and subvalvular obstructions. In 3DE, there are no limits to the alignment of the cross-sectional plane, regardless of the orientation in space of the aortic root, overcoming the problems derived from the longitudinal movement of the heart during the entire cardiac cycle.

Calibration of the gains and filters allows an accurate delineation of anatomical details of the valve, while the addition of colored tissue maps increases the perception of depth in 3D. The transesophageal approach with scans from the mid-upper

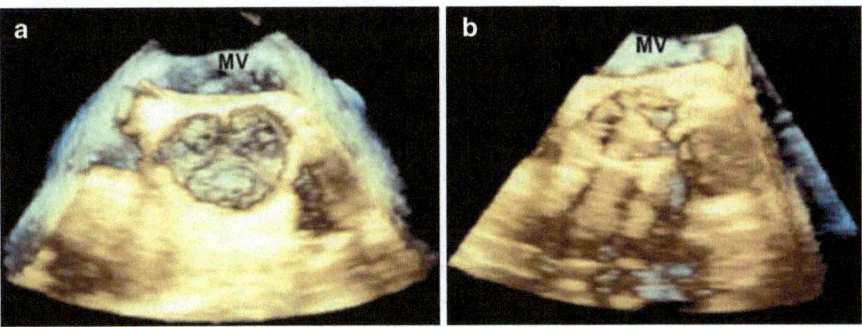

**Fig. 15.8** Three-dimensional transesophageal echocardiography showing (**a**) normal aortic valve in diastole from aortic view and (**b**) calcific aortic stenosis (aortic view). *MV* mitral valve

portion of the esophagus affords a better spatial resolution and, therefore, a better image quality for a 3D evaluation of the aortic valve.

The addition of color Doppler imaging can help to overcome the inaccuracy of spectral Doppler ultrasound for SV calculation. By providing a direct measure of the actual flow, color 3DE does not need nonsimultaneous measurements of the time-velocity integral and cross-sectional area of the LV outflow tract, thereby reducing the potential for errors. The measurement of stroke volume with color 3DE has proven to be more accurate than the two-dimensional continuity equation, even in situations with altered geometry of the outflow tract, such as in basal septum hypertrophy in the elderly.

Another method for the 3D calculation of LV stroke volume is that derived from 3D volume calculation, by subtracting the end-systolic volume from end-diastolic volume and adding the result to the numerator of the usual CE.

3DE allows better identification of the minimum orifice, especially in the case of commissural fusion or a valve with dome-shaped appearance. The planimetric area, measured by transesophageal 3D (3D TEE), has been shown to have a high correlation with the AVA derived from the continuity equation or calculated with Gorlin formula at catheterization. Furthermore, direct planimetry at 3D TEE has shown a higher accuracy compared with 2D TEE, which significantly overestimates the AVA. The superior ability of 3D TEE to better outline aortic valve morphology and measure the contours of cusps and commissures is the real advantage to 3D TEE over 2D TEE imaging. Nevertheless, the presence of calcification may make it difficult to trace the planimetry of the orifice area, due to masking phenomena and glare caused by calcification. In addition, as for 2DE, planimetry can overestimate the severity of aortic stenosis in patients with low stroke volume, due to reduced opening of the valve's anatomic area.

*An exercise test* is contraindicated in symptomatic patients with AS owing to a high risk of complications, including syncope, ventricular tachycardia, and death. In asymptomatic patients, it can be performed under close monitoring and has great prognostic value [21, 22]. Reduced tolerance to effort, onset of symptoms, and abnormal blood pressure response, such as an increase of less than 20 mmHg or a fall below baseline, are associated with an unfavorable outcome, so these patients should be considered symptomatic. In these cases, aortic valve replacement seems to be associated with a better outcome compared with medical treatment. ST segment depression is commonly seen and is nonspecific for CAD. Exercise stress echocardiography is challenging and seldom necessary. However, it may provide prognostic information in asymptomatic severe AS by assessing the increase in mean pressure gradient and the systolic pulmonary arterial pressure and change in LV function [23–25].

*Multislice computed tomography (MSCT) and Cardiac magnetic resonance (CMR)* imaging are increasingly used in patients with AS and can complement echocardiography in the diagnostic evaluation and monitoring of patients with asymptomatic severe AS, affecting treatment decisions. Both techniques provide detailed information of valve, aortic root, and aortic morphology and are useful for preprocedural assessment before surgical or transcatheter AV replacement (SAVR or TAVI).

MSCT has the capability of quantifying the degree and severity of aortic valve calcification (AVC) (Fig. 15.9). AVC is expressed in Agatston units (AU). The calcium score correlates strongly with actual aortic valve calcium weight, as measured postmortem, with the echocardiographic hemodynamic severity of AS (Vmax and AVA), and with clinical outcomes. Recent studies have shown that a calcium score <800 AU excluded severe AS with a high negative predictive value, while a score >1600 AU suggested severe AS. A threshold of 1651 AU provided the best combination of sensitivity and specificity, particularly for patients with depressed EF. However, a steeper slope of AS severity increase, with any given AVC load increase, in women than in men has been demonstrated. Hence, for diagnostic purposes, the AVC load linked to severe AS should be lower for women (severe AS very likely: men≥3000; women≥1600; severe AS likely: men≥2000; women≥1200) [4, 26–30].

MSCT measurement of the elliptical LVOT can bring incremental value to 2D echocardiography and improve AS severity assessment; however, given that CT measures a larger LVOT cross-sectional area compared with 2D echocardiography, larger cut-point values of AVA (<1.2 vs. 1.0 cm$^2$) should be used to identify severe AS and predict adverse events if a "hybrid CT-echocardiography method" is used to estimate AVA [31]. CT has gained prominence recently in the treatment of AS with the use of TAVI.

CMR is an effective tool in assessing cardiac anatomy and function [4, 32–34]. It allows a careful measuring of end-systolic and end-diastolic LV chamber volumes and resulting SV, which is of the outmost importance in the presence of suspected low-flow conditions, unless associated. SV measured by CMR can be used in the calculation of the CE-AVA, overcoming the limits of the 2D Doppler method. The AVA calculated from CMR-derived SV is often larger than traditional 2D Doppler CE-AVA. Moreover, CMR can quantify the degree of interstitial fibrosis, as detected with late gadolinium enhancement. Interstitial fibrosis is an important feature of the pathological hypertrophic remodeling that the LV undergoes in response to the elevated afterload in severe AS. A silent myocardial infarction can also be detected. These findings have been associated with a worse prognosis in general and after AVR [35, 36].

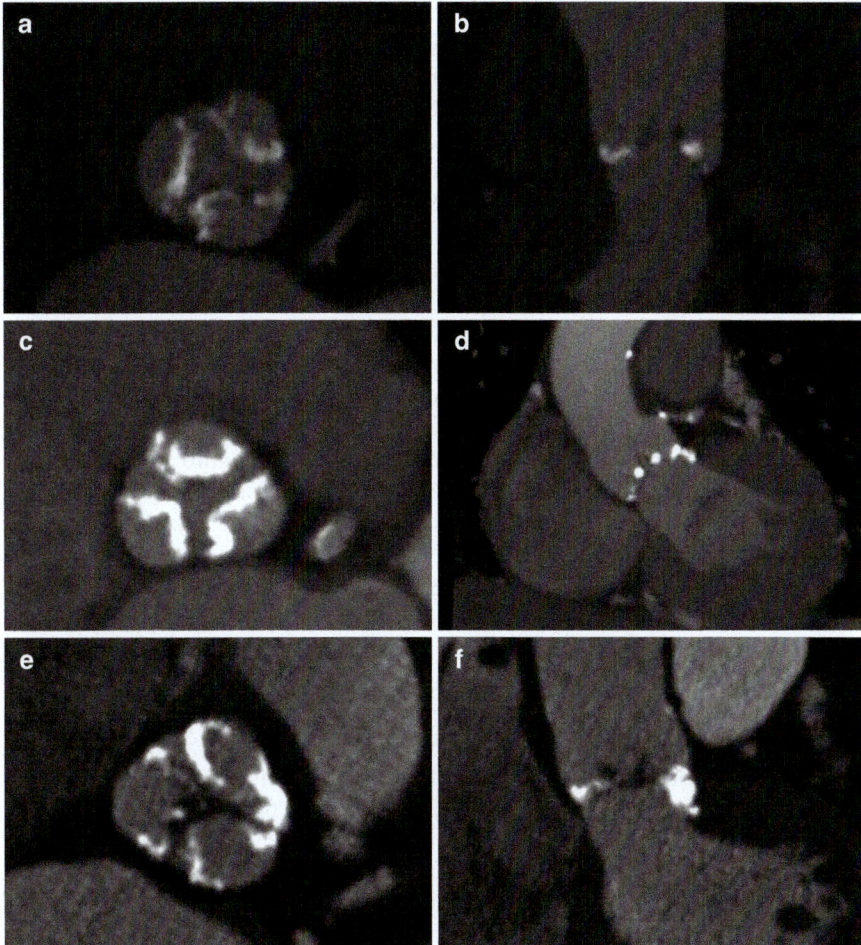

**Fig. 15.9** Images illustrating the aortic valve calcium score of three patients with increasing calcification grades. (**a, b**) Mild calcification, (**c, d**) intermediate calcification, and (**e, f**) severe calcification, involving also the LVOT

Nonetheless, the lack of thorough clinical validation of these modalities, paired with economic considerations, has slowed their widespread use in the detection and risk stratification of AS.

## 15.2 Invasive Diagnosis

At present, the principal role of cardiac catheterization in AS patients consists of determining whether there is concurrent coronary artery disease to be treated surgically or percutaneously for valve disease. The modern catheterization laboratory has become the place to solve the difficult diagnostic challenges that arise in patients with structural heart diseases when answers are not apparent through the clinical examination and noninvasive testing. Thus, the remaining questions are complex and pose difficult diagnostic dilemmas. Careful hemodynamic study to determine the severity of AS is indicated when echocardiography data leave doubts or are of nonoptimal quality, when there is a discrepancy between clinical information and echocardiographic findings, and when AS is associated with low cardiac output or altered LV function [4, 37, 38].

Assessment of AS relies on measurement of the valve gradient and calculation of valve area.

The optimal technique to assess aortic valve gradient is to record simultaneously left ventricular and ascending aortic pressures (Fig. 15.10). The peak-to-peak gradient has been the conventional measurement in the past. However, it is a nonphysiological parameter. Instead, it is recommended that the mean aortic valve gradient be used, which is the integrated gradient throughout the entire systolic ejection period and the optimal indicator of severity of obstruction. Most catheterization laboratories can now use computer analysis of the mean gradient, facilitating attainment of this measurement.

Assessment of AVA relies on the Gorlin formula, in which cardiac output is determined by the Fick principle. Most laboratories now use thermodilution (a derivation of the Fick principle) to measure cardiac output. In low-output conditions (cardiac output <2.5 L/min), the Gorlin equation overestimates the severity of valve stenosis. In these cases, the hemodynamic assessment of AS severity at rest and during maneuvers to increase the flow through the aortic valve (e.g., by infusing dobutamine) can provide crucial information [15]. The simplified Hakki method (valve area = cardiac output/square root of the gradient) differs from the Gorlin method by

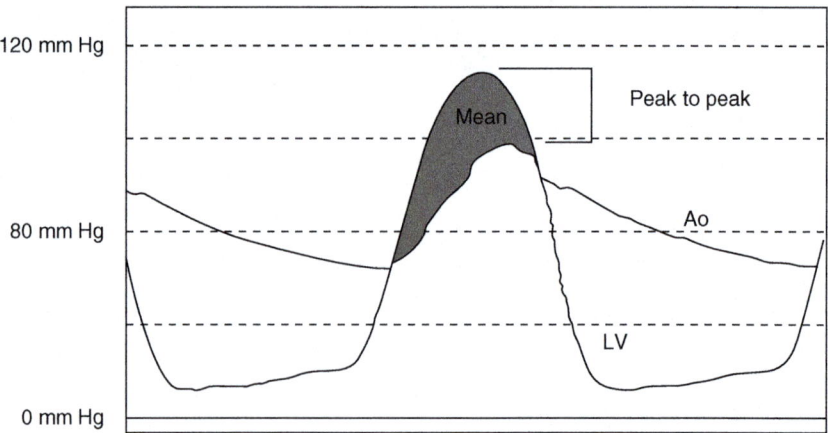

**Fig. 15.10** Simultaneous left ventricular (LV) and central aortic (Ao) pressures in a patient with aortic stenosis. The peak-to-peak gradient is the difference between the peak left ventricular and peak aortic pressures. The mean pressure gradient is the integrated gradient between the left ventricular and aortic pressure throughout the entire systolic ejection period

$18 \pm 13\%$ in patients with bradycardia (<65/m) or tachycardia (>100/m) [37, 39]. It can be used to ensure that the more complex Gorlin equation has been calculated with the proper data input. In the growing population of patients who have PLFLGAS, further evaluation may be indicated, perhaps with vasodilators, such as nitroprusside, to lower the high additional afterload resulting from a noncompliant aortic system. Patients with true severe AS may be able to be identified by demonstrating an increase in aortic valve gradient and a fixed valve area [37].

However, despite their proven effectiveness, AVA measurements have both practical and theoretical limits. The area is a planar measurement, which does not consider mitral inflow with its funnel shape or aortic outflow with a tubular shape. AVA calculation is based on a laminar flow of a noncompressible fluid. Turbulence is hence not considered. As a result, valve areas <0.7 cm$^2$ are almost always associated with clinical symptoms, and areas >1.1 cm$^2$ are not usually associated with symptoms, but the intermediate areas are in a gray zone. Another hemodynamic parameter that has proven its clinical utility is the calculation of valve resistance, though it is a complementary index that cannot be used instead of valve area assessment. Based on these considerations, according to current guidelines, hemodynamic assessment of AS on a routine basis is not necessary.

## 15.3 Timing of Interventions

AS is a disease with a variable and unpredictable rate of hemodynamic progression. The average annual increase in aortic jet velocity and AVA has been estimated to be 0.3 m/s and 0.1 cm$^2$, respectively [40]. Advanced age, male gender, and the presence of risk factors of atherosclerotic disease have been reported as predictors of a rapid progression, but to what extent these factors contribute to AS progression is unknown.

As many as 50% of patients with severe AS report no symptoms at the time of diagnosis. Patients with asymptomatic severe AS have a better prognosis than those with symptomatic severe AS. In patients with asymptomatic severe AS, 1-year and 5-year survival rates have been reported to range from 67% to 97% and 38% to 83%, respectively. The risk of sudden death has been reported to be approximately 1–1.5% per year. The median time to symptom onset, AVR, or death ranges between 1 and 4 and 5 years, respectively, after receiving the diagnosis. Approximately two-thirds of conservatively managed patients with asymptomatic AS will develop symptoms. As soon as even mild symptoms occur, the prognosis of severe AS is dismal, with survival rates of only 15–50% at 5 years. As many as 3% of patients can die suddenly—within 3–6 months—and as many as 6.5% of symptomatic patients can die while awaiting AVR. Importantly, ~70% of sudden deaths in patients with asymptomatic severe AS are not preceded by any of the classical AS symptoms [5, 6, 40–46].

A comparative summary of the intervention timing reported in the new guidelines for the management of patients with valvular heart disease issued by AHA/ACC and ESC/EACTS [5, 6] is given in Table 15.3.

**Table 15.3** Comparative summary of the intervention timing according to AHA/ACC and ESC/EACTS guidelines

| Timing of intervention in aortic stenosis | ESC | AHA/ACC |
|---|---|---|
| Severe AS and any related symptoms by history | IB | IB |
| Severe AS and any related symptoms on exercise testing | IC | IB |
| Asymptomatic severe AS and LVEF <50% not due to another cause | IC | IB |
| Asymptomatic severe AS when undergoing other cardiac surgery | IC | IB |
| Asymptomatic severe AS and decreased exercise tolerance or abnormal blood pressure response (fall or <20 mm Hg increase) | IIaB | IIaB |
| Symptomatic severe low-flow/low gradient AS with reduced LVEF confirmed by low-dose dobutamine stress test | IIaC | IIaB |
| Moderate AS when undergoing other cardiac surgery | IIaC | IIaC |
| Symptomatic severe low-flow/low-gradient AS with normal LVEF only after careful evaluation | IIaC | IIaC |
| Asymptomatic very severe AS with peak velocity ≥5.0–5.5 m/s when surgical risk is low | IIaC | IIaB |
| Asymptomatic severe AS with severe calcification and fast peak velocity progression ≥0.3 m/s/year when surgical risk is low | IIaC | IIbC |
| Symptomatic severe LF/LG AS with reduced LVEF without evidence of flow reserve by low dose dobutamine stress test | IIbC | N/A |
| Asymptomatic severe AS and one or more of the following findings, when surgical risk is low<br>– markedly elevated natriuretic peptides levels without other explanations<br>– increase of mean pressure gradient with exercise by ≥20 mmHg<br>– excessive LV hypertrophy in the absence of hypertension | IIbC | N/A |

In the absence of serious comorbid conditions that limit life expectancy or quality of life, aortic valve replacement (SAVR or TAVI) is indicated in virtually all symptomatic patients with severe AS and should be performed promptly after onset of symptoms. Age alone is not a contraindication for surgery. As long as the $\Delta P_{mean}$ remains >40 mmHg, there is virtually no lower EF limit for surgery [5, 6].

The management of patients with classical LFLGAS is more difficult. If depressed EF is predominantly caused by afterload mismatch, LV function usually improves after surgery. In this setting, the evidence of flow reserve is predictive of a better long-term outcome after AVR in most patients. Conversely, improvement in LV function after AVR is uncertain if the primary cause is scarring due to extensive myocardial infarction or cardiomyopathy. The outcome of patients without flow reserve is subject to a higher operative mortality. However, AVR can still improve EF, clinical status, and long-term survival in select patients [5, 6, 47–49]. The newly recognized entity of PLFLGAS requires special attention because of the limited amount of data on the natural history and outcome after surgery [5–14, 50]. In such cases, surgery should be performed only after a comprehensive evaluation.

Management of asymptomatic severe AS remains controversial. An active surveillance strategy (watchful waiting) is adopted for the vast majority of cases, with the unquestionable exception of patients with symptoms or abnormal findings on exercise test (who should be basically considered as symptomatic), patients still asymptomatic in spite of the presence of an LV dysfunction, and patients who need to undergo other cardiac surgery [5, 6, 21–25]. Given the current low periprocedural mortality rates for isolated SAVR and TAVI, earlier intervention has been increasingly advocated in asymptomatic severe AS patients in order to overcome the practical challenges of the watchful waiting strategy: interpreting symptoms or the lack thereof is notoriously difficult, particularly in elderly sedentary patients. Because AS progression is highly variable and unpredictable, rapid deterioration can occur. A standardized algorithm for active surveillance has not been defined or validated; approximately 15% of patients will not be able to perform an exercise test, a proportion that increases with age. Adherence to surveillance can be poor; late symptom reporting can result in irreversible myocardial damage, with worsened prognosis, despite AVR. Operative risk increases with patient age and LV dysfunction; the risk of sudden death is low but not negligible, and sudden death can be the first symptom of the disease.

A limited amount of data shows a better long-term outcome with an initial AVR strategy than with a watchful waiting strategy. Nonetheless, such a strategy could expose a number of patients to an unnecessary, expensive procedure and to its long-term complications [51–58].

Many attempts have been made to select patients in the pool of truly asymptomatic severe AS at higher risk for early symptoms onset and events and with greater prospect of improvement after an initial AVR.

Several specific predictors have been reported and already acknowledged by the new guidelines, mainly in Europe [5, 6]:

- Fast disease progression: increase in Vmax $\geq$0.3 m/s/year [59]
- Severe AS: Vmax $\geq$5.0 or 5.5 cm/s [57, 60, 61]
- Increase in $\Delta P_{mean} > 20$ mmHg or systolic pulmonary arterial pressure $> 60$ mmHg with exercise [23–25]
- Severe aortic valve calcification by MSCT [26–30]
- Excessive LV hypertrophy in the absence of hypertension [62]
- BNP level at rest or during exercise (no standardized data available, but outcomes progressively correlated with BNP ratio at rest and $\Delta$BNP with exercise) [63–65]

Indexed left atrial area [52], Zva [8, 52, 53, 66], and global longitudinal strain by speckle tracking [52, 53, 67–69] are other predictors that could in the near future refine the management of asymptomatic severe AS patients.

In general, surgical replacement allows for a marked improvement in clinical symptoms and in long-term survival in most patients, with an intraoperative mortality of 2–5% for patients below 70 years of age undergoing aortic valve replacement alone for the first time; this percentage rises to 5–15% in patients older than 70 [70].

The risk of operative mortality is increased by the following factors: advanced age, comorbidities, female gender, advanced New York Heart Association (NYHA) functional class, LV dysfunction, pulmonary hypertension, coronary artery disease, and prior cardiac surgery.

The predictors of intraoperative mortality have been identified based on a long series of cardiac surgery patients and have been correlated with cardiac diseases, patient age, comorbidity, and type of surgical procedure [71].

In this regard, there are two main models utilized to evaluate surgical risk, the Society of Thoracic Surgery Predicted Risk of Mortality (STS-PROM) [72] and the European System for Cardiac Operative Risk Evaluation (EuroSCORE) [73], recently updated to version II [74]. These systems are based on the assessment of cardiac and extracardiac factors. Though these represent the sole objective methods to estimate short-term mortality after surgical aortic valve replacement, they have several limitations. Nevertheless, the STS-PROM seems to reproduce more closely the operative and 30-day mortality for the highest-risk patients having AV replacement. These score systems are not specifically designed for AS and tend to overestimate or sometimes underestimate the real risk. Also, they are not widely applicable, as it is now well accepted that the risk is also related to the particular surgical team. Moreover, there are a series of clinical conditions (porcelain aorta, previous chest wall radiation, liver failure, chest wall malformation, frailty, active endocarditis, active cancer, low-flow low-gradient AS) that have not been taken into account in these risk scores but which very often are a contraindication or make surgery particularly risky. In addition, there are also conditions that can increase surgical risk for various reasons, such as left ventricular hypertrophy, left ventricular dilation, diastolic dysfunction, preoperative 6-min walking test, hypoalbuminemia/poor nutritional status, anemia, morbid obesity, and right ventricular dysfunction [75].

Nevertheless some authors have identified specific predictors with TAVI of early mortality and have developed simple scores using preprocedural variables, such as age >90 years, frailty, assisted living, NYHA class IV, pulmonary hypertension, diabetes mellitus, glomerular filtration rate < 45 mL/min, or dialysis, to predict 30-day or in-hospital mortality after TAVI. These simple scoring systems may facilitate identifying particularly high-risk patients who may require more intensive screening by a heart team [76–78].

In clinical practice, there is a tendency to consider patients over 80 years of age as inoperable *tout court*. The EuroHeart Survey [79], a prospective study, published in 2001 and carried out in over 5000 patients affected with moderate-to-severe valve diseases enrolled in 92 centers in 25 European countries, showed that while there is general agreement between the decision to intervene surgically and existing guidelines on the treatment of symptomatic patients, recourse to surgery in patients with serious symptoms is less frequent for several, often groundless, reasons. In the EuroHeart Survey, at least one-third of the elderly patients with comorbidities and AS were not considered operable. The reasons for nonintervention were, in 31% of patients with only severely diseased aortic valve, patient refusal to undergo surgery, regression of symptoms with medical therapy (about 39%) and end-stage disease in 18%, and symptoms ascribed to a concurrent coronary artery pathology (14%) with recent myocardial infarction in 7%.

Alongside the cardiac causes, the presence of at least one extracardiac condition was considered a contraindication for surgery in 55.3% of cases. The most frequent reasons reported were advanced age (27.6%, sole reason in 1.3% of cases), chronic obstructive pulmonary disease (13.6%), kidney failure (6.1%), patient refusal (16%), and low life expectancy (19.3%).

Clearly, the use of the EuroSCORE and STS score to quantify surgical risk is just one of the means of assessing the therapeutic approach; it must be corroborated by other essential elements, such as the patient's life expectancy and quality of life, as well as requests and expectations of patients and their families.

It has been proven that, despite high surgical risk, patients over 80 years of age have a much better prognosis after surgery compared with medical therapy alone.

Therefore, the development of a less invasive treatment to reduce the cardiovascular complications due to general anesthesia, thoracotomy, and extracorporeal circulation, to a minimum, has become essential for elderly patients affected with severe AS associated with comorbidities, who, without adequate treatment, would inevitably die in just a few months.

Therefore, given the complexity of patients affected with AS, in the patient selection phase, the European Working Group recommends that all "currently available risk scores should not be used as an isolated decision tool but as part of an integrated approach, which includes complete clinical evaluation, reference to local resources and surgical results, and the preferences of the patient and their family. Risk scores are not a substitute for clinical experience in the management of patients with valvular heart disease" [75].

# References

1. Dalla Volta S, Daliento L, Rozzolini R. Malattie del cuore e dei vasi (terza edizione). Libri Italia SRL: Mc Graw-Hill; 2005.
2. Baumgartner H, Hung J, Bermejo J, et al. Echocardiographic assessment of valve stenosis: EAE/ASE recommendations for clinical practice. Eur J Echocardiogr. 2009;10:1–25.
3. Chambers BJ. Aortic stenosis. Eur J Echocardiogr. 2009;10:11–9.
4. Saikrishnan N, Kumar G, Sawaya FJ, et al. Accurate assessment of aortic stenosis: a review of diagnostic modalities and hemodynamics. Circulation. 2014;129:244–53.
5. Nishimura R, Otto C, Bonow R, et al. AHA/ACC guideline for the management of patients with valvular heart disease: a report of the American College of Cardiology/American Heart Association Task Force on Practice Guidelines. Circulation. 2014;129:e521–643.
6. Vahanian A, Alfieri O, Andreotti F, et al. Guidelines on the management of valvular heart disease: the joint task force on the management of valvular heart disease of the European Society of Cardiology (ESC) and the European Association for Cardio-Thoracic Surgery (EACTS). Eur J Cardiothorac Surg. 2012;42:S1–S44.
7. Bach DS. Echo/Doppler evaluation of hemodynamics after aortic valve replacement: principles of interrogation and evaluation of high gradients. JACC Cardiovasc Imaging. 2010;3(3):296–304.
8. Hachicha Z, Dumesnil J, Bogaty P, et al. Paradoxical low-flow, low-gradient severe aortic stenosis despite preserved ejection fraction is associated with higher afterload and reduced survival. Circulation. 2007;115:2856–64.
9. Dumesnil J, Pibarot P, Carabello B. Paradoxical low flow and/or low gradient severe aortic stenosis despite preserved left ventricular ejection fraction: implication for diagnosis and treatment. Eur Heart J. 2010;31:281–9.
10. Awtry E, Davidoff R. Low-flow/low—gradient aortic stenosis. Circulation. 2011;124:739–41.

11. Lancellotti P. Grading aortic stenosis severity when the flow modifies the gradient-valve area correlation. Cardiovasc Diagn Ther. 2012;2(1):6–9.
12. Jander N, Minners J, Holme I, et al. Outcome of patients with low-gradient "severe" aortic stenosis and preserved ejection fraction. Circulation. 2011;123(8):887–95.
13. Dayan V, Vignolo G, Magne J, et al. Outcome and impact of aortic valve replacement in patients with preserved LVEF and low-gradient aortic stenosis. J Am Coll Cardiol. 2015;66(23):2594–603.
14. Clavel M, Berthelot-Richer M, Le Ven F, et al. Impact of classic and paradoxical low flow on survival after aortic valve replacement for severe aortic stenosis. J Am Coll Cardiol. 2015;65(7):645–53.
15. De Filippi CR, DuWayne LW, Brickner ME, et al. Usefulness of Dobutamine echocardiography in distinguishing severe from nonsevere valvular aortic stenosis in patients with depressed left ventricular function and low transvalvular gradients. J Am Cardiol. 1995;75:192–4.
16. Dahou A, Bartko P, Capoulade R, et al. Usefulness of global left ventricular longitudinal strain for risk stratification in low ejection fraction, low-gradient aortic stenosis. Circ Cardiovasc Imaging. 2015;8(3):e002117.
17. Ge S, Warner JB Jr, Abraham TP, et al. Three-dimensional surface area of the aortic valve orifice by three dimensional echocardiography: clinical validation of a novel index for assessment of aortic stenosis. Am Heart J. 1998;136:1042–50.
18. Poh K, Levine RA, Solis J, et al. Assessing aortic valve area in aortic stenosis by continuity equation: a novel approach using real-time three- dimensional echocardiography. Eur Heart J. 2008;29:2526–35.
19. Gutierrez-Chico JL, Zamorano JL, Prieto-Moriche E, et al. Real-time three-dimensional echocardiography in aortic stenosis: a novel, simple, and reliable method to improve accuracy in area calculation. Eur Heart J. 2008;29:1296–306.
20. Ng AC, Delgado V, Van der KF, et al. Comparison of aortic root dimension and geometries before and after transcatheter aortic valve implantation by 2- and 3-dimensional transesophageal echocardiography and multislice computed tomography. Circ Cardiovasc Imaging. 2010;3:94–102.
21. Das P, Rimington H, Chambers J. Exercise testing to stratify risk in aortic stenosis. Eur Heart J. 2005;26:1309–13.
22. Dhoble A, Sarano ME, Kopcky SL, et al. Safety of symptom-limited cardiopulmonary exercise testing in patients with aortic stenosis. Am J Med. 2012;125(7):704–8.
23. Maréchaux S, Hachicha Z, Bellouin A. Usefulness of exercise-stress echocardiography for risk stratification of true asymptomatic patients with aortic valve stenosis. Eur Heart J. 2010;31(11):1390–7.
24. Lancellotti P, Lebois F, Simon M, et al. Prognostic importance of quantitative exercise Doppler echocardiography in asymptomatic valvular aortic stenosis. Circulation. 2005;112:I377–82.
25. Lancellotti P, Magne J, Donal E, et al. Determinants and prognostic significance of exercise pulmonary hypertension in asymptomatic severe aortic stenosis. Circulation. 2012;26:851–9.
26. Cueff C, Serfaty J, Cimadevilla C, et al. Measurement of aortic valve calcification using multislice computed tomography: correlation with haemodynamic severity of aortic stenosis and clinical implication for patients with low ejection fraction. Heart. 2010;2011(97):721–6.
27. Clavel M, Messika-Zeitoun D, Pibarot P, et al. The complex nature of discordant severe calcified aortic valve disease grading: new insights from combined Doppler ecocardiographic and computed tomographic study. JACC. 2013;62:2329–38.
28. Aggarwal SR, Clavel M, Messika-Zeitoun D, et al. Sex differences in aortic valve calcification measured by multidetector computed tomography in aortic stenosis. Circ Cardiovasc Imaging. 2013;6:40–7.
29. Clavel M, Pibarot P, Messika-Zeitoun D, et al. Impact of aortic valve calcification, as measured by MDCT, on survival in patients with aortic stenosis. J Am Coll Cardiol. 2014;64(12):1202–13.
30. Clavel M, Pibarot P. Assessment of low-flow, low-gradient aortic stenosis: multimodality imaging is the key to success. EuroIntervention. 2014;10:U52–60.

31. Clavel M, Malouf J, Messika-Zeitoun D, et al. Aortic valve area calculation in aortic stenosis by CT and Doppler echocardiography. JACC Cardiovasc Imaging. 2015;8:248–57.
32. Chin CW, Khaw HJ, Luo E, et al. Echocardiography underestimates stroke volume and aortic valve area: implications for patients with small-area low-gradient aortic stenosis. Can J Cardiol. 2014;30(9):1064–72.
33. Clavel M, Dusmesnil JG, Pibarot P, et al. Discordant grading of aortic stenosis using echocardiography and what it means: new insights from magnetic resonance imaging. Can J Cardiol. 2014;30:959–61.
34. Wong S, Spina R, Toemoe S, et al. Is cardiac magnetic resonance imaging as accurate as echocardiography in the assessment of aortic valve stenosis? Interact Cardiovasc Thorac Surg. 2016;22:480–6.
35. Dweck MR, Joshi S, Murigu T, et al. Midwall fibrosis is an independent predictor of mortality in patients with aortic stenosis. J Am Coll Cardiol. 2011;58:1271–9.
36. Barone-Rochette G, Pièrard S, De Meester de Ravestein C, et al. Prognostic significance of LGE by CMR in aortic stenosis patients undergoing valve replacement. J Am Coll Cardiol. 2014;58:1271–9.
37. Nishimura RA, Carabello BA. Hemodynamics in the cardiac catheterization laboratory of the 21st century. Circulation. 2012;125:2138–50.
38. Grossman & Baim's Cardiac Catheterization. Angiography and intervention. 8th ed. Philadelphia: Lippincott Williams and Wilkins; 2013.
39. Hakki AH. A simplified valve formula for the calculation of stenotic valve areas. Circulation. 1981;63:1050–5.
40. Otto CM, Burwash IG, Legget ME, et al. Prospective study of asymptomatic valvular aortic stenosis. Clinical, echocardiographic, and exercise predictors of outcome. Circulation. 1997;95:2262–70.
41. Lund O, Nielsen TT, Emmertsen K, et al. Mortality and worsening of prognostic profile during waiting time for valve replacement in aortic stenosis. Thorac Cardiovasc Surg. 1996;44:289–95.
42. Rosenhek R, Binder T, Porenta G, et al. Predictors of outcome in severe, asymptomatic aortic stenosis. N Engl J Med. 2000;343:611–7.
43. Pellikka PA, Sarano ME, Nishimura RA, et al. Outcome of 622 adults with asymptomatic, hemodynamically significant aortic stenosis during prolonged follow-up. Circulation. 2005;111:3290–5.
44. Taniguchi T, Morimoto T, Shiomi H, et al., CURRENT AS Registry Investigators. Initial surgical versus conservative strategies in patients with asymptomatic severe aortic stenosis. J Am Coll Cardiol. 2015;66:2827–38.
45. Pellikka PA. Observation for mildly symptomatic normal-flow, low-gradient severe aortic stenosis: caution advised. Heart. 2015;101:1349–50.
46. Généreux P, Stone GW, O'Gara PT, et al. Natural history, diagnostic approaches and therapeutic strategies for patients with asymptomatic severe aortic stenosis. J Am Coll Cardiol. 2016;67:2263–88.
47. Monin JL, Quere JP, Monchi M, et al. Low gradient aortic stenosis: operative risk stratification and predictors for long-term outcome: a multicenter study using dobutamine stress hemodynamics. Circulation. 2003;108:319–24.
48. Levy F, Laurent M, Monin JL, et al. Aortic valve replacement for low-flow/low-gradient aortic stenosis: operative risk stratification and long-term outcome: a European multicenter study. J Am Coll Cardiol. 2008;51:1466–72.
49. Tribouilloy C, Lévy F, Rusinaru D, et al. Outcome after aortic valve replacement for low-flow/low-gradient aortic stenosis without contractile reserve on dobutamine stress echocardiography. J Am Coll Cardiol. 2009;53:1865–73.
50. Pibarot P, Dumesnil J. Low-flow, low- gradient aortic stenosis with normal and depress left ventricular ejection fraction. Am J Cardiol. 2012;60(19):1845–53.
51. Brown ML, Pellikka PA, Schaff HV, et al. The benefits of early valve replacement in asymptomatic patients with severe aortic stenosis. J Thorac Cardiovasc Surg. 2008;135:308–15.

52. Monin J, Lancellotti P, Monchi M, et al. Risk score for predicting outcome in patients with asymptomatic aortic stenosis. Circulation. 2009;120:69–75.
53. Lancellotti P, Donal E, Magne J, et al. Risk stratification in asymptomatic moderate to severe aortic stenosis: the importance of the valvular, arterial and ventricular interplay. Heart. 2010;96:1364–71.
54. Eleid MF, Pellikka PA. Asymptomatic severe aortic stenosis: what are we waiting for? J Am Coll Cardiol. 2015;66:2842–3.
55. Bonow RO. Asymptomatic aortic stenosis: it is not simple anymore. J Am Coll Cardiol. 2015;66:2839–41.
56. Pai RG, Kapoor N, Bansal RC, et al. Malignant natural history of asymptomatic severe aortic stenosis: benefit of aortic valve replacement. Ann Thorac Surg. 2006;82:2116–22.
57. Kang DH, Park SJ, Rim JH, et al. Early surgery versus conventional treatment in asymptomatic very severe aortic stenosis. Circulation. 2010;121:1502–9.
58. Lancellotti P, Magne J, Donal E, et al. Clinical outcome in asymptomatic severe aortic stenosis: insights from the new proposed aortic stenosis grading classification. J Am Coll Cardiol. 2012;59:235–43.
59. Kamath AR, Pai RG. Risk factors for progression of calcific aortic stenosis and potential therapeutic targets. Int J Angiol. 2008;17:63–70.
60. Rosenhek R, Zilberszac R, Schemper M, et al. Natural history of very severe aortic stenosis. Circulation. 2010;121:151–6.
61. Kitai T, Honda S, Okada Y, et al. Clinical outcomes in non-surgically managed patients with very severe versus severe aortic stenosis. Heart. 2011;97:2029–32.
62. Cioffi G, Faggiano P, Vizzardi E, et al. Prognostic value of inappropriately high left ventricular mass in asymptomatic severe aortic stenosis. Heart. 2011;97:301–7.
63. Nessmith MG, Fukuta H, Brucks S, et al. Usefulness of an elevated B-type natriuretic peptide in predicting survival in patients with aortic stenosis treated without surgery. Am J Cardiol. 2005;96(10):1445–8.
64. Clavel MA, Malouf J, Michelena HI, et al. B type natriuretic peptide clinical activation in aortic stenosis: impact on long-term survival. J Am Coll Cardiol. 2014;63:2016–25.
65. Capoulade R, Magne J, Dulgheru R, et al. Prognostic value of plasma B-type natriuretic peptide levels after exercise in patients with severe asymptomatic aortic stenosis. Heart. 2014;100(20):1606–12.
66. Banovic M, Brkovic V, Vujisic-Tesic B, et al. Valvulo-arterial impedance is the best mortality predictor in asymptomatic aortic stenosis patients. J Heart Valve Dis. 2015;24:156–63.
67. Lancellotti P, Donal E, Magne J, et al. Impact of global left ventricular afterload on left ventricular function in asymptomatic severe aortic stenosis: a two-dimensional speckle-tracking study. Eur J Echocardiogr. 2010;11:537–43.
68. Yingchoncharoen T, Gibby C, Rodriguez L, et al. Association of myocardial deformation with outcome in asymptomatic aortic stenosis with normal ejection fraction. Circ Cardiovasc Imaging. 2012;5:719–25.
69. Nagata Y, Takeuchi M, Wu VC, et al. Prognostic value of LV deformation parameters using 2D and 3D speckle-tracking echocardiography in asymptomatic patients with severe aortic stenosis and preserved LV ejection fraction. J Am Coll Cardiol Img. 2015;8:235–45.
70. Astor BC, Kaczmarek RG, Hefflin B, et al. Mortality after aortic valve replacement: results from a nationally representative database. Ann Thorac Surg. 2000;70:1939–45.
71. Culliford AT, Galloway AC, Colvin SB, et al. Aortic valve replacement for aortic stenosis in persons aged 80 years and over. Am J Cardiol. 1991;67:1256–60.
72. Shroyer AL, Coombs LP, Peterson E, et al. The society of thoracic surgeons: 30-day operative mortality and morbidity risk models. Ann Thorac Surg. 2003;75:1856–65.
73. Roques F, Nashef SA, Michel P, et al., Euro SCORE Study Group. Risk factors for early mortality after valve surgery in Europe in the 1990s: lessons from the Euro SCORE Pilot Program. J Heart Valve Dis. 2001;10:572–77.
74. http://www.euroscore.org/calc.html.

75. Rosenhek R, Iung B, Tornos P, et al. ESC Working Group on Valvular Heart Disease Position Paper: assessing the risk of interventions in patients with valvular heart disease. Eur Heart J. 2012;33(7):822–8.
76. Iung B, Laouénan C, Himbert D, et al. Predictive factors of early mortality after transcatheter aortic valve implantation: individual risk assessment using a simple score. Heart. 2014;14:1142–3.
77. Capodanno D, Barbanti M, Tamburino C, et al; OBSERVANT Research Group. A simple risk tool (the OBSERVANT score) for prediction of 30-day mortality after transcatheter aortic valve replacement. Am J Cardiol. 2014;113:1851–8.
78. Hermiller JB, Yakubov SJ, Reardon MJ, et al. Predicting early and late mortality after transcatheter aortic valve replacement. J Am Coll Cardiol. 2016;68(4):343–52.
79. Iung B, Baron G, Butchart EG, et al. A prospective survey of patients with valvular heart disease in Europe: the Euro Heart Survey on Valvular Disease. Eur Heart J. 2003;24:1231–43.

# Computed Tomography Imaging for Aortic Valve Disease

# 16

Mickaël Ohana, Anthony Shaw, Romi Grover,
John Mooney, Jonathon Leipsic, and Philipp Blanke

Transthoracic echocardiography remains the first-line modality when assessing aortic valve disease: its high temporal resolution and the hemodynamic data made available by the Doppler analysis are essential for an accurate diagnosis, risk stratification, and follow-up of these pathologies. However, in the context of a comprehensive imaging work-up before an aortic valve percutaneous intervention, a precise, 3D and, above all, reproducible morphological characterization of the aortic valve and the aortic root anatomy is needed [1].

Extensive research on the place of computed tomography (CT) in this interventional cardiology setting has been done in recent years, particularly with the rise of transcatheter aortic valve implantation (TAVI), and the literature has established computed tomography angiography (CTA) as the reference imaging modality to screen these patients and plan their procedures, with a direct benefit in terms of reduction of adverse effects [2]. All the expertise gained with these procedures has also brought new insights into the initial diagnosis, as well as the evaluation of stenosis severity, and risk stratification of the congenital and acquired aortic valve diseases. Consequently, CTA increasingly appears to be a comprehensive imaging examination able to diagnose, classify, and help plan the interventional procedure in simple, as well as in the more complex, cases.

In this chapter, and after a practical review of the technical aspects of aortic valve CTA, we will describe the CT imaging characteristics of the main aortic valve diseases, with emphasis on the key components of patient screening and procedural planning.

M. Ohana • A. Shaw • R. Grover • J. Mooney • J. Leipsic (✉) • P. Blanke
Department of Radiology, Centre for Heart Valve Innovation St Paul's Hospital, University of British Columbia, Vancouver, BC, Canada
e-mail: jleipsic@providencehealth.bc.ca

© Springer International Publishing AG 2018
C. Tamburino et al. (eds.), *Percutaneous Treatment of Left Side Cardiac Valves*,
https://doi.org/10.1007/978-3-319-59620-4_16

277

## 16.1  Aortic Valve CTA Technique

Acquisition protocols of straightforward examinations, such as non-contrast head CT, aortoiliac CTA, or CT pulmonary angiography, are largely standardized across vendors and institutions, so as to offer a constant and reliable image quality. On the contrary, acquisition protocols of complex examinations vary quite significantly among vendors and centers [3]. Cardiac CT is the most complicated of CT acquisitions, in which scanning equipment, technological choices, operator training, and patient characteristics directly influence the outcome [4]. The expertise gained from the wider use of coronary CTA has been translated into valve CT imaging, and the technology can actually be considered robust, if this modality is carried out by a dedicated cardiac imaging team.

### 16.1.1  CT Acquisition

Acquisition is a critical step in CTA, since it determines the image quality and, therefore, the reliability of the examination [5]. Besides advanced technical adjustments such as tube potential, tube current, reconstruction algorithm, or temporal enhancement software, physicians supervising and interpreting cardiac CT for valve disease must be experts in both data acquisition and interpretation.

#### 16.1.1.1  ECG Synchronization

In order to freeze cardiac motion and obtain a clear depiction of the aortic valve anatomy, a synchronization of the acquisition with the cardiac cycle is mandatory. As for coronary CTA, this is achieved though electrocardiogram (ECG) triggering and requires a 64-row scanner.

Two major synchronization modes [6] are available (Fig. 16.1):

- Prospective triggering, in which only a single portion of the cardiac cycle, usually either end diastole or end systole, is acquired. In this mode, the scanner focuses on a specific part of the cardiac cycle, and X-rays are triggered only during this predetermined period of interest. The major strength of this mode is its low radiation dosage; the disadvantages lies in its susceptibility to cardiac arrhythmia and high heart rates, the misalignment artifacts on 64- and 128-row scanners (Fig. 16.2), and in the static aspect of the images, as only one phase of the cardiac cycle is obtained.
- Retrospective ECG synchronized acquisitions, in which the entire cardiac cycle is acquired. In this mode, X-rays are emitted continuously over a certain number of heart beats (one to ten, depending on the scanner model and on the patient's heart rate), and any cardiac cycle time point can be reconstructed later. The main advantages of this mode are the possibility of studying valve motion via cine images, since the whole cycle is available for review, and a relative insensitivity to cardiac arrhythmia with ECG editing possibilities; the negative point is a significantly increased radiation dose.

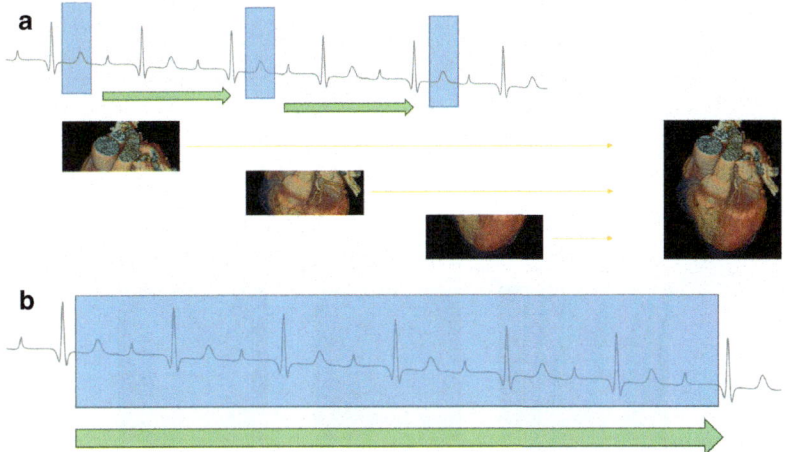

**Fig. 16.1** Cardiac CT acquisition. In prospective (**a**) ECG-triggered mode, one sequential acquisition (*blue* bar) is made every other heartbeat in the same cardiac phase, with table movement (*green arrows*) in between. Based on the number of rows, the coverage of each stack varies between 2.5 and 16 cm, meaning that 1–7 piles are required to cover the entire heart and the ascending aorta. They are subsequently merged (*orange arrows*) to form the volume of interest. In retrospective (**b**) ECG synchronized mode, the RX emission is constant over a definite number of heartbeats, and the table moves continuously

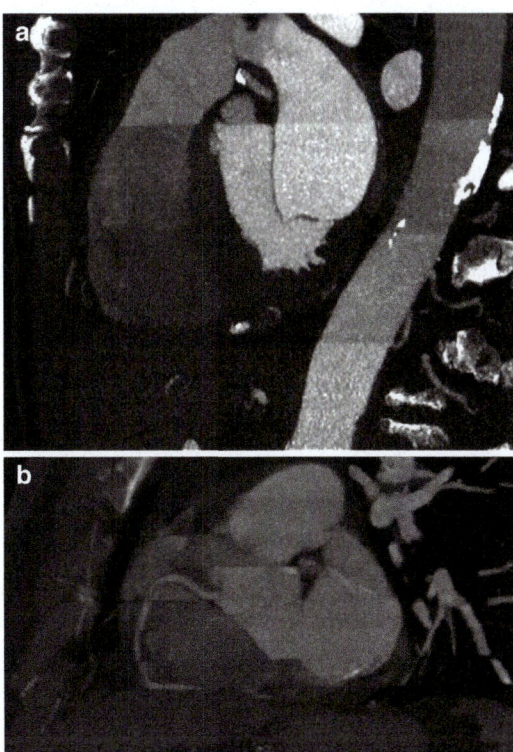

**Fig. 16.2** Misalignment artifacts on a cardiac CTA acquired with a 64-row scanner. (**a**) The misalignment is minimal; the piles can be differentiated only by the intensity of the blood pool enhancement. (**b**) The misalignment is severe, and that drastically limits the evaluation of the right coronary artery

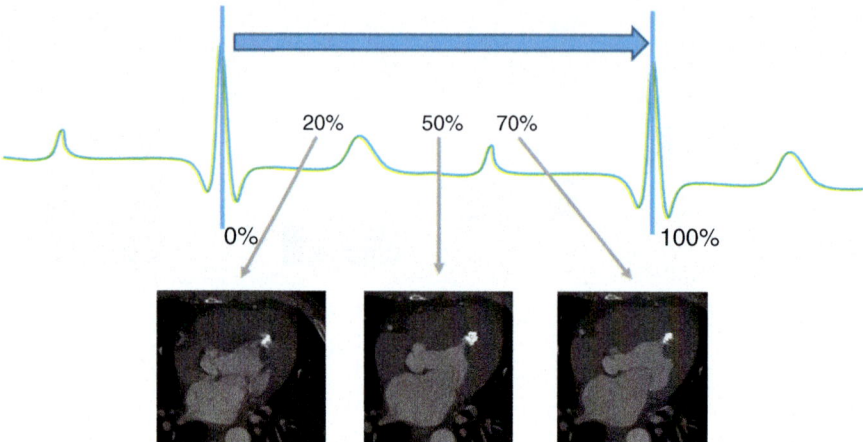

**Fig. 16.3** Reconstruction of phases after CT acquisition. R-R interval is by convention labeled from 0 to 100%. In this example, reconstructions were made at 20% (systole), 50% and 70% (diastole). Note how the right coronary artery is blurred at 20% and clear at 70%

With a prospective acquisition, only a single phase is obtained, while in a retrospective acquisition any phase can be reconstructed a posteriori. The reconstruction of the cardiac images with respect to the cardiac cycle follows a standardized rule: each cardiac cycle begins with an R wave and ends with an R wave, as detected by the scanner on the patient's ECG. A time point in the cardiac cycle is designated by its relative position in the R-R interval, expressed in percentage of the whole interval (Fig. 16.3). Usually, examinations acquired in retrospective mode are reconstructed from 0 to 90% every 10%, with ten phases covering the entire heart cycle.

### 16.1.1.2  Iodine Contrast Injection

Adequate luminal enhancement is essential in clearly depicting the valve morphology and requires a high concentration of iodine within the arterial lumen at the time of acquisition. This is obtained through

- The use of a high concentration iodine contrast media, equal to or above 320 mg/mL, with about 60–100 mL needed for an examination. Usual contraindications are renal failure, with an eGFR lower than 30 mL/min, and proven allergy to iodine contrast media.
- A high injection rate (4–6 mL/s) using an automatic power injector with saline flush; this requires a good caliber IV line.
- A bolus tracking technique to monitor the arrival of contrast media using serial axial slices repeated through the ascending aorta to follow, in real time, the progressive arterial uptake, until a predefined threshold (100–250 Hounsfield units) is reached and triggers the acquisition.

The arterial phase, in which the arterial luminal enhancement is maximum, is mandatory. Other phases such as the non-contrast or the late venous are optional. The non-contrast phase is used for measuring the burden of aortic valve calcification (i.e., calcium scoring), while the late venous phase is helpful when assessing the contrast uptake of a lesion.

### 16.1.1.3    Field of View and Slice Thickness

A coronary CTA always encompasses the aortic valve, but does not include the ascending aorta and the aortic arch. Dedicated aortic valve imaging should, in addition to the entire heart, routinely include the tubular portion of the aorta, as valvular pathologies (e.g., aortic stenosis, bicuspid valve) or originate (e.g., aortic dissection) from it.

In the axial plane, the field of view must be narrowed so as to center the image on the heart (Fig. 16.4) and gain some spatial resolution.

Slice thickness may vary among vendors, but must remain below 1 mm (usually between 0.5 and 0.625 mm) so as to obtain isotropic volumes suitable for the tridimensional posttreatment [7].

## 16.1.2  CT Posttreatment

Once the acquisition has been carried out, a first quality check is done to ensure the diagnostic quality of the examination, before releasing the patient from the CT scanner.

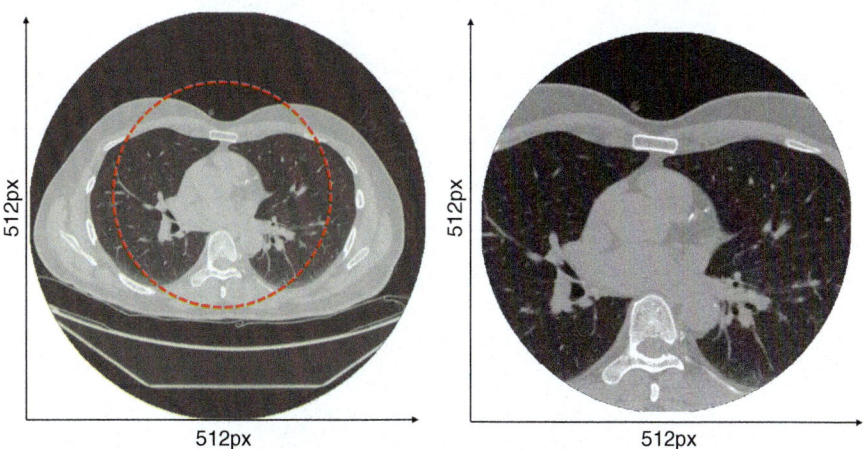

**Fig. 16.4**  Field of view. In a chest CT, the field of view is large, so as to encompass the entire chest (*left*): 36 cm are fitted in the 512 pixels of the image matrix. In a valve CT, the field of view must be limited to the area of interest (*right*): only 25 cm are fitted in 512 pixels, consequently increasing the spatial resolution

On a dedicated aortic valve CTA, one has to make sure that the following conditions are fulfilled (Fig. 16.5):

– Coverage of the left ventricular outflow tract (LVOT), the aortic sinus and the initial part of the ascending aorta
– Sufficient arterial enhancement, with a luminal density above 250 HU in the ascending aorta
– Absent or minimal motion artifacts and misregistration artifacts between the annulus and the sinus

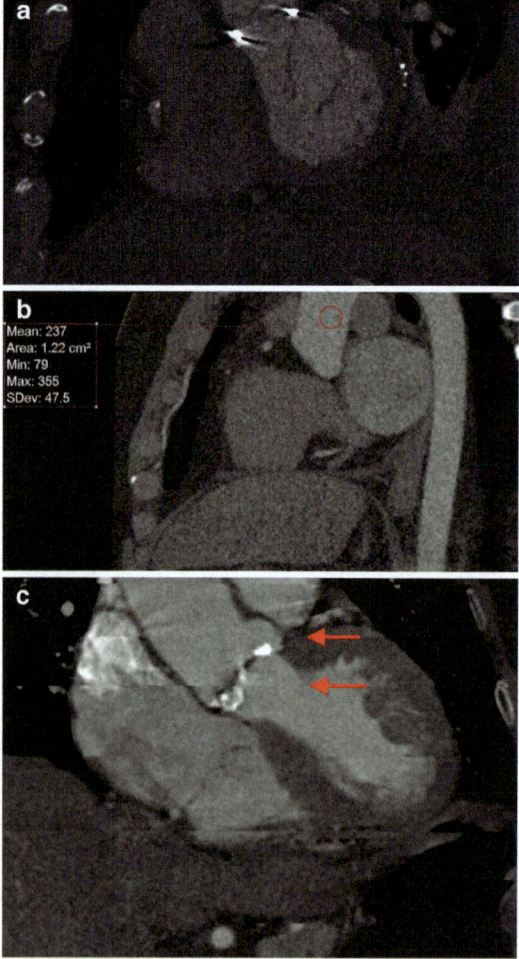

**Fig. 16.5** Valve CT image quality criteria. (**a**) The field of view is inadequate, with default of coverage of the aortic root. (**b**) The arterial enhancement is insufficient, with a density of only 237 HU in the ascending aorta. (**c**) Major misalignment artifacts hinder the proper evaluation of the annulus in this 64-row acquisition

### 16.1.2.1   Qualitative Analysis

Even though the axial slices remain at the basis of the radiological interpretation, standard and advanced image post processing [3] are needed to accurately depict the valve anatomy.

*Multiplanar reconstructions* (MPRs) are the most useful tool. Because images are isotropic, reconstructions in other planes, i.e., coronal, sagittal, or oblique, can be achieved while keeping the exact same image quality. Double obliquity allows the reader to simultaneously tilt a plane in reference to two perpendicular slices and is of paramount importance in achieving adequate measurements of vessels and other structures.

MPR views can be combined, in examinations acquired in retrospective mode, with a cine mode review of the different reconstructed phases covering the entire heart cycle. This allows a 4D navigation of the dataset, where the user can scroll between the phases (i.e., between systole and diastole) and the acquired volume.

*Maximum intensity projection* (MIP) reconstructions are obtained by summing the densest voxels over a pre-definite thickness, usually 3–10 mm. In CTA, brighter voxels correspond to iodine contrast, calcifications, and bones: raw MIP reconstructions will therefore bring out these structures, and the reader can adjust the MIP thickness so as to keep the bony structures out.

*Volume rendering* (VR) is another post-processing method based on voxel density using a specific 3D shading algorithm to create an impression of volume. Dedicated cardiac VR requires the suppression of the surrounding structures, such as the ribs, the lungs, or the abdominal organs, which can be time consuming. Limitations of MIP and VR are encountered with highly calcified structures and with stents, where the dense materials hinder the evaluation of the underlying opacified lumen. Ultimately, one has to keep in mind that VR and MIP are only reconstructions, and as such are prone to various computer and user generated artifacts. Consequently, any lesion detected over the VR or the MIP images has to be verified on the MPR slices.

### 16.1.2.2   Quantitative Analysis

Distance measurements can be obtained in two different ways on a dedicated workstation (Fig. 16.6):

- Linear measurements are the base and are made on a strictly perpendicular-to-the-flow axial view (utility of double obliquity MPR). When measuring a vessel, the smallest and largest diameters are drawn from lumen to lumen.
- Double oblique transverse imaging along the center line of any vascular structure is essential to ensure accurate measurements. This can be done semiautomatically with secondary manual adjustments. A contour-smoothing algorithm is used to flatten the small irregularities. Once the lumen is segmented, a perimeter and a surface are obtained, from which a mean diameter can be computed. The surface-based mean diameter is the most reproducible one. This tool is also used to measure the surface of the valve opening/closing.

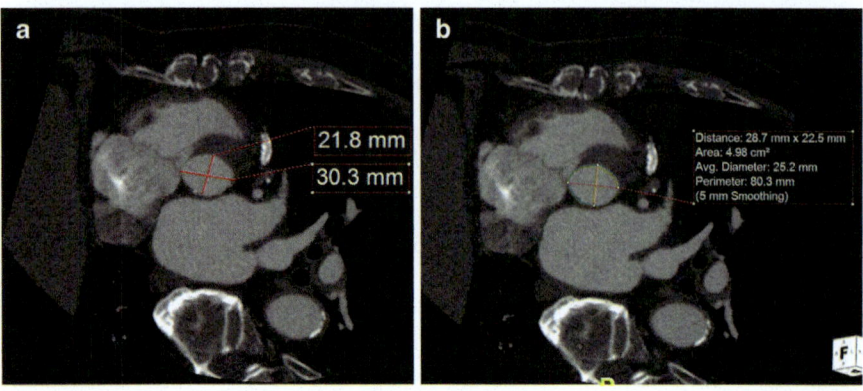

**Fig. 16.6** CT distance measurements. (**a**) Linear measurements are drawn by the reader from lumen to lumen. (**b**) The lumen contour is semiautomatically segmented, with a 5 mm smoothing to flatten the small irregularities, and the minimum diameter, maximum diameter, area, and area-based diameter and perimeter are automatically computed. Note the variation in the maximum diameter between both types of measures

### 16.1.3 Radiation Dose

A retrospective CTA for an aortic valve study delivers from 5 up to 15 mSv, depending on the scanner used (the more recent, the less the dose) and on the patient (the more thin and the more bradycardic, the less the dose) [8], which is reasonable when compared to a diagnostic coronary catheter angiogram (around 5 mSv) or to the mean annual natural radiation dose (around 2.5 mSv per year).

## 16.2   Aortic Stenosis

### 16.2.1 CT Diagnosis

Diagnosis of AS using CT takes advantage of the high spatial resolution and of the excellent calcium depiction of the technique [9]. AS displays fairly classic imaging findings on CT, including leaflet thickening, leaflet calcifications (typically involving the noncoronary cusp in priority), and restricted leaflet motion on the cine images with decreased opening of the valve, and can be accompanied with ascending aorta dilatation and concentric left ventricular hypertrophy [10].

A non-contrast ECG-gated phase can be used to accurately quantify the burden of calcification of the aortic valve in a fashion similar to that done for scoring of calcium in the coronary arteries. The aortic valve score obtained (Agatston) is a reproducible marker of the severity of the calcification and has been shown to correlate well with the severity of AS. A threshold of 1651 has been proposed [11] to differentiate non-severe from severe AS, with a 82% sensitivity and a 80%

specificity, and appears robust even when the left ventricular ejection fraction is severely decreased. It has also been suggested that different thresholds should be used for women (>1274) and men (>2065) [12]. Interestingly, an Agatston score of less than 700 excludes severe AS, with a high negative predictive value.

The high spatial resolution of CT is also efficient in measuring the geometric orifice area of a stenotic aortic valve, which is the area formed by the free sides of the aortic valve leaflets at peak systole. This requires a retrospective acquisition, with careful review of all available phases in order to determine the phase in which the valve opening seems to be the largest (usually end systole, i.e., between 20 and 40%). Once the correct phase is selected, the annulus plane is determined using MPR (cf. TAVI work-up below) and is shifted up to the valve to encompass the free sides of the leaflets. A freehand segmentation tool is then used to draw the valvular orifice, with exclusion of calcium and leaflet thickening, to obtain an aortic valve area expressed in square centimeters (Fig. 16.7). It is commonly recommended that minimum intensity projection reconstruction (minIP) be used to help mitigate the impact of calcification on the planimetric assessment of the geometric valve area. This measure is systematically larger than the one derived from echocardiography data, with an overall difference between 0.12 [13] and 0.6 cm$^2$ [14]. This can be explained by the fact that echocardiography relies on gradient and therefore calculates an effective valve area, while CT relies on morphology and gives an anatomic/geometric valve area [15]. Aortic valve area thresholds to differentiate severe AS vary among authors [13, 16, 17]; however, 1.2 cm$^2$ is an accepted cutoff. Consequently, CT can be helpful particularly when Doppler estimation of the aortic valve gradient is unreliable.

## 16.2.2  Before Transcatheter Aortic Valve Implantation

CT plays a central role in the selection of patients suitable for TAVI and is the reference method [2] for the aortic annulus and aortic root sizing, assessing the coronary ostia position, and predicting the appropriate angiography projection angles [18, 19]. CTA is also essential in defining iliac vessels tortuosity, stenosis, and severity of calcified atherosclerosis, in order to plan the safest access route and minimize vascular complications [20]. Using a 64- or 128-row single source scanner, a comprehensive TAVI planning protocol often requires two consecutive steps: first, a retrospectively ECG-gated aortic root CTA followed by an ungated aortoilio-femoral CTA [21] (Fig. 16.8).

Prosthesis selection relies on the measurement of the virtual basal ring of the aortic valve ventricular plane, which determines the aortic annulus. This is defined as the ring formed by the junction of the hinge point of each cusp. The measurements need to be done in end systole, in which the annulus size is the greater [22]; this usually corresponds to the 20–40% phases. Once the correct phase is identified and selected, a double-oblique MPR is used to align all three hinge points of the aortic cusps: one can begin with aligning the crosshair on the right coronary cusp on

**Fig. 16.7** Aortic valve area CT measurement. The opening surface of the aortic valve is segmented manually, with careful exclusion of the calcium and the leaflet thickening. (**a**) We have an example of a valve area measured at 1.57 cm$^2$, indicating a moderate stenosis. (**b, c**) One can see the positive effect of thick-slice minIP reconstruction (**b**) on the leaflet free sides, conspicuity, compared with the MIP image (**c**), where the valve calcifications can render an accurate delineation of the orifice difficult

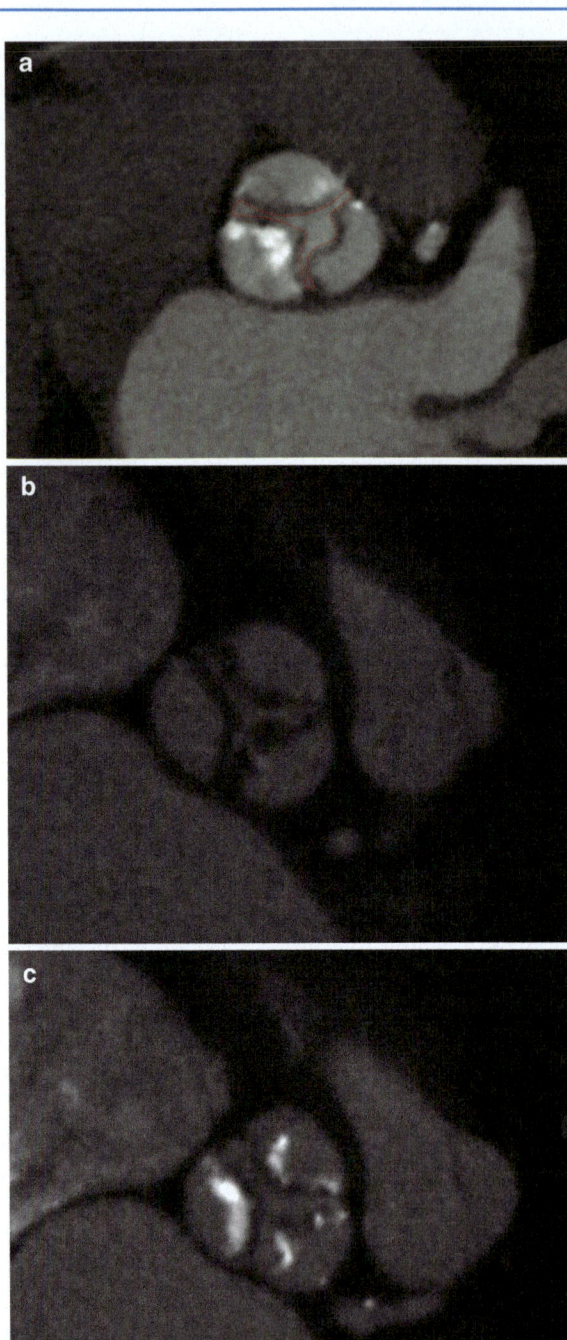

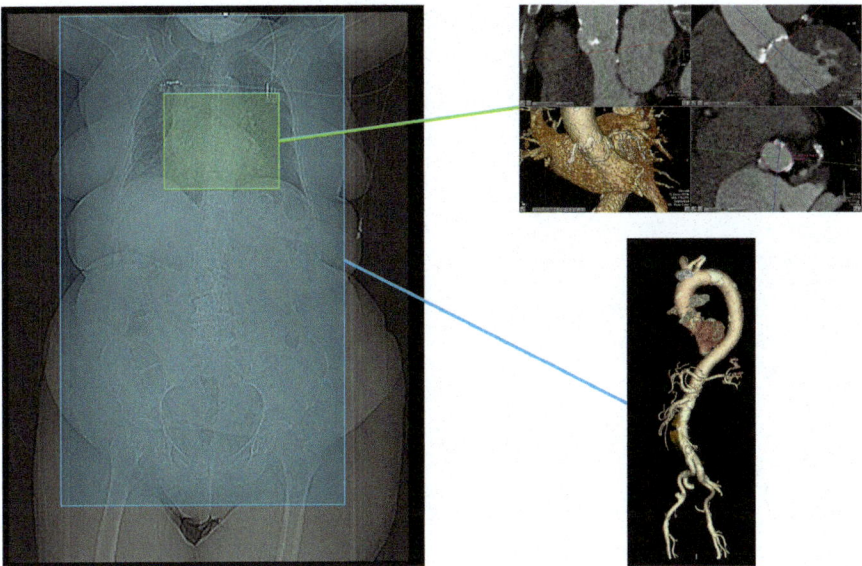

**Fig. 16.8** Classical TAVI planning CTA acquisition protocol. First, the aortic valve and the aortic root are acquired with ECG synchronization, and then the CAP aorta CTA is acquired

an axial view, then rotate the sagittal oblique axis to align with the left coronary cusp, and finally rotate the coronal oblique to align with the noncoronary cusp (Fig. 16.9). Once the annulus plane is defined, one can position the crosshair in the middle of it, and rotate either the sagittal oblique or the coronal oblique in a turn-around fashion to ensure that the hinge point of each cusp is indeed in plane.

With the annular plane defined, the following measurements (Fig. 16.10) can be made:

– Annulus size: Various CT measurements have been used to help guide annulus sizing and device selection, with reliance now being almost exclusively on annular area and perimeter. Area was initially favored owing to the fact that it was highly reproducible across workstation platforms. Perimeter is now commonly used as well, particularly for self-expandable devices, as all CT workstations have now begun to integrate perimeter smoothing algorithms to improve reproducibility [23]. At present, area remains the measurement of choice for balloon-expandable prostheses. This is likely wise as it is a more conservative measurement than perimeter: the aortic annulus is commonly noncircular and the perimeter of a noncircular structure is always greater than the perimeter of a circular structure of the same size. Sizing algorithms have been developed on the basis of both of these measurements of the annulus, with the most common goal being to place a transcatheter heart valve larger than the native annulus by a pre-specified percentage of either the annular area or perimeter. The self-expandable devices with lower radial forces need greater degrees of oversizing to reduce the

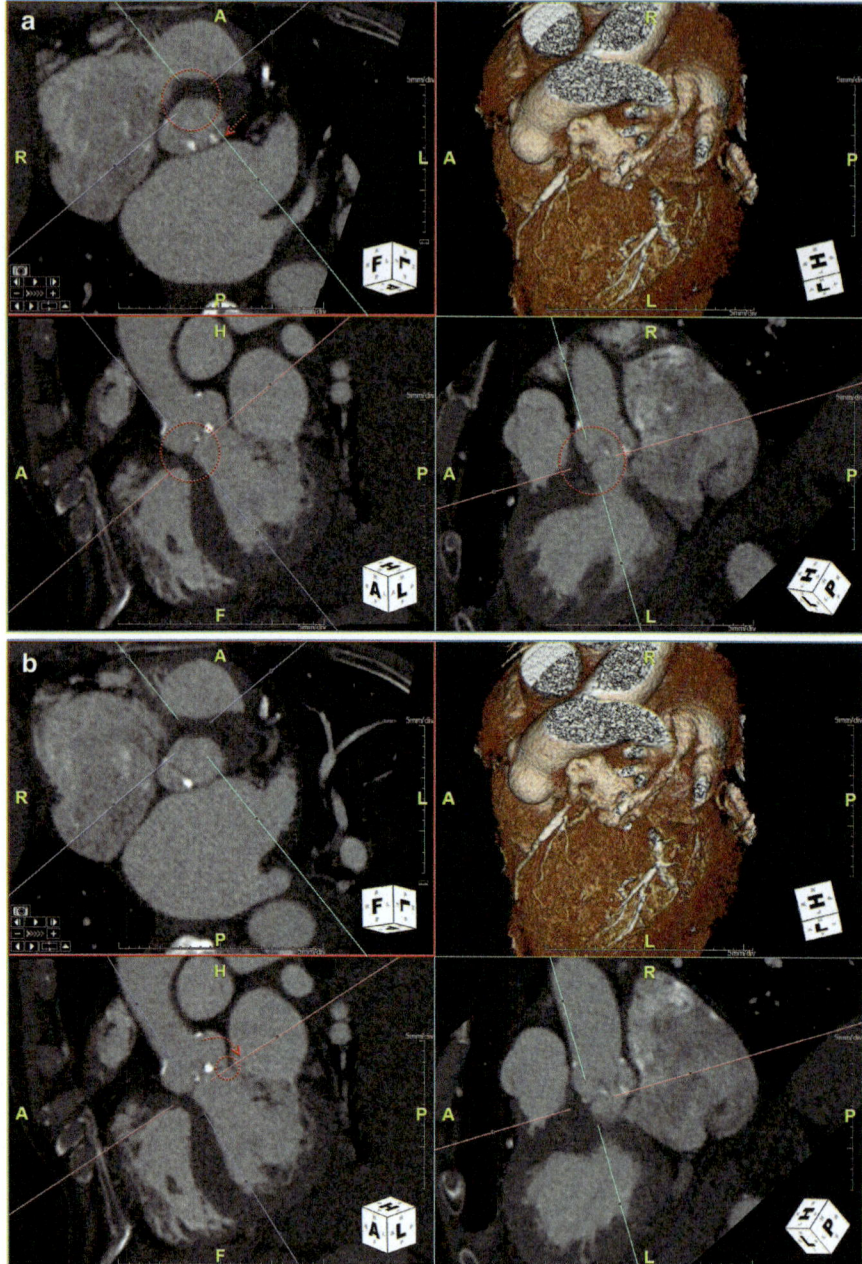

**Fig. 16.9** Annulus definition using CTA. First, one has to align the MPR crosshair on the right coronary cusp hinge point (**a**—*red circle*), then align one of the sagittal oblique plane on the left coronary cusp plane (**a**—*red arrow*). Second, the axial plane is tilted (**b**—*red arrow*) so as to align with the hinge point of the left cusp (**b**—*red circle*). Third, the noncoronary cusp is aligned (**c**) and the axial plane is again tilted (**d**—*red arrow*) to attain the hinge point of the last cusp (**d**—*red circle*). Finally, a turnaround check is done (**e**—*red arrow*) to confirm the alignment of the hinge points (**e**—*red circles*)

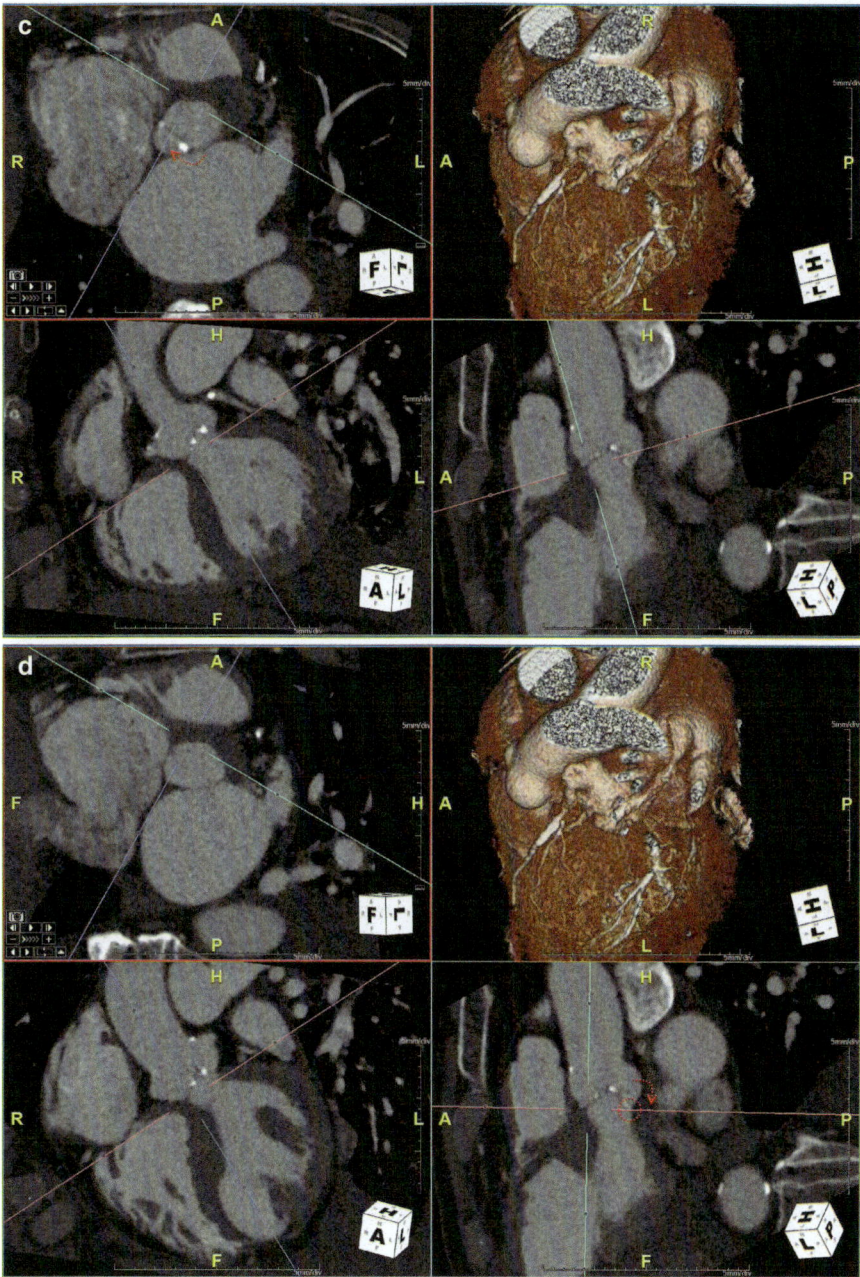

**Fig. 16.9** (continued)

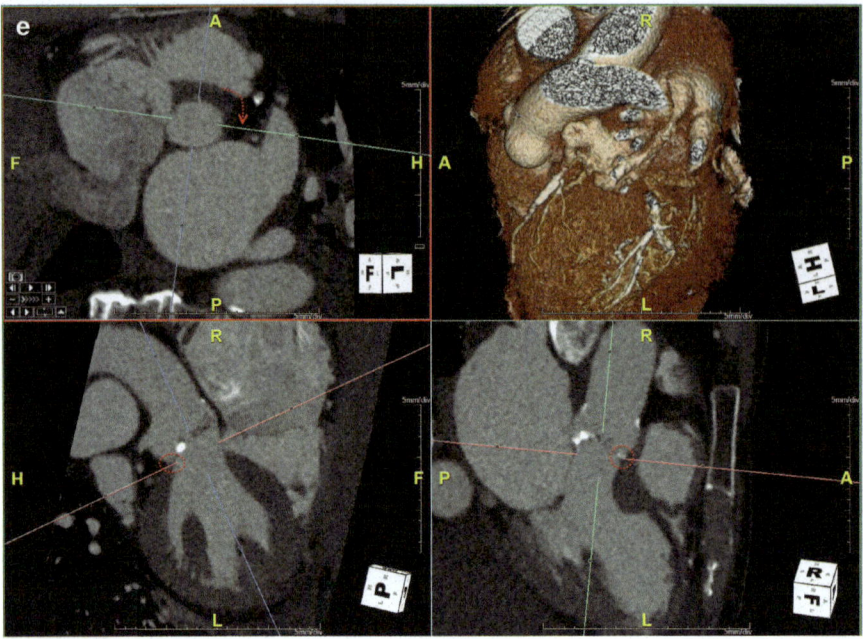

**Fig. 16.9** (continued)

    risk of paravalvular leak compared with balloon-expandable prostheses, for which annular rupture is a risk with excessive oversizing.

– Coronary ostial height: the orthogonal distance between the annulus plane and the ostium of the left main and the right coronary artery is measured on the sagittal or the coronal oblique plane.

– Coplanar projection angle: fluoroscopy arm positioning for optimal annulus alignment can be derived from the CT, providing that the software used has this specific capability.

    Other required measures are:

– Sinus of Valsalva: three diameters, from the bottom of the cusp to the opposite commissure

– The minimal luminal diameter of the iliac arteries for sheath accessibility

### 16.2.3 Before Open Surgery

The role of CT before open aortic valve surgery is limited to the search for extensive ascending aorta wall calcifications ("porcelain aorta") (Fig. 16.11) that could render impossible its cannulation [24], and the prediction of suitable anatomy for a mini-invasive procedure [25].

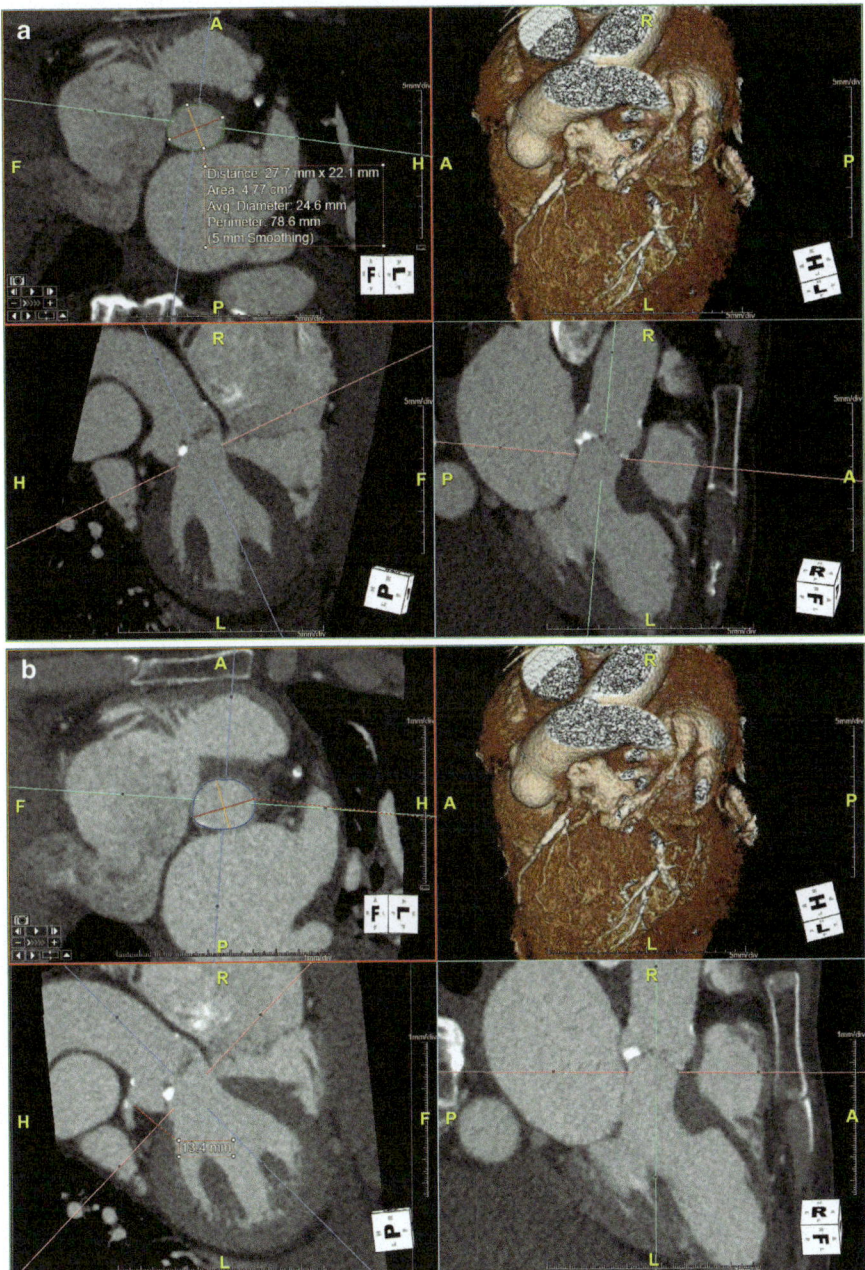

**Fig. 16.10**  Measurements for TAVI work-up. Once the annulus plane is defined, its area and perimeter are measured by segmentation (**a**). The coronary ostial height is measured as the orthogonal distance between the ostium and the annulus plane (**b**—left main, **c**—right coronary artery)

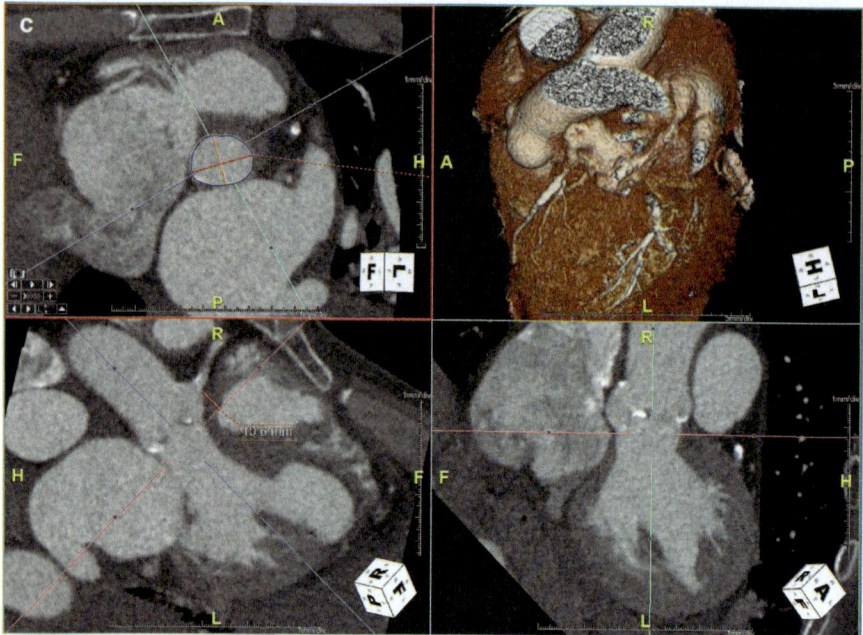

**Fig. 16.10** (continued)

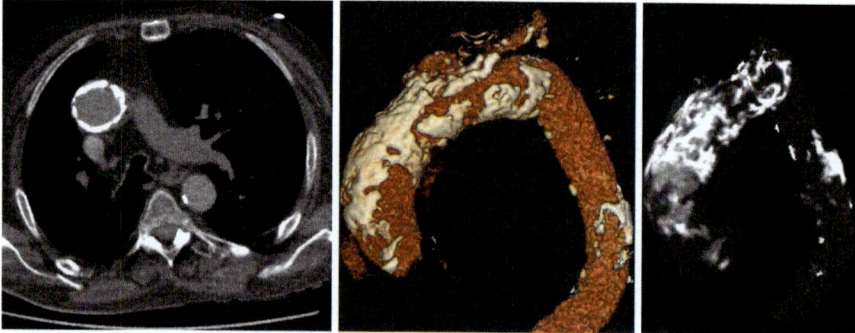

**Fig. 16.11** Porcelain aorta. Almost circumferential ascending aortic wall calcifications (*left*), which are well depicted on the VR (*middle*) and MIP (*right*) reconstructions

## 16.3 Aortic Regurgitation

The role of CT in the diagnosis of aortic regurgitation is less well established, though the technique and the posttreatment are quite similar. When aortic regurgitation is secondary to an intrinsic valve disease, CT can show retraction of the leaflets, and thickening and/or calcifications. On the contrary, when aortic regurgitation is passive, leaflet anatomy is normal, and the main role of CT is to precisely measure the aortic root.

Visual assessment of the valve residual opening in end diastole has shown a good correlation with echocardiography for grading the severity of the regurgitation [26]. Indeed, a normal coaptation of the leaflets in end diastole is sufficient to rule out a moderate or severe regurgitation. However, mild aortic regurgitation can exhibit normal CT leaflet coaptation and therefore be missed. This is a particular issue in the setting of aortic valve calcification because the more the valve is calcified, the more the visualization of the regurgitant orifice can be easily obscured. It has been suggested that when the valve calcium scoring is greater than 937, the risk of false negatives with CT is high [27].

To measure the regurgitant orifice area, one has to select the correct CT phase corresponding to end diastole. It is important to recognize that this does not correspond to a pre-specified percentage of the R-R interval and requires adjudication through interrogation of the mitral valve. In practice, we select the phase immediately before the closure of the mitral valve. Once selected, the annulus plane is determined and is shifted up to the valve at the level of the leaflets to best visualize the leaflet malcoaptation. A freehand tool is then used to obtain the planimetry of the regurgitant orifice. In a large study, moderate aortic regurgitation had a valve area of about 0.37 cm², while severe patients had an area of 0.81 cm², though with some overlap between groups [27]. It has been proposed to use a threshold of 0.25 cm² valve opening for moderate AR, and 0.75cm² for severe AR [28].

## 16.4  Leaflet Anomalies

CT is an excellent tool for a positive diagnosis and classification of leaflet anomalies, particularly the bicuspid aortic valve (BAV). Identification of the various BAV phenotypes with CT is more reliable than with echocardiography [29], yielding a sensitivity of 94% and a specificity of 100%, compared with 71% and 71% for ultrasound [30]. Identification of BAV is of paramount importance in a pre-TAVI work-up, as this affects the device selection, the procedure, and the prognosis [31], though the 30-day mortality, the rate of paravalvular leak, and the incidence of annular rupture have been shown to be somewhat comparable between BAV and tricuspid AV [29].

The normal tricuspid appearance is essentially defined by the presence of three commissures, each located between the free sides of two AV cusps, and giving the orifice a triangular appearance in peak systole.

There are several classifications of BAV morphology, and are of various complexity; they have historically relied on either pathology or echocardiography [32]. The most common classification system used clinically is one proposed by Sievers, in 2007 [33]. In this seminal work, a classification system was proposed after examination of 304 surgically excised bicuspid aortic valves. Three factors were defined as essential for the diagnosis. The two less emphasized elements referenced were the spatial location of the raphe and the functional status of the aortic valve. The most important characterizing feature was the number of raphes—designating three "types": a Type 0 BAV with no raphe, a Type 1 BAV with a single raphe, and a Type 2 BAV with two raphes. The location of the valve opening in a Type 0 valve is either anterior-posterior or lateral, while in Type 1 or 2 BAVs the raphe is located between the left (L) and right (R) cusps (L-R, 71%), between the right and noncoronary cusps (N) (R-N, 15%), or between the left and noncoronary cusps (N-L, 3%). These anatomical findings described by Sievers are easily characterized on CT, given its strong spatial resolution and its multiplanar imaging capabilities.

More recently, it has become increasingly clear that MDCT can provide insight into the morphological changes that exist across the spectrum of bicuspid valve disease. A new MDCT-based classification (Fig. 16.12) has been proposed by Jilaihawi et al. [34], with the advantage of being anatomically based and designed to be relevant in the era of TAVI. In this classification, an entity known as a tricommissural bicuspid valve, which was previously referred to as a functional or acquired bicuspid valve, is described. There is increasing data in the pathology literature suggesting that this subtype is congenital in nature, but manifests later in life. To make this diagnosis with CT, the first step of the analysis should be to define the annulus plane, bearing in mind that in BAV patients the virtual basal ring is commonly located higher in position. Once in the annulus plane, the second step is to count the number of hinge points to determine if there are two or three points. When three points are encountered, it is a tricommissural BAV, and a bicommissural if only two points are present.

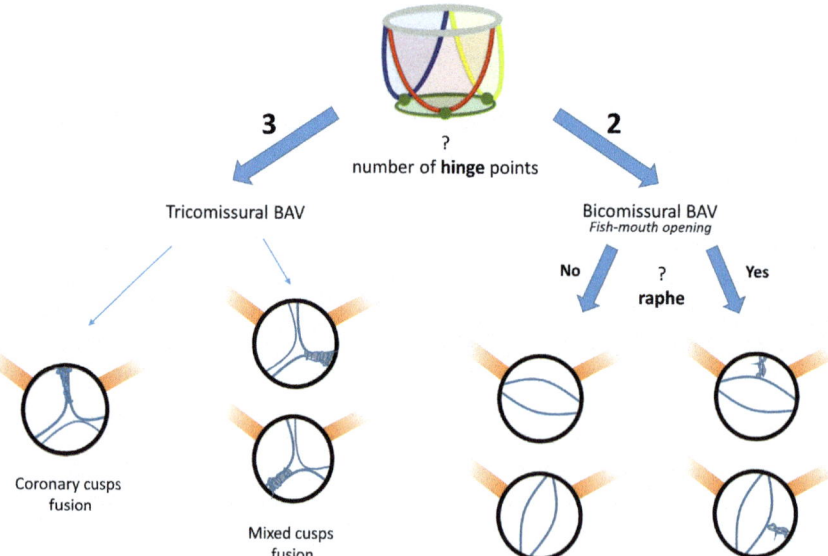

**Fig. 16.12** Bicuspid valve classification

The tricommissural type accounts for 23% of cases. In this morphology, the bicuspid aspect is secondary to a complete fusion of two cusps at the commissural level. This fusion can occur either between the coronary cusps (62% of cases) or either between a coronary cusp and the noncoronary (38% of cases). Of importance, this fusion exhibits the same cephalad extent as the two other commissures.

The bicommissural type, in which only two hinge points are present, can be found with (56%) or without (21%) a raphe. When a raphe is present, two cusps are fused by a fibrous or calcified ridge, which however does not reach the height of the commissure fusion. In bicommissural BAV, the valve opening can be made between the coronary cusps (mixed cusp fusion, accounting for 12% of cases in the raphe type, and 79% of cases in the non-raphe type) or between the coronary and the noncoronary cusps (88% of cases for the raphe type, and 21% for the non-raphe type).

## 16.5 Infective Endocarditis

Evidence of endocardial involvement with echocardiography (valve vegetation, perivalvular abscess, new dehiscence of a prosthetic valve) is one of the major criteria for a positive diagnosis of infective endocarditis [35]. However, vegetations as well as perivalvular abscesses can be difficult to detect even with TEE, with a sensitivity ranging between 48 and 100% [36]. ECG-gated CTA has demonstrated an overall 97% sensitivity and 88% specificity for the detection of valvular lesions, with a 96% sensitivity and 97% specificity for >4 mm vegetations, and a 100% sensitivity and specificity for the abscesses/pseudoaneurysms [37].

On CT, vegetations are seen as irregularly shaped hypodense masses (Fig. 16.13) that are oscillating and adherent to the endocardium. Abscesses are heterogeneous paravalvular masses typically located in the paravalvular space, but which can also extend to the myocardium. A pseudoaneurysm is a lesion filled with contrast media, with a direct continuity with the aortic root or the cardiac chambers; CT appears to be superior to TEE for showing the perivalvular extent of these lesions, particularly the annulus involvement.

In addition to these direct findings, cardiac CTA has also the advantage of showing the coronary artery anatomy, which could be useful in ruling out coronary artery disease before surgery and/or anticipating potential surgical difficulties when septic lesions are close to the coronary arteries [37].

## 16.6 Tumors

The most common valve tumor is the papillary fibroelastoma, which is a benign lesion involving predominantly the aortic valve, and is usually discovered incidentally or secondary to distal embolization [38]. Papillary fibroelastomas are small tumors, usually <1 cm and ranging from 0.2 to 5 cm [39], and are seen on CT as

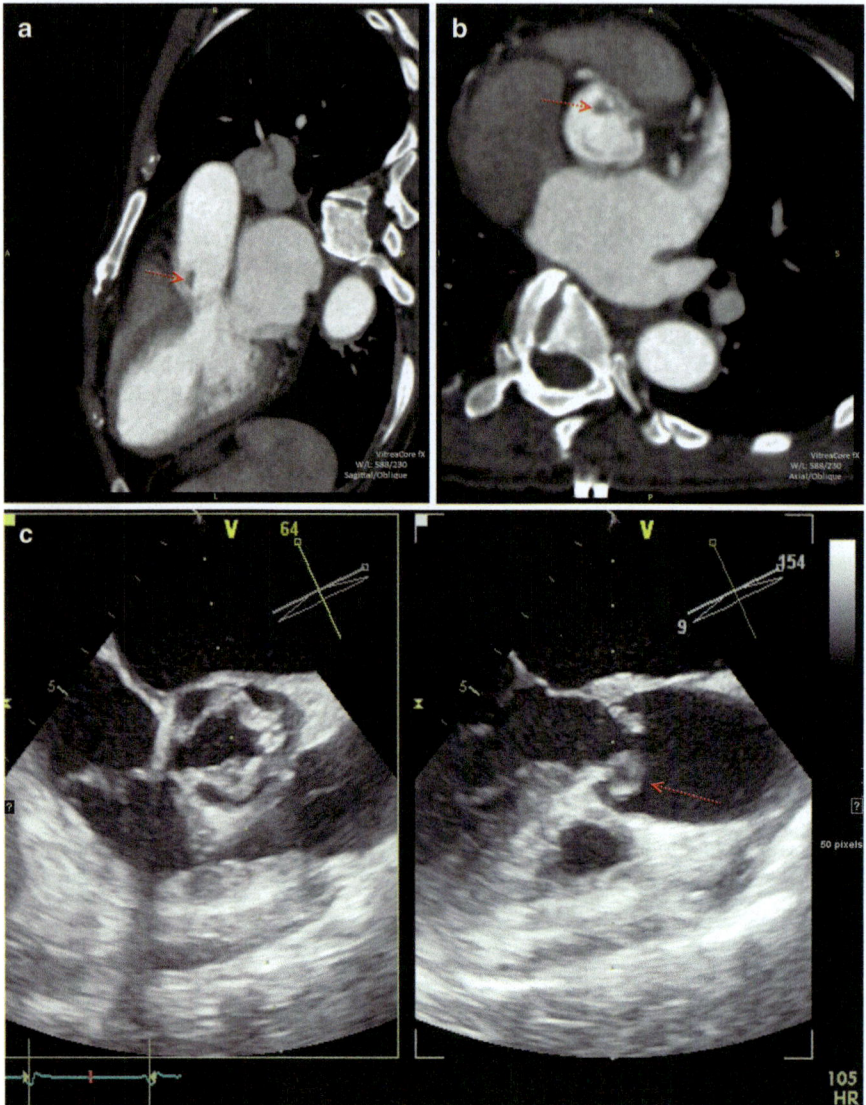

**Fig. 16.13** Infective endocarditis. CTA example (**a**, **b**, *red arrows*) of a vegetation in an infective aortic endocarditis in a 62-year-old man, and correlation with transesophageal echocardiography (**c**)

well-circumscribed round or oval hypodense lesions. They are attached to the valve more frequently in its upstream side, commonly through a pedicle.

Other aortic valve primary tumors are extremely rare, and the major differential is an infective endocarditis vegetation, which usually destroys the valve anatomy and exhibits a different clinical presentation [40].

## 16.7    Postoperative Follow-Up and Complications

### 16.7.1  After Surgical Aortic Valve Replacement

Complications after surgical AV replacement can be, in some cases, diagnosed with CT [41].

Valvular regurgitation is defined by an abnormal regurgitant volume and can affect biological or mechanical prosthetic valves, provided an impingement of the leaflet/disk closure is present.

This can be secondary to infective endocarditis, the CT appearance of which is similar to that on the native valve (i.e., small round hypodense lesions), and are usually located on the ventricular surface of the prosthesis.

Thrombosis and pannus can also cause valvular destruction and regurgitation/obstruction. Pannus usually develops on the ventricular side of the valve; on the contrary, thrombus tends to develop on the aortic side. Pannus is seen on CT as a hypodense structure extending from the ventricular wall to the valve surface, and the attenuation of which is similar to that of the ventricular septum; CT can help in identifying a resulting flow limitation [42]. Thrombus is also seen as an hypodense structure [43], but usually less dense than the ventricular septum.

Structural failure can also be at the origin of valvular regurgitation. For biological valves, CT can help in identifying insufficient leaflet coaptation, with measurement of the valve residual opening area in end systole [44], and identification of leaflet thickening or leaflet calcifications. Indeed, cusp calcifications has been linked to bioprosthetic valve failure, and can also be quantified with a calcium score [45], as for native valves. Cine CT of prosthetic valves, provided a retrospective ECG-gated acquisition has been used, can detect prosthetic valve dysfunction [46], such as incorrect leaflet opening.

Paravalvular regurgitation is defined by an abnormal retrograde blood flow around the valve between the prosthesis and the annulus. It can be directly recognized on CT as an enhancing structure adjacent to the valve and linking the LVOT with the ascending aorta. Differential with valve dehiscence is difficult. Valve dehiscence is secondary to suture breakdown and is favored by infective endocarditis, ascending aorta dilatation, and native valve calcifications. On CT, dehiscence is seen as a complete gap between the margin of the prosthetic valve and the annulus, with leakage of contrast flowing from the LVOT to the aortic sinus. It is usually bigger and larger than a simple paravalvular regurgitation.

### 16.7.2  After TAVI

CT follow-up of TAVI patients is only done in cases of new onset of symptoms suggestive of valve dysfunction, or in cases of discordant/equivocal echocardiography findings [21]. Normal post-deployment appearance varies between valve models; one must ascertain a good positioning (i.e., a lower part of the prosthesis located in the LVOT below the annulus plane, and an upper part located in the aortic root

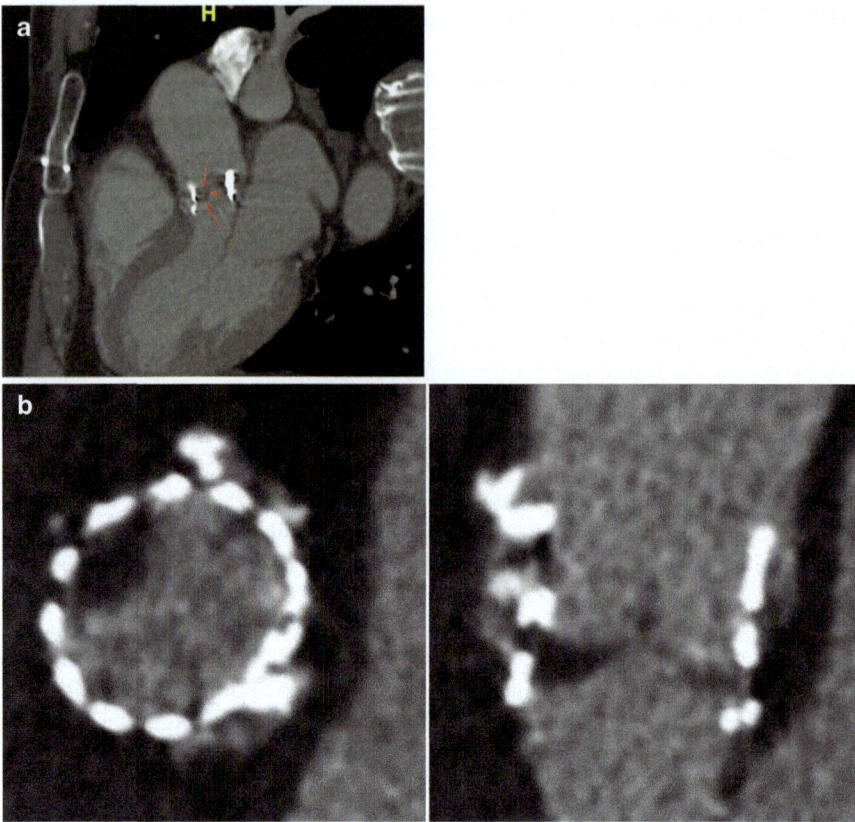

**Fig. 16.14** TAVI complications. Follow-up CTA performed 40 days after TAVI in a patient with progressively increasing mean transaortic gradient. (**a**) Low-attenuation thickening of the right coronary leaflet (*red arrows*) consistent with thrombus. Follow-up CTA done 30 days after TAVI in an asymptomatic patient. (**b**) Hypodense thickening of the prosthetic leaflets corresponding to HALT

beyond the distal portion of the native cusps), and a good expansion with displacement of the native leaflets up in the aortic sinus.

CT is the reference modality for a diagnosis of acute post-procedural complications: aortic dissection, annular and aortic root rupture, cardiac tamponade, contained rupture with pseudoaneurysm formation, and valve thrombosis (Fig. 16.14a) [47]. Valve migration, as well as valve integrity, can also be analyzed with CT: aspect of the stent and the prosthetic leaflets can reveal stent fracture or leaflet degeneration. More recently, a new entity described as early hypo-attenuated leaflet thickening (HALT), and corresponding to a hypodense thickening of the prosthetic leaflets (Fig. 16.14b) combined with reduced valve motion, has been described [48, 49]. This finding has recently been shown to resolve after oral anticoagulation, and not seen in those on anticoagulation, suggesting that it relates to subclinical valve thrombus formation. However, the importance of this finding is unknown.

## Conclusion

Thanks to its high spatial resolution and its excellent calcium depiction, CT is particularly suited for the exploration of calcified AS, mainly for the pre-TAVI work-up, and for a positive diagnosis and grading in patients in whom echocardiography is non-conclusive. Other CT applications for aortic valve pathologies are emerging, but for now remain a second-line option, limited to specific indications and patients.

## References

1. Hoey ET, Ganeshan A. Multi-detector CT angiography of the aortic valve-part 1: anatomy, technique and systematic approach to interpretation. Quant Imaging Med Surg. 2014;4(4):265–72.
2. Binder RK, Webb JG, Willson AB, et al. The impact of integration of a multidetector computed tomography annulus area sizing algorithm on outcomes of transcatheter aortic valve replacement: a prospective, multicenter, controlled trial. J Am Coll Cardiol. 2013;62(5):431–8.
3. Ohana M, Georg Y, Lejay A, et al. Current optimal morphological evaluation of peripheral arterial diseases. J Cardiovasc Surg. 2015;56(2):287–97.
4. Leipsic J, Abbara S, Achenbach S, et al. SCCT guidelines for the interpretation and reporting of coronary CT angiography: a report of the Society of Cardiovascular Computed Tomography Guidelines Committee. J Cardiovasc Comput Tomogr. 2014;8(5):342–58.
5. Abbara S, Arbab-Zadeh A, Callister TQ, et al. SCCT guidelines for performance of coronary computed tomographic angiography: a report of the Society of Cardiovascular Computed Tomography Guidelines Committee. J Cardiovasc Comput Tomogr. 2009;3(3):190–204.
6. Earls JP, Berman EL, Urban BA, et al. Prospectively gated transverse coronary CT angiography versus retrospectively gated helical technique: improved image quality and reduced radiation dose. Radiology. 2008;246(3):742–53.
7. Machida H, Tanaka I, Fukui R, et al. Current and novel imaging techniques in coronary CT. Radiographics. 2015;35(4):991–1010.
8. Halliburton SS, Abbara S, Chen MY, et al. SCCT guidelines on radiation dose and dose-optimization strategies in cardiovascular CT. J Cardiovasc Comput Tomogr. 2011;5(4):198–224.
9. Saikrishnan N, Kumar G, Sawaya FJ, Lerakis S, Yoganathan AP. Accurate assessment of aortic stenosis: a review of diagnostic modalities and hemodynamics. Circulation. 2014;129(2):244–53.
10. Hoey ET, Ganeshan A. Multi-detector CT angiography of the aortic valve-part 2: disease specific findings. Quant Imaging Med Surg. 2014;4(4):273–81.
11. Cueff C, Serfaty JM, Cimadevilla C, et al. Measurement of aortic valve calcification using multislice computed tomography: correlation with haemodynamic severity of aortic stenosis and clinical implication for patients with low ejection fraction. Heart. 2011;97(9):721–6.
12. Clavel MA, Messika-Zeitoun D, Pibarot P, et al. The complex nature of discordant severe calcified aortic valve disease grading: new insights from combined Doppler echocardiographic and computed tomographic study. J Am Coll Cardiol. 2013;62(24):2329–38.
13. Clavel MA, Malouf J, Messika-Zeitoun D, Araoz PA, Michelena HI, Enriquez-Sarano M. Aortic valve area calculation in aortic stenosis by CT and Doppler echocardiography. JACC Cardiovasc Imaging. 2015;8(3):248–57.
14. Halpern EJ, Mallya R, Sewell M, Shulman M, Zwas DR. Differences in aortic valve area measured with CT planimetry and echocardiography (continuity equation) are related to divergent estimates of left ventricular outflow tract area. AJR Am J Roentgenol. 2009;192(6):1668–73.
15. Flachskampf FA. Stenotic aortic valve area: should it be calculated from CT instead of echocardiographic data? JACC Cardiovasc Imaging. 2015;8(3):258–60.

16. Pouleur AC, le Polain de Waroux JB, Pasquet A, Vanoverschelde JL, Gerber BL. Aortic valve area assessment: multidetector CT compared with cine MR imaging and transthoracic and transesophageal echocardiography. Radiology. 2007;244(3):745–54.

17. Anger T, Bauer V, Plachtzik C, et al. Non-invasive and invasive evaluation of aortic valve area in 100 patients with severe aortic valve stenosis: comparison of cardiac computed tomography with ECHO (transesophageal/transthoracic) and catheter examination. J Cardiol. 2014;63(3):189–97.

18. Al-Hassan D, Blanke P, Leipsic J. Multidetector computed tomography in transcatheter aortic valve implantation. Where we stand. Minerva Cardioangiol. 2013;61(4):407–27.

19. Naoum C, Blanke P, Leipsic J. Computed tomography imaging prior to transcatheter aortic valve replacement. Curr Radiol Rep. 2015;3(5):1–7.

20. Lejay A, Caspar T, Ohana M, et al. Vascular access complications in endovascular procedures with large sheaths. J Cardiovasc Surg. 2016;57(2):311–21.

21. Blanke P, Schoepf UJ, Leipsic JA. CT in transcatheter aortic valve replacement. Radiology. 2013;269(3):650–69.

22. Murphy DT, Blanke P, Alaamri S, et al. Dynamism of the aortic annulus: effect of diastolic versus systolic CT annular measurements on device selection in transcatheter aortic valve replacement (TAVR). J Cardiovasc Comput Tomogr. 2016;10(1):37–43.

23. Blanke P, Willson AB, Webb JG, et al. Oversizing in transcatheter aortic valve replacement, a commonly used term but a poorly understood one: dependency on definition and geometrical measurements. J Cardiovasc Comput Tomogr. 2014;8(1):67–76.

24. Rajiah P, Schoenhagen P. The role of computed tomography in pre-procedural planning of cardiovascular surgery and intervention. Insights Imaging. 2013;4(5):671–89.

25. Loor G, Desai MY, Roselli EE. Pre-operative 3D CT imaging for virtual planning of minimally invasive aortic valve surgery. JACC Cardiovasc Imaging. 2013;6(2):269–71.

26. Feuchtner GM, Dichtl W, Schachner T, et al. Diagnostic performance of MDCT for detecting aortic valve regurgitation. AJR Am J Roentgenol. 2006;186(6):1676–81.

27. Feuchtner GM, Dichtl W, Muller S, et al. 64-MDCT for diagnosis of aortic regurgitation in patients referred to CT coronary angiography. AJR Am J Roentgenol. 2008;191(1):W1–7.

28. Alkadhi H, Desbiolles L, Husmann L, et al. Aortic regurgitation: assessment with 64-section CT. Radiology. 2007;245(1):111–21.

29. Hayashida K, Bouvier E, Lefevre T, et al. Transcatheter aortic valve implantation for patients with severe bicuspid aortic valve stenosis. Circ Cardiovasc Interv. 2013;6(3):284–91.

30. Alkadhi H, Leschka S, Trindade PT, et al. Cardiac CT for the differentiation of bicuspid and tricuspid aortic valves: comparison with echocardiography and surgery. AJR Am J Roentgenol. 2010;195(4):900–8.

31. Rubin JM, Avanzas P, del Valle R, et al. Atrioventricular conduction disturbance characterization in transcatheter aortic valve implantation with the Core valve prosthesis. Circ Cardiovasc Interv. 2011;4(3):280–6.

32. Popma JJ, Ramadan R. CT imaging of bicuspid aortic valve disease for TAVR. JACC Cardiovasc Imaging. 2016;9(10):1159–63. doi:10.1016/j.jcmg.2016.02.028.

33. Sievers HH, Schmidtke C. A classification system for the bicuspid aortic valve from 304 surgical specimens. J Thorac Cardiovasc Surg. 2007;133(5):1226–33.

34. Jilaihawi H, Chen M, Webb J, et al. A bicuspid aortic valve imaging classification for the TAVR era. JACC Cardiovasc Imaging. 2016;9(10):1145–58. doi:10.1016/j.jcmg.2015.12.022.

35. Durack DT, Lukes AS, Bright DK. New criteria for diagnosis of infective endocarditis: utilization of specific echocardiographic findings. Duke Endocarditis Service. Am J Med. 1994;96(3):200–9.

36. Mylonakis E, Calderwood SB. Infective endocarditis in adults. N Engl J Med. 2001;345(18):1318–30.

37. Feuchtner GM, Stolzmann P, Dichtl W, et al. Multislice computed tomography in infective endocarditis: comparison with transesophageal echocardiography and intraoperative findings. J Am Coll Cardiol. 2009;53(5):436–44.

38. Takeuchi N, Takada M, Fujita K, Nishibori Y, Maruyama T, Naba K. Aortic valve papillary fibroelastoma associated with acute cerebral infarction: a case report. Case Rep Cardiol. 2013;2013:485029.
39. Darvishian F, Farmer P. Papillary fibroelastoma of the heart: report of two cases and review of the literature. Ann Clin Lab Sci. 2001;31(3):291–6.
40. Sparrow PJ, Kurian JB, Jones TR, Sivananthan MU. MR imaging of cardiac tumors. Radiographics. 2005;25(5):1255–76.
41. Pham N, Zaitoun H, Mohammed TL, et al. Complications of aortic valve surgery: manifestations at CT and MR imaging. Radiographics. 2012;32(7):1873–92.
42. Han K, Yang DH, Shin SY, et al. Subprosthetic pannus after aortic valve replacement surgery: cardiac CT findings and clinical features. Radiology. 2015;276(3):724–31.
43. Chan J, Marwan M, Schepis T, Ropers D, Du L, Achenbach S. Images in cardiovascular medicine. Cardiac CT assessment of prosthetic aortic valve dysfunction secondary to acute thrombosis and response to thrombolysis. Circulation. 2009;120(19):1933–4.
44. Chenot F, Montant P, Goffinet C, et al. Evaluation of anatomic valve opening and leaflet morphology in aortic valve bioprosthesis by using multidetector CT: comparison with transthoracic echocardiography. Radiology. 2010;255(2):377–85.
45. Mahjoub H, Mathieu P, Larose E, et al. Determinants of aortic bioprosthetic valve calcification assessed by multidetector CT. Heart. 2015;101(6):472–7.
46. Tsai IC, Lin YK, Chang Y, et al. Correctness of multi-detector-row computed tomography for diagnosing mechanical prosthetic heart valve disorders using operative findings as a gold standard. Eur Radiol. 2009;19(4):857–67.
47. Leetmaa T, Hansson NC, Leipsic J, et al. Early aortic transcatheter heart valve thrombosis: diagnostic value of contrast-enhanced multidetector computed tomography. Circ Cardiovasc Interv. 2015;8(4):e001596.
48. Pache G, Schoechlin S, Blanke P, et al. Early hypo-attenuated leaflet thickening in balloon-expandable transcatheter aortic heart valves. Eur Heart J. 2016;37(28):2263–71.
49. Makkar RR, Fontana G, Jilaihawi H, et al. Possible subclinical leaflet thrombosis in bioprosthetic aortic valves. N Engl J Med. 2015;373(21):2015–24.

# Echocardiographic Imaging for Transcatheter Aortic Valve Replacement

# 17

Wanda Deste, Denise Todaro, and Gerlando Pilato

Echocardiography plays an important role in the percutaneous procedure of transcatheter aortic valve replacement (TAVR), starting with pre-implant screening, choosing the correct size of the valve device, in the case of complications during implantation, and in post-implant and follow-up assessment.

## 17.1 Pre-implant Screening and Evaluation

In patients with aortic stenosis (AS), transthoracic echocardiography (TTE) allows an overall assessment of morphology and valve function, as well as left ventricular functionality, in terms of the wall thickness, cavitary volumes, and overall contractility. In addition to conventional parameters to be assessed in AS patients set out by the guidelines of the American Society of Echocardiography (Table 17.1) [1, 2], in the case of patients undergoing TAVR, particular attention is to be paid to some additional parameters, which are peculiar to the procedure.

The aortic valve complex comprises the left ventricular outflow tract (LVOT), which is composed of the basal septum of the ventricle and the mitral-aortic junction, the aortic annulus, the aortic cusps, the sinuses of Valsalva, and the sinotubular junction (Fig. 17.1).

Correct sizing of the annulus, as well as a correct characterization of periannular region (cusps, LVOT, and proximal aortic ring), will allow the correct choice of the transcatheter heart valve (THV), and to anticipate and prevent possible complications, such as perivalvular regurgitation, occlusion of the coronary ostia, or rupture of the annulus [3–6].

W. Deste, M.D. (✉) • D. Todaro, M.D. • G. Pilato, M.D.
Division of Cardiology, Ferrarotto Hospital, University of Catania, Catania, Italy
e-mail: wandadeste@virgilio.it

© Springer International Publishing AG 2018
C. Tamburino et al. (eds.), *Percutaneous Treatment of Left Side Cardiac Valves*,
https://doi.org/10.1007/978-3-319-59620-4_17

**Table 17.1** Pre-procedural transthoracic assessment

| Pre-procedural echocardiographic imaging |
| --- |
| Aortic valve and root |
|   • Aortic valve morphology |
|   • Bicuspid versus tricuspid |
|   • Degree and location of calcium |
| Annular dimensions |
|   • Minimum and maximum diameters |
|   • Perimeter |
|   • Area |
| Aortic valve hemodynamics |
|   • Aortic valve gradients and area |
|   • Stroke volume |
|   • Impedance |
| Left ventricular outflow tract |
|   • Extent and distribution of calcium |
|   • Presence of sigmoid septum |
| Aortic root dimensions and calcification |
|   • Sinus of Valsalva diameter |
|   • Sinotubular junction diameter and calcification |
|   • Location of coronary ostia and risk of obstruction |
| Mitral valve |
|   • Severity of mitral regurgitation |
|   • Presence of mitral stenosis |
|   • Severity of ectopic calcification |
|   • Anterior leaflet calcification |
| Left ventricular size and function |
|   • Wall motion assessment/exclude intracardiac thrombus |
|   • Left ventricular mass/hypertrophy and septal morphology |
|   • Assessments of function: ejection fraction, strain and torsion, diastolic function |
| Right heart |
|   • Right ventricular size and function |
|   • Tricuspid valve morphology and function |
|   • Estimate of pulmonary artery pressures |

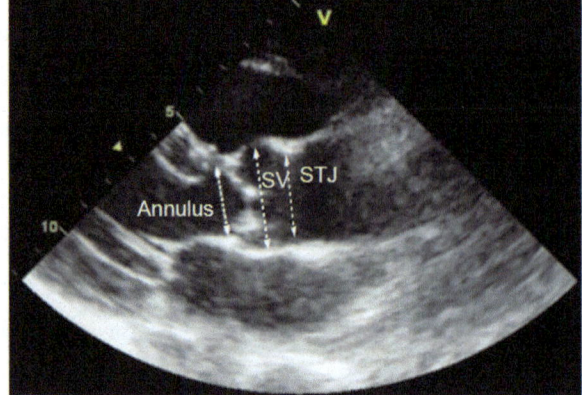

**Fig. 17.1** The aortic valve complex: aortic annulus; SV, sinuses of Valsalva; STJ, sinotubular junction (parasternal long-axis TTE view)

### 17.1.1 Aortic Annulus

The most important measure currently used for the choice of the prosthesis is the annulus, i.e., the virtual plane at the level of the hinge point, i.e., the lowest attachment site of the three aortic cusps [7].

The measurement of the diameter of this virtual ring is difficult because the annulus is often asymmetric and oval, with a larger annular diameter on the coronal plane and a smaller diameter on the sagittal plane [8–10]. In addition, in the case of the tricuspid valve, any plane passing through the bisector of a cusp at the level of the hinge point on one side does not project on the hinge point of the other side but in a region of fibrous tissue between the valve leaflets (Fig. 17.2).

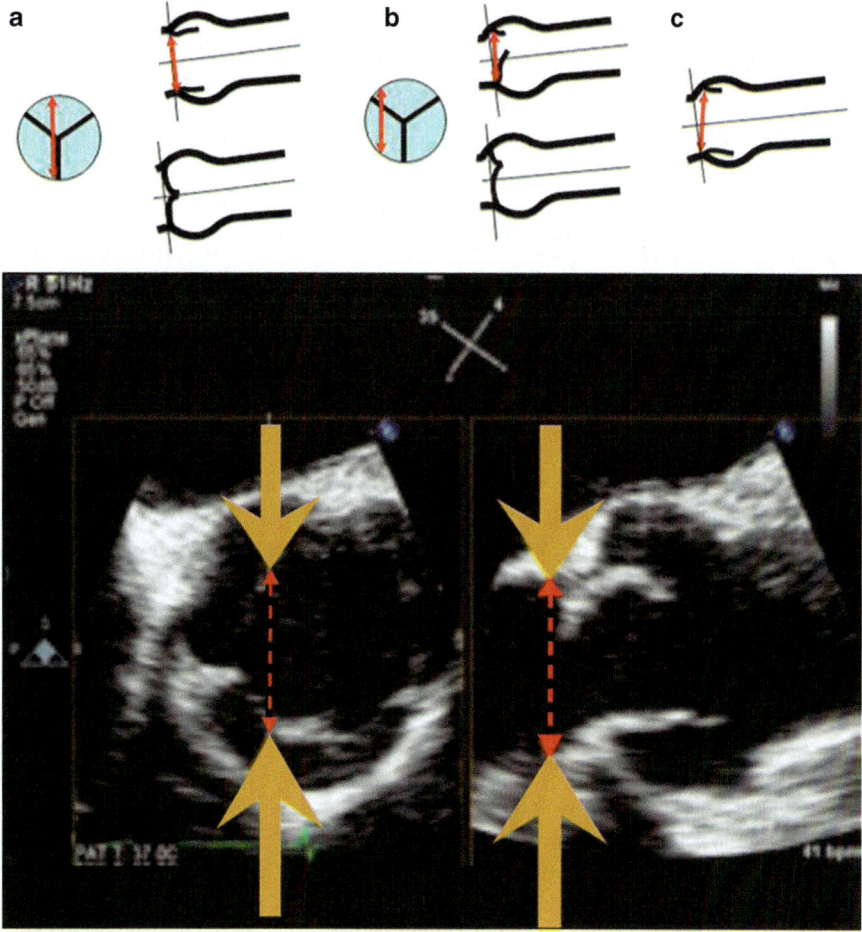

**Fig. 17.2** Measurement of the aortic annulus. (**a**) Correct: centrally positioned diameter and central closure of leaflets. (**b**) Incorrect: eccentric annular measurement. The hinge points are slightly displaced upward and do not correspond to the nadir of the cusp attachments, with incomplete opening and closing of leaflets. (**c**) Incorrect: oblique annular measurement. *Thin lines* correspond to the long axis of the ascending aorta and, orthogonally, correct orientation of the annular diameter. In the image below echo views of incorrect measurement

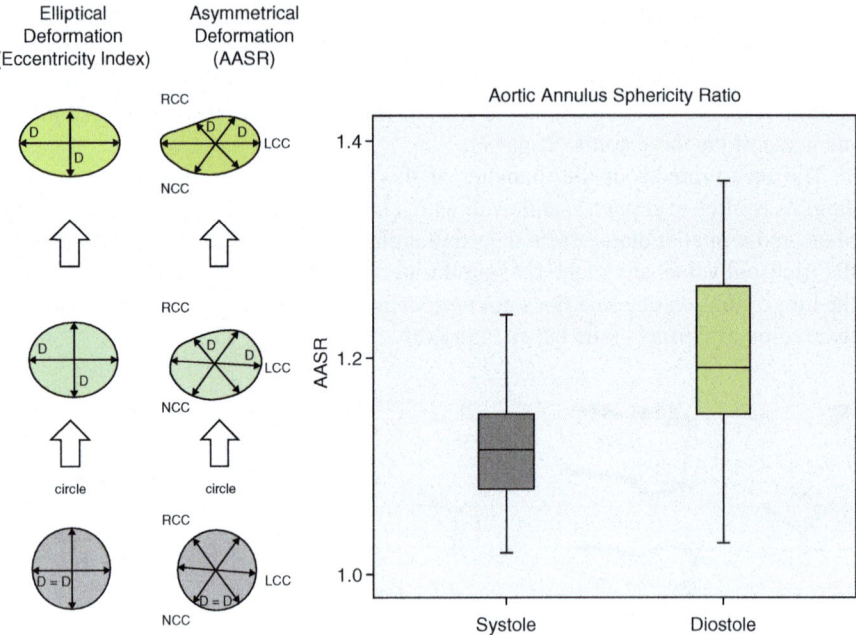

**Fig. 17.3** Deformation of the aortic annulus shape in systole and diastole. Note the difference of the eccentricity index (EI) and the aortic annulus sphericity ratio (AASR): an EI and AASR of 1.0 correspond to an ideal circle. An AASR higher than 1.0 indicates increasing asymmetrical deformation. In the image below are examples of asymmetrical deformation of the aortic annulus. Adapted by Lehmkuhl et al. Intern J Cardiovasc Imaging 2013

Conventionally, this diameter is measured in long axis (sagittal plane) during systole, and though it is no longer indicated for sizing, this measurement can be considered valid in most cases, provided that an appropriate algorithm for oversizing is used [6]. It is also important that this measurement is carried out in systole since at this stage the annulus is less elliptical, due to the dynamic nature of the shape of the annulus [11], thus making it possible to obtain greater measures compared with diastole (Fig. 17.3). The correct long-axis window should divide the maximum diameter of the aorta in two, and simultaneous use of 3D multislice technology will allow imaging of both the short axis and long axis, thus ensuring the imaging of the correct annular plane. In this condition, the hinge point of the right coronary cusp is displayed anteriorly and the fibrous trigone posteriorly. Since there are no anatomical markers for the virtual annular plane within the fibrous trigone, the correct annular diameter is calculated assuming that the virtual annulus is perpendicular to the long axis of the aorta, taking care not to mistake the calcifications of the attachment of the valve leaflets inside of the sinuses of Valsalva for the hinge point of the aortic cusp. This measurement certainly cannot be the only one used for sizing, but it can be used as an initial confirmation of the size of the prosthesis, as it represents the shorter diameter of the oval annulus. Moreover, it remains relevant to optimize the measurements of the LVOT used in the continuity equation.

For a more correct measurement of the aortic annulus, 3D transesophageal echocardiography (TEE) is useful (Fig. 17.4). As shown by numerous studies, it provides

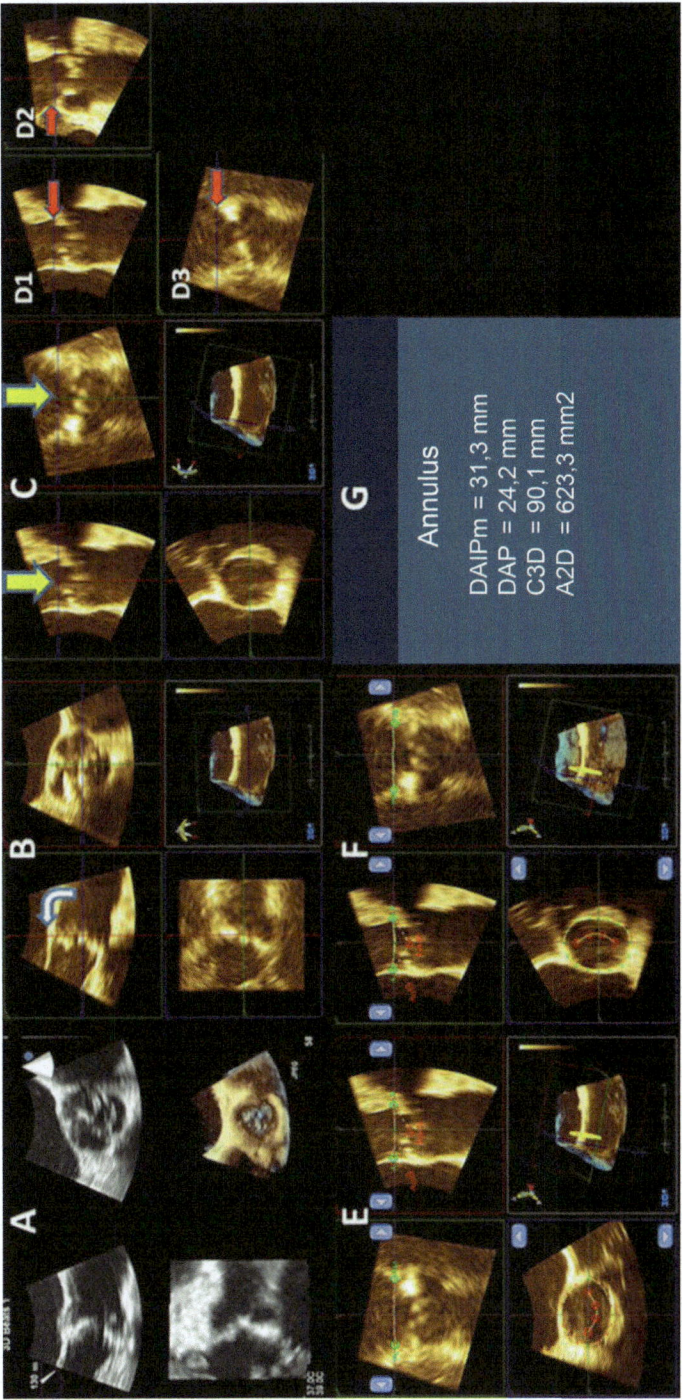

**Fig. 17.4** Determination of annulus size by 3D-TEE MVQ software. (**a**) Acquisition of 3D volume set from a long-axis 2D-TEE view. (**b**) Midsystole: identification of the transverse plane of the annulus by alignment of the two orthogonal long-axis views. (**c**) The location of the two orthogonal long-axis views (in the *green* and *red panels, yellow arrows*) can be seen in the transverse plane (*blue panel*) to confirm that this transverse plane is at the virtual annulus. To confirm this, (**D1–D3**) the hinge point of the cusps (*red arrows*) should be imaged in the orthogonal long-axis views during this rotation. (**e, f**) Four points, which define two orthogonal planes of the annulus, are placed along the maximum and minimum diameters of the annulus in the three orthogonal long-axis views. All points lie at the blood-tissue interface and at the annulus and can be adjusted manually if needed. (**g**) Once all points have been confirmed, perimeter, area, and maximum and minimum diameters are then automatically determined by the MVQ package. Adapted by Khalique et al. Circ Cardiovasc Imaging 2014

accurate and highly reproducible measurements that are comparable to those obtained by standard multislice computed tomography (MSCT) [12–19]. Altiok et al. [10] found a high correspondence between 3D TTE and MSCT for the coronal and sagittal diameters, the perimeter of the annulus, and area. The advantages of 3D technology include real-time imaging of the hinge points and elimination of errors due to manual tracing of the planes. Nevertheless, 3D TTE too is unable to overcome the physical limitations of ultrasounds, which create blooming and artifacts in the lateral lobe, as well as acoustic drops.

The measurement of the annulus by 3D TTE is possible in two modes: direct planimetry and indirect planimetry.

Direct planimetry employs commercial software that manipulates the 3D volume using a multislice approach. The transverse annular plane (short axis) is obtained using the orthogonal views to the long axis (sagittal and coronal) as a guide, thus allowing the direct measurement of the annulus (by manual tracing), and of the maximum and minimum diameters [20]. With this method, Jilaihawi et al. [18] found that 3D TEE significantly underestimates MSCT measurements of the aortic annulus, while still outperforming 2D TTE in predicting significant paravalvular regurgitation (PVR).

Indirect planimetry, instead, avoids the direct planimetry of the transverse plane, eliminating errors due to manual tracing. By means of specific software originally designed for the mitral valve [12], it employs the planes of the long axis and identifies the annulus by means of neighboring anatomical structures, such as the mitral flaps, the aortic root, and the septum. In this way, the artifacts due to the lateral lobes are identifiable on the axis and are not mistaken with the annulus. Acoustic shadows can be managed using the annular plane of the short axis as a reference, while being sure to take the annular points consistently with the neighboring points, and reflecting the shape of the virtual annulus. Validations of this method have been described in studies, which found no significant differences in the measurement of the area and perimeter compared with MSCT [19].

Echocardiography offers several advantages with respect to MSCT. The first and foremost is certainly the absence of the use of contrast agent, which allows it to be used also in patients with chronic kidney failure. In addition, the analysis of a large number of cardiac cycles, of which an average is calculated, allows use in patients with significant arrhythmias. In these cases, MSCT, which creates a composite image of multiple cardiac cycles, is limited by the generation of jump or movement artifacts. Echo 3D provides real-time imaging of the hinge points, eliminating errors due to manual tracing of the direct planimetry of the annulus by MSCT. Though echocardiographic imaging (both 2D and 3D) can be limited by blooming and lateral lobe artifacts, as well as by the acoustic drop, MSCT is also affected by artifacts generated from calcification of the annulus and valve. Finally, new software packages are being developed that are able to further automate acquisition and reduce operator-dependent variability in the measurement of the aortic annulus.

## 17.1.2 LVOT

The calculation of the aortic valve effective orifice area (EOA) with the continuity equation requires the measurement of the diameter of the LVOT at the same level of pulsed Doppler of the velocity-time integral (VTI), since both are combined to calculate the stroke volume.

In patients with aortic stenosis, the LVOT sample volume must be taken apically to the flow convergence region, and the LVOT systolic diameter must be measured at maximum 5 mm from the aortic annulus (between 1 and 2 mm of the annular plane), avoiding excessively apical measurements and, in particular, those at the level of the sigmoid septum (Fig. 17.5). In this way the systolic diameter of the LVOT should be 1 or 2 mm smaller than the annular diameter, and a difference of >2 mm should point to an error in the measurement of the LVOT or annulus. Moreover, the hypertrophy of the basal septum can be found in about 25% of patients with aortic stenosis and impairs the measurement of the LVOT. In these patients, the measurement of the LVOT should be carried out closer to the annulus to prevent the projection of the septum. Numerous studies have shown that the LVOT is often elliptical [21–23] if observed at the level of the long axis (sagittal), thus determining an underestimation of its actual area. In addition, comparative studies between standard 2D measurements (TTE or TEE) and the 3D planimetry of the LVOT area have shown that cardiac output [24] or EOA [25, 26] is underestimated by 10–23% using the 2D.

Despite these results, an EOA of <1 cm² calculated with the conventional method is associated with a higher mortality (risk ratio 1.78%, 95% confidence interval: 1.33-2.35, $p < 0.001$) even in the absence of symptoms (risk ratio 1.65;

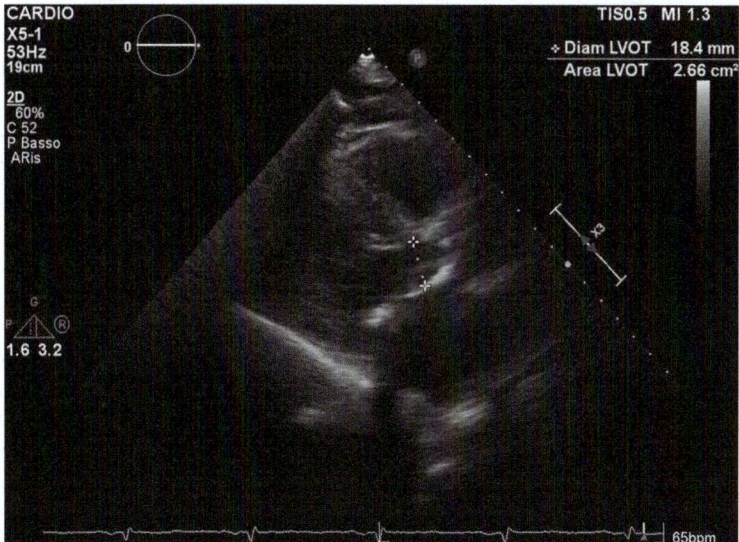

**Fig. 17.5** LVOT measurement (parasternal long-axis TTE view)

95% confidence interval: 1.05–2.47; $p = 0.02$) [27]. The 2014 guidelines of the American Heart Association/American College of Cardiology [28] continue to recommend the use of standard measurements for the assessment of the severity of AS [1].

In addition to the diameter of the LVOT, in the pre-TAVR evaluation, a key role is played by the qualitative characteristics of the LVOT and by the geometry of the septum. Marked septal hypertrophy could indeed make it difficult to position and implant the THV because of the sharp angle of the LVOT and the difficulty of maintaining a coaxial alignment of the guide and the delivery system. This may be particularly evident during the transapical approach, in which the position of the apical cannula is fixed. A hypertrophic and hyperdynamic septum could also result in an upward displacement of the prosthesis during implantation. In contrast, a particularly thin membranous septum with dystrophic calcifications may involve other complications, such as an interventricular defect [29]. Calcium at the level of the LVOT is also an important predictor of paravalvular leaks [30, 33] and rupture of the annulus.

### 17.1.3 Aortic Valve

Valve anatomy, the severity and localization of calcifications, and the symmetrical opening of the valve must be carefully assessed.

The extent and distribution of calcification is correlated with an excessive movement of the THV during implantation [32] and with paravalvular regurgitation [31, 33–35]. It also increases the risk of embolization of calcified nodules in the coronary ostia, ruptures of the annulus, perforations of the root, periaortic hematomas, and aortic dissection [3, 36, 37].

The valvular opening must be evaluated to identify any asymmetries that would make the alignment of the THV difficult during the release and onset of PVR. One extreme example of asymmetry in valve opening is a bicuspid aortic valve. Despite two TAVR reports in a series of patients with bicuspid aortic valve have shown results comparable with patients with tricuspid aortic valve in terms of acute procedural success, valve hemodynamics, and short-term survival [29, 38], many case reports of THV implanted in patients with congenital abnormalities of the aortic valve have limited their use in this population since significant residual aortic regurgitation or suboptimal flow characteristics have been reported [39–41].

The most recent retrospective multicenter analysis of 139 patients has shown a mortality rate of 3.9%, with a rate of embolization of the prosthesis and conversion in cardiac surgery in 2.2%. In this case, procedural mortality is higher than that reported in TAVR in tricuspid valves with balloon-expandable prostheses (0.9%), although the embolization rate of the prosthesis and the rate of conversion to an open surgical procedure are comparable [42]. A greater incidence of periprosthetic regurgitation has also been reported in bicuspid valves ≥2: 28.4% in total, 17.4% when sizing was done by MSCT. There are no differences in terms of PVR between the self-expanding valve and balloon-expandable valve ($p = 0.99$).

Applying the classification of Sievers et al. [43] for the bicuspid aortic valve, an increased rate of post-implant residual aortic regurgitation can also be noted in patients with bicuspid aortic valve type 1 (with single raphe) compared to those with type 0 (no raphe) (34.2% vs. 13.3%, respectively, $p = 0.03$) [44]. This may be related to the thick calcification often along the raphe that hinders adequate stent implantation at the level of the LVOT.

### 17.1.4 Aortic Root

Safe and successful implantation of the THV finally requires an overall assessment of the "neighboring zone": the diastolic diameter of the sinuses of Valsalva and their height, the diastolic diameter of the sinotubular junction, and the height of the coronary ostia can affect the choice of the THV size and the decisions concerning valve implantation.

The localization of the coronary ostia is of primary importance since their occlusion can determine a catastrophic ventricular dysfunction. In particular, the complications related to the occlusion of the ostium of the right coronary artery are significantly less frequent than those of the occlusion of the left coronary artery. A meta-analysis of 18 studies showed that coronary obstruction is the result of the displacement of the calcified left coronary cusp and not of the THV stent and that the factors typically associated with the obstruction of the coronary ostia include female gender, small aortic root diameter (mean diameter 27.8 ± 2.8 mm), and height of the left coronary ostium (mean height 10.3 ± 1.6 mm) [5].

Though MSCT is often employed for these measurements [45, 46], 3D TTE allows the rapid acquisition of the coronary plane for the measurement of the distance between the annulus and the ostium of the left coronary artery, as well as of the length of the coronary cusp during the procedure. The comparison of the measurements of the implantation height of the left coronary artery obtained by 3D TTE and MSCT has shown a great degree of concordance (13.47 ± 1.67 mm vs. 13.64 ± 1.82 mm) with a better correlation than between angiography and MSCT [10]. In addition, real-time imaging of the ostium of the left coronary artery during valvuloplasty or during TAVR can help to predict and prevent coronary obstruction.

## 17.2 Follow-Up

Together with clinical medicine, TTE plays a leading role in post-TAVI medium- and long-term follow-up, allowing the assessment of the outcome of the procedure, with early detection of restenosis or residual regurgitation.

The evaluation of stenosis of the prosthetic valve is a process composed of various assessment parameters and is the result of their integration. The conventional parameters used to determine aortic stenosis of prosthetic valves are those published in guidelines, which take into account flow-dependent and flow-independent parameters [47] (Table 17.2).

**Table 17.2** Doppler echocardiographic evaluation of prosthetic aortic valves

| Parameter | Normal | Possible stenosis | Suggest significant stenosis |
|---|---|---|---|
| Peak velocity (m/s) | <3 | 3–4 | >4 |
| Mean gradient (mmHg) | >20 | | >35 |
| Contour of the jet velocity | Triangular, early peaking | Triangular to intermediate | Rounded, symmetrical contour |
| DVI | ≥0.30 | | <0.25 |
| EOA (cm²) | >1.2 | 1.2–0.8 | <0.8 |
| AT (ms) | <80 | 80–100 | >100 |

*DVI* Doppler velocity index, *EOA* effective orifice area, *AT* acceleration time

The limit of flow-dependent parameters, such as the peak velocity and mean gradient, is inherent in the variability of this measurement in relation to the preload at that given moment. The flow-independent parameters, i.e., the EOA and the Doppler velocity index (DVI), have limits: the EOA does not take into account the cardiac output in relation to the body surface of the patient (there are several cutoffs of stenosis severity for patients with BSA > 1.6 m$^2$ and those with BSA < 1.6 m$^2$), and DVI is dependent on the size of the LVOT, which, as seen above, may be subject to measurement errors. In particular, the measurement of LVOT velocity must be measured at the level of the apical margin of the prosthesis. In the case of a stent protruding from the LVOT into ventricle, it must be measured at the level of the proximal portion of the stent [48].

According to the Valve Academic Research Consortium (VARC)-2 criteria, it is necessary to consider initially a flow-dependent parameter (mean gradient) and a flow-independent parameter (EOA). If these parameters are discordant, the calculation of the DVI is advised. If it is abnormal, one can assume that there is valve dysfunction; if it is normal, possible LVOT calculation errors or a mismatch should be taken into consideration. Furthermore, it is not recommended to use acceleration time, a parameter that depends on ventricular function and heart rate [49].

The evaluation of post-TAVI aortic regurgitation is extremely important, and several studies have confirmed the association between moderate and/or severe aortic regurgitation and mortality [50]. Moreover, aortic regurgitation is one of the VARC-2 criteria to determine prosthetic dysfunction (Fig. 17.6).

The conventional evaluation parameters mentioned in the guidelines include both quantitative and semiquantitative criteria (Table 17.3). Though all echocardiographic projections are useful for an overview of aortic regurgitation, the short-axis parasternal view is instrumental in locating the leak and distinguishing intraprosthetic from periprosthetic aortic regurgitation [51].

One of the semiquantitative methods employed to quantity regurgitation is based on the percentage of color of the jet that covers the circumference between the stent of the prosthesis and the native valve. A value of less than 10% indicates mild regurgitation; a value between 10 and 20% moderate regurgitation; and a value of over 20% severe regurgitation. The vena contracta, which is an estimate of the effective regurgitant orifice area, is not one of the evaluation parameters for post-TAVI regurgitation because it often features multiple and eccentric jets.

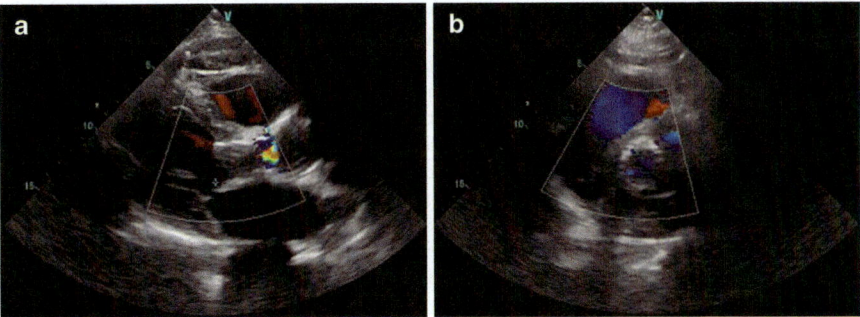

**Fig. 17.6** Mild PVL after TAVR. (**a**) Parasternal long-axis TTE view. (**b**) Parasternal short-axis TTE view

**Table 17.3** Prostetic aortic valve regurgitation

|  | Mild | Moderate | Severe |
| --- | --- | --- | --- |
| Semi-quantitative parameters |  |  |  |
| Diastolic flow reversal in the descending aorta | Absent or brief early diastolic | Intermediate | Prominent, holodiastolic |
| Circumferential exent of PVL (%) | <10 | 10–29 | 30 |
| Quantitative parameters |  |  |  |
| Regurgitant volume (mL) | <30 | 30–59 | 60 |
| Regurgitant fraction (%) | <30 | 30–49 | 50 |
| EROA (cm$^2$) | 0.10 | 0.10–0.29 | 0.30 |

*PVL* paravalvular leak, *EROA* effective regurgitant orifice area

# References

1. Baumgartner H, Hung J, Bermejo J, et al. Echocardiographic assessment of valve stenosis: EAE/ASE recommendations for clinical practice. J Am Soc Echocardiogr. 2009;22:1–23, quiz 101–2.
2. Zoghbi WA, Enriquez-Sarano M, Foster E, et al. Recommendations for evaluation of the severity of native valvular regurgitation with two-dimensional and Doppler echocardiography. J Am Soc Echocardiogr. 2003;16:777–802.
3. Barbanti M, Yang TH, Rodès Cabau J, et al. Anatomical and procedural features associated with aortic root rupture during balloon-expandable transcatheter aortic valve replacement. Circulation. 2013;128:244–53.
4. Athappan G, Patvardhan E, Tuzcu EM, et al. Incidence, predictors, and outcomes of aortic regurgitation after transcatheter aortic valve replacement: meta-analysis and systematic review of literature. J Am Coll Cardiol. 2013;61:1585–95.
5. Barbanti M, Webb JG, Gilard M, Capodanno D, Tamburino C. Transcatheter aortic valve implantation in 2017: state of the art. EuroIntervention. 2017;13:AA11–21.
6. Detaint D, Lepage L, Himbert D, et al. Determinants of significant paravalvular regurgitation after transcatheter aortic valve: implantation impact of device and annulus discongruence. J Am Coll Cardiol Intv. 2009;2:821–7.
7. Piazza N, de Jaegere P, Schultz C, Becker AE, Serruys PW, Anderson RH. Anatomy of the aortic valvar complex and its implications for trans-catheter implantation of the aortic valve. Circ Cardiovasc Interv. 2008;1:74–81.

8. Tzikas A, Schultz CJ, Piazza N, et al. Assessment of the aortic annulus by multislice computed tomography, contrast aortography, and trans-thoracic echocardiography in patients referred for transcatheter aortic valve implantation. Catheter Cardiovasc Interv. 2011;77:868–75.

9. Koos R, Altiok E, Mahnken AH, et al. Evaluation of aortic root for definition of prosthesis size by magnetic resonance imaging and cardiac computed tomography: implications for transcatheter aortic valve implantation. Int J Cardiol. 2012;158:353–8.

10. Altiok E, Koos R, Schroder J, et al. Comparison of two-dimensional and three-dimensional imaging techniques for measurement of aortic annulus diameters before transcatheter aortic valve implantation. Heart. 2011;97:1578–84.

11. Hamdan A, Guetta V, Konen E, et al. Deformation dynamics and mechanical properties of the aortic annulus by four-dimensional computed tomography insights into the functional anatomy of the aortic valve complex and implications for transcatheter aortic valve therapy. J Am Coll Cardiol. 2012;59:119–27.

12. Hahn RT, Khalique O, Williams MR, et al. Predicting paravalvular regurgitation following transcatheter valve replacement: utility of a novel method for three-dimensional echocardiographic measurements of the aortic annulus. J Am Soc Echocardiogr. 2013;26:1043–52.

13. Santos N, de Agustin JA, Almeria C, et al. Prosthesis/annulus discongruence assessed by three-dimensional transesophageal echocardiography: a predictor of significant paravalvular aortic regurgitation after transcatheter aortic valve implantation. Eur Heart J Cardiovasc Imaging. 2012;13:931–7.

14. Janosi RA, Kahlert P, Plicht B, et al. Measurement of the aortic annulus size by real-time three-dimensional transesophageal echocardiography. Minim Invasive Ther Allied Technol. 2011;20:85–94.

15. Tsang W, Bateman MG, Weinert L, et al. Accuracy of aortic annular measurements obtained from three-dimensional echocardiography, CT and MRI: human in vitro and in vivo studies. Heart. 2012;98:1146–52.

16. Gripari P, Ewe SH, Fusini L, et al. Intra-operative 2D and 3D transesophageal echocardiographic predictors of aortic regurgitation after transcatheter aortic valve implantation. Heart. 2012;98:1229–36.

17. Smith LA, Dworakowski R, Bhan A, et al. Real-time three-dimensional transesophageal echocardiography adds value to transcatheter aortic valve implantation. J Am Soc Echocardiogr. 2013;26:359–69.

18. Jilaihawi H, Doctor N, Kashif M, et al. Aortic annular sizing for transcatheter aortic valve replacement using cross-sectional 3-dimensional transesophageal echocardiography. J Am Coll Cardiol. 2013;61:908–16.

19. Khalique OK, Kodali SK, Paradis JM, et al. Aortic annular sizing using a novel three-dimensional echocardiographic method: use and comparison with cardiac computed tomography. Circ Cardiovasc Imaging. 2014;7:155–63.

20. Kasel AM, Cassese S, Bleiziffer S, et al. Standardized imaging for aortic annular sizing: implications for transcatheter valve selection. J Am Coll Cardiol Img. 2013;6:249–62.

21. Burgstahler C, Kunze M, Loffler C, Gawaz MP, Hombach V, Merkle N. Assessment of left ventricular outflow tract geometry in non-stenotic and stenotic aortic valves by cardiovascular magnetic resonance. J Cardiovasc Magn Reson. 2006;8:825–9.

22. Doddamani S, Bello R, Friedman MA, et al. Demonstration of left ventricular outflow tract eccentricity by real time 3D echocardiography: implications for the determination of aortic valve area. Echocardiography. 2007;24:860–6.

23. De Vecchi C, Caudron J, Dubourg B, et al. Effect of the ellipsoid shape of the left ventricular outflow tract on the echocardiographic assessment of aortic valve area in aortic stenosis. J Cardiovasc Comput Tomogr. 2014;8:52–7.

24. Montealegre-Gallegos M, Owais K, Hess P, Jainandunsing JS, Matyal R. Cardiac output calculation and three-dimensional echocardiography. J Cardiothorac Vasc Anesth. 2014;28:547–50.

25. Saitoh T, Shiota M, Izumo M, et al. Comparison of left ventricular outflow geometry and aortic valve area in patients with aortic stenosis by two-dimensional versus three-dimensional echocardiography. Am J Cardiol. 2012;109:1626–31.

26. Gaspar T, Adawi S, Sachner R, et al. Three-dimensional imaging of the left ventricular outflow tract: impact on aortic valve area estimation by the continuity equation. J Am Soc Echocardiogr. 2012;25:749–57.
27. Malouf J, Le Tourneau T, Pellikka P, et al. Aortic valve stenosis in community medical practice: determinants of outcome and implications for aortic valve replacement. J Thorac Cardiovasc Surg. 2012;144:1421–7.
28. Nishimura RA, Otto C. 2014 ACC/AHA valve guidelines: earlier intervention for chronic mitral regurgitation. Heart. 2014;100:905–7.
29. Masson JB, Kovac J, Schuler G, et al. Trans-catheter aortic valve implantation: review of the nature, management, and avoidance of procedural complications. J Am Coll Cardiol Intv. 2009;2:811–20.
30. Ewe SH, Ng AC, Schuijf JD, et al. Location and severity of aortic valve calcium and implications for aortic regurgitation after transcatheter aortic valve implantation. Am J Cardiol. 2011;108:1470–7.
31. Khalique OK, Hahn RT, Gada H, et al. Quantity and location of aortic valve complex calcification predicts severity and location of paravalvular regurgitation and frequency of post-dilation after balloon-expandable transcatheter aortic valve replacement. J Am Coll Cardiol Intv. 2014;7:885–94.
32. Dvir D, Lavi I, Eltchaninoff H, et al. Multicenter evaluation of Edwards SAPIEN positioning during transcatheter aortic valve implantation with correlates for device movement during final deployment. J Am Coll Cardiol Intv. 2012;5:563–70.
33. Haensig M, Lehmkuhl L, Rastan AJ, et al. Aortic valve calcium scoring is a predictor of significant paravalvular aortic insufficiency in transapical aortic valve implantation. Eur J Cardiothorac Surg. 2012;41:1234–40; discussion 1240–1.
34. Feuchtner G, Plank F, Bartel T, et al. Prediction of paravalvular regurgitation after transcatheter aortic valve implantation by computed tomography: value of aortic valve and annular calcification. Ann Thorac Surg. 2013;96:1574–80.
35. Colli A, D'Amico R, Kempfert J, Borger MA, Mohr FW, Walther T. Transesophageal echocardiographic scoring for transcatheter aortic valve implantation: impact of aortic cusp calcification on postoperative aortic regurgitation. J Thorac Cardiovasc Surg. 2011;142:1229–35.
36. Genereux P, Reiss GR, Kodali SK, Williams MR, Hahn RT. Periaortic hematoma after transcatheter aortic valve replacement: description of a new complication. Catheter Cardiovasc Interv. 2012;79:766–76.
37. Leber AW, Kasel M, Ischinger T, et al. Aortic valve calcium score as a predictor for outcome after TAVI using the CoreValve revalving system. Int J Cardiol. 2013;166:652–7.
38. Kochman J, Huczek Z, Scislo P, et al. Comparison of 1- and 12-month outcomes of transcatheter aortic valve replacement in patients with severely stenotic bicuspid versus tricuspid aortic valves (results from a multicenter registry). Am J Cardiol. 2014;114:757–62.
39. Wijesinghe N, Ye J, Rodés-Cabau J, et al. Transcatheter aortic valve implantation in patients with bicuspid aortic valve stenosis. J Am Coll Cardiol Intv. 2010;3:1122–5.
40. Ferrari E, Locca D, Sulzer C, et al. Successful transapical aortic valve implantation in a congenital bicuspid aortic valve. Ann Thorac Surg. 2010;90:630–2.
41. Chiam PT, Chao VT, Tan SY, et al. Percutaneous transcatheter heart valve implantation in a bicuspid aortic valve. J Am Coll Cardiol Intv. 2010;3:559–61.
42. Smith CR, Leon MB, Mack MJ, et al. Transcatheter versus surgical aortic-valve replacement in high-risk patients. N Engl J Med. 2011;364:2187–98.
43. Sievers HH, Schmidtke C. A classification system for the bicuspid aortic valve from 304 surgical specimens. J Thorac Cardiovasc Surg. 2007;133:1226–33.
44. Mylotte D, Lefevre T, Sondergaard L, et al. Transcatheter aortic valve replacement in bicuspid aortic valve disease. J Am Coll Cardiol. 2014;64:2330–9.
45. Barbanti M, Leipsic J, Binder R, et al. Underexpansion and ad hoc post-dilation in selected patients undergoing balloon-expandable transcatheter aortic valve replacement. J Am Coll Cardiol. 2014;63:976–81.
46. Leipsic J, Gurvitch R, Labounty TM, et al. Multidetector computed tomography in transcatheter aortic valve implantation. J Am Coll Cardiol Img. 2011;4:416–29.

47. Zoghbi WA, Chambers JB, Dumesnil JG, et al. Recommendations for evaluation of prosthetic valves with echocardiography and Doppler ultrasound: a report from the American Society of Echocardiography's guidelines and Standards Committee and the Task Force on Prosthetic Valves, developed in conjunction with the American College of Cardiology Cardiovascular Imaging Committee, Cardiac Imaging Committee of the American Heart Association, the European Association of Echocardiography, a Registered Branch of the European Society of Cardiology, The Japanese Society of Echocardiography and the Canadian Society of Echocardiography, endorsed by the American College of Cardiology Foundation, American Heart Association, European Association of Echocardiography, a registered branch of the European Society of Cardiology, The Japanese Society of Echocardiography, and Canadian Society of Echocardiography. J Am Soc Echocardiogr. 2009;22:975–1014; 1082–4.
48. Clavel MA, Webb JG, Pibarot P, et al. Comparison of the hemodynamic performance of percutaneous and surgical bioprostheses for the treatment of severe aortic stenosis. J Am Coll Cardiol. 2009;53:1883–91.
49. Ben Zekry S, Saad RM, Ozkan M, et al. Flow acceleration time and ratio of acceleration time to ejection time for prosthetic aortic valve function. JACC Cardiovasc Imaging. 2011;4:1161–70.
50. Kodali SK, Williams MR, Smith CR, et al. Two-year outcomes after transcatheter or surgical aortic-valve replacement. N Engl J Med. 2012;366:1686–95.
51. Zamorano JL, Badano LP, Bruce C, et al. EAE/ASE recommendations for the use of echocardiography in new transcatheter interventions for valvular heart disease. J Am Soc Echocardiogr. 2011;24:937–65.

# Vascular Access Management in Transcatheter Aortic Valve Implantation

# 18

Marco Barbanti, Gerlando Pilato, and Carmelo Sgroi

Though transcatheter aortic valve implantation (TAVI) has given ample proof of being a safe procedure, it is not devoid of complications. Peripheral vascular complications and bleeding at the access site are still among the problems most frequently associated with transfemoral TAVI. The transfemoral route is the access of first choice, and the improvement of TAVI devices has made it possible to reduce the size of introducers and delivery systems from the initial 22–24 Fr of the early devices to 18 Fr, first, and now to the 14–16 Fr of many new-generation devices. This has made it possible to broaden the range of indications treated with the transfemoral approach to serve a larger number of patients.

Vascular access management involves a comprehensive approach that includes the assessment of vascular anatomy through different imaging tools (angiography, computed tomographic angiography, magnetic resonance imaging, and ultrasound) and knowledge of materials and techniques designed to reduce the risk of vascular complications to a minimum (Tables 18.1 and 18.2).

## 18.1 Screening

### 18.1.1 Anatomy of the Iliofemoral Axis

The abdominal aorta bifurcates into the right and left common iliac artery, which in turn bifurcates into the external and internal iliac arteries. Once it crosses the inguinal ligament, the external iliac artery takes the name of common femoral artery.

M. Barbanti (✉) • G. Pilato • C. Sgroi
Ferrarotto Hospital, University of Catania, Catania, Italy
e-mail: mbarbanti83@gmail.com

© Springer International Publishing AG 2018
C. Tamburino et al. (eds.), *Percutaneous Treatment of Left Side Cardiac Valves*,
https://doi.org/10.1007/978-3-319-59620-4_18

**Table 18.1** Valve Academic Research Consortium (VARC)-2 classification of vascular access site and access-related complications

*Major vascular complications*

Any aortic dissection, aortic rupture, annulus rupture, left ventricle perforation, or new apical aneurysm/pseudoaneurysm OR

Access site or access-related vascular injury (dissection, stenosis, perforation, rupture, arteriovenous fistula, pseudoaneurysm, hematoma, irreversible nerve injury, compartment syndrome, percutaneous closure device failure) leading to death, life-threatening or major bleeding, visceral ischemia, or neurological impairment OR

Distal embolization (non-cerebral) from a vascular source requiring surgery or resulting in amputation or irreversible end-organ damage OR

The use of unplanned endovascular or surgical intervention associated with death, major bleeding, visceral ischemia, or neurological impairment OR

Any new ipsilateral lower extremity ischemia documented by patient symptoms, physical exam, and/or decreased or absent blood flow on lower extremity angiogram OR

Surgery for access site-related nerve injury OR

Permanent access site-related nerve injury

*Minor vascular complications*

Access site or access-related vascular injury (dissection, stenosis, perforation, rupture, arteriovenous fistula, pseudoaneurysms, hematomas, percutaneous closure device failure) not leading to death, life-threatening or major bleeding, visceral ischemia, or neurological impairment OR

Distal embolization treated with embolectomy and/or thrombectomy and not resulting in amputation or irreversible end-organ damage OR

Any unplanned endovascular stenting or unplanned surgical intervention not meeting the criteria for a major vascular complication OR

Vascular repair or the need for vascular repair (via surgery, ultrasound-guided compression, transcatheter embolization, or stent graft)

Percutaneous closure device failure

Failure of a closure device to achieve hemostasis at the arteriotomy site, leading to alternative treatment (other than manual compression or adjunctive endovascular ballooning)

The common femoral artery bifurcates again into the superficial and deep femoral artery (Figs. 18.1 and 18.2).

## 18.1.2 Pre-TAVI Assessment of the Femoral-Iliac Axis

In the overall assessment of the iliofemoral axes of a transfemoral TAVI candidate, three main factors need to be considered:

– Lumen diameter
– Wall plaques
– Vessel tortuosity

Ideally, the minimum lumen diameter should be greater than the diameter of the introducer that will be used. This will be measured at the puncture site (common femoral artery), at the external iliac artery, and at the common iliac artery

**Table 18.2** Comparison between transfemoral and transapical aortic valve implantation

| | Transfemoral (TF) | Transapical (TA) |
|---|---|---|
| Access | Femoral artery | Left ventricular apex |
| Access mode | Retrograde | Antegrade |
| Incision length [cm] | 1–2 | ~5 |
| Distance to aortic valve [cm] | ~70–100 | ~7–10 |
| Wire insertion | Through the aortic arch, retrograde | Through the aortic arch, antegrade |
| Wire positioning | Arbitrary, across iliac vessels and aortic arch, irregularities, slack | Coaxial, straight |
| Valve insertion | Through the aortic arch, retrograde | Does not touch aorta |
| Valve orientation | Arbitrary | Commissural (anatomical) alignment possible |
| Valve implantation | Some mobility during implantation | Little mobility, stepwise and controlled implantation usually feasible |
| Application system retrieval | Across the aortic arch, relatively long distance | Direct and straight |
| Access closure | Complication rates as high as 10% | Very low complication rate, ~1% |
| Perspectives | Smaller systems will become available | Allows access to almost any diameter of the devices—this may lead to potentially better tissue longevity |
| Future developments | Improved vascular closure systems | Percutaneous access and closure systems |

(Fig. 18.3). The presence of vascular sections with a diameter smaller than the outer diameter of the introducer is a contraindication to the procedure via the transfemoral route. In fact, a sheath/femoral artery ratio of 1.05 or higher has proven to predict both vascular complications and 30-day mortality. However, in the case of short stenotic segments without calcification, balloon angioplasty before inserting the introducer is a valid and safe alternative (Fig. 18.4). It should be noted however that in the absence of severe calcification, bulky atheromatous burden, or severe tortuosity, short segments of relatively compliant artery can be up to 1 mm smaller in diameter than the intended sheath, allowing it to be safely cannulated.

During the screening phase, the assessment of the degree of calcification and vessel tortuosity requires a great deal of attention by operators. An important feature of calcification is its distribution around the perimeter of the artery; calcification of the vessel is commonly defined as concentric if it spans beyond 270° around the circumference of the artery. This is the most adverse condition in the transfemoral approach, especially when vessel diameter is borderline. In these cases, the artery is not distensible, and it can be difficult or, at times, even impossible to advance the introducer. Another aspect to be considered is when a plaque is present at the puncture site. On the one hand, the presence of calcification on the anterior wall of the

**Fig. 18.1** 3D CT reconstruction of the iliofemoral axis. *CIA* common iliac artery, *IIA* internal iliac artery, *EIA* external iliac artery, *CFA* common femoral artery, *SFA* superficial femoral artery, *DFA* deep femoral artery

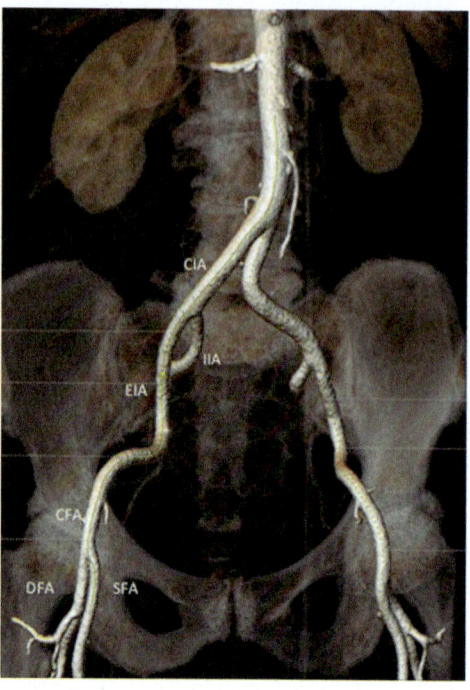

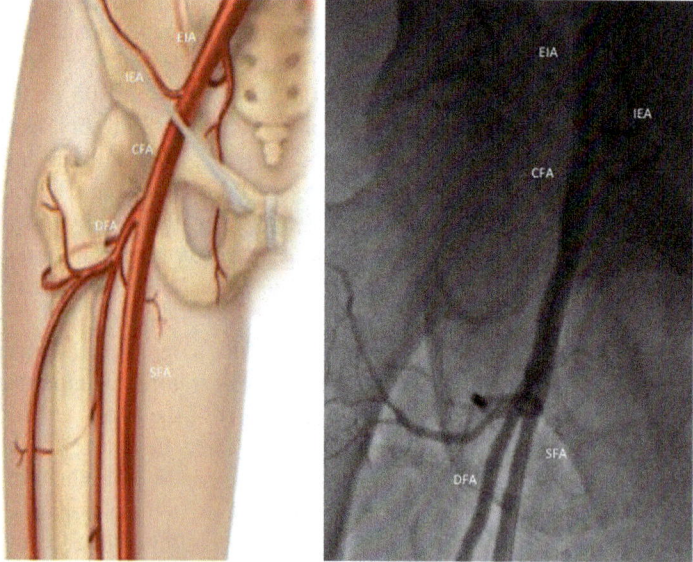

**Fig. 18.2** Illustration of the iliofemoral axis (*left*). Angiographic view of the iliofemoral axis (*right*): *EIA* external iliac artery, *CFA* common femoral artery, *SFA* superficial femoral artery, *DFA* deep femoral artery

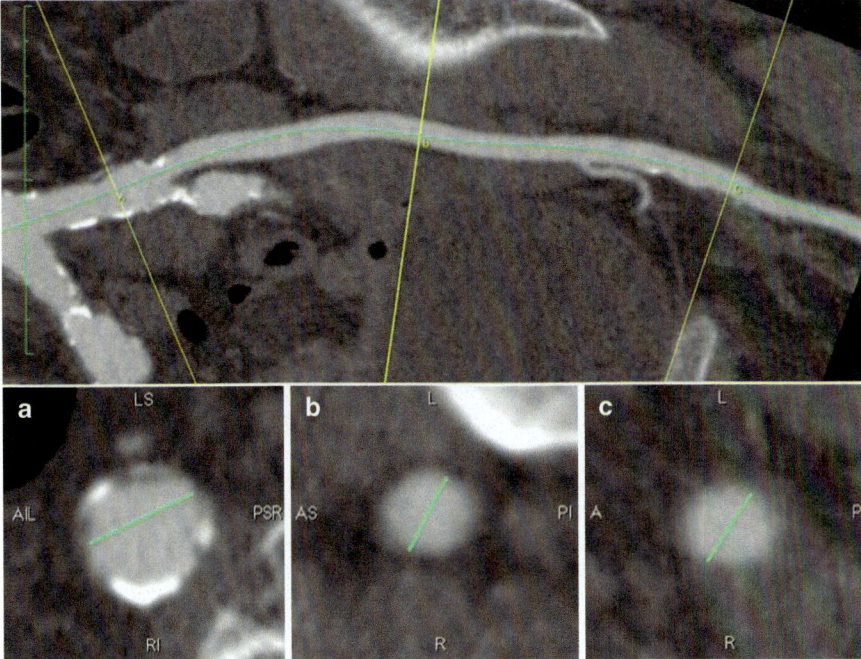

**Fig. 18.3** CT reconstruction of the right iliofemoral artery with curved multiplanar reformats. Measurement (*green line*) of the common iliac artery (**a**) of the external iliac artery (**b**) and common femoral artery (**c**)

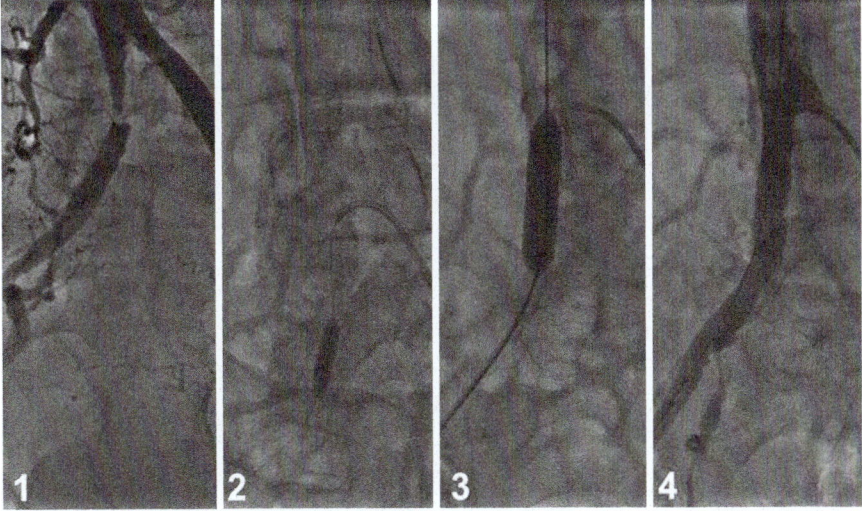

**Fig. 18.4** Treatment of severe right common iliac stenosis in a patient indicated for transfemoral TAVR. After pre-dilatation with a 5.0 mm balloon catheter, a 9.0 × 25-mm balloon-expandable Express stent (Boston Scientific, Natick, MA) was deployed with good final result. Eight days later patients underwent transfemoral TAVR uneventfully

common femoral artery (Fig. 18.5) could compromise the effectiveness of the percutaneous closure systems (Prostar or ProGlide), and it may be necessary to surgically isolate the femoral artery. On the other, the presence of plaques located solely on the posterior wall generally has a marginal impact on the effectiveness of the closure systems (Fig. 18.6).

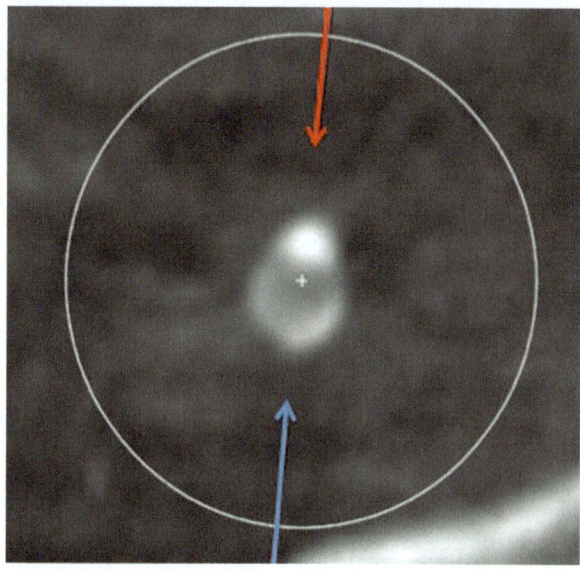

**Fig. 18.5** CT image of the common femoral artery with calcification of the anterior wall (*red arrow*). The posterior section shows mild calcification (*blue arrow*)

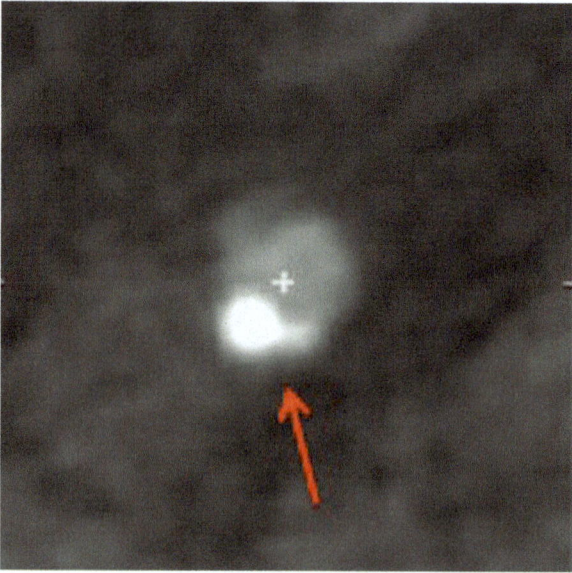

**Fig. 18.6** CT image of the common femoral artery with calcification of the posterior wall (*red arrow*)

Vessel tortuosity is not generally a concern when it is not associated with wall calcification, since simply introducing a guidewire is enough to straighten the vessel. When, instead, major wall calcifications are present, the iliofemoral axis is stiffer and the insertion of the introducer may be unsafe.

There are various classifications of the degree of calcification and tortuosity of the iliofemoral axis. Those most frequently adopted are the following: calcifications are broadly defined as 0, no calcifications; 1, mild calcifications; 2, moderate calcifications; and 3, severe calcifications (Fig. 18.7).

Tortuosity is defined as follows: 0, no tortuosity; 1, mild tortuosity (angles from 30 to 60°); 2, moderate tortuosity (angles from 61 to 90°); and 3, severe tortuosity (angles >90°) (Figs. 18.8 and 18.9).

## 18.1.3 Angiography

Pre-procedure screening of patients often starts with conventional angiography. Angiography provides a basic assessment of luminal size but offers a very limited evaluation of the presence of atherosclerosis and plaque burden, as well as of the degree of vessel tortuosity.

A calibrated pigtail catheter is placed in the abdominal aorta just above the iliac bifurcation. Both the iliac and femoral arteries are visualized by injecting 20–35 mL of contrast medium. The common femoral artery and the level of the femoral bifurcation compared with the head of the femur are to be assessed. The diameter of the lumen of the iliac and femoral arteries can be measured with the calibration device of the catheter. The advantages of angiography are high spatial resolution and the possibility of assessing the course of the vessel and plaque burden. A limited movement of the vessel may indicate a stiffer and more calcified artery. Angiography provides

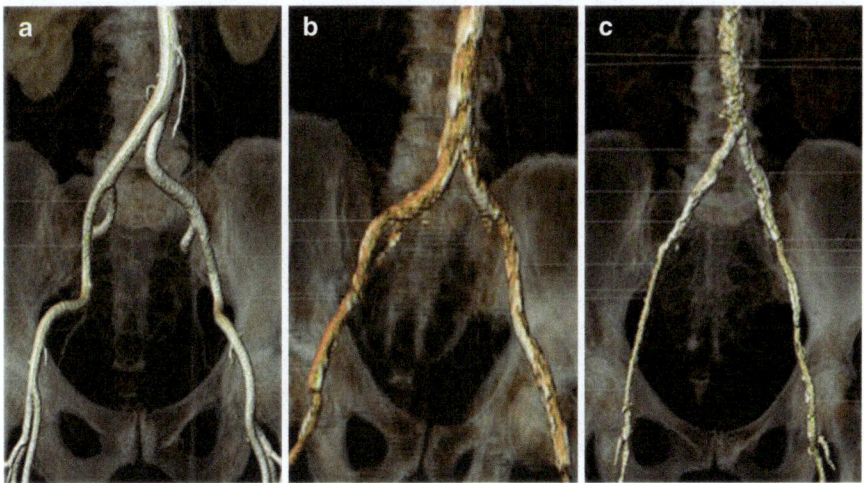

**Fig. 18.7**   3D CT reconstruction with mild (**a**), moderate (**b**), and severe (**c**) calcifications

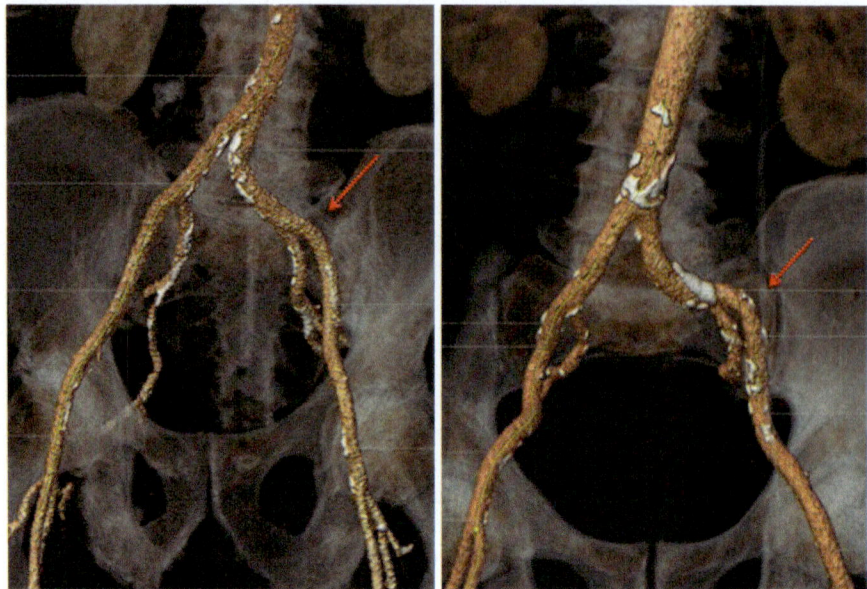

**Fig. 18.8** 3D CT reconstruction of the iliofemoral axis with no tortuosity (*left*) and mild tortuosity (*right*)

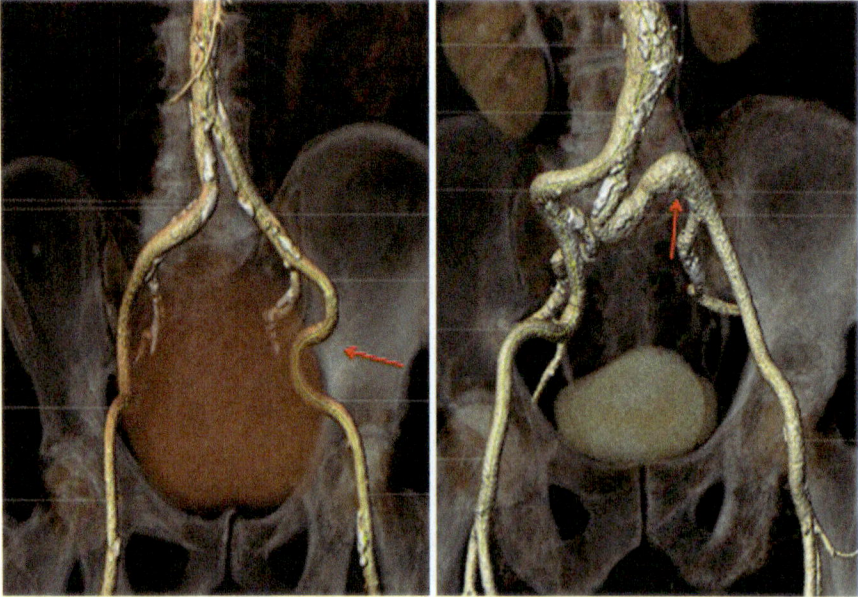

**Fig. 18.9** 3D CT reconstruction of the iliofemoral axis with moderate tortuosity (*left*) and severe tortuosity (*right*)

only a limited assessment of the degree of atherosclerosis and of tortuosity. Digital subtraction angiography (DSA) is still considered the gold standard because of its higher spatial resolution. However, both angiography and DSA show arterial anatomy in 2D. It follows that a stenosis that is visible only in 3D cannot be viewed [1].

### 18.1.4 Multidetector Computed Tomography

Because of the limitations of angiography, multidetector computed tomography (MDCT) has become the single most important imaging modality for the examination of the abdominal and iliofemoral arteries. There are major differences among protocols in terms of radiation dose and the amount of contrast medium administered. The latter is particularly important considering the possible risk of contrast-induced nephropathy (CIN) in the TAVI population.

Zemedkun M. et al. studied the feasibility and reproducibility of an MDCT protocol that involved the administration of low doses of contrast medium. The low-dose patients ($n = 16$) received 80% less contrast in volume than those studied with the standard protocol ($n = 17$) ($23 \pm 10$ vs. $125 \pm 23$ mL, $p < 0.001$). There were no significant differences in terms of quality of the obtained image ($3.8 \pm 0.4$ vs. $3.9 \pm 0.3$, $p = 0.76$) and of interpretability (100% for each $P = 1.0$) between the groups of patients who received the lower dose of contrast medium and those who received the normal protocol. There were no significant differences in terms of CIN rates after MDCT between the standard protocol and low-dose groups [2] (10% vs. 3%; $p = 0.55$).

Other studies have shown that 10% of elderly patients with aortic stenosis who received a pre-TAVI CT scan develop acute kidney injury (AKI). It has also been found that intravenous administration of <90 mL of contrast medium reduces this risk in patients with and without kidney injury. However, in the majority of patients, kidney function is recovered prior to TAVI.

A standardized approach reduces morbidity and mortality rates from vascular injury and includes a number of reconstructions, including three-dimensional (3D) rendered volume imaging, curved multiplanar reformats, and maximum intensity projection images [3]. Employing a centerline approach to elongate the vessel image, multiple luminal measurements should be made in a plane orthogonal to the vessel rather than in the transverse axial plane. With this approach, MDCT can evaluate vessel size, degree of calcification, minimal luminal diameter, plaque burden, and vessel tortuosity and also identify high-risk pathologies, including dissections and complex atheroma (Fig. 18.10).

### 18.1.5 Intravascular Ultrasound

In the evaluation process of the iliofemoral axes prior to TAVI, intravascular ultrasound (IVUS) can be a valid alternative. It has the advantage of high resolution and affords 3D vision. It also allows analysis of the composition and thickness of plaque, avoiding artifacts due to calcifications, which at times reduce the quality of MDCT.

**Fig. 18.10** CT image of
the aorta with severe
atheroma and presence of
circumferential
calcifications

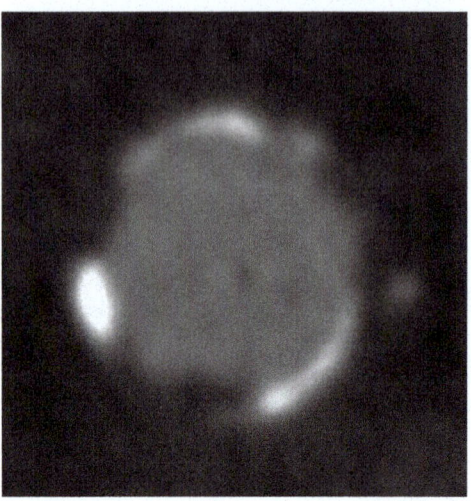

It is also possible to distinguish between concentric and nonconcentric plaques. In a study comparing IVUS and angiography, there were no significant differences in terms of evaluation of the diameter of the lumen and the extent of stenosis [4]. The limits are the invasiveness and cost of ultrasound probes.

### 18.1.6 Magnetic Resonance Imaging

As regards the evaluation of aortic anatomy, magnetic resonance imaging (MRI) is a valid option. It has the advantage of vascular screening with a low risk of nephrotoxicity, though the resolution is lower than that of CT imaging. A recent meta-analysis has shown that MRI is very accurate in detecting stenosis of over 50%, with a median sensitivity of 95% and a median specificity of 97%. MRI without contrast agent may be a promising alternative, especially in those patients with renal insufficiency of stage 6 kidney failure (GFR < 30 mL/min), to help reduce the potential risk of terminal AKI/dialysis. A recent study has shown that MRI without contrast agent correlates well with MRI with contrast agent in the measurement of the aortic annulus [5] (MR image of the iliofemoral axes, Fig. 18.11).

### 18.2    Vascular Access Management

### 18.2.1 Puncture

Ideally, a femoral arterial puncture should be above the most inferior border of the inferior epigastric artery and above the femoral bifurcation (Fig. 18.12), on the

**Fig. 18.11** 2D MRI reconstruction of the iliofemoral axis. *CIA* common iliac artery, *IIA* internal iliac artery, *EIA* external iliac artery, *CFA* common femoral artery, *SFA* superficial femoral artery, *DFA* deep femoral artery

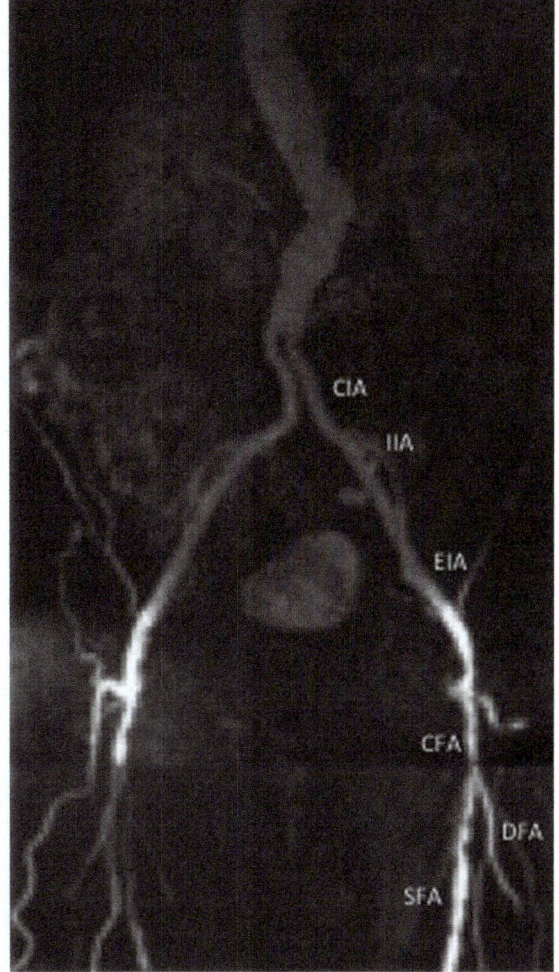

vessel's anterior wall, with an angle of 45–60° compared with the plane of the vessel wall to minimize the path between the skin and the artery wall and facilitate percutaneous closure. A number of techniques can be used to ensure an optimal puncture.

The puncture can be made under angiographic guidance (anteroposterior view at 0°) with injections of contrast agent through a pigtail catheter positioned just above the iliac crest. Alternatively, dye injection can be administered with a Judkins right catheter (preferably 5 Fr), inserted in a crossover fashion from the contralateral artery and placed a few centimeters above the site puncture. On occasion, it may be helpful to place a contralateral catheter and use this as a fluoroscopic landmark, aiming at an eyelet of the pigtail. This can facilitate extremely accurate anterior wall

**Fig. 18.12** Angiography of the femoral artery. The space between the *white line* above and the *white line* below indicates the ideal puncture site of the artery. *EIA* external iliac artery, *CFA* common femoral artery, *SFA* superficial femoral artery, *PFA* profunda femoris artery

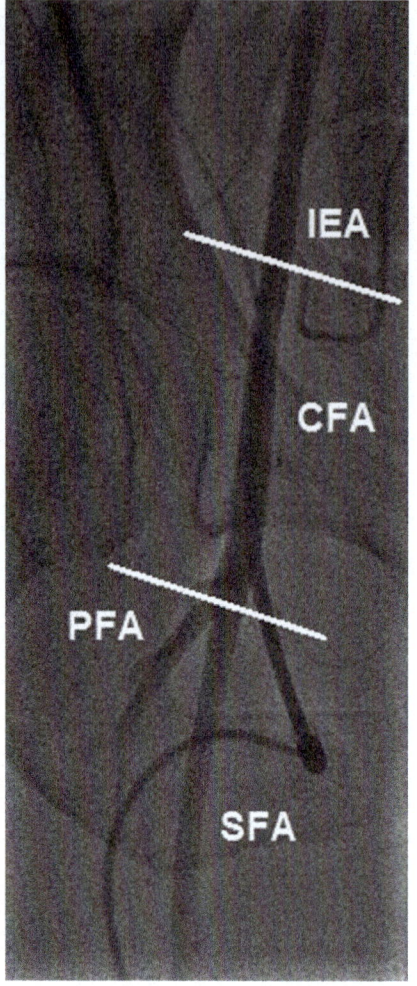

puncture without contrast, even in obese patients (Fig. 18.13). Ultrasound guidance with a sterile, packed 5–10 MHz linear array transducer can also be extremely helpful in assuring accurate front wall puncture and avoiding plaque.

Before placing the sutures with Prostar or ProGlide, a 0.018" hydrophilic wire (V-18 Control Wire Guide Wire, Boston Scientific Corporation) guidewire can be positioned at the periphery of the superficial femoral artery, advanced in crossover from the contralateral femoral artery, and kept in place until the end of the procedure, so as to be ready to intervene in case of dissection and/or rupture of the common femoral artery where the large-bore introducer is inserted. Alternatively, particularly in the case of difficult crossover approach, the superficial femoral artery can be cannulated with a 4 Fr sheath, and a 0.018" wire can be placed in ascending aorta.

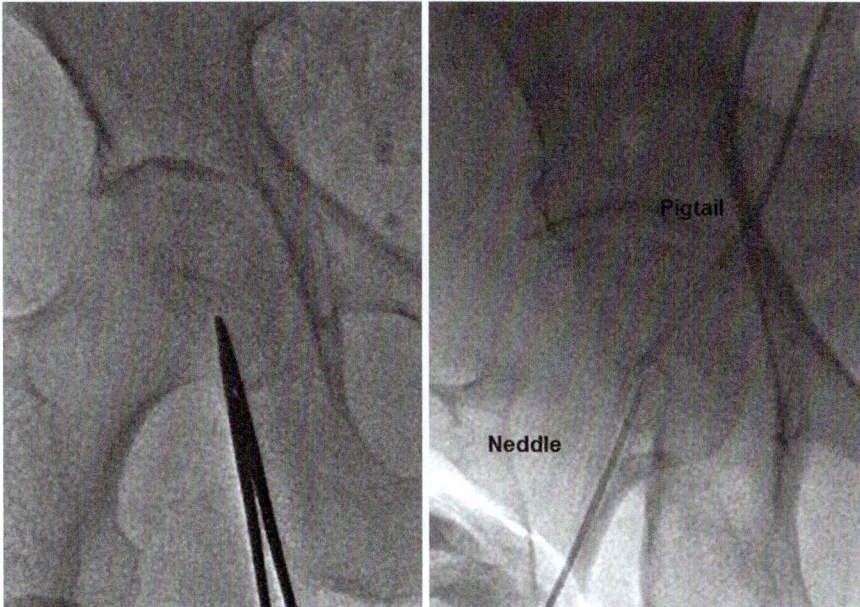

**Fig. 18.13** Useful techniques to guide the femoral puncture. To determine the exact puncture site, a radiopaque object can be placed over the femoral head (*left*). Alternatively, a catheter can be introduced through the contralateral femoral artery and used as a target or for contrast injections to facilitate puncture under fluoroscopy (*right*)

## 18.2.2  Surgical Isolation and Closure Systems

### 18.2.2.1   Surgical Cutdown

During early experiences with TAVI via the transfemoral route, due to the large size of the introducers, surgical cutdown and isolation of the common femoral artery was the standard approach [6]. Surgical cutdown can be performed at the beginning of the procedure to allow visualization and selection of the ideal puncture site and control of the artery above and below the puncture site. Alternatively, the artery is exposed only for closure after the percutaneous puncture. Though most transfemoral procedures are now performed percutaneously, surgical cutdown is useful in very obese patients, and when a high puncture is needed due to a high femoral bifurcation [7], or in the case of lengthy calcifications along the anterior wall of the common femoral artery.

## 18.2.3  Percutaneous Closure Systems

There are no available percutaneous devices specifically intended for large vessel closure. However, preclosure with either the Prostar XL 10 Fr device or two ProGlide 6 Fr devices is commonly used for this purpose.

### 18.2.3.1    Perclose ProGlide

Introduced in 1997, the Perclose device was the first suture-based vascular closure device on the market. The 6 Fr device, intended for use with 5–8 Fr sheaths and routinely used for femoral access site closure after coronary angiography and intervention, places a suture through the arterial wall like a stapler (i.e., from the outside in) and uses a pre-tied self-locking surgical sliding knot for hemostasis. Initially, a braided polyester suture was used but has been replaced in the current device generation by a monofilament polypropylene suture, which provides more tensile strength and elicits less inflammatory tissue response. The current generation Perclose ProGlide device is composed of a plunger, handle, guide, and sheath. The Perclose ProGlide tracks over a standard 0.038" (or smaller) guidewire. A hemostasis valve restricts the blood flow through the sheath with or without the guidewire in place. The guide houses the needles, and the foot, and precisely controls the placement of these needles around the puncture site. The handle is used to stabilize the device during use. The plunger advances the needles and is used to retrieve the suture. A marker lumen is contained within the guide, with the intraluminal port of the lumen positioned at the distal end of the guide. Proximally, the marker lumen exits from the body of the device. The marker lumen allows a pathway for back bleeding (obtaining mark) from the femoral artery to ensure proper device positioning. Knot pusher and/or suture trimmer are included and are designed to position the tied suture knot to the top of the arteriotomy.

Percutaneous closure with two ProGlides is depicted in Fig. 18.14. Usually, the femoral artery is punctured and dilated with a standard arterial 6 Fr sheath, as described above. The ProGlide device is then advanced over a 0.035" guidewire, and the first suture is deployed slightly angulated at 10 o'clock. Guidewire access is maintained, and a second ProGlide device is inserted and deployed at 2 o'clock. After this device is removed, a larger dilator is inserted. The regular 0.035" J-tip wire is now exchanged to a stiffer wire, and the large sheath is advanced under fluoroscopy. After conclusion of the procedure, the introducer sheath is slowly removed, but the stiff wire is left to maintain access. The sutures are tightened. In the case of sufficient hemostasis, the wire can be removed, and the sutures further tightened using the knot pusher to ensure approximation of the knot to the vessel wall. Should hemostasis fail, it is possible to implant a third (or even more) ProGlide over the guidewire. Recently, Kahlert et al. reported a series of 94 TAVI patients in whom preclosure of the arterial access site was accomplished with a single 6 Fr ProGlide; an efficient hemostasis with cessation of any bleeding within 10 min of final knot tying was obtained in 83 of the 94 patients, and there was only one closure failure, with continuous bleeding despite prolonged manual compression requiring endovascular treatment [8].

### 18.2.3.2    Prostar

The first cases of percutaneous closure using the Prostar device were reported in 1996. Later, in order to reduce the invasiveness of endovascular aortic aneurysm repair, the Prostar and Perclose devices were utilized off-label to preclose the femoral artery. This was initially done with surgical exposure and direct visualization of

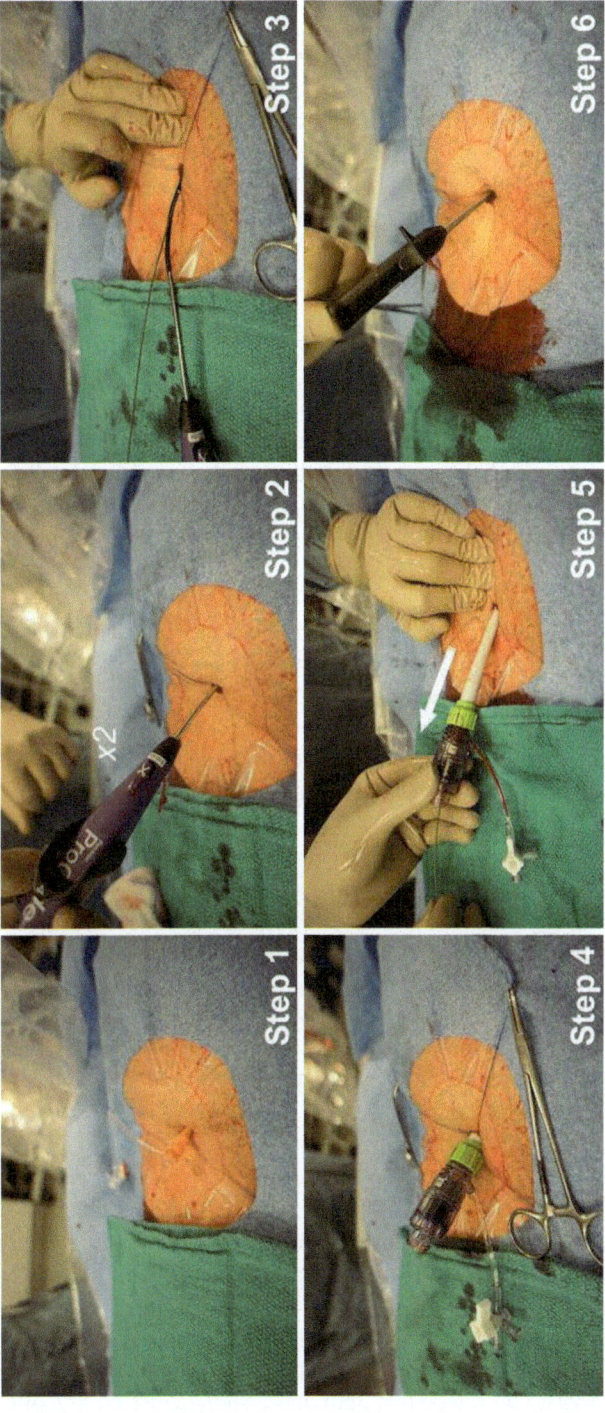

**Fig. 18.14** Steps of percutaneous closure with two ProGlides. After a regular 7-F is introduced (*Step 1*), sutures are deployed at 10 and 2 o'clock (*Steps 2 and 3*). After the 16-F dilator is inserted, a regular J wire is exchanged for a stiffer wire, and the large sheath is inserted under fluoroscopy (*Step 4*). After implantation of the valve, the sheath is retrieved (*Step 5*) and the sutures are tightened (*Step 5*). The wire is removed if sufficient hemostasis is achieved and the sutures are further tightened using the knot pusher (*Step 6*)

the femoral artery using two Prostar devices and later without a cutdown, resulting in totally percutaneous aortic aneurysm repair. Totally percutaneous endovascular aneurysm repair was found to be associated with a lower rate of late groin complications, shorter procedure time, and less severe scar tissue formation.

Compared with the ProGlide, the Prostar device requires a few minor procedures: a transversal incision at the puncture site with a length 8–10 mm is necessary; the subcutaneous tissue should be also separated with forceps with rounded tips both above and below the introducer, mounting the dilator and guidewire, or by using a finger. The latter maneuver may be preferred because it is less traumatic and allows optimal subcutaneous tissue separation around the femoral artery. When inserting the Prostar, it is important to ensure that the tip of the device does not engage the renal artery. Therefore, this maneuver should be performed under fluoroscopy guidance. Once the Prostar is inserted, and also during needle extraction, make sure that the blood jet exiting the posterior straight cannula is pulsatile (Fig. 18.15). Optimal subcutaneous preparation is confirmed by obtaining a good pulsatile flow without forcing the insertion of the device within the artery. It is recommended to make sure that the system rests against the artery wall using your left hand and slowly pulling back the four needles with your right hand. A nonpulsatile flow can be caused by:

1. The occlusion of the lumen of the cannula by clots or debris of subcutis tissue; in this case the Prostar should be retrieved and the cannula flushed with saline to ascertain the patency of the cannula.
2. The anterior hole of the cannula located in the shaft of the device is not in the lumen; at this point it is extremely important to recognize whether the Prostar has passed through the posterior wall of the artery or is still confined proximally the anterior wall.
3. Less likely, low flow is caused by the presence of an obstructive lesion localized proximally in the iliofemoral artery or systemic low cardiac output.

After needle deployment, if one or more needles do not come out, it means that they are deflected into the subcutis (Fig. 18.16). This situation often occurs when not all the components of the device are correctly aligned or in the presence of heavy calcifications. In such cases the needles should be repositioned in the Prostar device. This can be done with the aid of a surgical needle holder, taking care not to bend the needles (Fig. 18.17).

### 18.2.3.3   MANTA

The MANTA vascular closure device (VCD) (Essential Medical Inc., Malvern, PA, USA) is a novel collagen-based closure device that specifically targets arteriotomies. The MANTA VCD has a closure unit, a delivery system, and a dedicated sheath with introducer. There is also a separate 8 Fr puncture location dilator (Fig. 18.18). The puncture location dilator and the MANTA sheath both have a visible metric ruler for assessing the adequate depth. The closure unit comprises the following components: a resorbable polymer (poly-lactic-co-glycolic acid)

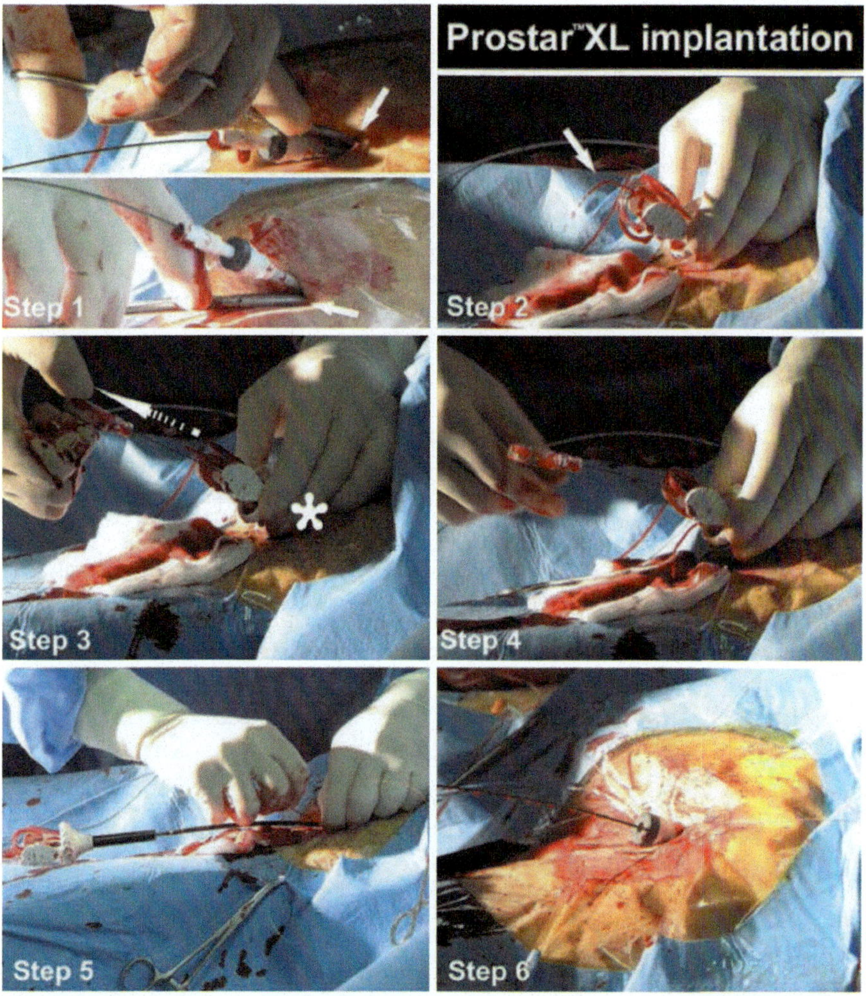

**Fig. 18.15** Prostar insertion. After dissecting the subcutaneous upper and lower part of the introducer (*white arrow*) (*Step 1*), the Prostar is inserted until a pulsatile blood flow comes out of the straight tube (*white arrow*) (*Step 2*), maintaining the position with the left hand (*Step 3\**) and using the right hand to pull out the needles (*Step 4*), and, once removed, the suture lines are cut (*Step 5*). At this point, the Prostar is pulled out, and the guidewire is reinserted, with repositioning of the 9-F introducer (*Step 6*)

intra-arterial toggle, an extravascular hemostatic bovine collagen pad, a connecting non-resorbable polyester suture, and a stainless steel suture lock (Fig. 18.2). The delivery system has a tube containing the closure unit and a device handle with a tension gauge to release the closure unit from the tube. The MANTA system comes in a 14 Fr or 18 Fr size. The 14 Fr MANTA VCD is indicated for closing punctures of 10–14 Fr and the 18 Fr MANTA VCD for punctures of 15–22 Fr.

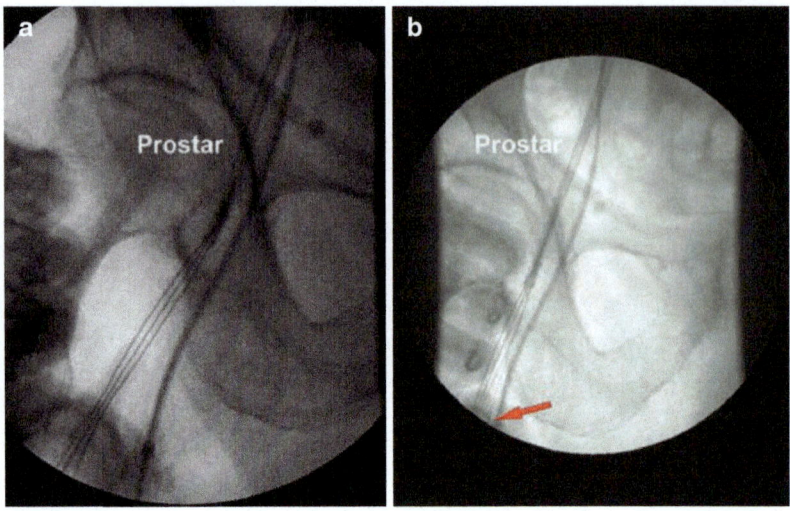

**Fig. 18.16** Maneuver to retract the needle of the 10-F Prostar XL showing the correct position of the four needles. The image to the right (**a**) shows a deviation of one of the medial needles located in the subcutaneous tissue. Needle deviation during extraction (**b**). One of the needles can be deviated by calcification or an incorrect position of the Prostar. The first maneuver is to reinsert all the needles with the help of a Klemmer to retract the entire system

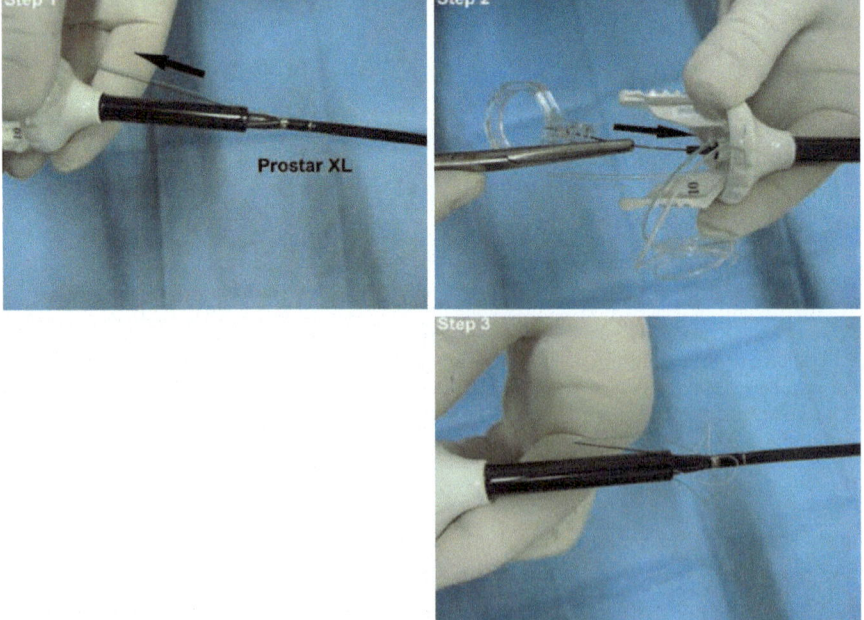

**Fig. 18.17** Needle deviation during extraction. One of the needles can be deviated by calcification or an incorrect position of the Prostar. The first maneuver is to reinsert all the needles with the help of a Klemmer to retract the entire system

**Fig. 18.18**  Graphical
representation of the Manta
closure device (Essential
Medical Inc., Malvern, PA,
USA)

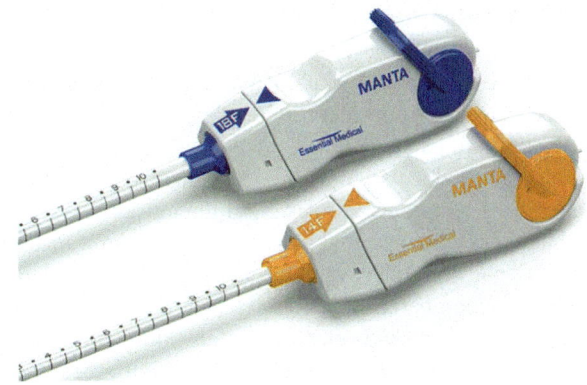

**Fig. 18.18**  Graphical representation of the Manta closure device (Essential Medical Inc., Malvern, PA, USA)

After a 0.035″ guidewire and 6 Fr sheath are introduced into the common femoral artery, the sheath is exchanged for the 8 Fr puncture location dilator to measure the length of the subcutaneous track from the skin to the endovascular lumen. Pulsatile blood emerges when the dilator tip is in the arterial vessel. The dilator is then pulled back until the blood flow ceases and the depth of the vessel lumen can be read from the metric ruler. Empirically 2 cm is added to assure endoluminal deployment of the toggle during the actual MANTA delivery. The arterial access is then upscaled to the proper sheath size to perform the index procedure. At the end of the index procedure, significant subcutaneous blood collection should be excluded before using the MANTA VCD because significant hematoma could alter the puncture depth relative to the state at baseline. The procedural sheath is exchanged over a 0.035″ guidewire for the dedicated MANTA sheath. The sheath introducer is removed and the MANTA closure unit is advanced over the wire into the sheath until the MANTA delivery hub snaps the sheath hub and a clicking sound will be heard. The MANTA sheath closure unit assembly is then slowly withdrawn at a 45° angle with the right hand while providing slight left hand counter push to the skin level to avoid skin tenting. At the predetermined deployment level, the toggle is released by rotating the lever of the MANTA delivery handle in a clockwise direction. The assembly is then slowly and gently withdrawn from the patient. Pulling force can be monitored by a color code. When excessive force is applied, the color code will switch from green to red, accompanied by an audible "click." As the MANTA sheath clears the skin layer, a blue tamper tube emerges from the deployment tube. Digital left hand pressure around the puncture site is released to advance the tamper tube down along the suture line and secure the stainless steel lock onto the vessel to compact the collagen pad further. The black suture marker becomes visible to indicate full compaction of the collagen. At this point, the arterial wall is sandwiched between toggle and collagen. Tension on the assembly is released, and the tamper is slid up the suture line out of the puncture tract. When hemostasis is confirmed, the guidewire is removed. If needed, a final tamp with tension on the handle and monitored pressure on the tamper (green color at tension gauge) can be performed to ensure complete hemostasis. The suture is cut above the blue tamper and at skin level.

## 18.2.4 Introducers

In the presence of very calcified arteries, expandable introducers are an instrument to be taken into consideration to decrease the number of vascular complications. Two types of expandable introducers are most commonly used. One is the Edwards eSheath introducer, which provides a mechanism for the mechanical expansion that allows the temporary expansion of the introducer when it is inserted into the valve. Once the release system passes through the introducer, it returns to its initial diameter. Expansion reduces the force needed to insert and move the release system to a minimum compared with non-expandable introducers. It also reduces the time during which the artery is expanded, thus minimizing the risk of vascular trauma.

Then there is the 14 Fr SoloPath® introducer (Terumo Corporation, Tokyo, Japan). It is an expandable device with a central balloon on which the introducer is mounted. Its end is reinforced and has a smaller diameter to allow the passage also through calcified and tortuous arteries. Once it is inserted into the femoral artery and reaches the abdominal aorta, the balloon is inflated for 60 s and then deflated and removed leaving a central lumen that reaches 21 Fr [9].

## 18.2.5 Large Caliber Sheath Management

Large sheaths should always be advanced while being observed fluoroscopically with the support of a stiff guidewire, such as the Amplatz Extra or Super Stiff wire. When there is extreme tortuosity, even stiffer wires, such as the Meier wire (Boston Scientific, Natick, MA) or the Lunderquist wire (Cook Medical Inc., Bloomington, IN), can be helpful.

The bulk of experience with transfemoral TAVI has been with the balloon-expandable Edwards-type valves (Edwards Lifesciences, Irvine, CA) and the self-expanding CoreValve (Medtronic, Minneapolis, MN). Over time, the delivery profile of both valve systems has been modified dramatically. The Edwards SAPIEN valve required a 22/24 Fr sheath, while the newer Edwards SAPIEN XT valves can be introduced through 18/19 Fr sheaths and even smaller expandable sheaths. The last-generation Edwards SAPIEN 3 valve is delivered through a 14 Fr expandable sheath. Similarly, the Medtronic CoreValve saw a gradual decrease in sheath size from 25 Fr (first generation) to 18 Fr (third generation). The last-generation Evolut R (Medtronic Inc., Galway, Ireland) is delivered through a 14 Fr delivery system.

Early procedures utilized large sheaths originally designed for endovascular aortic procedures. Currently the 18 Fr Cook introducer is currently used for implantation of the CoreValve device and many of the newer valves from other manufacturers. Several manufacturers are developing new and improved sheath systems compatible with their delivery catheters, while others are incorporating sheaths into the delivery system itself.

The expandable Edwards eSheath features a dynamic expansion mechanism that allows for transient sheath expansion during valve delivery. The trauma of dilatation during sheath insertion is greatly reduced. Immediately after the transcatheter heart valve passes, the sheath returns to a low profile diameter. This reduces the time the access vessel is expanded, thereby hypothetically minimizing the risk of vascular trauma (Fig. 18.19). Since the sheath transiently expands and then contracts, there is the possibility of incomplete arterial sealing. To avoid this it is best to advance the sheath all the way into the patient, where the larger and non-expandable strain relief portion of the sheath provides reliable sealing.

The SoloPath sheath (Terumo, Japan) has been widely used with CoreValve and Symetis ACURATE neo implantation devices, though a SAPIEN XT compatible system has also been available. This introducer consists of a flexible, reinforced polymer sheath mounted over a central balloon dilatation catheter (the expander). The folded distal region of the sheath is 14 Fr in diameter, facilitating passage through small-diameter and tortuous arteries. Once inserted through the femoral artery and into the abdominal aorta, the SoloPath expander is briefly inflated, deflated, and then removed, leaving a large central lumen (up to 21 Fr) (Fig. 18.20).

Though sheath diameters continue to become smaller, femoral access may still be limited by atherosclerotic stenosis. Balloon angioplasty can often facilitate sheath insertion, though stent implantation can be problematic if these are not adequately sized and expanded. Alternatively, direct surgical access to the iliac artery is often a reasonable option.

After sheath removal, it is prudent to leave a guidewire in place until hemostasis is confirmed. Should this fail, a sheath can be reinserted, or an occlusion balloon advanced proximal to the bleeding site to allow surgical closure. Blood pressure

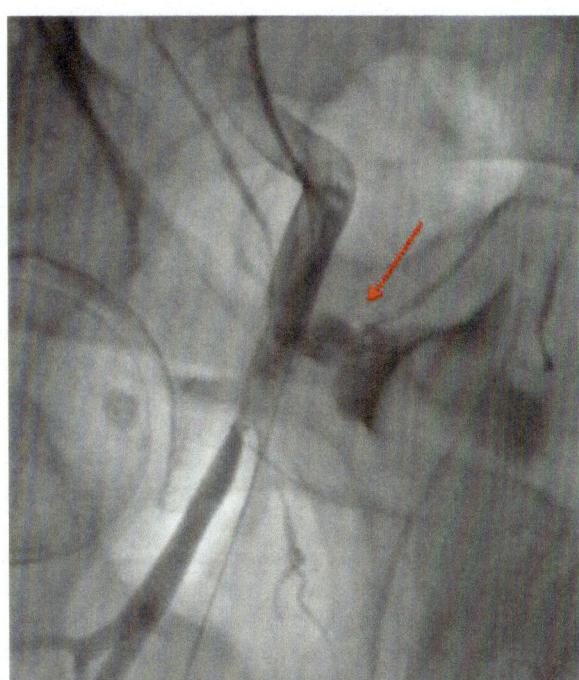

**Fig. 18.19** Selective angiography of the right femoral artery with spreading of contrast medium (*red arrow*) in the common femoral artery

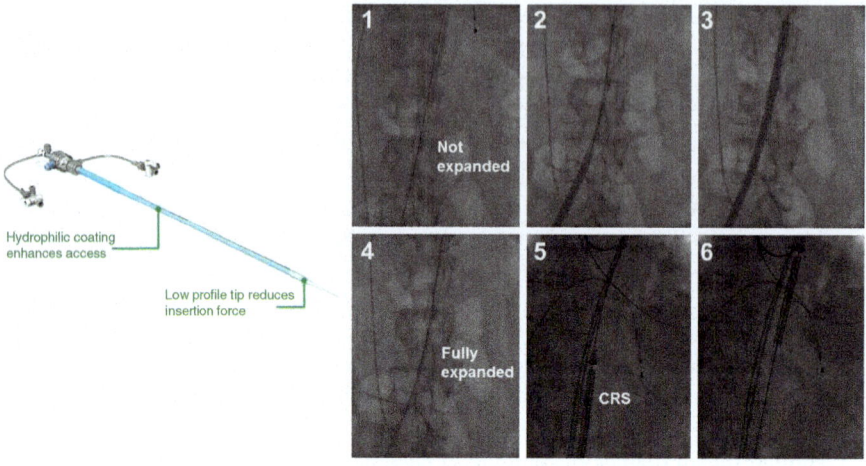

**Fig. 18.20** SoloPath expandable sheath (*left*). On the *right*, the unexpanded sheath is advanced over a stiff wire (*1*). The sheath is then expanded (*2–4*). The self-expanding CoreValve prosthesis can easily navigate through the expanded sheath (*5, 6*)

should be monitored for rapid detection of signs of perforation, such as hypotension and/or tachycardia. Once the sheath is removed, the ProGlide or Prostar sutures are tightened. If hemostasis is achieved, the wire is removed and the sutures are further tightened. Completion angiography from the contralateral side can be done to rule out residual internal leaks or stenosis.

As long as wire access to the access artery is maintained, problematic bleeding can be managed with reinsertion of the sheath. Alternatively, placement of a dedicated occlusion balloon proximal to the perforation from the ipsilateral or contralateral artery can provide reliable temporary hemostasis and hemodynamic stability while the bleeding site is appropriately managed. Some groups have advocated routine use of a balloon advanced to the external femoral artery and inflated in order to block the blood flow down to the in situ puncture and avoid bleeding during knot tightening. On occasion, substitution of heparin with protamine can be helpful, particularly if there is persistent oozing. However, this is not generally necessary and can increase the risk of femoral artery thrombosis, particularly when femoral compression is also utilized.

## 18.3    Alternatives to the Transfemoral Approach

Today, the retrograde transfemoral route is the standard approach for most biological devices that have been developed for TAVI, as it is less invasive, feasible under mild sedation, and completely percutaneous. Despite the significantly smaller profile of the delivery systems of new-generation TAVI devices, the transfemoral approach is still contraindicated when the minimum diameter of the vessel is less than 5.5 mm and in the case of tortuosity or severe calcifications of the femoral or iliac arteries or of the distal aorta [10–12]. In addition, the transfemoral approach should be considered with caution in patients with aneurysms at the level of the thoracic and/or abdominal aorta. It is for this reason that over the years alternative approaches have been developed. The most used today are:

- Subclavian approach
- Transapical approach
- Transaortic approach

### 18.3.1 Subclavian Approach (Fig. 18.21)

In the trans-subclavian approach, the presence of a vascular surgeon is essential to isolate the subclavian artery and insert the dedicated introducer (usually the puncture site is slightly lateral to the outer edge of the first rib, i.e., where the subclavian artery becomes the axillary artery).

Routinely, this approach is well tolerated with local anesthesia and mild sedation. The conventional Seldinger technique is the most used for the puncture of the

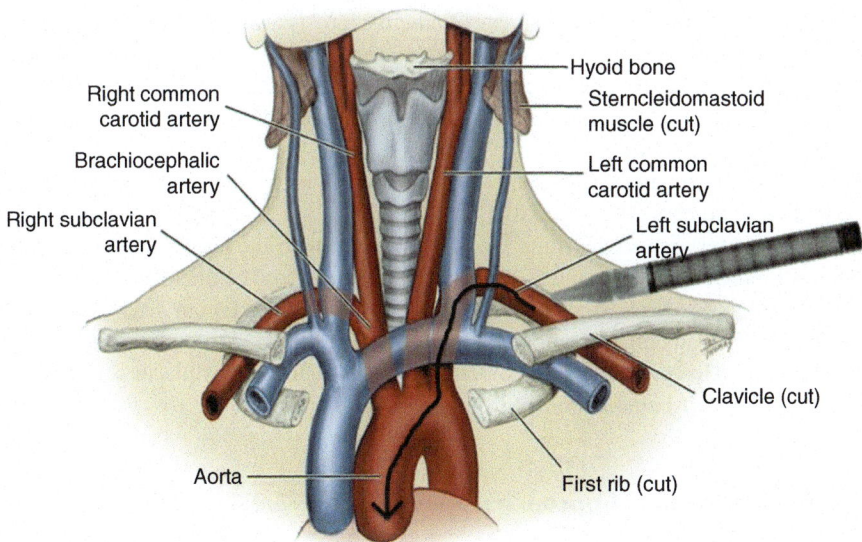

**Fig. 18.21** Representation of the arterial system (ascending aorta, brachiocephalic trunk, left carotid artery, and left subclavian artery) and of the venous system (superior vena cava, brachiocephalic trunk, and left subclavian vein) of the large vessels in the upper chest. The image on the *right* shows the delivery system whose tip is directed toward the access site in the left subclavian artery. The *black arrow* indicates the course of the device inside the arterial system to the aortic valve

artery after preparing a tobacco pouch. However, some operators prefer an arteri-otomy or positioning a graft. At this point, the standard introducer used for the transfemoral approach is advanced on a stiff guidewire through the subclavian artery in the aortic arch and then in the ascending aorta, blocking it just below the origin of the brachiocephalic artery. From this point on, TAVI is performed with the same technique used for the transfemoral approach. At the end of the proce-dure, hemostasis is obtained simply by tightening the tobacco-pouch sutures, and the layers of the skin are sutured conventionally; a drainage tube is seldom needed. During the procedure, the activated clotting time must be kept between 200 and 250 s.

The insertion of the large introducer into the subclavian artery may seem puz-zling since it is often considered more fragile than the common femoral artery, and its anatomical position makes the management of bleeding in the event of a vessel rupture challenging. Moreover, the subclavian artery in elderly patients is often the site of calcifications and tortuosity. In this respect, attentive pre-procedure screen-ing of the anatomy of the artery in terms of vessel diameter, degree of tortuosity, and the presence and extent of calcification is imperative [13, 14].

One particular condition is the presence of the left internal mammary artery graft to the left anterior descendent coronary artery, since the introduction of the large caliber introducer could put the patency of the vessel at risk and cause ischemia [15]. In order to avoid this, screening by imaging should be carried out before the procedure to ensure that the minimum diameter is sufficient to accommodate the introducer, and that there are no areas of atherosclerosis around the grafts, or severe tortuosity. Once the introducer is inserted, an injection of contrast agent should be given to ensure that it is not occlusive. Moreover, immediately after the release of the valve, the introducer should be withdrawn to avoid covering the ostium of the graft before being removed.

Access via the subclavian route is also feasible in patients with a pacemaker permanently positioned in the axillary region. In fact, surgical cutdown to access the subclavian artery is usually quite medial compared with the pacemaker pouch and does not interfere with the pulse generator and the electrode catheters.

The left subclavian artery is preferable to the right subclavian artery for TAVI because it generally allows a more axial orientation of the device with the aortic root and annulus. However, the right subclavian access can be feasible in select cases and only if the vascular anatomy allows it.

## 18.3.2 Transapical Approach (Figs. 18.22 and 18.23)

The transapical approach is used for TAVR and provides for a surgical minithoraco-tomic incision at the apex of the heart. This technique should be avoided in patients who have undergone prior cardiac surgery due to the increased risk of bleeding from previous adhesions. It is contraindicated in patients with a recent history of throm-bus at the apex of the left ventricle and with large-sized aneurysm of the cardiac apex.

**Fig. 18.22** Representation of the transapical access. The image shows the Sapien (balloon-expandable valve) at the time of balloon inflation and release of the prosthesis. On the tip of the heart it is possible to see tobacco pouch which is used to close the breach at the entry point of the device in the heart

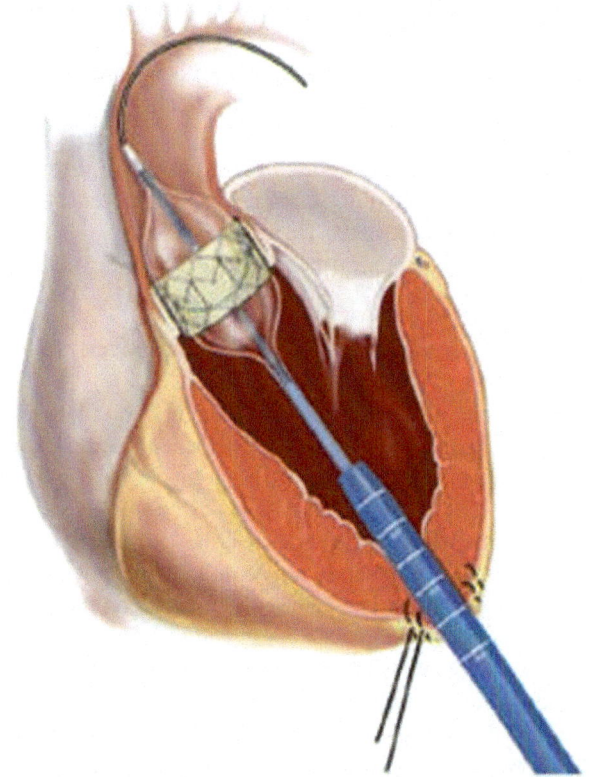

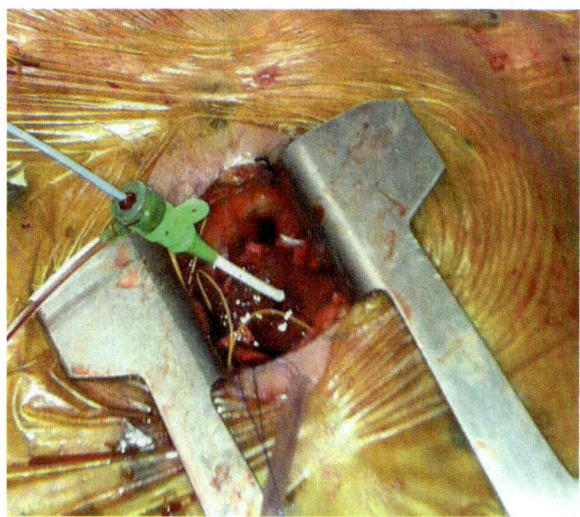

**Fig. 18.23** Photo taken during the transapical TAVI procedure. The retractor allows the operator to expose a greater surface area

### 18.3.3 Imaging: Procedural Planning and Guidance

The transthoracic or transesophageal echocardiogram is useful both to locate the cardiac apex before incision and to monitor any pericardial effusions. CT is useful in pre-procedure screening especially to the 3D volume-rendered reconstructions that allow the identification of the extension of the pulmonary tissue above the cardiac apex, location of the cardiac apex and coronary arteries, and even the anatomy of the papillary muscles. The distance from the skin to the LV apex, optimal intercostal space, and appropriate angle for entry can all be obtained from the CTA [16].

### 18.3.4 Transapical Left Ventricular Access Technique

The procedures are carried out in a hybrid cath lab room under general anesthesia, with a surgical team on standby. The patient should be prepped and draped in a sterile fashion from the clavicles to the groin, in case emergent thoracotomy is needed. Once the transapical puncture site has been selected, left anterolateral thoracotomy is performed first. In general, it is best to perform a lower incision rather than a higher one, since the apex can be pulled down by traction on the pericardial sutures. The pericardium is opened longitudinally, and the placement of stable sutures provides good exposure of the apex. The next step is to identify the location of the left anterior descending artery. Two tobacco-pouch sutures are placed (Prolene 2-0, large needle with interrupted Teflon pledgets; Ethicon Inc., Somerville, NJ, USA) deep enough in the myocardial wall, without penetrating the left ventricular cavity, near the apex, and laterally to the left anterior descending artery. The apex is then pierced with a needle, and a soft guidewire is inserted and advanced through the native aortic valve in the antegrade direction. Once the implantation procedure is completed, both the catheter and stiff guidewire are withdrawn simultaneously. The apex is closed with the sutures previously implanted. Sometimes more sutures can be needed (usually for reinforcement in Teflon; Ethicon Inc) to achieve complete hemostasis. Sutures are also applied to close the pericardium, and a drainage tube is positioned.

### 18.3.5 Transaortic Approach (Figs. 18.24 and 18.25)

The transaortic approach was initially utilized as an alternative when conventional approaches were not possible. With increasing experience in many centers, it is now being used as a preferred approach in non-transfemoral patients.

### 18.3.6 Patient Selection

Two important points when considering suitability of the approach for a patient are:

1. Access point: This represents the area where tobacco pouch is made and through which the introducer is advanced. This area should be free of calcifications and allow an optimal alignment of the release system with the aortic annulus for

**Fig. 18.24** Representation of transaortic access with the entry site of the delivery system at the level of the ascending aorta. The image shows the Sapien delivery system (balloon-expandable valve) at the time of balloon inflation and release of the prosthesis

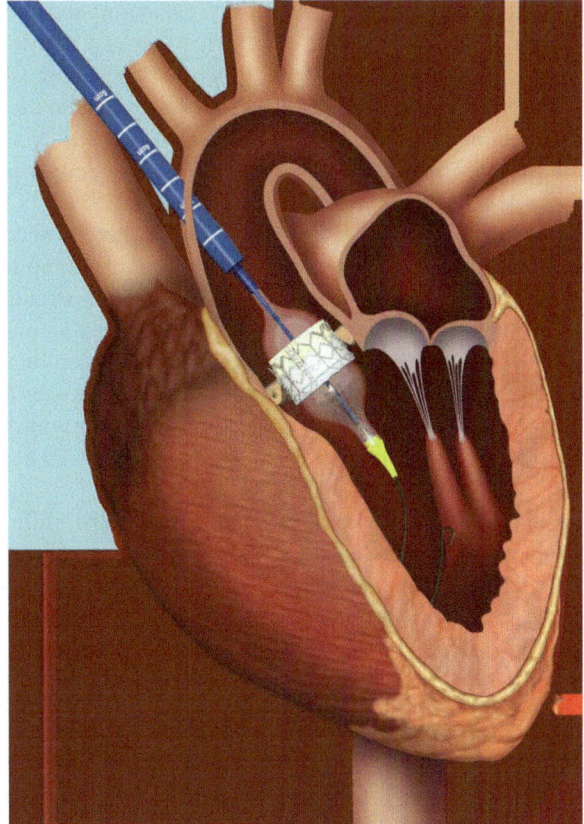

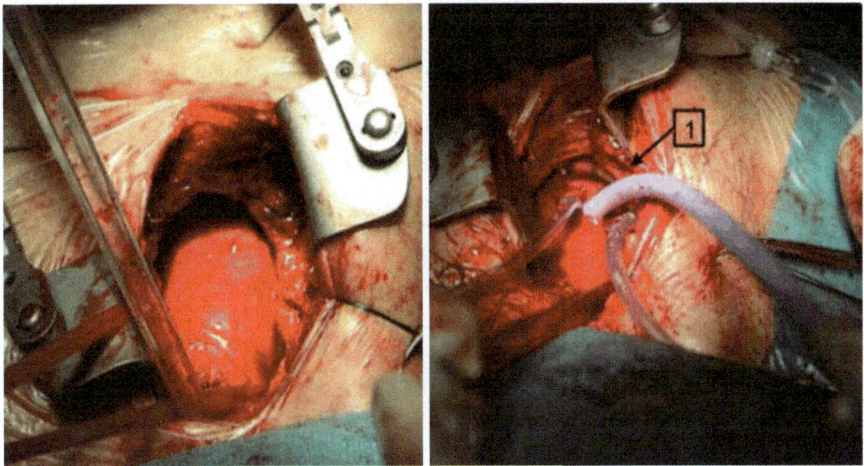

**Fig. 18.25**  Photo taken during the transaortic TAVI procedure. The image on the *left* shows the exposure of the post-ministernotomy ascending aorta. The image on the *right* shows the site

correct positioning of the valve. Considering the elderly age of patients undergoing TAVI, the presence of calcifications is a fairly common event, though these often spare the ideal area for the transaortic approach access. Also in porcelain aortas, transaortic TAVI is feasible provided that the access point is free of calcifications. For this purpose, CT and its reconstructions are of fundamental importance to identify calcifications and the correct puncture site so that it is aligned as best as possible with the aortic annulus.

2. Reoperation: In the case of cardiac surgery reoperation, CT and angiography are of great support in preventing possible complications, e.g., damage to the grafts implanted in the aorta or damage to structures such as the brachiocephalic artery and the aorta, which can have an unconventional anatomy after the closure of the previous sternotomy. Depending on the position taken after the procedure, it is necessary to consider whether to choose the approach with ministernotomy or right anterior thoracotomy in the case of structures adhering to the sternum.

In the case of prior CABG, the course of the graft must be thoroughly investigated both in the case of implantation of the left internal mammary artery for the left anterior descending artery and in the case of the right internal mammary artery. In these cases, the safest approach is right anterior thoracotomy to avoid damaging the grafts.

### 18.3.7 Options for the Transaortic Approach

Exposure of the ascending aorta can be carried out either through a ministernotomy or a right anterior thoracotomy:

1. Ministernotomy can be performed either with a J-shaped incision through the second or third intercostal space or with a T-shaped incision through the second intercostal space. The advantages of ministernotomy are that it is a more familiar technique to cardiac surgeons and does not require opening the pleura. It allows a rapid conversion to conventional open sternotomy in case of complications. Usually it is better tolerated by patients in terms of post-procedure recovery.

2. Right anterior thoracotomy is carried out through the second intercostal space but can also be performed through the first intercostal space. This technique does not provide for the incision of the bone and is the approach of choice in patients with aortocoronary bypass.

In general, the approach with right anterior thoracotomy is preferable if the aorta is on the right side of the median line and not very far from the rib cage or in the case of prior bypass. Ministernotomy is preferred if the aorta is on the median line or deeper.

# References

1. Owen AR, Roditi GH. Peripheral arterial disease: the evolving role of non-invasive imaging. Postgrad Med J. 2011;87:189–98.
2. Zemedkun M, LaBounty TM, Bergman G, Wong SC, Lin FY, Reynolds D, Gomez M, Dunning AM, Leipsic J, Min JK. Effectiveness of a low contrast load CT angiography protocol in octogenarians and nonagenarians being evaluated for transcatheter aortic valve replacement. Clin Imaging. 2015;39(5):815–9.
3. Toggweiler S, Gurvitch R, Leipsic J, Wood DA, Willson AB, Binder RK, Cheung A, Ye J, Webb JG. Percutaneous aortic valve replacement: vascular outcomes with a fully percutaneous procedure. J Am Coll Cardiol. 2012;59:113.
4. Arthurs ZM, Bishop PD, Feiten LE, Eagleton MJ, Clair DG, Kashyap VS. Evaluation of peripheral atherosclerosis: a comparative analysis of angiography and intravascular ultrasound imaging. J Vasc Surg. 2010;51:933–8.
5. Collins R, Burch J, Cranny G, Aguiar-Ibáñez R, Craig D, Wright K, Berry E, Gough M, Kleijnen J, Westwood M. Duplex ultrasonography, magnetic resonance angiography, and computed tomography angiography for diagnosis and assessment of symptomatic, lower limb peripheral arterial disease: systematic review. BMJ. 2007;334:1257.
6. Webb JG, Altwegg L, Boone RH, Cheung A, Ye J, Lichtenstein S, Lee M, Masson JB, Thompson C, Moss R, Carere R, Munt B, Nietlispach F, Humphries K. Transcatheter aortic valve implantation: impact on clinical and valve-related outcomes. Circulation. 2009;119:3009–16.
7. Toggweiler S, Webb J. Challenges in transcatheter aortic valve implantation. Swiss Med Wkly. 2012;142:w13735.
8. Barbash IM, Barbanti M, Webb J, Molina-Martin De Nicolas J, Abramowitz Y, Latib A, Nguyen C, Deuschl F, Segev A, Sideris K, Buccheri S, Simonato M, Rosa FD, Tamburino C, Jilaihawi H, Miyazaki T, Himbert D, Schofer N, Guetta V, Bleiziffer S, Tchetche D, Immè S, Makkar RR, Vahanian A, Treede H, Lange R, Colombo A, Dvir D. Comparison of vascular closure devices for access site closure after transfemoral aortic valve implantation. Eur Heart J. 2015;36:3370–9.
9. Barbanti M, Binder RK, Freeman M, Wood DA, Leipsic J, Cheung A, Ye J, Tan J, Toggweiler S, Yang TH, Dvir D, Maryniak K, Lauck S, Webb JG. Impact of low-profile sheaths on vascular complications during transfemoral transcatheter aortic valve replacement. EuroIntervention. 2013;9:929–35.
10. Grube E, Schuler G, Buellesfeld L, Gerckens U, Linke A, Wenaweser P, Sauren B, Mohr FW, Walther T, Zickmann B, Iversen S, Felderhoff T, Cartier R, Bonan R. Percutaneous aortic valve replacement for severe aortic stenosis in high-risk patients using the second- and current third-generation self-expanding CoreValve prosthesis: device success and 30-day clinical outcome. J Am Coll Cardiol. 2007;50:69–76.
11. Piazza N, Grube E, Gerckens U, den Heijer P, Linke A, Luha O, Ramondo A, Ussia G, Wenaweser P, Windecker S, Laborde JC, de Jaegere P, Serruys PW. Procedural and 30-day outcomes following transcatheter aortic valve implantation using the third generation (18 Fr) CoreValve revalving system: results from the multicentre, expanded evaluation registry 1-year following CE mark approval. EuroIntervention. 2008;4:242–9.
12. Thomas M, Schymik G, Walther T, Himbert D, Lefevre T, Treede H, Eggebrecht H, Rubino P, Colombo A, Lange R, Schwarz RR, Wendler O. One-year outcomes of cohort 1 in the edwards SAPIEN aortic bioprosthesis European outcome (SOURCE) registry: the European registry of transcatheter aortic valve implantation using the Edwards SAPIEN valve. Circulation. 2011;124:425–33.
13. Petronio AS, De Carlo M, Bedogni F, Maisano F, Ettori F, Klugmann S, Poli A, Marzocchi A, Santoro G, Napodano M, Ussia GP, Giannini C, Brambilla N, Colombo A. 2-year results of CoreValve implantation through the subclavian access: a propensity-matched comparison with the femoral access. J Am Coll Cardiol. 2012;60:502–7.

14. Muensterer A, Mazzitelli D, Ruge H, Wagner A, Hettich I, Piazza N, Lange R, Bleiziffer S. Safety and efficacy of the subcla- vian access route for TAVI in cases of missing transfemoral access. Clin Res Cardiol. 2013;102(9):627–36.
15. Modine T, Sudre A, Collet F, Delhaye C, Lemesles G, Fayad G, Koussa M. Transcutaneous aortic valve implantation using the axillary/subclavian access with patent left internal thoracic artery to left anterior descending artery: feasibility and early clinical outcomes. J Thorac Cardiovasc Surg. 2012;144:1416–20.
16. Kliger C, Jelnin V, Sharma S, Panagopoulos G, Einhorn BN, Kumar R, Cuesta F, Maranan L, Kronzon I, Carelsen B, Cohen H, Perk G, Van Den Boomen R, Sahyoun C, Ruiz CE. CT angiography-fluoroscopy fusion imaging for percutaneous transapical access. JACC Cardiovasc Imaging. 2014;7:169–77.

# Preparation for Transcatheter Aortic Valve Implantation

# 19

Marco Barbanti, Claudia Ina Tamburino,
and Simona Gulino

## 19.1 Finding the Optimal Coplanar View

Finding the optimal coplanar view of the aortic annulus is of paramount importance when performing transcatheter aortic valve implantation (TAVI). During TAVI, the aortic root and the prosthetic valve delivery catheter should both be visualized in an optimal angulation. Planar structures, such as the aortic annular plane, and the tip of the delivery catheter, are optimally visualized when they are perpendicular to the source-to-detector direction.

The valve apparatus is a three-dimensional (3D) anatomic structure, which limits angiographic capabilities to find the ideal alignment between cusps properly.

In a given patient, there are infinite fluoroscopic projections in which the three aortic cusps are located on the same plane. These projections follow a sigmoid (line of perpendicularity) in which the layout of the cusps at angiography is different: toward the right anterior oblique (RAO), the three cusps will be arranged with the non-coronary cusp to the left and the right and left coronary cusps superimposed to the right; in anteroposterior projections (~RAO 10°, left anterior oblique [LAO] 10°), the non-coronary cusp will be located on the left, the right coronary cusp at the center, and the left coronary cusp to the left; in the left anterior oblique (LAO) projections, the non-coronary and right coronary cusps will be overlapped on the left and the left cusp on the right (Fig. 19.1).

Different strategies to accomplish this key step during TAVI have been proposed:

- Fluoroscopy/angiography-based approach ("follow the right cusp") [1]
- Angiographic 3D reconstruction
- Multidetector computed tomography (MDCT)-based approach

M. Barbanti (✉) • C.I. Tamburino • S. Gulino
Ferrarotto Hospital, University of Catania, Catania, Italy
e-mail: mbarbanti83@gmail.com

© Springer International Publishing AG 2018
C. Tamburino et al. (eds.), *Percutaneous Treatment of Left Side Cardiac Valves*,
https://doi.org/10.1007/978-3-319-59620-4_19

347

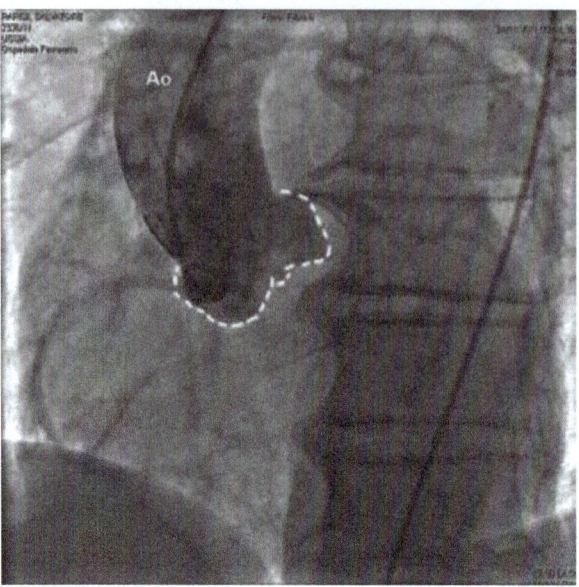

**Fig. 19.1** Fluoroscopy of the aortography in left anterior oblique projection. The dotted line indicates the aotic cusps aligned in the same plane. *Ao* aorta

## 19.2 Fluoroscopy/Angiography-Based Approach

In the case of TAVI patients with normal anatomy of the aortic root, the first step is to identify the right coronary cusp, which will serve as a landmark. If the right cusp is positioned below the non-coronary cusp or left cusp, the C-arm must be rotated to a RAO or LAO angulation, respectively.

If the right cusp appears to be higher or lower than the ideal intercept plane with the other cusps, the X-ray beam should be angulated cranially (CRA) or caudally (CAU), respectively. In general, the angle change on a single plane (RAO-LAO or CRA-CAU) generates, at an angiographic level, a shift of the right cusp on both planes by following these rules:

- By rotating the C-arm in the LAO direction, the right cusp will tend to move to the left (in the direction of the non-coronary cusp) and upward (Fig. 19.2).
- By rotating the C-arm in the RAO direction, the right cusp will tend to move to the right (in the direction of the left cusp) and downward (Fig. 19.2).
- By rotating the C-arm in the CRA direction, the right cusp will tend to move to the left (in the direction of the non-coronary cusp) and downward (Fig. 19.2).
- By rotating the C-arm in the CAU direction, the right cusp will tend to move to the right (in the direction of the left cusp) and upward (Fig. 19.2).

A step-by-step approach would be as follows: a pigtail catheter is placed in the right cusp as a reference and an aortogram anteroposterior view (0°–0°). If the right cusp is located on the "right" side behind the non-coronary cusp, the C-arm must be

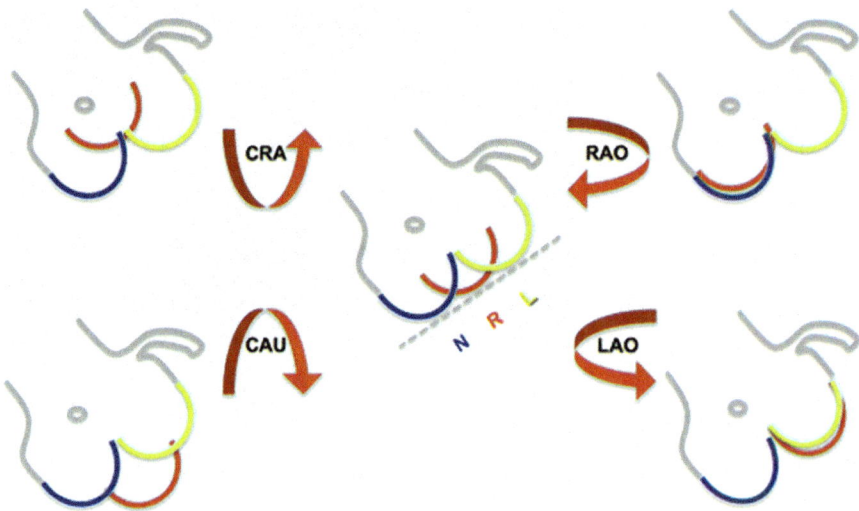

**Fig. 19.2** Schematic illustration of the "follow the right cusp" rule pointing to the proper alignment in the case of normal aortic root anatomy (Adapted from Kasel AM, et al.)

led to a RAO projection in order to follow the right cusp. After the projection view
has been changed, the right cusp will appear in the middle, but still deeper than the
other cusps. Once again, follow the right cusp by turning the C-arm clockwise to the
CAU direction. After alignment is obtained, providing that the most caudal attachments of all three of the aortic leaflets result in one axial image, a final angiogram
can be performed to confirm the working projection.

## 19.3    Angiographic 3D Reconstruction

Before being applied in the field of TAVI, 3D angiographic reconstructions of the
aortic root captured from rotational C-arm fluoroscopic images were evaluated in
different interventional settings, for example, in endovascular aortic aneurysm
repair [2] and catheter ablation procedures [3].

3D angiographic reconstructions are generated from images of a C-arm rotational aortic root angiography (220°). Radiographic contrast is injected through a
pigtail catheter placed in the non-coronary cusp (32 mL at 8 mL/s or 20 mL diluted
with 40 mL normal saline injected at 15 mL/s). Immediately before and during
contrast injection, rapid ventricular pacing must be instituted at a rate of 160–180
beats per minute. In the case of general anesthesia and endotracheal intubation, a
ventilator breath-hold can be also used during the injection to reduce respiratory
motion. Acquisition is achieved in approximately 4 s, and the volume set is reconstructed on a commercially available, dedicated workstation. After automatic depiction of the aortic valve cusps, a circle is generated indicating the aortic valve plane.
The reconstruction is then rotated until the circle appears as a straight line, indicating a view perpendicular to the valve (Fig. 19.3).

**Fig. 19.3** Three-dimensional aortic root reconstruction. The red circle below the annular plane, becoming a straight line, indicates that the projection is perpendicular to the valve

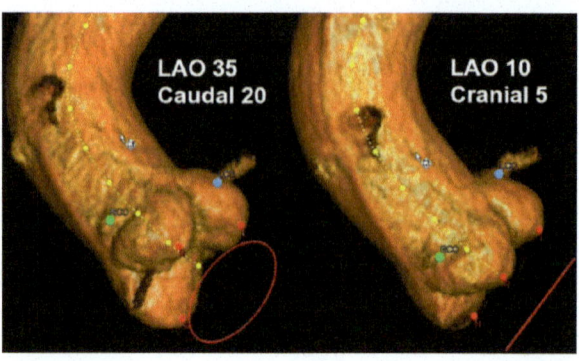

## 19.4    MDCT-Based Approach

The technique that is most widely used today for determining the release projection involves the use of MDCT (Fig. 19.4). Assuming that the patient will take the same position on the table of the MDCT and in the cath lab, it is in fact possible to calculate the projection that allows viewing the three aortic cusps on the same plane in an extremely accurate manner.

MDCT imaging in double-oblique position allows identification of the three aortic cusps. By rotating the axis on sagittal and coronal views, one is able to obtain the perfect position of the aortic virtual ring, with the nadir of the three cusps on the same plane. Points are then placed at the most inferior aspects of the valve cusps, and angles are determined by manually rotating the 3D aortic reconstructions to discern the appropriate projection.

Even when the coplanar view has been identified on MDCT scan, a check during the index procedure before proceeding with valve implantation is recommended.

## 19.5    Crossing of the Stenotic Aortic Valve

There are various techniques for crossing the aortic valve, each depending on the experience of the operator. The preferred technique is the one that allows optimal orientation of the catheter tip in order to direct the guide wire toward the aortic orifice.

The most frequently used materials are the soft tip straight standard guide and the Amplatz catheter (AL-1/AL-2) for the left coronary artery. The AL-1 is preferable in case of small or vertical aorta and the AL-2 in the case of aortic ectasia and horizontal aorta (Fig. 19.5). Other catheters that can be used for this purpose are standard pigtail (or angled pigtail in case of dilated aorta), the Judkin catheter (JR) for right coronary artery or small aorta, or a multipurpose catheter (MP) (Fig. 19.6).

Choosing the guide wire is also important, since it can facilitate the procedure. Hydrophilic guides or Teflon-coated straight-tipped guide wires are available. Among these, the straight-tipped guide wire (PTFE Guidewire Medtronic, Medtronic Vascular, Danvers, Massachusetts, USA) is usually preferred because it is easily

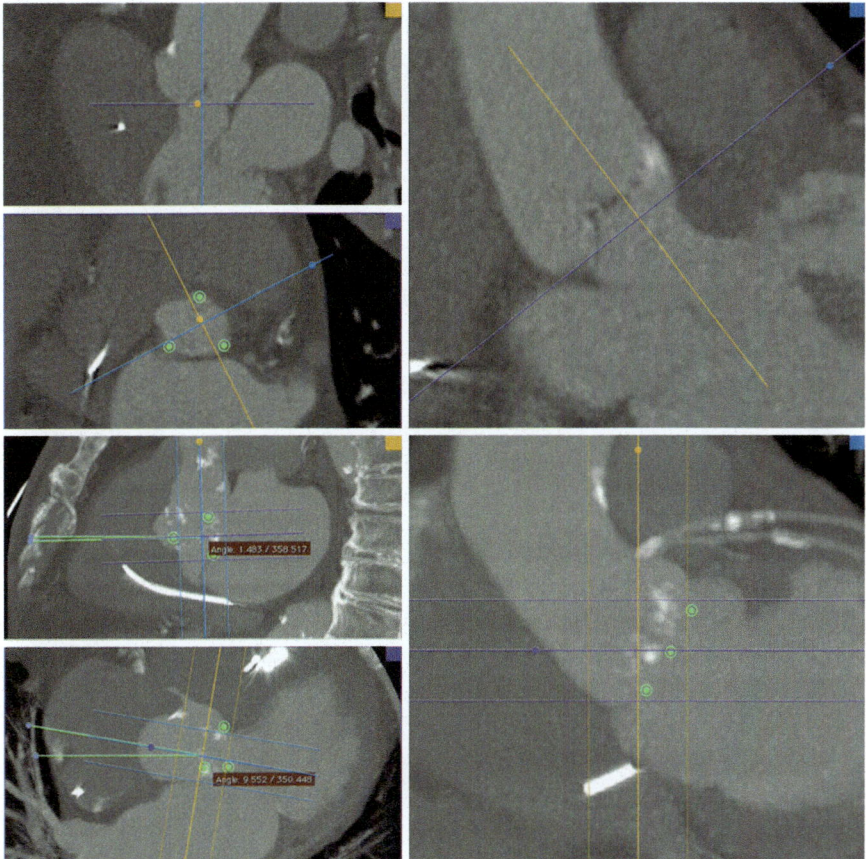

**Fig. 19.4** Identify aortic cusps and place points on them. *Step* 1: by rotating the axis on sagittal and coronal views, one is able to obtain the perfect position of the aortic virtual ring with the nadir of the three cusps on the same plane. *Step* 2: place a point on each cusp in double oblique view. *Step* 3: find the widest dimension of aortic root in the coronal view and increase. *Step* 4: rotate both sagittal and double oblique axis tool until the three points appear aligned with equal distances between them in the coronal oblique view. This is the optimal position of the aortic cusps. *Step* 5: finally, in order to determine C-arm angles, we use the sagittal oblique view for cranial-caudal, and the double oblique view for lateral positioning of C-arm. Note that angles formed below and above the horizontal reference line in the sagittal oblique view indicate, respectively, caudal and cranial angulations of the C-arm, while in the double oblique view they indicate right and left angulations, respectively

maneuverable; also, the hydrophilic properties of the Terumo guide wire (Radiofocus, Terumo, Tokyo, Japan) do not facilitate its handling.

Before starting crossing maneuvers, it is necessary to make sure that the patient is properly decoagulated, and 50 UI/Kg of unfractionated heparin should be administered to achieve an activated clotting time of 200 s.

The first step consists of finding the best view. This is usually obtained with computed tomography. However, when this is not available, operators often use the anteroposterior view, or a left-anterior oblique view (20°–40°), with the tip of the

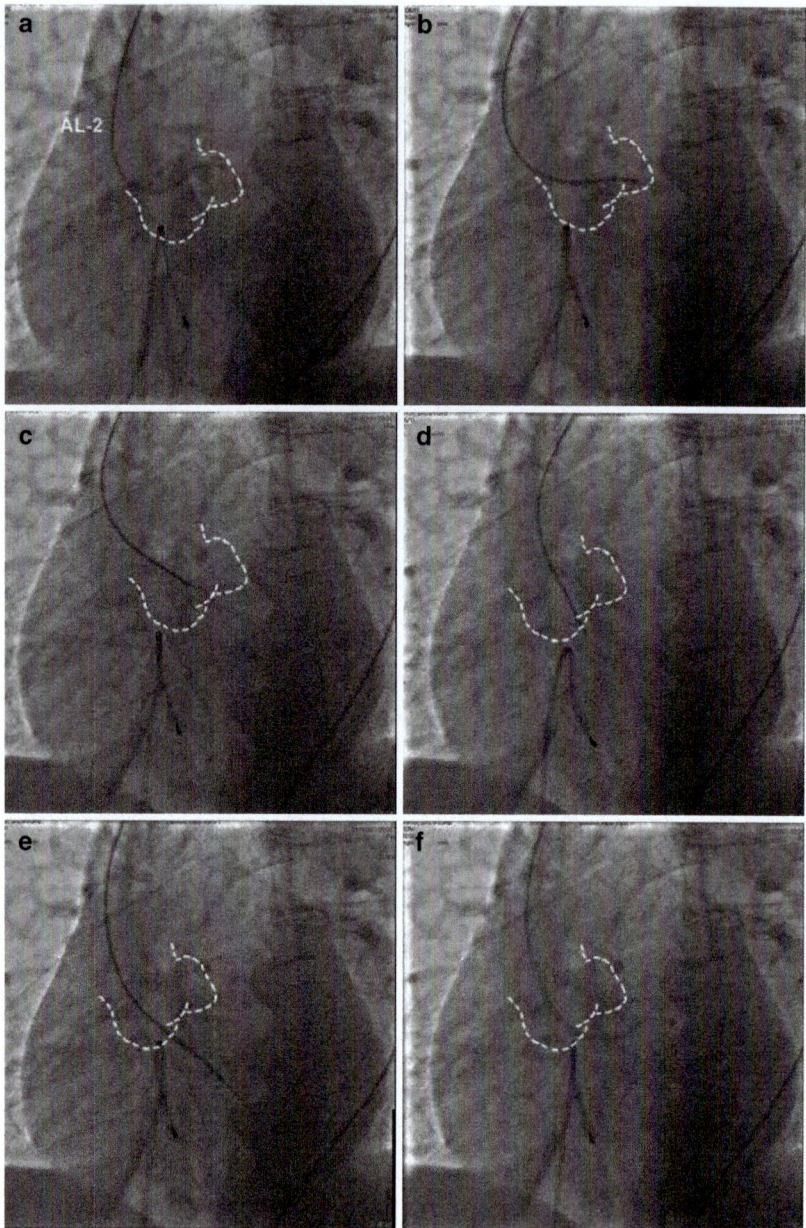

**Fig. 19.5** Fluoroscopy showing all the steps in aortic valve crossing using a 6-Fr Amplatz Left curve 2 (AL-2) catheter and the straight guidewire. The dotted line indicates the edge of the aortic root

catheter directed toward the left main. The distribution of the cusp calcifications should be assessed in order to locate, or at least hint at, where the valve opens. An orthogonal view helps to guide the catheter, especially in bicuspid valves. Aortography (contrast flow 15 mL/s, volume 20–30 mL, injection pressure 900–1000 psi) can come in handy in identifying the latter.

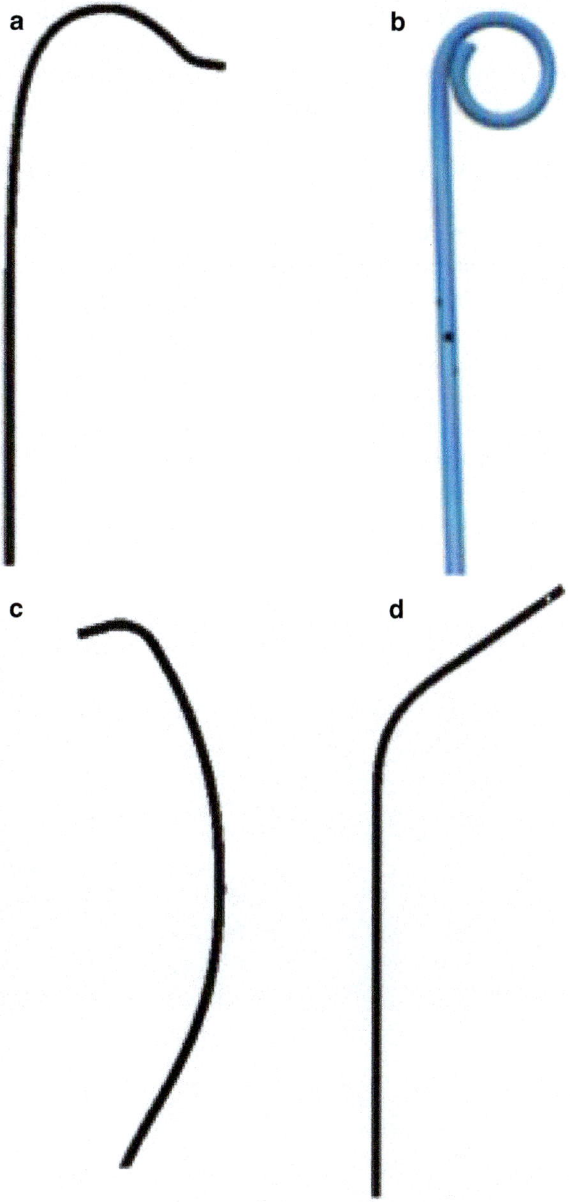

**Fig. 19.6** Catheters
commonly used to cross
the aortic valve; (**a**)
Amplatz Left curve 1 or 2;
(**b**) Pig tail catheter; (**c**)
Judkins right (JR) 6-Fr
catheter; (**d**) multi purpose
catheter (MP)

When the AL catheter and the straight-tipped guide wire are used, the catheter is then withdrawn slowly with the left hand by slightly rotating it clockwise so that the tip of the catheter is pointed to the center of the valvular plane, while the guide wire is advanced and pulled back in sequence for no more than 3 cm using the right hand, in order to probe the aortic plane until you manage to cross the orifice. The length of the soft tip can be adjusted, depending on the operator's choice or based on the grade of calcification of the valve. The straight guide with mobile core is used to adjust the system's stiffness and to change direction of the catheter.

Another technique for crossing the native aortic valve provides for positioning the catheter (AL, JR, or MP) at the level of the ascending aorta and using a straight-tipped hydrophilic wire, which is gently advanced and pulled back in sequence until crossing of the aortic valve.

When performing this maneuver, the operators need to be careful not to enter the left main with the guide wire and, also, not to puncture the cusps because this can lead to complications while delivering the prosthesis and to its under-expansion.

Once the AL catheter crosses through the valve and enters the left ventricle (LV), a right-anterior oblique view must be gained to follow the path of the catheter through the LV and to check for its optimal positioning, close to the apex of the ventricle, and to position the stiff guide wire. The change in view is intended to reduce the risk of injuring the LV free wall (Fig. 19.7).

In some cases, the AL can be trapped among mitral chordae tendineae; this is a suboptimal position, and it is suggested to either reposition the catheter or to recross the valve in order to avoid the chordae.

It is good practice to measure the LV pressure, once the catheter is inserted, both to confirm the transvalvular pressure gradient and to register protodiastolic and

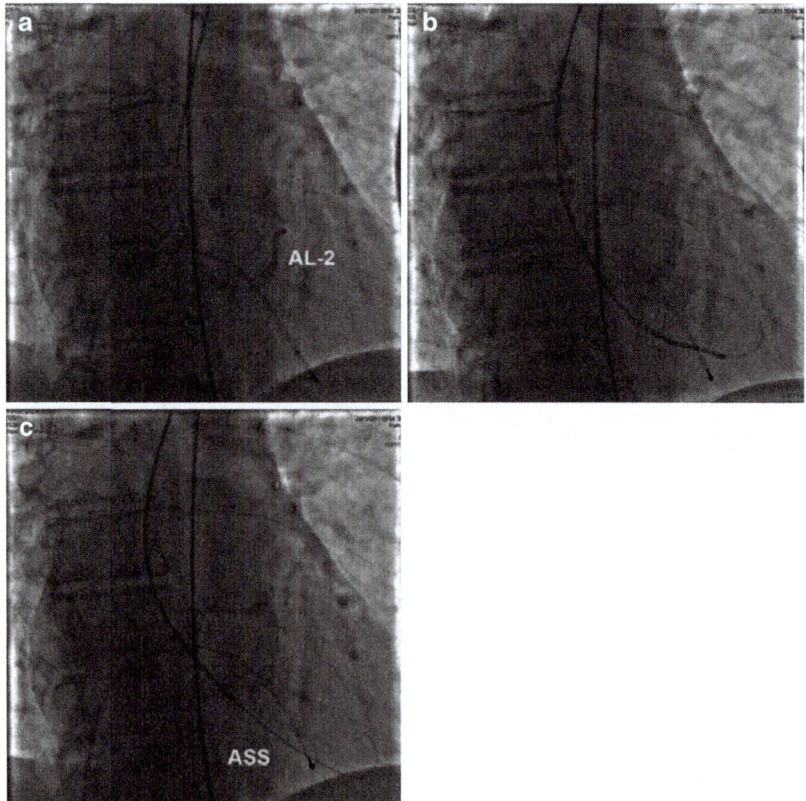

**Fig. 19.7** Fluoroscopy showing the placement of an Amplatz Super Stiff (ASS) guidewire with the 6-Fr Amplatz Left curve 2 (AL-2) catheter

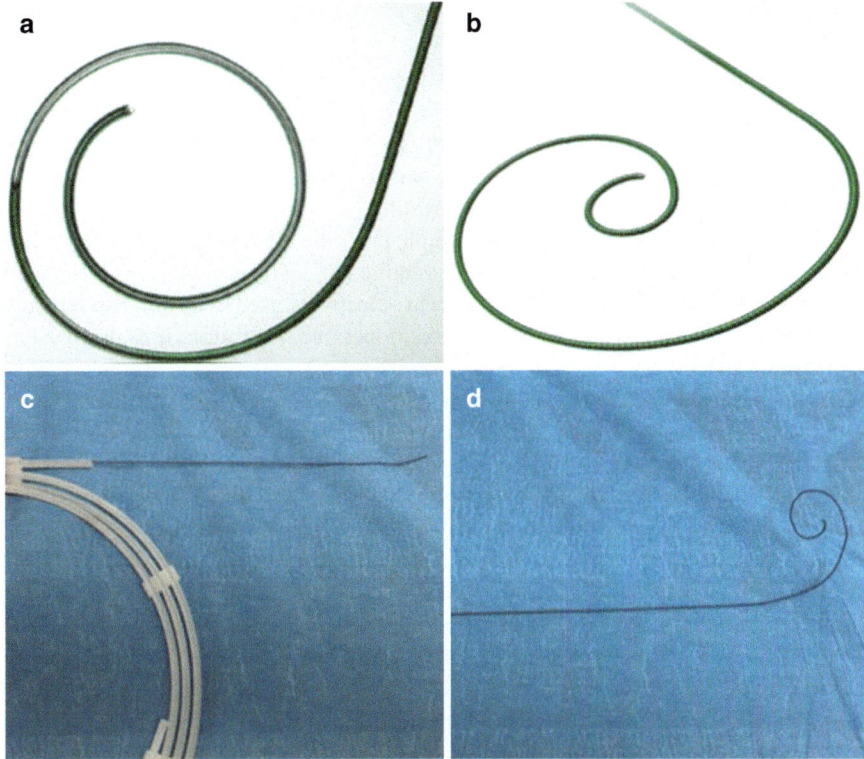

**Fig. 19.8** Most frequently used guidewires to cross the aortic valve; (**a**) Confida (Medtronic); (**b**) Safari (Boston Scinetific); (**c**) Amplatz Super Stiff (Boston Scinetific) straight tip or (**d**) with manually curved tip

telediastolic pressure of the LV. This information is important, especially compared with the transvalvular pressure at the end of the procedure, after valve release, to assess whether the implantation is hemodynamically effective.

When the Amplatz super stiff is used, a small curve is formed on the soft distal part (1 or 3 cm) of the guide wire; alternatively, the pre-shaped Safari™ (Boston Scientific) or Confida (Medtronic) (Fig. 19.8) can be used and is positioned at the apex of the LV.

In experienced hands, this step has a low incidence of complications; the most frequent are:

– Ventricular arrhythmias; these can be due to the mechanical stimulation by the catheter or the guide wire.
– Coronary artery dissection while probing the valvular plane with the straight-tipped or hydrophilic guide wire.
– Cardiac perforation, which can occur during the positioning of the guide wire in the LV.
– Cerebral embolization of calcium fragments; this can be a consequence of probing the valvular plane with the straight-tipped or hydrophilic guide wire.

## 19.6 Balloon Valvuloplasty

Percutaneous balloon valvuloplasty (BAV) was first described in 1984 by Lababidi and Neuhaus [4] and was reported for the treatment of congenital aortic stenosis (AS) in children and young adults. In 1986, Cribier was the first to perform BAV in adults with calcific AS [5]. The procedure was so successful so that it led to the birth of registries [6, 7] for the analysis of the results.

Aortic valvuloplasty proved to be a simple procedure, but with a high occurrence of restenosis at 6 and 12 months and with a limited effect on disease progression and survival [8, 9]. Therefore, this procedure was selectively used as a palliative remedy, in cases of patients with severe AS deemed inoperable. Nowadays it is also used as a bridge to TAVI.

Balloon dilatation creates a modest and temporary improvement of valvular function, symptoms, and outcomes. Aortic valve area increases by an average 0.3–0.4 cm$^2$ and results in a reduction of the average gradient of about 50% [8–10]. Early experience with this technique had a 30% rate of in-hospital complications and, though procedural mortality was only about 3%, mortality at 30 days was about 14% [9]. Most recent series have shown a reduction in acute mortality and complications. Ben-Dor et al. [11], in a cohort of 262 patients who underwent a total of 301 BAV procedures, found that serious adverse events occurred in 15.6% (47) of patients, intraprocedural death in 1.6% (5), stroke in 1.99% (6), coronary occlusion in 0.66% (2), severe aortic regurgitation (AR) in 1.3% (4), resuscitation/cardioversion in 1.6% (5), cardiac tamponade in 0.33% (1), and permanent pacemaker implantation in 0.99% (3).

At present, BAV is not considered the standard of care for AS, but, as mentioned, is increasingly being used in patients affected with degenerative valve disease that present with severe comorbidities and a severely impaired hemodynamic clinical picture as a bridge to surgical [12] or transcatheter valve replacement [13–17].

In patients with low flow-low gradient AS and low LV ejection fraction, BAV can also have a diagnostic/prognostic role in assessing improvement in LV function after the reduction of the transaortic gradient [15]. In patients with severe functional mitral regurgitation or pulmonary hypertension, BAV has the potential of reducing the degree of mitral regurgitation and pulmonary pressure with the possibility of improving procedural and short-term outcomes.

Based on the up-to-date data available, the best candidates for BAV are elderly patients, those with severe LV impairment, as a bridge to TAVI, extremely ill patients in whom even TAVI could be futile or an overtreatment, due to the short life expectancy.

## 19.7 Mechanism of Dilatation and Restenosis

BAV acts on calcific aortic valve and AS by increasing leaflet mobility and enlarging the valve orifice. The predominant mechanism of dilatation is the fracture of calcified nodules and elastic expansion of the aorta [18]. Other possible mechanisms include the separation of fused commissures in rheumatic valve disease and microfractures along stromal cleavage planes. Restenosis has been correlated, instead, with remodeling, with fibrotic scarring of the fissures created by the balloon on calcified nodules, with a mechanism of heterotopic ossification, and with the elastic rebound of the previously dilated aortic annulus. Histopathological studies have found the presence of immature scar tissue composed of fibroblasts, capillaries, and inflammatory infiltrate, inside small torn areas in the collagenous stroma or in fractures in calcified nodules [18–20].

## 19.8   Description of Procedure

The procedure can be performed using the retrograde or antegrade approach, with single- or double-balloon technique (the latter being less frequently used). The approach most commonly used is the retrograde, performed through the left or right femoral artery, in which a sheath is placed. The size of the sheath varies from 8 to 12 Fr, depending on the balloon used (Table 19.1, Fig. 19.9). The procedure

**Table 19.1** Most frequently used balloons for aortic balloon valvuloplasty and corresponding sheaths

| Balloon | Size (diameter in mm) | Length (mm) | Sheath diameter (Fr) |
|---|---|---|---|
| NuMED | 16 (pediatric) | 30–40–50–60 | 9 |
| NuCLEUS™ | 18 | 40 | 10 |
| | 20, 22, 25, and 28 | 40 | 12 |
| | 28 and 30 | 40 | 14 |
| | 22 and 25 | 50 | 12 |
| NuMED Tyshak II™ | 16 and 17 | All from 20 to 60 | 7 |
| | 18, 20, and 22 | All from 20 to 60 | 8 |
| | 23 and 25 | All from 20 to 60 | 9 |
| | 30 | All from 20 to 60 | 10 |
| NuMED Z-MED | 16 | 30, 40, and 60 | 7 |
| | 17 | 30 and 60 | 7 |
| | 18 | 20, 30, 40, and 60 | 10 |
| | 19 | 60 | 11 |
| | 20 and 22 | 30, 40, 50, 60, and 80 | 12 |
| | 23 | 20, 30, 40, and 50 | 12 |
| | 24 | 20, 40 | 12 |
| | 25 | 30, 40, 50, 60, and 80 | 12 |
| | 26 | 20, 30, and 40 | 12 |
| | 28 | 20, 30, and 40 | 12 |
| | 30 | 20, 30, 40, 60, and 80 | 14 |
| Edwards Lifesciences | 20, 23, and 25 | 40 | 12 |
| V8™ InterValve | 17, 19, 21, 23 mm at waist 22, 24, 25.5, 27.5 mm at bulbous segments | 66, 68, 70, and 70 respectively | 12 |
| True dilatation™ | 20 | 45 | 11 |
| Endotech | 22 and 24 | 45 | 12 |
| | 26 | 45 | 13 |
| Osypka VACS II | 16 and 17 | All from 30 to 60 mm | 7 |
| | 18, 20, and 22 | All from 30 to 60 mm | 8 |
| | 24 and 26 | All from 30 to 60 mm | 9 |
| | 28 and 30 | All from 30 to 60 mm | 10 |
| Cristal Balloon | 18 | 40 | 7 |
| | 20 | 45 | 7 |
| | 23 | 45 | 9 |
| | 25, 28, and 30 | 50 | 9 |

Fig. 19.9 Balloons used to perform aortic valvuloplasty. (**a**) NuMED NuCLEUS™; (**b**) NuMED Tyshak II™; (**c**) NuMED Z-MED™; (**d**) V8™ InterValve; (**e**) True dilatation™ Endotech; (**f**) Opsyka VACS II; (**g**) Cristal balloon

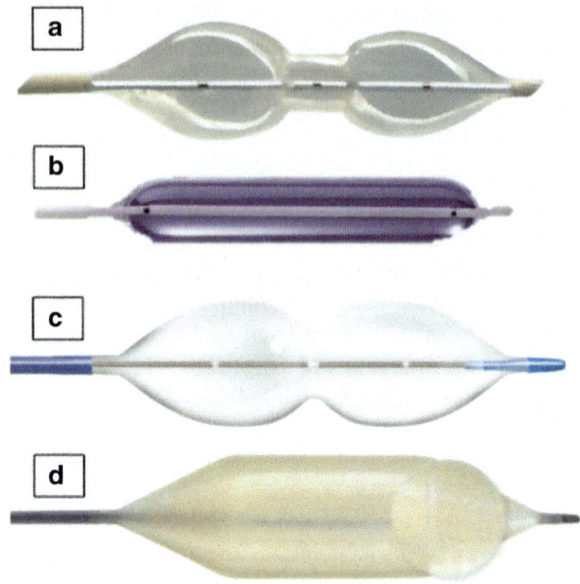

can be also performed without a sheath. After the sheath placement and the crossing of the valve (see section above), the stiff guide wire is placed in the LV, and the balloon is advanced and placed across the aortic valve, at the level of the aortic annulus.

The balloon size of choice is usually dependent on the native valve area and perimeter, which can be accurately calculated if an angio-CT scan is done, or can be approximately decided based on aortography (Table 1). When palliative BAV is performed, the size of the balloon is usually small (e.g., 18 mm diameter) in order to avoid possible complications such as severe aortic regurgitation or annulus rupture.

The balloon is then inflated, with a solution of normal saline water and contrast medium with a 4:1 ratio, and left inflated for a few seconds (3–5 s usually) in order to crush the cusps against the walls of the aorta (Fig. 19.10). When performing BAV during the TAVI procedure, it can be useful to inject some contrast medium (contrast flow 10 mL/s, volume 10 mL, injection pressure 400 psi) with a pigtail placed above the inflated balloon [21]. This can show if the balloon makes a perfect sealing or if there are leaks and in this case of what degree; this step can help to confirm once again the size of the prosthesis chosen (Fig. 19.11).

When performing the retrograde approach, which is the most frequently used, operators can encounter some difficulties, especially in crossing severely stenotic valves, and, though rarely, it can result in vascular complications at the insertion site of large-gauge catheters [9].

More recently, the use of an antegrade approach through femoral vein access has been described, even if the rate of performance of this technique is not high. In detail, after performing a standard transseptal puncture with a Brockenbrough

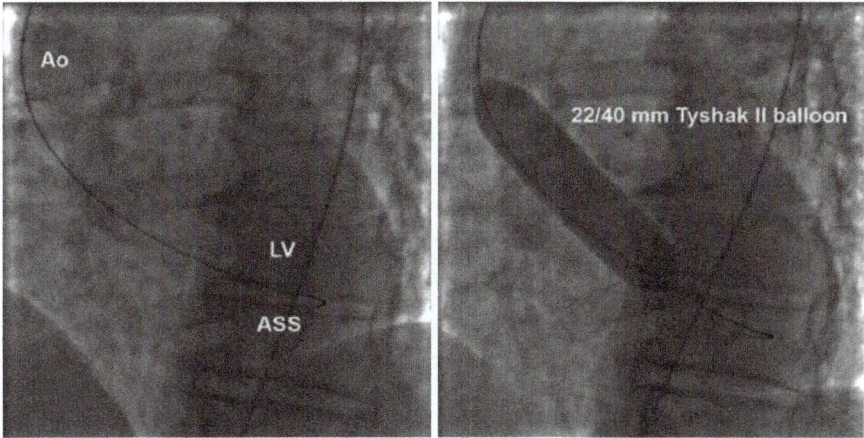

**Fig. 19.10** Standard aortic vslvuloplasty performed with low profile Tyshak II balloon (NuMed, Ca, USA) without right ventricular rapid pacing. *Ao* aorta; *LV* left ventricle; *ASS* Amplatz Super Stiff

**Fig. 19.11** Balloon aortic valvuloplasty with simultaneous aortography performed during rapid pacing

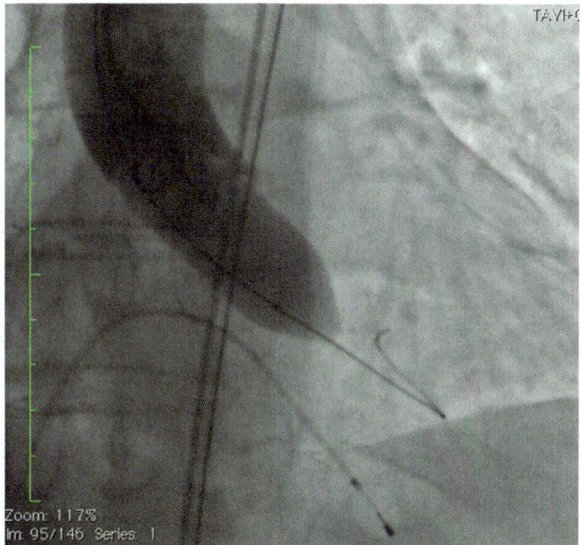

needle (St. Jude Medical, Sylmar, CA, USA) advanced through an 8 Fr catheter for transseptal approach, a floating balloon catheter is advanced in the left atrium, LV, and aorta, and a stiff guide wire is inserted until it reaches the descending aorta. Using a goose neck catheter (Amplatz Goose Neck Snare, ev3 Endovascular Inc., Plymouth, MN, USA) inserted though the right or left femoral artery, the guide wire in descending aorta is snared and pulled out on the arterial side to stabilize the system. The balloon is then advanced from the venous side, positioned at the calcific aortic valve, and inflated [18].

Antegrade BAV can be done with a conventional or Inoue balloon (Toray, Japan), which is typically used for mitral valvuloplasty, and is geometrically well suited for the anatomy of the aortic valve and sinuses of Valsalva. It also has a faster "inflation-deflation" kinetic compared with conventional balloons, thus reducing the risk of hemodynamic instability during the procedure. The antegrade approach is technically more complex, but has the considerable advantage of eliminating the arterial puncture in the large arteries, using larger balloons, allowing greater balloon stability, and reducing the risk of peripheral embolization [11, 18].

In order to obtain a more stable balloon position and prevent its movement during inflation, rapid pacing of the right ventricle can be performed at a frequency between 180 and 220 bpm during the balloon inflation phase. This is a very important step since ventricular systole, especially in patients with preserved contractile function, can lead to a rapid and uncontrollable movement of the balloon during its inflation if rapid pacing is not performed. High-frequency pacing drastically reduces LV stroke volume and allows to optimally and to stably position the balloon prior to its inflation. In doing so, smaller balloons can be used, thus reducing the time of "inflation-deflation" [18].

Potential complications of BAV are generally aortic regurgitation, in most cases mild, and the onset of ventricular arrhythmias, such as atrioventricular block or left bundle branch block. For this reason, in addition to technical reasons, the use of temporary pacemaker in the right ventricle is important during the procedure. Other serious complications include vascular access site lesions, cardiac perforation and tamponade, coronary artery dissection, cerebrovascular events and systemic embolization, and, most frequently when performing the retrograde approach, damage to the mitral valve [11–17].

## 19.9    Echocardiographic Guidance During TAVI

Echocardiography is an integral part of every aspect of the TAVI procedure. TEE can be used pre-procedurally for 3D annular sizing, as well as for the assessment of risk for complications. Intra-procedural TEE can assist in wire placement and heart valve position. Finally, the rapid assessment of cardiac and valvular function following implantation can improve response time in critical but treatable hemodynamic emergencies (Table 19.2).

Consensus papers and guidelines confirm these important aims of echocardiography. However, as TAVI has become standardized, with high procedural success and reduced complications, the focus has shifted toward a "minimalist" strategy, with conscious sedation and without routine use of intraprocedural TEE guidance [21–23]. The role of TEE, however, is not negligible.

The use of 3D TEE has significantly improved the accuracy of valve assessment, particularly the measurement of the aortic annular area and perimeter, as well as the coronary ostial height, helping in the prosthesis choice and size. This assessment is useful for all patients with kidney failure for which a CT evaluation is not available. Moreover, the assessment of the transcatheter heart valve landing zone (including the left ventricular outflow tract, the aortic annulus, aortic cusps, and sinuses of Valsalva, coronary ostia, and sinotubular junction) is extremely useful, particularly

**Table 19.2** Intraprocedural TEE recommendations

---

**THV choice and sizing**

- Improve the accuracy of valve assessment, particularly in patients with renal insufficiency for whom MDTC evaluation is not available
- Allow assessment of the THV landing zone, particularly in patients at risk for coronary occlusion or anulus rupture

---

**Wire placement (pacing wire and left ventricular stiff wire)**

- Guide the position of pacing wire in the right ventricle and ensure stable position of stiff wire in the apex without entanglement in mitral apparatus/worsening mitral regurgitation.
- Exclude perforation and pericardial effusion.

---

**BAV**

- Detect uncommon complications such as valve rupture and severe aortic regurgitation
- Predict coronary occlusion
- Size the annulus

---

**Positioning of THV**

- Confirm the ideal location within the aortic landing zone
- Rapid assessment of fully-repositionable THV position

---

**Post-implant assessment of THV**

- Assess THV positioning, shape, and leaflet motion; perform comprehensive hemodynamic measurement
- Assess paravalvular regurgitation relying on short-axis images of the LVOT just apical to the inflow edge of the THV (and gastric views for confirmation)
- Assess coronary artery patency and ventricular function
- Assess mitral valve morphology and function.
- Assess TR velocities and estimate pulmonary artery pressures.
- Exclude perforation and pericardial effusion.

---

**Continuous monitoring of all aspects of the procedure**

- Reduce contrast media use
- Consente la diagnosi immediata delle complicanze

---

**Optimal transapical cannulation site**

- Avoid right ventricular or interventricular septal perforation

---

| Complications of TAVR causing hemodynamic instability, assessed by TEE |
| --- |
| Severe transvalvular or paravalvular aortic regurgitation |
| Severe mitral regurgitation |
| Pericardial effusion and possible etiology |
| Aortic rupture or dissection |
| Complications related to BAV (severe AR, periaortic hematoma, aortic dissection, or rupture) |
| Ventricular dysfunction |
| Suicide ventricle |

for patients deemed at high risk of coronary occlusion and annulus rupture, in order to clarify the treatment plans or help the operator in the correct valve sizing in problematic cases.

Secondly, the significant advantage of real-time TEE imaging is the continuous monitoring of all aspects of the procedure. Instead of limiting procedural assessment to bursts of fluoroscopic visualization or injection of contrast, TEE allows a safe, continuous imaging of all cardiac structures, as well as the aorta. In cases without adequate radiographic imaging, TEE has been successfully used with equivalent short- and midterm outcomes, with reduced contrast media use.

Once the pre-implant assessment is complete, intra-procedural imaging of wire placement (pacing wire and left ventricular stiff wire) and balloon aortic valvuloplasty are also performed. Wire and cannulation position and complications can easily be evaluated, avoiding incorrect stiff wire placement in the left ventricle, which is responsible for acute mitral regurgitation or instability/mal-positioning of the THV. Ideal pacemaker tip location in the right ventricle should be confirmed. Excluding entanglement of wires in the mitral apparatus may prevent acute mitral regurgitation. Optimal transapical cannulation site should be routinely assessed (either from mid-esophageal views or transgastric views). Optimal position will avoid the right ventricle and be angulated away from the interventricular septum.

Imaging of the balloon aortic valvuloplasty procedure can rapidly detect uncommon complications, such as severe aortic regurgitation, but can also be used diagnostically to size the annulus or predict coronary occlusion. Checking valve position during the pacing run can be particularly useful in avoiding malpositioning of the valve.

During the percutaneous aortic valve implantation procedure, live 3D (narrow sector) can be useful in positioning the bioprosthesis across the annulus. The 2D TEE long-axis view (about 120°) is usually sufficient to guide proper placement of the percutaneous valve (figure), but at times the presence of severe calcification of the native valve and anterior mitral leaflet can be made for significant acoustic shadowing that interferes with precise echocardiographic visualization of the bioprosthesis, thus making it difficult to distinguish between the valve and balloon. However, live 3D imaging increases the field of view and frequently improves localization of the crimped valve margins within the aortic valve apparatus. The biplane orthogonal view (x-plane), which provides complementary 2D planes, can also be useful in monitoring valve positioning and deployment.

The commercially available self-expanding valve has in the past been performed under fluoroscopic guidance with little need for TEE assistance; however, the second-generation, fully repositionable valves can be most efficiently implanted using echocardiographic guidance. Because of the curvature of the aorta, the self-expanding valve will initially be non-coaxial with the long axis of the aorta, the tip pointing posteriorly and to the left. Because of the posterolateral orientation of the valve, when initial deployment begins, the posterior edge of the THV is "higher" (more aortic) than the anterior edge. Imaging should confirm that this edge is at least 4 mm (but typically not more than 10 mm) below the annulus for the first-generation valve and 3–5 mm below the annulus for the second-generation valve. As the valve is deployed, it will typically "pivot" on the posterior end, causing the anterior edge of the THV to move more superiorly; this is the justification for positioning the valve initially based on the location of this posterior THV edge. Because the second-generation valve is fully repositionable, a rapid assessment of position and paravalvular aortic regurgitation (PAR) can be made with TEE imaging. Moreover, valve positioning with the assistance of TEE imaging can reduce contrast load or fluoroscopic time.

Post-implant assessment of valve size, shape, and function can be performed rapidly using the orthogonal biplane view with color Doppler ultrasound, which provides a quick and accurate assessment of the final result, thanks to the simultaneous presence of a long-axis and short-axis view (Fig. 19.12).

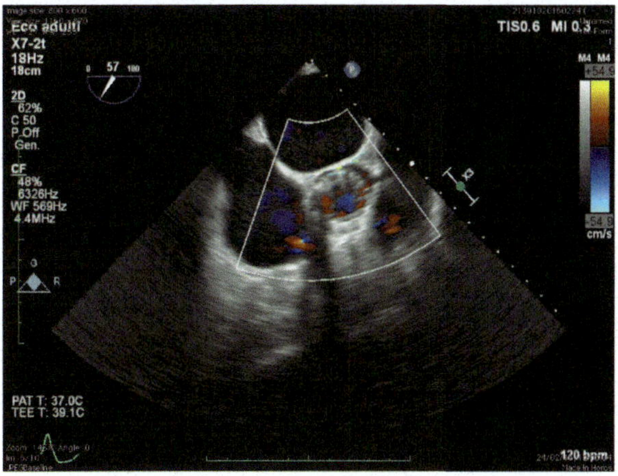

**Fig. 19.12** Post-TAVI prosthesis assessment of the paravalvular leak

Finally, the 3D color Doppler volume obtained from a deep gastric and/or mid-esophageal view enables direct planimetric determination of any regurgitant orifices in the case of residual aortic insufficiency. At the end of the procedure, it is also important to confirm that all the device cusps move well, that the valve stent has a circular shape derived from a proper expansion of the device, and that there is no interference with other adjacent structures, above all the anterior leaflet of the mitral valve.

When assessing for PAR using TEE, color Doppler evaluation should be performed just below the lower border of the transcatheter valve (within the left ventricular outflow tract) and should not be confused with flow within the sinus of Valsalva. The latter flow is frequently between the sinus and the native cusps and does not typically communicate with the ventricle. In addition, some paravalvular leaks fail to reach the left ventricular outflow tract because of the fabric skirt seal at the lower border of the THV. Central regurgitation should be evaluated at the coaptation point of the leaflets.

The causes of hemodynamic collapse, such as annular or ventricular rupture, severe aortic regurgitation, or many other intra-procedural complications (Table 19.2), can be diagnosed within seconds, allowing quick and likely lifesaving intervention, thus adding safety to the TAVR procedure.

## References

1. Kasel A, Cassese S, Leber A, von Scheidt W, Kastrati A. Fluoroscopy-guided aortic root imaging for TAVR-"follow the right cusp" rule. J Am Coll Cardiol Img. 2013;6:274–5.
2. Rabitsch E, Celedin S, Kau T, Illiasch H, Hausegger K. Flat-panel CT as a new perinterventional imaging modality in aortic stent graft procedures: work in progress. Rofo. 2008;180:127–33.
3. Nolker G, Asbach S, Gutleben KJ, Rittger H, Ritscher G, Brachmann J, Sinha AM. Image-integration of intraprocedural rotational angiography-based 3D reconstructions of left atrium

and pulmonary veins into electroanatomical mapping: accuracy of a novel modality in atrial fibrillation ablation. J Cardiovasc Electrophysiol. 2010;21:278–83.

4. Lababidi Z, Wu JR, Walls JT. Percutaneous balloon aortic valvuloplasty: results in 23 patients. Am J Cardiol. 1984;53:194–7.

5. Cribier A, Sasin T, Saondi N, et al. Percutaneous transluminal valvuloplasty of acquired aortic stenosis in elderly patients: an alternative of valve replacement? Lancet. 1986;1:63–7.

6. Samin M, Stella P, Agostoni P, Kluin J, Ramjankhan F, Budde R, Sieswerda G, Algeri E, van Belle C, Elkalioubie A, Juthier F, Belkacemi A, Bertrand M, Doevendans P, van Belle E. Automated 3D analysis of pre-procedural MDCT to predict annulus plane angulation and C-arm positioning: benefit on procedural outcome in patients referred for TAVR. JACC Cardiovasc Imaging. 2013;6:238–48.

7. Immè S, Attizzani GF, Sgroi C, et al. Pre-defining optimal C-arm position for TAVI with CT-scan using free software. Euro Intervention. 2013;9(7):878–9.

8. Otto CM, Mickel MC, Kennedy JW, et al. Three-year outcome after balloon aortic valvulo-plasty. Insights into prognosis of valvular aortic stenosis. Circulation. 1994;89:642–50.

9. NHLB Balloon Registry Partecipants. Percutaneous balloon aortic valvuloplasty. Acute and 30-day follow-up results in 674 patients from the NHLBI Balloon Valvuloplasty Registry. Circulation. 1991;84:2383–7.

10. Ragimtoola SH. Catheter balloon valvuloplasty for severe calcific aortic stenosis: a limited role. J Am Coll Cardiol. 1994;23:1076–8.

11. Ben-Dor I, Pichard AD, Salter LF, et al. Complications and outcome of balloon aortic valvulo-plasty in high-risk or inoperable patients. JACC Cardiovasc Interv. 2010;3:1150–6.

12. Johnson RG, Dhillon JS, Thurer RL, et al. Aortic valve operation after percutaneous aortic balloon valvuloplasty. Ann Thorac Surg. 1990;49:740–4.

13. Ussia GP, Capodanno D, Barbanti M, et al. Balloon aortic valvuloplasty for severe aortic stenosis as a bridge to high-risk transcatheter aortic valve implantation. J Invasive Cardiol. 2010;22:394–9.

14. Doguet F, Godin M, Lebreton G, et al. Aortic valve replacement after percutaneous valvulo-plasty—an approach in otherwise inoperable patients. Eur J Cardiothorac Surg. 2010;38:394–9.

15. Hamid T, Eichhofer J, Clarke B, et al. Aortic balloon valvuloplasty: is there still a role in high-risk patients in the era of percutaneous aortic valve replacement? J Interv Cardiol. 2010;23:358–61.

16. Tissot CM, Attias D, Himbert D, et al. Reappraisal of percutaneous aortic balloon aortic valvu-loplasty as a preliminary treatment strategy in the transcatheter aortic valve implantation era. EuroIntervention. 2011;7:49–56.

17. Saia F, Marrozzini C, Moretti C, et al. The role of percutaneous balloon aortic valvuloplasty as a bridge for transcatheter aortic valve implantation. EuroIntervention. 2011;7:723–9.

18. Baim DS. Grossman's cardiac catheterization, angiography and intervention. 7th ed. Philadelphia: Lippincott Williams and Wilnkins; 2006.

19. Safian RD, Mandell VS, Thurer RE, et al. Post-mortem and intra-operative balloon valvulo-plasty of calcific aortic stenosis in elderly patients: mechanism of successful dilatation. J Am Coll Cardiol. 1987;9:665–70.

20. Pedersen WR, Van Tassel RA, Pierce TA, et al. Radiation following percutaneous balloon aortic valvuloplasty to prevent restenosis (RADAR pilot trial). Catheter Cardiovasc Interv. 2006;68:183–92.

21. Barbanti M, Sgroi C, Immè S, et al. Usefulness of contrast injection during balloon aortic valvuloplasty before transcatheter aortic valve replacement: a pilot study. Eurointervention. 2014;10:241–7.

22. Barbanti M, Capranzano P, Ohno Y, et al. Early discharge after transfemoral transcatheter aortic valve implantation. Heart. 2015;101:1485–90.

23. Barbanti M, Todaro D, Costa G, et al. Optimized screening of coronary artery disease with invasive coronary angiography and ad hoc percutaneous coronary intervention during transcatheter aortic valve replacement. Circ Cardiovasc Interv. 2017;10(8). pii: e005234. doi: 10.1161/CIRCINTERVENTIONS.117.005234.

# Transcatheter Aortic Valve Implantation: Edwards SAPIEN 3

# 20

Marco Barbanti, Martina Patanè, and Ketty La Spina

## 20.1 Introduction

Transcatheter aortic valve implantation (TAVI) has been accepted as a treatment option for symptomatic severe aortic stenosis in inoperable patients [1, 2] and a reasonable alternative to conventional surgical aortic valve replacement in intermediate and high surgical risk patients [3–7]. After the first in-human TAVI more than 10 years ago [8], this technology continues to be developed and refined. One of the latest generations of the transcatheter heart valve (THV) is the Edwards SAPIEN 3 (Edwards Lifesciences, Irvine, CA, USA), a new balloon-expandable THV, which incorporates features to reduce vascular complications and paravalvular regurgitation (PVR) and to improve precise and easy positioning.

## 20.2 Evolution of Balloon-Expandable Transcatheter Heart Valves

The clinical experience with balloon-expandable T    he deployment balloon was incorporated in a deflectable  guiding catheter. Subsequent improvements in the valve and delivery system resulted in the second-generation balloon-expandable

M. Barbanti (✉) • K. La Spina
Ferrarotto Hospital, University of Catania, Catania, Italy
e-mail: mbarbanti83@gmail.com

M. Patanè
Centro Cuore Morgagni, Pedara (CT), Italy

© Springer International Publishing AG 2018
C. Tamburino et al. (eds.), *Percutaneous Treatment of Left Side Cardiac Valves*,
https://doi.org/10.1007/978-3-319-59620-4_20

THV, the Edwards SAPIEN THV (Edwards Lifesciences, Irvine, CA, USA) (Fig. 20.1). The stent remained basically unchanged, though the leaflets were made of bovine pericardial tissue, which is pretreated to decrease valve calcification. Moreover, the fabric skirt, which is made of polyethylene terephthalate (PET), extends further to improve sealing and potentially reduce PVR. Together with improvements in the valve design, several modifications were also made to the delivery systems, i.e., the tip of the balloon catheter (nose cone), the system profile, and controllability. The SAPIEN XT valve (Edwards Lifesciences, Irvine, CA, USA) is the third-generation balloon-expandable THV and also consists of treated bovine pericardial leaflets; however, the stent material was changed to cobalt-chromium (Fig. 20.1). Changes in the design as well as the materials have led to low-profile THVs, which further reduced the risk of vascular complications [9]. While the 23 mm and 26 mm Cribier-Edwards and Edwards SAPIEN valves required 22 Fr and 24 Fr sheaths, respectively, the SAPIEN XT valve is implanted via the trans-femoral approach using the NovaFlex delivery system (Edwards Lifesciences, Irvine, CA, USA), which is delivered through 16 Fr (20, 23 mm valves), 18 Fr (26 mm valve), or 20 Fr (29 mm valve) expandable sheaths (eSheath, Edwards Lifesciences).

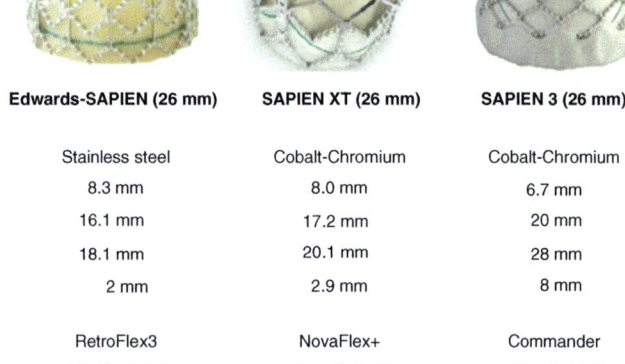

|  | Edwards-SAPIEN (26 mm) | SAPIEN XT (26 mm) | SAPIEN 3 (26 mm) |
|---|---|---|---|
| Prosthetic material | Stainless steel | Cobalt-Chromium | Cobalt-Chromium |
| Crimped profile | 8.3 mm | 8.0 mm | 6.7 mm |
| Frame height (expanded) | 16.1 mm | 17.2 mm | 20 mm |
| Frame height (crimped) | 18.1 mm | 20.1 mm | 28 mm |
| Frame shortening (deployment) | 2 mm | 2.9 mm | 8 mm |
| Delivery system | RetroFlex3 | NovaFlex+ | Commander |
| Sheath model | Retroflex 24 Fr | eSheath 18 Fr | eSheath 14 Fr |
| Recommended minimum artery diameter | 7 mm | 6.5 mm | 5.5 mm |
| Sheath ID (unexpanded) | 7.9 mm | 6 mm | 4.7 mm |
| Sheath OD (unexpanded) | 9.2 mm | 7.2 mm | 6 mm |
| Sheath OD (expanded) |  | 8.9 mm | 8 mm |

**Fig. 20.1** Comparison of the balloon-expandable 26 mm SAPIEN valves, the delivery system, and the sheath sizes. Edwards SAPIEN, SAPIEN XT, and SAPIEN 3 valves. *ID* internal diameter, *OD* outer diameter

## 20.3   SAPIEN 3

The S3 THV incorporates a unique stent and leaflet design that allows a further lower profile compared with the SAPIEN XT valve.

The device consists of seven components:

- Percutaneous aortic valve device (Fig. 20.2)
- Commander delivery system consisting of a flexible catheter (Fig. 20.3)
- Z-MED II balloon (NuMed, Inc., Hopkinton, New York, USA) (16 x 40 mm for the 20 mm devices, 20 × 40 mm for 23 mm devices, 23 × 40 mm for 26 mm devices, 25 × 40 mm for the 29 mm device) (Fig. 20.4)
- Two inflation devices (Fig. 20.5)
- 14/16 Fr eSheath introducer for the transfemoral approach (Fig. 20.6) and 18/21 Fr for the transapical and transaortic approaches
- Device loading system ("Crimper") (Fig. 20.7)
- Device protective sponge ("Qualcrimp") (Fig. 20.8)

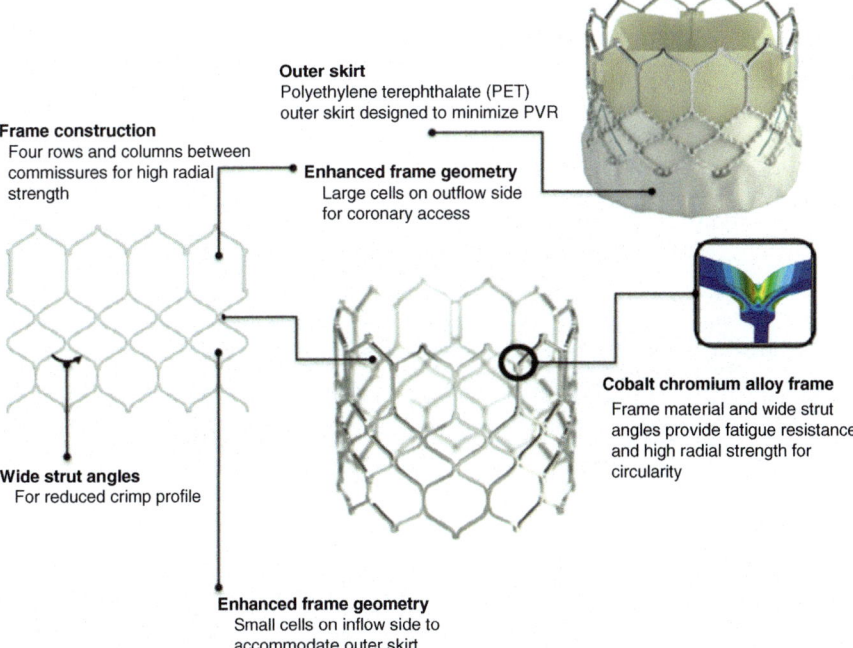

**Outer skirt**
Polyethylene terephthalate (PET) outer skirt designed to minimize PVR

**Frame construction**
Four rows and columns between commissures for high radial strength

**Enhanced frame geometry**
Large cells on outflow side for coronary access

**Cobalt chromium alloy frame**
Frame material and wide strut angles provide fatigue resistance and high radial strength for circularity

**Wide strut angles**
For reduced crimp profile

**Enhanced frame geometry**
Small cells on inflow side to accommodate outer skirt

**Fig. 20.2** The SAPIEN 3 transcatheter heart valve and the frame design. The SAPIEN 3 (Edwards Lifesciences, Irvine, CA, USA) is composed of a trileaflet bovine pericardial tissue valve with a balloon-expandable, radiopaque, cobalt-chromium frame, and inner and outer PET fabric. The inflow of the valve is covered by an outer PET cuff, which enhances paravalvular sealing. The cobalt-chromium alloy frame and wide strut angles provide fatigue resistance and high radial strength for circularity, while large cells on the outflow side make for easy coronary access

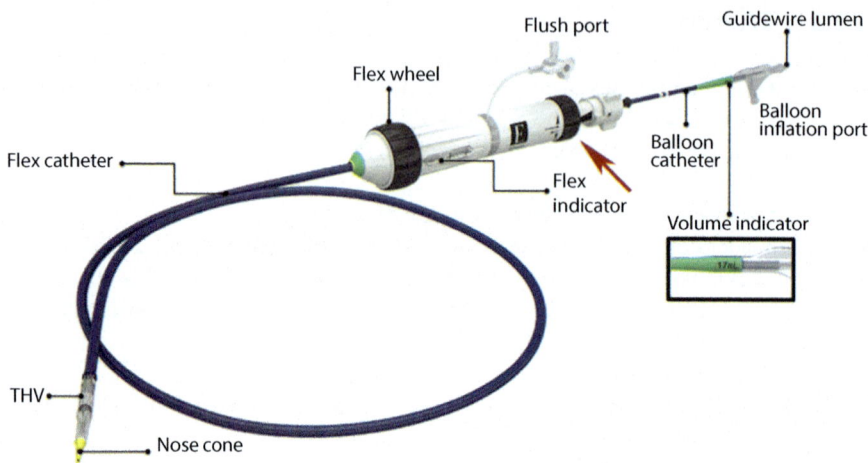

**Fig. 20.3** Features of the Commander delivery system: the handle contains a flexion indicator (rotating the blue wheel creates flexion), depicting to what degree or not the catheter is flexed, a fine adjustment wheel for fine adjustment of the transcatheter heart valve during valve alignment (black wheel) (*red arrow*), and a balloon lock knob (white wheel) to secure the balloon catheter to the flex catheter. Once the native valve is crossed, alignment of the crimped transcatheter valve in the aortic annulus is achieved by rotating the fine adjustment wheel at the back of the handle (*white arrows* on black wheel). Before deployment, the position of the valve can be precisely changed millimeter by millimeter more aortic or ventricular without having to push or pull the catheter

| THV Size | Edwards Balloon Catheter for Predilation | Guidewire Compatibility | Minimum eSheath Size | Nominal Volume | Rated Burst Pressure |
|---|---|---|---|---|---|
| 20 mm | 16 mm x 4 cm x 130 cm | 0.035" | 14 Fr | 10 mL | 6 atm |
| 23 mm | 20 mm x 4 cm x 130 cm | 0.035" | 14 Fr | 16 mL | 6 atm |
| 26 mm | 23 mm x 4 cm x 130 cm | 0.035" | 14 Fr | 21 mL | 6 atm |
| 29 mm | 25 mm x 4 cm x 130 cm | 0.035" | 16 Fr | 26 mL | 6 atm |

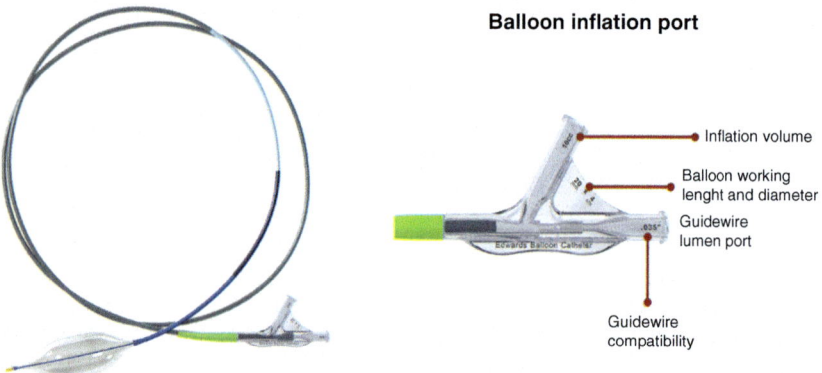

**Fig. 20.4** Z-MED II valvuloplasty balloon catheter for pre-dilation of the native stenotic valve

**Fig. 20.5** Atrion QL
inflation devices

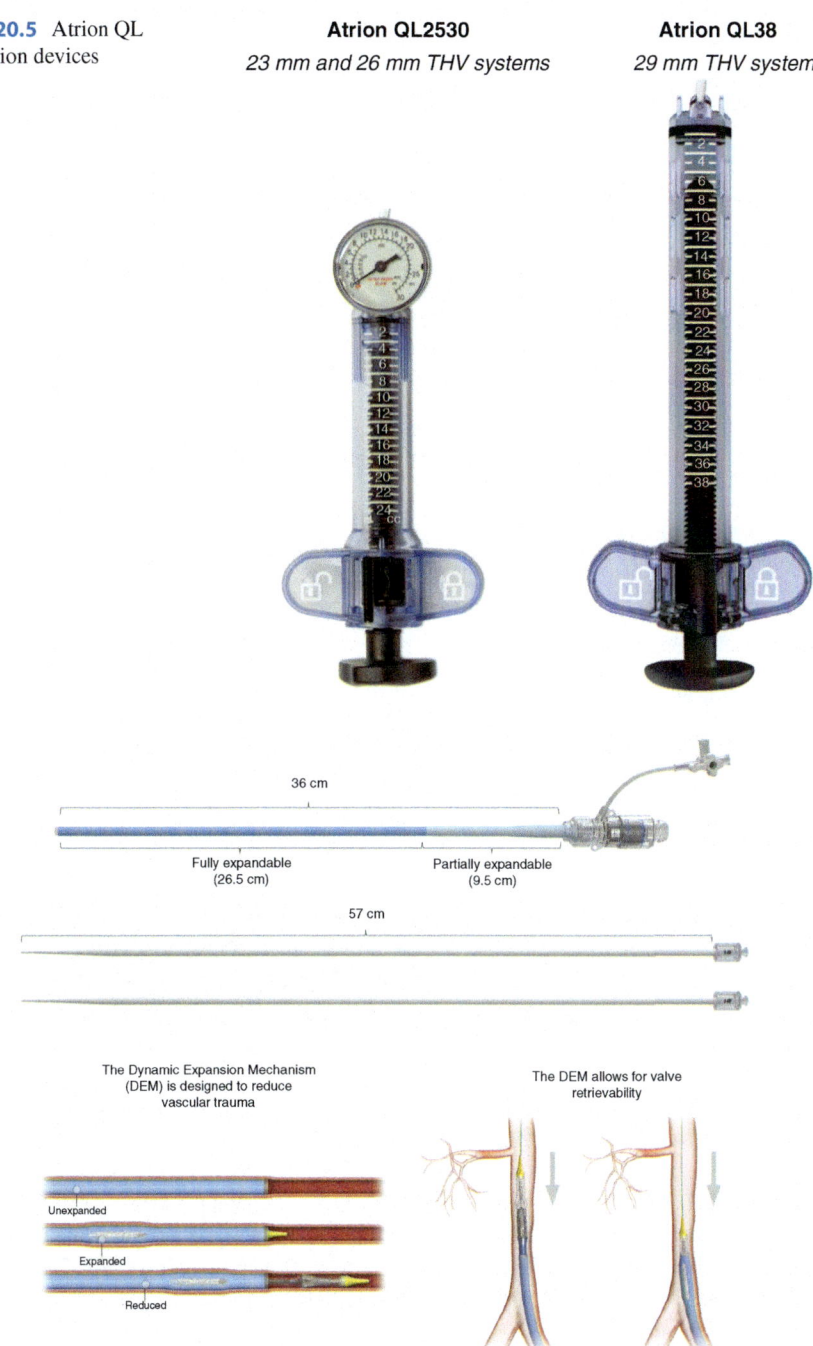

**Atrion QL2530**

*23 mm and 26 mm THV systems*

**Atrion QL38**

*29 mm THV system*

36 cm

Fully expandable
(26.5 cm)

Partially expandable
(9.5 cm)

57 cm

The Dynamic Expansion Mechanism
(DEM) is designed to reduce
vascular trauma

The DEM allows for valve
retrievability

Unexpanded

Expanded

Reduced

**Fig. 20.6** Edwards eSheath introducer set. For 20, 23 and 26 mm THV, no color coding for 14 Fr eSheath. For 29 mm THV, 16 Fr eSheath is color coded either green or no color. Sheath sizes are labeled on the sheath handle. The dynamic expansion mechanism (DEM) is designed to reduce vascular trauma, allowing for transient sheath expansion during delivery system passage and reducing the time the access vessel is expanded

Crimp stopper                                    Crimper

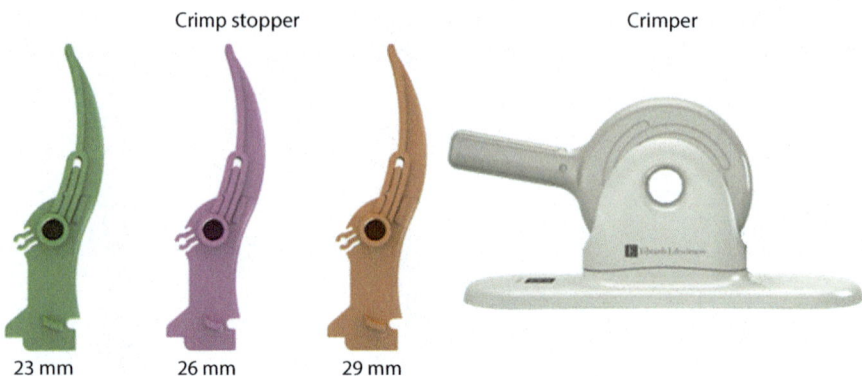

23 mm              26 mm              29 mm

**Fig. 20.7** Crimper system: the Crimper is the same for all THV sizes and is packaged separately. Color-coded two-piece crimp stopper is used during crimping and is packaged with the delivery system

**Fig. 20.8** The Qualcrimp crimping accessory is designed to protect the THV leaflets when crimping to a low profile, and is packaged with the delivery system

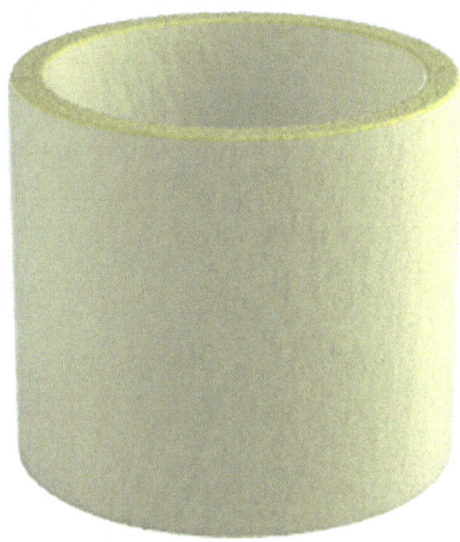

## 20.4 Transcatheter Heart Valve

Compared with the previous generation SAPIEN XT, the design of the SAPIEN 3 frame has been modified to enhance the geometry for ultralow delivery profile while maintaining the high radial strength for circularity and optimal hemodynamics (Fig. 20.2).

The frame has large cells on the outflow side for coronary access and small cells on the inflow side.

The height of the SAPIEN 3 valves is 3–4 mm longer than previous generation balloon-expandable valves; the 23, 26, and 29 mm SAPIEN 3 valves have expanded heights of 18, 20, and 22.5 mm, respectively (Table 20.1). As with earlier devices, the inflow of the SAPIEN 3 is covered by an internal PET skirt. In addition, the

**Table 20.1** SAPIEN 3 THV frame characteristics dimensions

|                   | 20 mm | 23 mm | 26 mm | 29 mm |
|-------------------|-------|-------|-------|-------|
| Tissue            | Bovine pericardium, ThermaFix tissue treatment | | | |
| Frame             | Cobalt-chromium alloy | | | |
| Crimped height    | 21    | 24.5  | 27    | 31    |
| Expanded height   | 15.5  | 18    | 20    | 22.5  |
| Foreshortening    | 5.5   | 6.5   | 7     | 8.5   |
| Inner skirt height | 7.9  | 9.3   | 10.2  | 11.6  |
| Outer skirt height | 5.2  | 6.6   | 7.0   | 8.1   |

outer one-third of the valve is covered by PET skirt in order to reduce PVR. Three sizes, 23, 26, and 29 mm, are currently available and are implanted via transfemoral, trans-subclavian, transapical, and transaortic approaches.

## 20.5   Delivery Systems

The transfemoral Commander delivery system (Edwards Lifesciences), which is advanced through 14 Fr (20, 23 mm valves) and 16 Fr (29 mm valve) expandable eSheaths, incorporates a nose-cone-tipped inner balloon catheter on which the prosthesis is crimped and an outer deflectable flex catheter (Fig. 20.3). It has the following features:

1. Improved distal flexing which enables crossing the aortic valve in challenging anatomies and controlled coaxial alignment (Fig. 20.9)
2. Precise positioning of the THV within the native valve (Fig. 20.10)
3. Decreased tapered tip length compared to the SAPIEN XT system

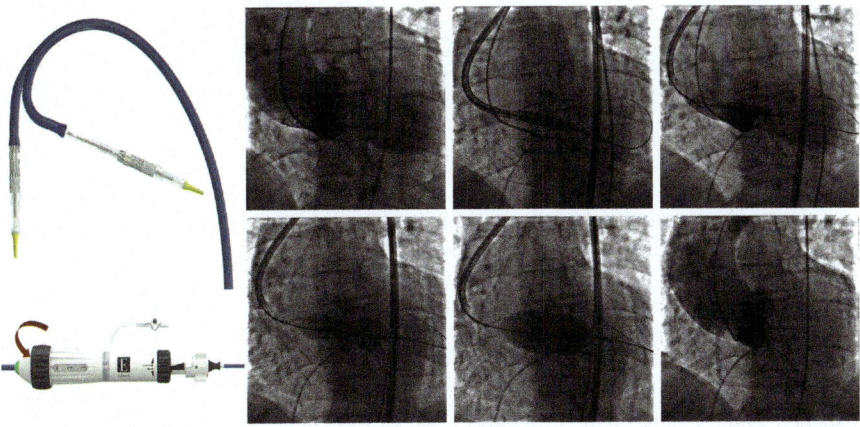

**Fig. 20.9** The Commander system ensures improved bending, thus allowing navigation, the crossing of the native aortic valve, and optimal alignment even in challenging anatomies. The panels on the left show an example of implantation of SAPIEN 3 26 mm prosthesis in a patient with horizontal aorta

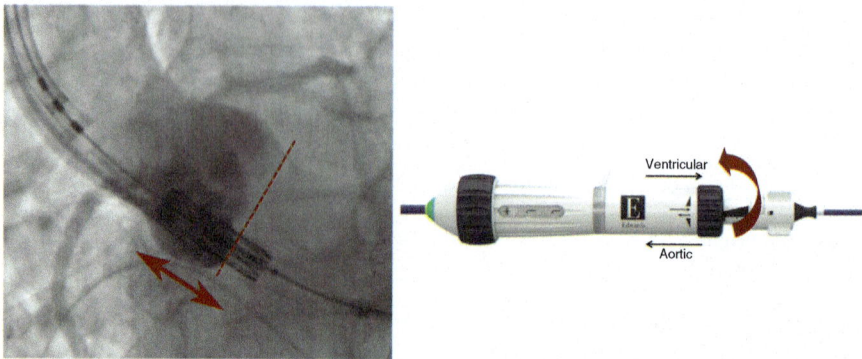

**Fig. 20.10** Rotating the fine alignment wheel allows the operator to advance or retract the balloon, which carries the valve several millimeters up or down within the annulus without pushing or pulling on the entire delivery system

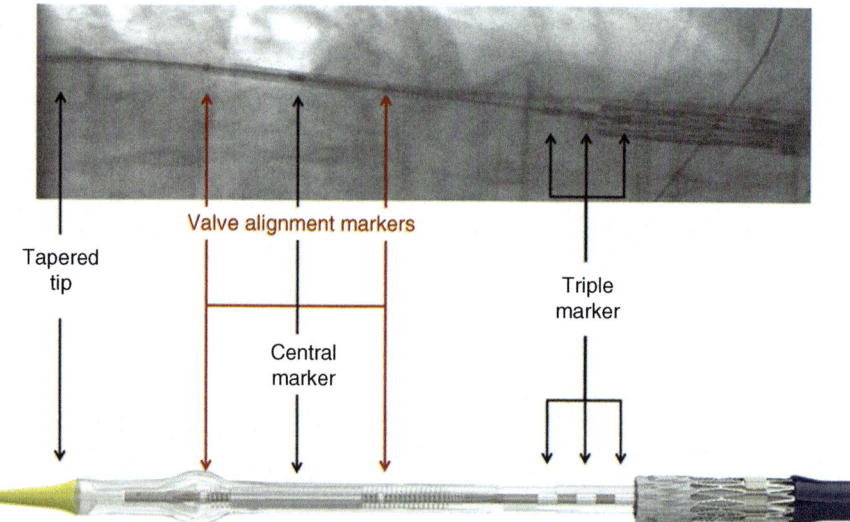

**Fig. 20.11** Fluoroscopic view of the Commander delivery system. The central radiopaque marker indicates the middle of the deployment balloon. The valve is flanked by two small markers, which assist in aligning the valve on the balloon. The three radiopaque markers (in a row) proximal to the valve indicate to where the flex catheter has to be pulled back to fully expose the deployment balloon

The balloon catheter has radiopaque valve alignment markers defining the valve position and the working length of the balloon. A central radiopaque marker in the balloon assists in valve positioning (Fig. 20.11). The outer deflectable flex catheter is attached to the handle, which includes a wheel to deflect the flex catheter tip, a flex indicator that shows the degree of tip flexion, a fine adjustment wheel for fine alignment of the THV during valve positioning, and a balloon lock knob to secure the balloon catheter to the flex catheter (Fig. 20.3). Rotating the fine alignment wheel allows the operator to advance or retract the balloon, which carries the valve several millimeters up or down within the annulus without pushing or pulling on the entire delivery system. The transapical/direct aortic Certitude (Edwards Lifesciences) delivery system has also been downsized to 18 Fr for 20, 23 and 26 mm valves and 21 Fr for a 29 mm valve.

## 20.6    Sizing of the SAPIEN 3

Paravalvular regurgitation (PVR) and aortic root injury are important complications during TAVI. Appropriate sizing of the THV is crucial to reduce the incidence of PVR, which has been shown to be associated with mortality [10, 11]. Multidetector computed tomography (MDCT) has been shown to be predictive of PVR due to its three-dimensional capabilities and better visualization of the noncircular annular geometry [12–14]. Indeed, integration of an MDCT annulus area sizing algorithm reduced PVR in patients who underwent TAVI with the SAPIEN XT in a prospective multicenter study [15].

The SAPIEN 3 THV is currently available with labeled diameters of 20, 23, 26, and 29 mm. When fully expanded with an appropriately sized balloon, these THVs have predicted diameters of 19.75, 22.75, 25.71, and 28.75 mm, with external valve areas of 314, 409, 519, and 649 mm$^2$, respectively (Fig. 20.5). Sizing recommendations were based on annular area measurements, with the percentage of oversizing (positive percentage) or undersizing (negative percentage) calculated using the formula: % oversizing = (THV nominal area/MDCT annular area − 1) × 100. It is important to select the appropriate size of THV based on the degree of oversizing since aggressive oversizing is strongly associated with an increased risk of aortic root rupture [16]. For the SAPIEN XT THV, 5–10% area oversizing was considered optimal; however, most patients would not meet this optimal zone due to the large increments among manufactured prosthesis sizes. Therefore, a range from 1 to 15% (20% in the absence of adverse root features, which includes more than minimal left ventricular outflow tract calcification, and shallow sinuses of Valsalva) was considered acceptable, with the integration of intentional balloon underfilling in those cases of calculated oversizing by area of more than 20% [17].

Because of the presence of the outer skirt, a lesser degree of area oversizing might be acceptable for the SAPIEN 3 THV than the previously recommended value for the SAPIEN XT THV (Table 20.1). This minimal area oversizing provides the great advantage of a lower risk of annulus injury, without an increased risk of PVR [18].

Looking at the sizing chart of the SAPIEN 3 THV, there are locations where two sizes are potentially indicated. In fact, either the smaller or the larger THV can be implanted (Table 20.2). In general, a larger THV should be preferred in consideration of better aortic valve orifice area. However, it may not always be possible to implant the larger THV size in borderline annulus diameters. In fact, the smaller THV size is recommended for borderline annulus diameters in special situations:

- Severe annulus calcification: use of a larger THV size can result in annular rupture.
- Left ventricular outflow tract and/or mitral annular calcification: use of a larger THV size can result in annular rupture.
- Narrow sinotubular junction: use of a larger THV size can result in ventricular shift of THV during deployment, or annular rupture.

**Table 20.2** Sizing guidance for the SAPIEN 3 transcatheter heart valve on the basis of 3-dimentional computed tomography measurements

| CT dimension | | | Area oversizing *% | | |
|---|---|---|---|---|---|
| | | | THV | | |
| 3D area-derived diameter (mm) | 3D annular area (mm²) | 20 mm | 23 mm | 26 mm | 29 mm |
| 18.0 | 254 | 29.1 | | | |
| 18.2 | 260 | 26.2 | | | |
| 18.5 | 270 | 21.5 | | | |
| 18.6 | 273 | 20.1 | | | |
| 18.9 | 280 | 17.1 | | | |
| 19.0 | 283 | 15.9 | | | |
| 19.2 | 290 | 13.1 | | | |
| 19.6 | 300 | 9.3 | | | |
| 19.9 | 310 | 5.8 | | | |
| 20.0 | 314 | 4.5 | 29.3 | | |
| 20.2 | 320 | 2.5 | 26.9 | | |
| 20.5 | 330 | −0.6 | 23.0 | | |
| 20.7 | 338 | −3.0 | 20.1 | | |
| 21.0 | 346 | −4.9 | 17.3 | | |
| 21.1 | 350 | −6.3 | 16.0 | | |
| 21.4 | 360 | −8.9 | 12.8 | | |
| 21.7 | 370 | | 9.7 | | |
| 22.0 | 380 | | 6.8 | | |
| 22.3 | 390 | | 4.1 | | |
| 22.6 | 400 | | 1.5 | 29.8 | |
| 22.8 | 410 | | −1.0 | 26.6 | |
| 23.0 | 415 | | −2.2 | 25.1 | |
| 23.1 | 420 | | −3.3 | 23.6 | |
| 23.4 | 430 | | −5.6 | 20.7 | |
| 23.7 | 440 | | −7.7 | 18.0 | |
| 23.9 | 450 | | −9.8 | 15.3 | |
| 24.0 | 452 | | | 14.8 | |
| 24.2 | 460 | | | 12.8 | |
| 24.5 | 470 | | | 10.4 | |
| 24.7 | 480 | | | 8.1 | |
| 25.0 | 490 | | | 5.9 | |
| 25.2 | 500 | | | 3.8 | 29.8 |
| 25.5 | 510 | | | 1.8 | 27.3 |
| 25.7 | 520 | | | −0.2 | 24.8 |
| 26.0 | 530 | | | −2.1 | 22.5 |
| 26.2 | 540 | | | −3.9 | 20.2 |
| 26.4 | 546 | | | −4.9 | 18.9 |
| 26.5 | 550 | | | −5.6 | 18.0 |
| 26.7 | 560 | | | −7.3 | 15.9 |
| 26.9 | 570 | | | −8.9 | 13.9 |
| 27.2 | 580 | | | | 11.9 |
| 27.4 | 590 | | | | 10.0 |
| 27.6 | 600 | | | | 8.2 |
| 27.9 | 610 | | | | 6.4 |
| 28.0 | 615 | | | | 5.5 |
| 28.1 | 620 | | | | 4.7 |
| 28.3 | 630 | | | | 3.0 |
| 28.5 | 640 | | | | 1.4 |
| 28.8 | 650 | | | | −0.2 |
| 29.0 | 660 | | | | −1.7 |
| 29.2 | 670 | | | | −3.1 |

**Table 20.2** (continued)

| | | | Area oversizing *% | | |
|---|---|---|---|---|---|
| CT dimension | | | THV | | |
| 3D area-derived diameter (mm) | 3D annular area (mm²) | 20 mm | 23 mm | 26 mm | 29 mm |
| 29.4 | 680 | | | | −4.6 |
| 29.5 | 683 | | | | −5.0 |
| 29.6 | 690 | | | | −5.9 |
| 29.9 | 700 | | | | −7.3 |

The percentage of over or under sizing can be determined based on a known annulus area. The recommended ranges for individual valves are highlighted. *% annular area over (+) or under (−) sizing as estimated by computed tomography (CT)

- Porcelain aorta: use of a larger THV size can result in aortic rupture of dissection.
- Narrow root and low coronary ostia: use of a larger THV size can impair coronary flow obstruction.
- Bulky leaflet and low coronary ostia: use of a larger THV size can impair coronary flow or obstruction.

Finally, it should be emphasized that the technique of underfilling the balloon used to implant the SAPIEN XT is not advisable for the SAPIEN 3 device due to the asymmetrical expansion of the frame during implantation. Reduced frame expansion results in the failure of the ventricular portion of the device to shorten, with potential negative consequences in terms of valve performance, and the development of conduction disorders.

## 20.7   Procedural Overview

### 20.7.1 Transfemoral Approach

The first steps of the TAVI procedure have been described in the previous chapters.

After valvuloplasty, the balloon is withdrawn and the Commander (in default position) is advanced with the device crimped on its distal end up into the descending aorta (Fig. 20.12). Under fluoroscopic guidance, the balloon, distally positioned and delimited by two radiopaque markers, is aligned inside the valve with two

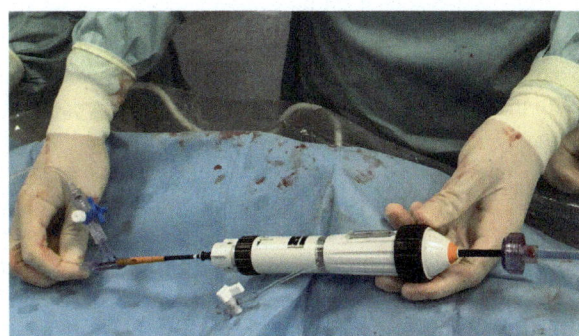

**Fig. 20.12** Framing of Commander delivery catheter after being inserted through the eSheath introducer

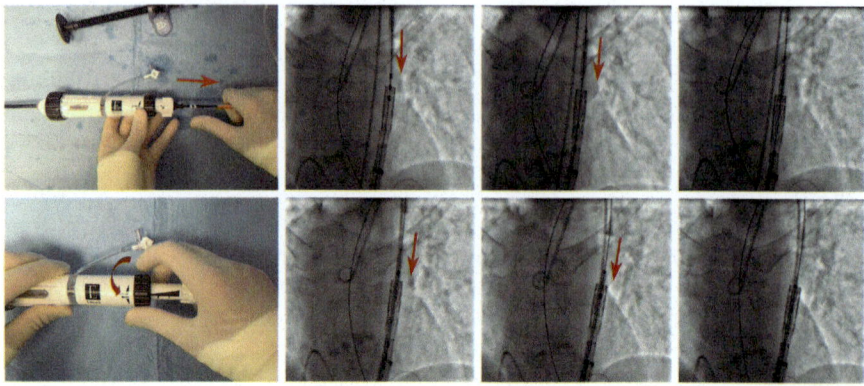

**Fig. 20.13** Maneuvers of balloon alignment inside the crimped prosthesis (see text for details)

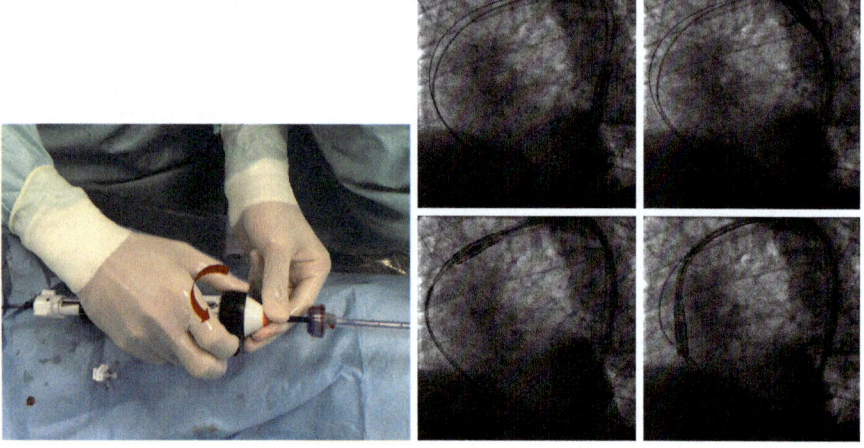

**Fig. 20.14** Pictures of the Commander delivery system while advancing through the aortic arch

maneuvers: withdrawing the shaft with the right hand while holding the delivery body with the left hand and ensuring that the stiff guidewire remains still into the left ventricle (Fig. 20.13) and then rotating the proximal knob of the delivery system to optimize alignment (fine tuning) (Fig. 20.13). Once this position is obtained, the Commander is advanced through the aortic arch by flexing it with the distal knob and placed on the aortic annulus (Fig. 20.14). Under fluoroscopic guidance, while holding the position of the shaft with the right hand, the Commander is withdrawn with the left hand to the right until the catheter reaches the two radiopaque markers (Fig. 20.15). At this point the device is placed at the right height and oriented orthogonally to the valve plane. By means of very short pacing intervals (few seconds) and injections of contrast medium, it is possible to check that the entire system is stable before inflation and that pacing is effective.

Once satisfied with the position, it is possible to proceed with implantation in four quick steps (Fig. 20.16):

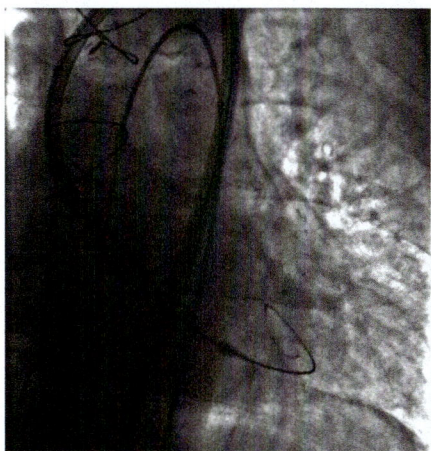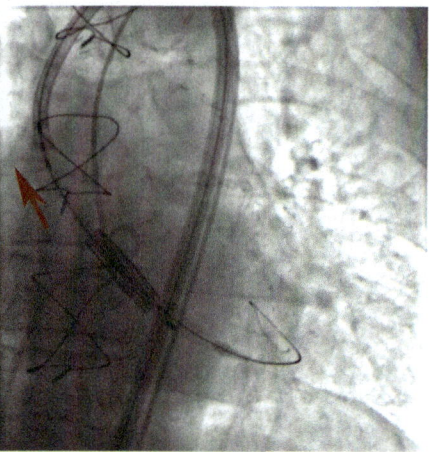

**Fig. 20.15** The Edwards SAPIEN 3 prosthesis is placed across the aortic annulus. And the flex catheter is pulled back to the middle of the triple marker. Particularly in patients with small ventricles, verify that the guidewire is properly looped in the ventricle prior to native valve crossing to avoid ventricular perforations. The stiff portion of the guidewire should extend beyond the distal end of the delivery system at all times

1. Pacing: typically 180–220 bpm, but in any case it must be sufficient to obtain a systolic pressure of <30 mmHg.
2. Angiography: makes it possible to check that the device is positioned correctly (central marker slightly above the annular plane). If the operator is not satisfied the height, it can be finely adjusted by rotating (clockwise or counterclockwise) the tuning knob (Fig. 20.10).
3. Inflation: the balloon should be inflated gently and progressively, injecting the entire volume present in the inflation device; the balloon is kept inflated for 5 s (Fig. 20.16b–e).
4. Deflation and end of pacing: the balloon is deflated and then, only once you are sure that it is completely deflated, pacing should be ended (Fig. 20.16f). It is important to point out that pacing must begin a few seconds before inflation and stop about 3 s after the balloon is completely deflated so as to minimize the risk of malpositioning. The Commander is removed from the left ventricle and realigned by returning it to the default position (Fig. 20.17).

## 20.7.2 Transapical Approach

If the arterial accesses are not deemed suitable (small vessels, major tortuosity, stenosis, or severe circumferential calcifications), the transcatheter apical approach is used. In this case, inserting the device requires the Certitude transapical delivery system (Edwards Lifesciences) (Fig. 20.18). The procedure is performed in the operating room with a beating heart, under general anesthesia and orotracheal intubation. The technique of the transapical approach has been detailed previously. Once the apex is pierced with a needle, and a soft guidewire is inserted and advanced through the native

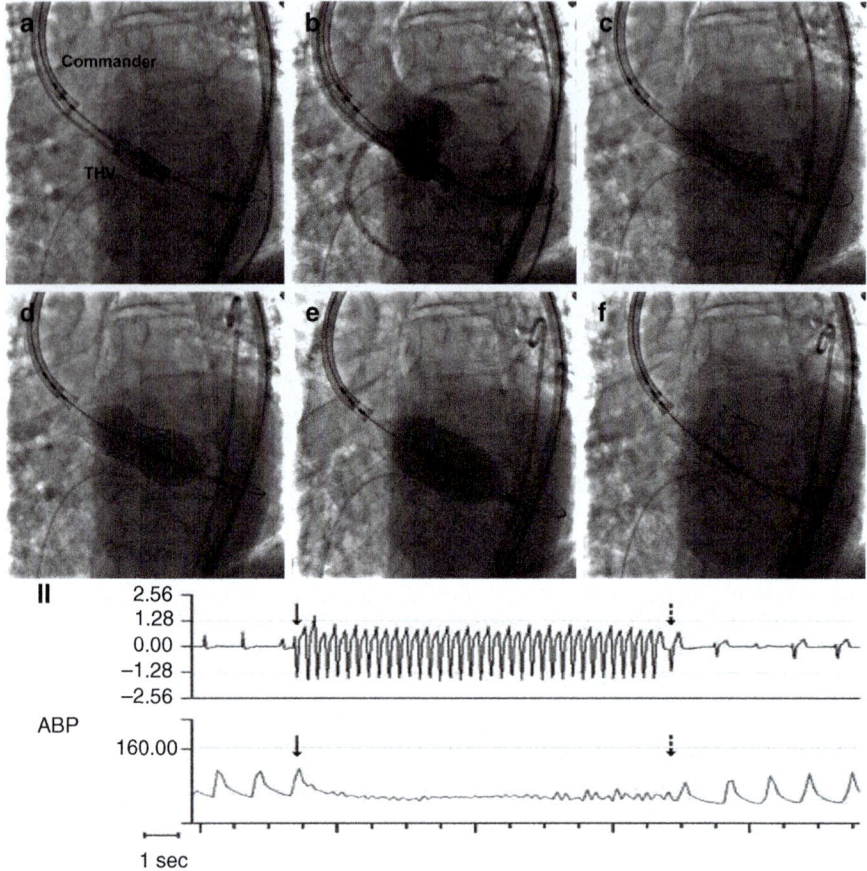

**Fig. 20.16** The balloon-mounted prosthetic valve is positioned adjacent to native valve calcification; position is checked with aortography; and under rapid pacing (180–220 bpm) the deployment balloon is inflated and deflated after 5 s. Pacing is then stopped once the balloon is completely deflated. *THV* transcatheter heart valve

aortic valve in the antegrade direction, a 7–8 Fr introducer is inserted through the aortic valve and then exchanged with a 260 cm × 0.035″ J-tip guidewire (Amplatz Super Stiff, Boston Scientific, Natick, MA), which is advanced through the aortic arch and into the descending aorta (Fig. 20.19b). The Edwards eSheath is then introduced (Fig. 20.19c). Depending on the size of the chosen valve (Z-Med II, Inc. Numed), a 16 × 40 mm, 20 × 40 mm, 23 × 40 mm, or 26 × 40 mm balloon is positioned over the stenotic valve. In this case as well, valvuloplasty is performed during pacing at 180–220 bpm; during the dilatation, blood pressure must be kept above 60 mmHg to avoid a hemodynamic worsening (valvuloplasty must not be performed if the pressure recorded before inflation is <100 mmHg). Once the balloon is withdrawn, the introducer is inserted and positioned 4–5 cm below the aortic annulus (Fig. 20.19d).

The prosthetic valve is then inserted and positioned through the annulus, and the pusher is withdrawn inside the introducer (Fig. 20.19e). Once the device is perfectly

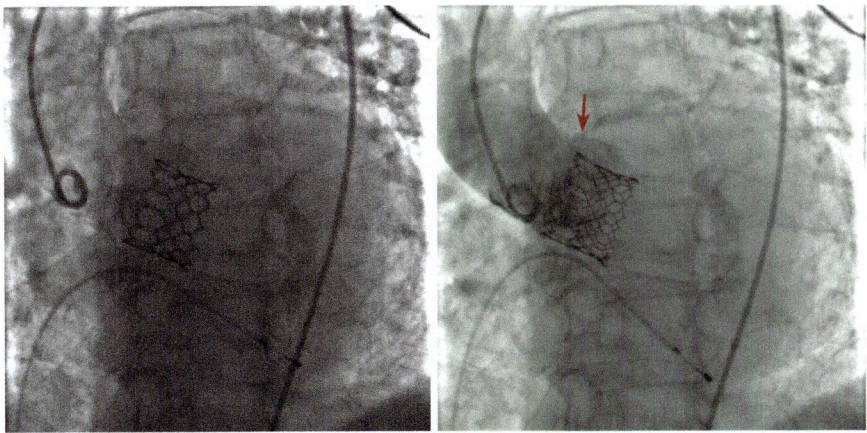

**Fig. 20.17** Angiographic check of the implantation height, aortic regurgitation, and patency of coronary ostia (*red arrow*)

**Fig. 20.18** Edwards Certitude transapical/ transaortic delivery system

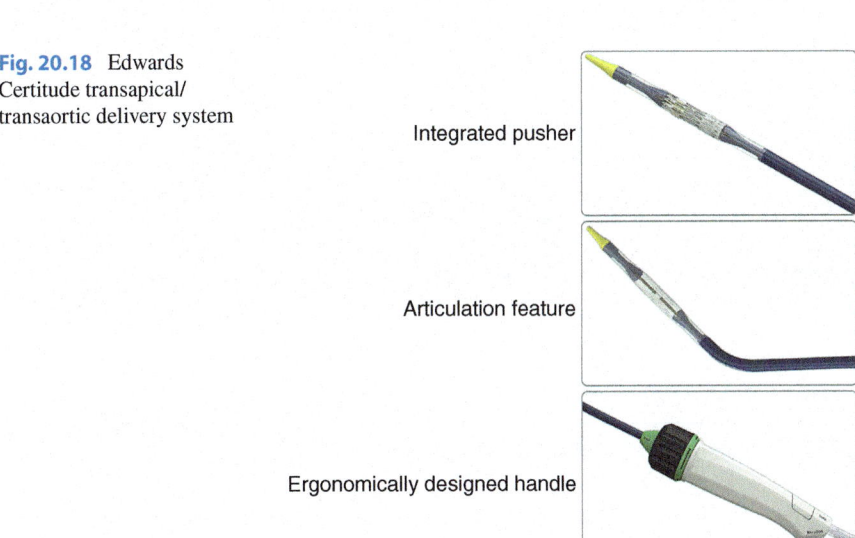

Integrated pusher

Articulation feature

Ergonomically designed handle

aligned, pacing and inflation of the balloon inside the device are done according to the technique described above (Fig. 20.19f–h). Once the device is implanted and the balloon is deflated, pacing is stopped, and the balloon withdrawn; aortography is usually performed to make sure that there are no periprosthetic leaks and that the coronary ostia are preserved (Fig. 20.19i).

Once the implantation procedure is completed, both the catheter and stiff guide-wire are withdrawn simultaneously. The apex is closed with the sutures previously implanted. Sometimes more sutures can be needed (usually for reinforcement in Teflon; Ethicon Inc.) to achieve complete hemostasis. Sutures are also applied to close the pericardium, and a drainage tube is positioned.

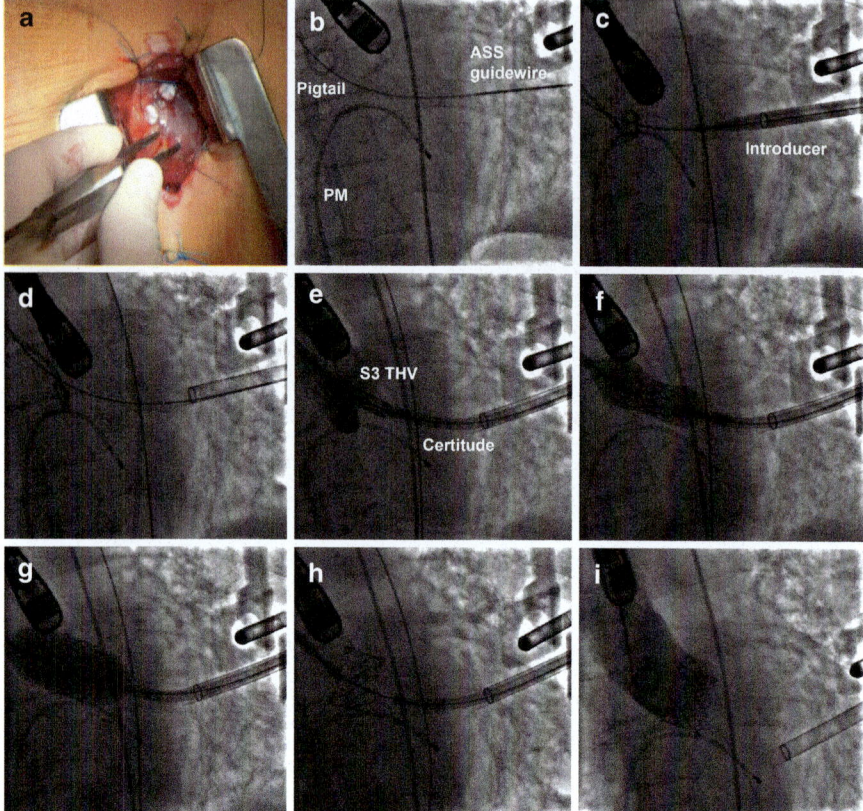

**Fig. 20.19** Example of the SAPIEN 3 transapical heart valve implantation

## 20.8    Procedural Details

In terms of implant technique, there are four main aspects of the SAPIEN 3 THV that should be underlined:

1. Pre-implant balloon dilation
2. Central marker positioning before THV deployment
3. The foreshortening of the frame
4. Balloon inflation technique

In the early years of TAVI, pre-dilation of the native aortic valve was a necessary step before implanting the device. This allowed crushing the calcified cusps to make the delivery system advance more easily and to obtain a better seal of the prosthetic valve. Today, an increasing number of operators prefer skipping this step. Considering the sharp reduction in the size of the crimped valve and of the release system, crossing the valve is no longer a challenge. When implanting the SAPIEN

3 valve, valvuloplasty is limited increasingly to those cases in which balloon sizing is needed (contrasting or unreliable CT or echocardiographic measurements) or in the case of extremely calcified valves in which difficult guidance of the delivery system through the aortic valve is expected [19].

At the beginning of the experience with the SAPIEN 3, it was suggested to proceed with valve deployment once this central marker has been aligned at the level of the annulus. This strategy usually resulted in around a 40/60 ventricular/aortic ratio. More recently, small modifications of the implantation technique have been adopted: indeed, before valve deployment, it is now indicated to place the bottom of the central marker of the crimped THV at the ideal line crossing the base of the cusps or slightly above, thus aiming at a higher implant (30/70 or 20/80 ventricular/aortic ratio) (Fig. 20.17 and 20.20). This new positioning guidance has been reported to further reduce the incidence of PVR and conduction disturbances [20].

As previously mentioned, the design of the SAPIEN 3 is asymmetrical, with large cells on the outflow side and small cells on the inflow side, in order to enable ultralow delivery profile. This particular frame conformation produces an asymmetrical shortening of the frame during implantation, which is much more pronounced at the ventricular side than the aortic side (Fig. 20.20).

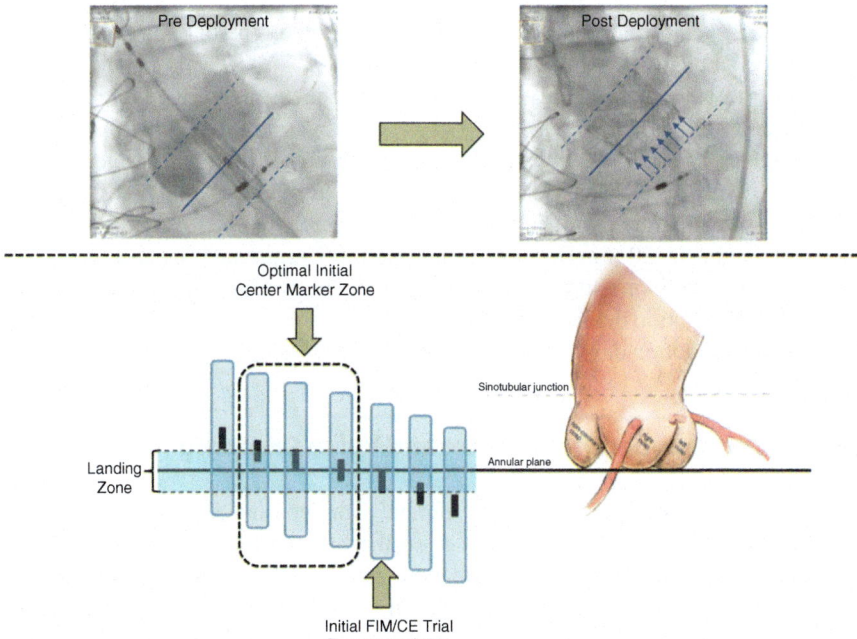

**Fig. 20.20** Edwards SAPIEN 3 valve foreshortening and recommended pre-deployment valve positioning. The upper panels depict the basal foreshortening of the SAPIEN 3 prosthesis after complete deployment (*blue arrows*). The lower figure represents the initial positioning guidance used in FIM & CE trial, based on SAPIEN XT experience and the current indication with the bottom of center marker position 1–3 mm higher than the base of cusps

Finally, balloon inflation has to be performed in a very slow and progressive manner in order to have a very stable system and predictable implant. Slow inflation has been established as the standard approach.

## 20.9    Device Preparation

It should be noted that the materials marked with the pink strip belong to the kit for the 20 mm valve, the green strip is part of the kit for the 23 mm valve, the purple strip is part of the kit for the 26 mm valve, while the orange strip is part of the kit for the 29 mm valve.

*Balloon Preparation*
1.  Flush the guidewire lumen with heparinized saline.
2.  Connect the inflation device filled with contrast mixture to the balloon valve and lumen.
3.  Fill the 50 mL Luer syringe with approximately 10 mL of contrast agent.
4.  Turn the valve to attach the syringe and balloon, excluding the inflation device.
5.  Draw air from the balloon by pulling the plunger to the end.
6.  Gently release the plunger in order to replace the air with the mixture.
7.  Eliminate the air trapped in the syringe and, if necessary, add contrast mixture.
8.  Repeat several times until air is no longer aspirated. The balloon is now properly debubbled.
9.  Turn the valve to exclude the balloon and connect the syringe and inflation device.
10. Eliminate any air in the inflation device by drawing it into the syringe.
11. If necessary, replenish the missing contrast mixture in the inflation device.
12. Once the inflation device is filled with the proper volume of contrast mixture (16 mL for the 20 mm balloon, 21 mL for the 23 mm balloon, and 61 mL for the 25 mm balloon), turn the valve to exclude the syringe, and connect the balloon and inflation device.
13. Lock the inflation device.

## 20.10  Commander Preparation and Valve Crimping

After thoroughly flushing the delivery lumen with heparinized saline, remove the "peel-away" balloon cover by pulling it on the blue portion of the catheter. The Commander is placed in the default position, and the proximal part of the loader is inserted from the distal end of the catheter. It must then be verified that the catheter's flex mechanism works properly. The balloon should be prepared following the same steps described for the valvuloplasty balloon; in this case, the 20 mm, 23 mm, 26 mm, and 29 mm device balloons should be filled with 11, 17, 23, and 33 mL, respectively, of saline and contrast medium mixture. In order to ensure that the system is debubbled well, the balloon can be inflated up to about 20% of its diameter, causing the bubbles to rise in its proximal portion, and then aspirated again. Once balloon preparation is completed, the device is then crimped. After rinsing the valve in three basins of nonheparinized saline solution (1 min per basin), crimp for the first time to reduce the diameter by about 20–30%. Place the valve in the Qualcrimp, ensuring to maintain the orientation (green stitching facing the ventricular side) and coaxiality, and perform a second crimping, by pushing the Crimper knob to the end. The Qualcrimp is removed, and other crimping operations are performed only when the operator is ready for implantation (the valve can be left completely crimped for no more than 15 min). Once the crimping phase is completed, the device is returned to the default position again, making sure that the catheter is in contact with the valve and that the valve is covered with the distal portion of the loader.

# References

1. Leon MB, Smith CR, Mack M, et al. Transcatheter aortic-valve implantation for aortic stenosis in patients who cannot undergo surgery. N Engl J Med. 2010;363:1597–607.
2. Makkar RR, Fontana GP, Jilaihawi H, et al. Transcatheter aortic-valve replacement for inoperable severe aortic stenosis. N Engl J Med. 2012;366:1696–704.
3. Smith CR, Leon MB, Mack MJ, et al. Transcatheter versus surgical aortic-valve replacement in high-risk patients. N Engl J Med. 2011;364:2187–98.
4. Barbanti M, Capranzano P, Ohno Y, et al. Early discharge after transfemoral transcatheter aortic valve implantation. Heart. 2015;101:1485–90.
5. Nishimura RA, Otto CM, Bonow RO, et al. 2014 AHA/ACC guideline for the management of patients with valvular heart disease: a report of the American College of Cardiology/American Heart Association Task Force on Practice Guidelines. Circulation. 2014;129:e521–643.
6. Tamburino C, Barbanti M, D'Errigo P, et al., OBSERVANT Research Group. 1-year outcomes after transfemoral transcatheter or surgical aortic valve replacement: results from the Italian observant study. J Am Coll Cardiol. 2015;66:804–12.
7. Leon MB, Smith CR, Mack MJ, et al., PARTNER 2 Investigators. Transcatheter or surgical aortic-valve replacement in intermediate-risk patients. N Engl J Med. 2016;374(17):1609–20.
8. Cribier A, Eltchaninoff H, Bash A, et al. Percutaneous transcatheter implantation of an aortic valve prosthesis for calcific aortic stenosis: first human case description. Circulation. 2002;106:3006–8.
9. Barbanti M, Binder RK, Freeman M, et al. Impact of low-profile sheaths on vascular complications during transfemoral transcatheter aortic valve replacement. EuroIntervention. 2013;9:929–35.
10. Hayashida K, Lefevre T, Chevalier B, et al. Impact of post-procedural aortic regurgitation on mortality after transcatheter aortic valve implantation. JACC Cardiovasc Interv. 2012;5:1247–56.
11. Kodali S, Pibarot P, Douglas PS, et al. Paravalvular regurgitation after transcatheter aortic valve replacement with the Edwards SAPIEN valve in the PARTNER trial: characterizing patients and impact on outcomes. Eur Heart J. 2015;36:449–56.
12. Hayashida K, Bouvier E, Lefevre T, et al. Impact of CT-guided valve sizing on postprocedural aortic regurgitation in transcatheter aortic valve implantation. EuroIntervention. 2012;8:546–55.
13. Jilaihawi H, Kashif M, Fontana G, et al. Cross-sectional computed tomographic assessment improves accuracy of aortic annular sizing for transcatheter aortic valve replacement and reduces the incidence of paravalvular aortic regurgitation. J Am Coll Cardiol. 2012;59:1275–86.
14. Willson AB, Webb JG, Labounty TM, et al. 3-Dimensional aortic annular assessment by multidetector computed tomography predicts moderate or severe paravalvular regurgitation after

transcatheter aortic valve replacement: a multicenter retrospective analysis. J Am Coll Cardiol. 2012;59:1287–94.

15. Binder RK, Webb JG, Willson AB, et al. The impact of integration of a multidetector computed tomography annulus area sizing algorithm on outcomes of transcatheter aortic valve replacement: a prospective, multicenter, controlled trial. J Am Coll Cardiol. 2013;62:431–8.

16. Barbanti M, Yang TH, Rodes Cabau J, et al. Anatomical and procedural features associated with aortic root rupture during balloon-expandable transcatheter aortic valve replacement. Circulation. 2013;128:244–53.

17. Barbanti M, Leipsic J, Binder R, et al. Underexpansion and ad hoc post-dilation in selected patients undergoing balloon-expandable transcatheter aortic valve replacement. J Am Coll Cardiol. 2014;63:976–81.

18. Yang TH, Webb JG, Blanke P, et al. Incidence and severity of paravalvular aortic regurgitation with multidetector computed tomography nominal area oversizing or undersizing after transcatheter heart valve replacement with the SAPIEN 3: a comparison with the SAPIEN XT. JACC Cardiovasc Interv. 2015;8:462–71.

19. Barbanti M, Sgroi C, Immè S, et al. Usefulness of contrast injection during balloon aortic valvuloplasty before transcatheter aortic valve replacement: a pilot study. EuroIntervention. 2014:10(2):241–7.

20. Barbanti M, Buccheri S, Rodés-Cabau J, et al. Transcatheter aortic valve replacement with new-generation devices: A systematic review and meta-analysis. Int J Cardiol. 2017;245:83–9.

# Transcatheter Aortic Valve Implantation: Medtronic CoreValve Evolut R

**21**

Sebastiano Immè, Denise Todaro, and Alessio La Manna

## 21.1 Characteristics of the Device vs. CoreValve®

The Evolut® R valve (Medtronic, Inc., Minneapolis, Minnesota, USA) represents the latest generation of Medtronic self-expanding aortic valve devices. It consists of a trileaflet valve made of porcine pericardial tissue and sutured in a supra-annular position on a compressible and self-expandable nitinol frame. The high radial force of the stent allows the self-expansion and the exclusion of native-calcified valve leaflets, which are pressed against the wall of the aortic root, while preventing the device from collapsing on itself (Fig. 21.1).

Over the years, the device has undergone several changes, which have increased efficiency and, at the same time, facilitated implantation. The first-generation device used bovine pericardial tissue and was implanted with the aid of 24 Fr guiding catheters [1]. The second generation of implants, consisting of porcine pericardial tissue, had a small profile so that they could be implanted using 21 Fr catheters and allow access through a vascular bed with a smaller diameter. Moreover, this device was characterized by a wider upper segment for more secure fastening to the wall of the ascending aorta to allow implantation even in patients with an ascending aortic diameter of over 45 mm. The implantation of this device was performed under general anesthesia, with extracorporeal support, using the retrograde approach. The third-generation device, the CoreValve ReValving System, further reduced the size of the guiding catheter to an 18 Fr device, allowing for a truly percutaneous approach for aortic valve replacement.

S. Immè, MD (✉)
Centro Cuore Morgagni, Pedara, CT, Italy
e-mail: sebastiano.imme@alice.it

D. Todaro, MD • A. La Manna, MD
Ferrarotto Hospital, University of Catania, Catania, Italy

© Springer International Publishing AG 2018
C. Tamburino et al. (eds.), *Percutaneous Treatment of Left Side Cardiac Valves*,
https://doi.org/10.1007/978-3-319-59620-4_21

**Fig. 21.1** The Evolut® R
valve (Medtronic, Inc.,
Minneapolis, Minnesota)

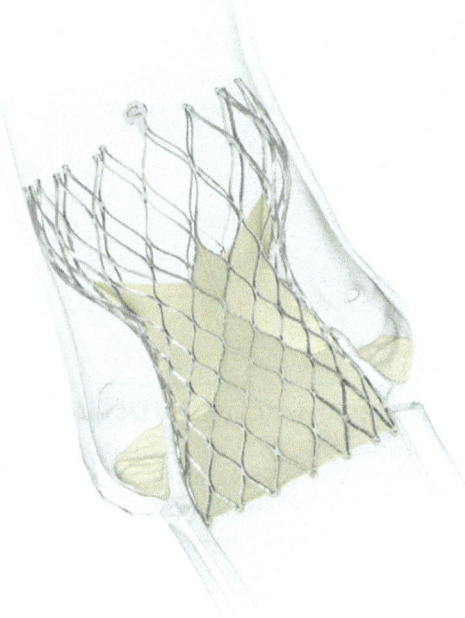

The introduction of the fourth-generation device, the Medtronic CoreValve Evolut R (Medtronic), provides several refinements to improve anatomical fit, annular sealing, and durability. In particular, the device is designed to enable recapturability and repositionability [2].

### 21.1.1  Transcatheter Valve

The Medtronic CoreValve Evolut R System is composed of the Evolut R valve and the EnVeo R Delivery Catheter System (DCS) with the InLine sheath (Fig. 21.2).

The trileaflet Evolut® R was created by suturing the three valve leaflets obtained from a single sheet of porcine pericardium, which is 50% thinner than bovine pericardium, on the Nitinol support, with the addition of a "skirt," which facilitates closure and is shaped to achieve better fluid dynamics.

The Evolut R frame is tailored to reduce the overall height, approximately 10% shorter than the original CoreValve® frame, while preserving the height of the pericardial skirt (12 mm) with an extended skirt of the inflow tract to provide a seal against

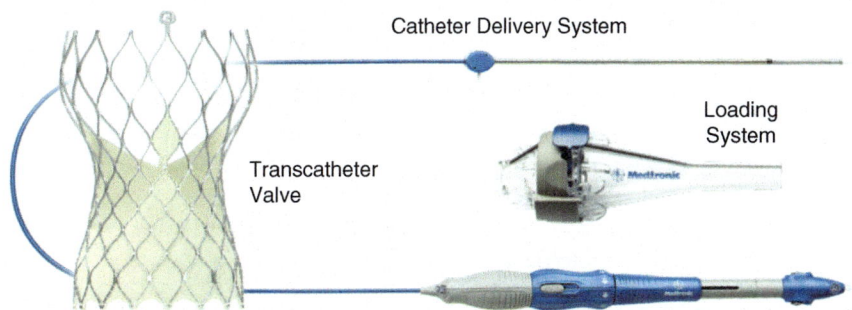

**Fig. 21.2** The Medtronic CoreValve® Evolut® R System (Medtronic, Inc., Minneapolis, Minnesota, USA): the Evolut R valve, the EnVeo R Delivery Catheter System (DCS), the InLine sheath

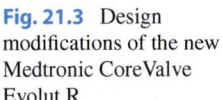

**Fig. 21.3** Design modifications of the new Medtronic CoreValve Evolut R

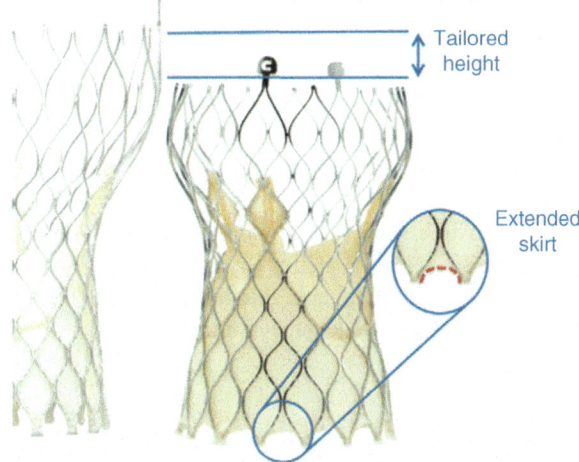

paravalvular leakage (Fig. 21.3). The shortened valve height is designed to optimize fit, particularly in angulated anatomy. The Evolut R maintains the cell geometry of the recent CoreValve prosthesis to optimize frame conformance to the native aortic annulus, especially in patients with noncircular or asymmetrically calcified annulus [2].

The self-expanding Nitinol stent with a diamond-shaped pattern has thermal memory characteristics, and its radiopacity allows the correct positioning of the bioprosthesis. Designed to have three levels of radial force, in particular in the left ventricular outflow tract, it allows the valve to adapt to the native annulus of the patient, to reduce paravalvular leaks, and to avoid the migration of the prosthesis.

The Evolut R valve maintains the supra-annular valve design of the CoreValve platform: the multilevel design of the stent allows intra-annular anchoring with supravalvular action to improve hemodynamic performance by maintaining leaflet functionality, which is not affected by the shape and size of the original annulus (Fig. 21.4). Furthermore, it delivers a constant radial force to mitigate the possible paravalvular regurgitation and to be the least invasive as possible on the conducting tissues.

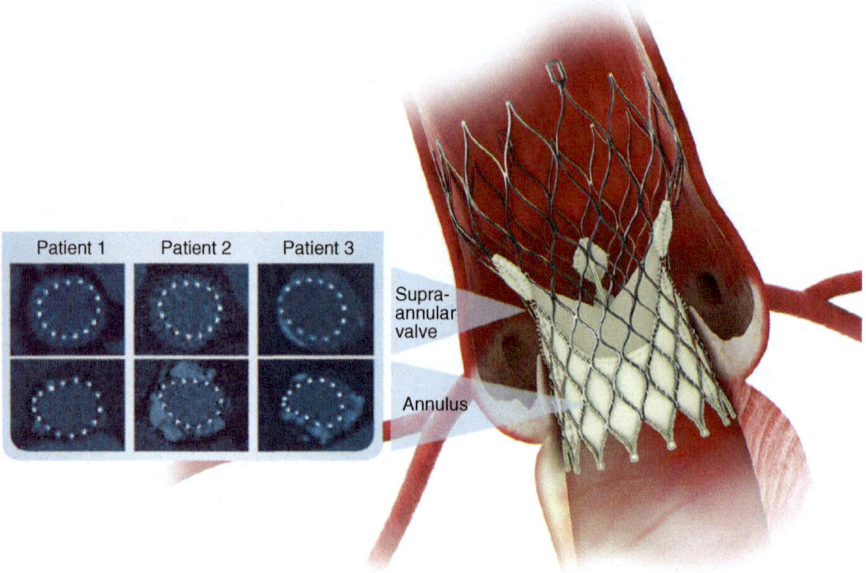

**Fig. 21.4** The supra-annular valve design of the Evolut R valve

The valve is fixed in a glutaraldehyde solution containing isopropyl acid. The bioprosthesis is also treated with alpha amino oleic acid, derived from oleic acid, a natural long-chain fatty acid that has an anticalcifying action that is able to reduce both early and late valve degeneration.

### 21.1.2 Delivery System

The Evolut R is delivered with the EnVeo R delivery system (Medtronic). This next-generation delivery system is designed to have a stable and predictable deployment, with proper implantation depth, and, especially when the valve is "flowering," will be more predictable through the EnVeo handle 1:1 response and an improved valve release mechanism.

The EnVeo R DCS with the InLine sheath enables the valve to be fully repositionable and recapturable before full deployment and allows for the whole system to be inserted into a patient without the need for a separate access sheath, reducing the overall profile of the system, equivalent to the outer diameter of a 14 Fr sheath, the lowest profile on the market for transarterial delivery. This improves access and reduces risk of major vascular complications. Furthermore, positioning accuracy is meant to reduce procedural complications, including reduced rates of paravalvular leak, valve malposition, and conduction disturbances [3, 4].

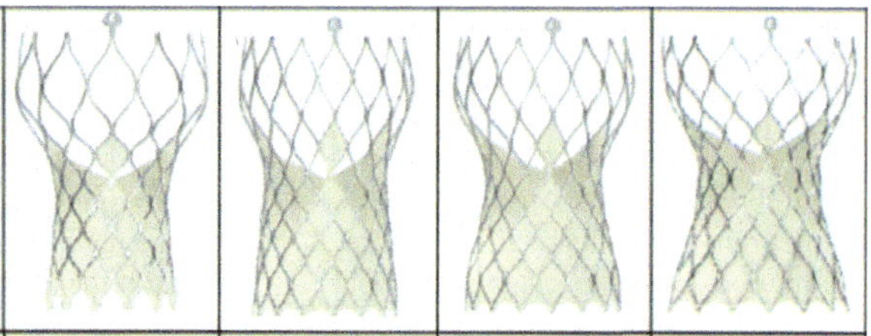

| Size | 23 mm | 26 mm | 29 mm | 34 mm |
|------|-------|-------|-------|-------|
| Annulus Diameter | 18 - 20 mm | 20 - 23 mm | 23 - 26 mm | 26 - 30 mm |
| Annulus Perimeter π x Diameter | 56.5 - 62.5 mm | 62.8 - 72.3 mm | 72.3 - 81.7 mm | 81.7 - 94.2 mm |
| Sinus of Valsalve (Mean) | ≥25 mm | ≥27 mm | ≥29 mm | ≥31 mm |
| SOV Height (Mean) | ≥15 mm | ≥15 mm | ≥15 mm | ≥16 mm |

**Fig. 21.5** Valve size selection

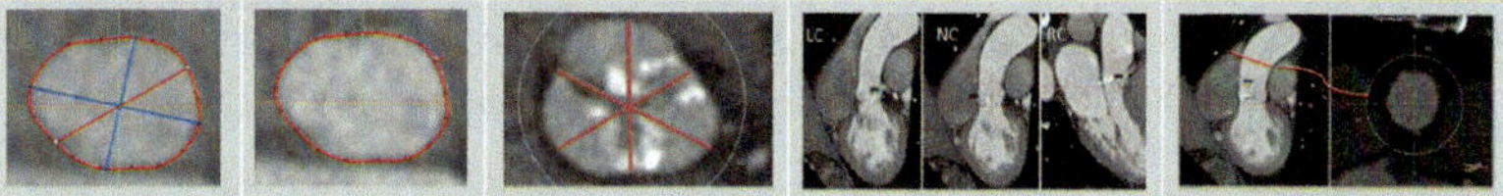

| | Aortic Annulus | | Sinus of Valsalva | | Ascending Aorta Diameter |
|--|----------------|--|-------------------|--|--------------------------|
| CT Image | | | | | |
| | Double oblique axial slice at the level of the nadirs of all 3 leaflets (aortic annulus plane) | Double oblique axial slice at the level of the nadirs of all 3 leaflets (aortic annulus plane) | Double-oblique axial slice at widest portion of the sinuses | Double-oblique axial image at aortic annulus: • LC & NC: oblique coronal image • RC: oblique sagittal image | Oblique coronal image at 30 mm from aortic annulus |
| Measure | Preferred: perimeter derived diameter Alternate: Calculated mean of major and minor diameters | Linear distance of tracing around the aortic annulus | Average Diameters from each commissure through the center to the opposite sinus | Average SoV height measured from annular plane to STJ | Maximum and orthogonal ascending aorta diameters on orthogonal image |

**Fig. 21.6** Multislice computed tomography anatomical measures

## 21.2 Patient Selection and Sizing

The CoreValve Evolut R prosthesis is available in four sizes: 23, 26, 29, and 34 mm (Fig. 21.5). In choosing the right bioprosthesis, a preliminary multislice computed tomography scan is recommended. It provides an accurate and reproducible assessment of the valve annulus (maximum and minimum diameter, perimeter), sinus of Valsalva, and minimum diameter of the vascular accesses. It also allows the operator to determine the angle of the aortic annulus in order to choose the most suitable vascular access (transfemoral, subclavian, or direct aortic) (Fig. 21.6, Table 21.1).

**Table 21.1** Access considerations

| Access consideration by MSCT | IFU guidance by MSCT |
|---|---|
| Minimum transarterial access vessel diameter | ≥5.0 mm (5.5 mm for Evolut R 34 mm) |
| Aortic root angulation, femoral access | Not recommended if >70° |
| Aortic root angulation, left subclavian | Not recommended if >70° |
| Aortic root angulation, right subclavian | Not recommended if >30° |
| Vascular access location, direct aortic access | Ascending aorta access site ≥60 mm from basal plane |

Specifically:

– Evolut R 23 mm is indicated in the case of an annulus with a perimeter ranging from 56.5 to 62.8 mm and sinuses of Valsalva with a mean diameter >25 mm.
– Evolut R 26 mm is indicated in the case of an annulus with a perimeter ranging from 62.8 to 72.3 mm and sinuses of Valsalva with a mean diameter >27 mm.
– Evolut R 29 mm is indicated in the case of an annulus with a perimeter ranging from 72.3 to 81.7 mm and sinuses of Valsalva with a mean diameter >29 mm.
– Evolut R 34 mm is indicated in the case of an annulus with a perimeter ranging from 81.7 to 94.2 mm and sinuses of Valsalva with a mean diameter >31 mm.

The height of the sinuses of Valsalva must be at least 15 mm (16 mm for the Evolut R 34 mm), and the minimum diameter of the vascular access must not be less than 5 mm (5.5 mm for the Evolut R 34 mm).

## 21.3  Evolut R System Loading Preparation

Once the right valve prosthesis has been chosen, it is possible to mount the valve on the delivery system, as instructed in the valve loading procedure [5].

The packaging of the delivery system can be used as a tray to mount the valve. The package also features a tray with three compartments for washing the prosthesis.

### 21.3.1  Step 1

By positioning the delivery system handle to the right, and removing the blue locking tabs that connect the distal to the proximal portion, the distal part of the tray can be rotated clockwise by 180° (Fig. 21.7a). During this operation, make sure that the stylet is fully inserted in the guidewire lumen of the nose cone (the stylet protects the catheter shaft within the capsule and must remain in the delivery system until loading of the valves is complete).

**Fig. 21.7** Evolut® R
System loading
preparation. (**a**) Initial
positioning, (**b**) washing of
the capsule

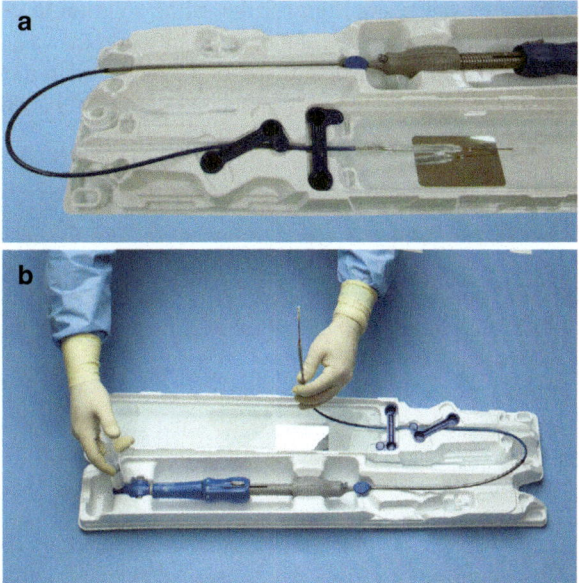

### 21.3.2   Step 2

Fill the bowl integrated into the tray up to the rim with cold sterile saline solution (between 0 and 8 °C [32 and 46 °F]) and the mounting trays with sterile saline solution at room temperature, i.e., between 15 and 25 °C (59 and 25 °F).

### 21.3.3   Step 3

The prosthesis is preserved in a glutaraldehyde solution; remove it from its container using round-tip tweezers, making sure not to touch the tissue part of valve. Check that the serial number on the container matches that on the label of the valve; remove the label and then wash the prosthesis.

### 21.3.4   Step 4

Rinse the prosthesis in the first of the washing bowls by gently stirring the prosthesis for 15 s to remove the glutaraldehyde. Then repeat for another 15 s in the second bowl, and then leave the prosthesis immersed in the third bowl up to the time of mounting.

### 21.3.5   Step 5

Wash the capsule: connect a 10-mL syringe full of cold saline solution to the capsule flush port at the proximal end of the handle. Gently lift the capsule in a vertical position and rotate the handle to expose the paddle attachment. Then wash slowly using the syringe, waiting for the saline solution to come out of the capsule, and then delicately immerse the capsule in the cold water bowl before the syringe is completely empty. Fasten the tip of the device with the locking clip to ensure complete immersion up to the complete mounting of the valve in order to prevent introducing air into the capsule (Fig. 21.7b).

### 21.3.6   Step 6

The EnVeo R system (Fig. 21.8) will allow easy and accurate assembly of the Evolut R TAV. A system of cones and tubes allows crimping the prosthesis (like the process for mounting the CoreValve).

Immerse the bioprosthesis and all the components of the mounting system in the incorporated bowl filled with cold water to prevent air from penetrating inside the capsule.

Ensure that the capsule of the delivery system is fully retracted and that the stylet is fully inserted into the guidewire lumen (to avoid damaging the catheter shaft during loading), and pull the capsule guide tube over the catheter shaft toward the handle until its elastic tip is completely proximal to the paddle attachment, without advancing flexible elastic tip over the capsule (Fig. 21.9a).

### 21.3.7   Step 7

Ensure that the backplate has been inserted into the inflow cone and the exposed part of the backplate is facing up. Insert the inflow portion of the bioprosthesis frame into the inflow cone, ensuring that the "C" paddle is facing up and is aligned with the paddle attachment pockets. Do not "hand crimp" or "pre-crimp" the TAV (Fig. 21.9b).

Secure the outflow cone onto the inflow cone until it locks, and ensure that all outflow crowns are captured by the outflow cone when attaching to the inflow cone.

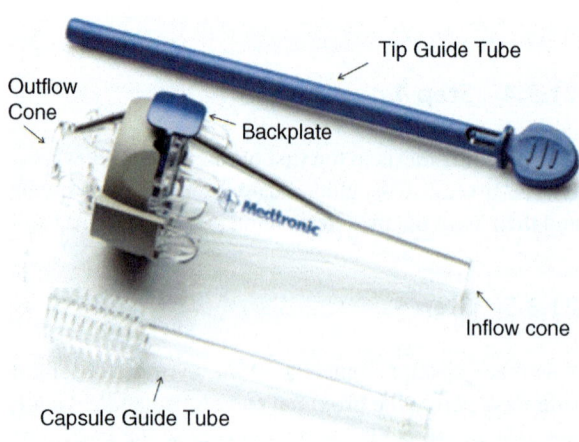

**Fig. 21.8** Loading system components

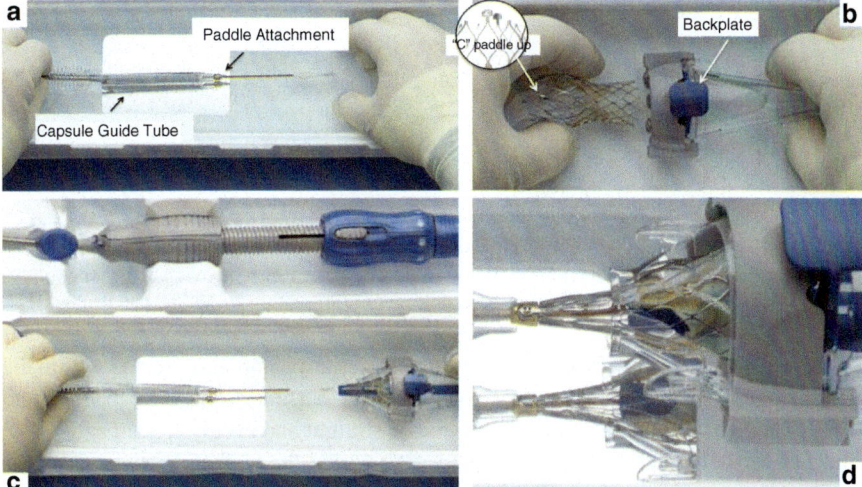

**Fig. 21.9** Evolut® R System loading preparation. (**a**) Step 6: paddle attachment and capsule guide tube. (**b**) Step 7: the "C" paddle. (**c**) Step 8. (**d**) Properly seated paddles

Then insert the catheter tip guide tube completely into the distal end of the inflow cone until the blue tip contacts the inflow cone. Inspect the outflow crowns of the TAV, and, if needed, manually move the outflow crowns so they are evenly spaced and the paddles are across from one another. Use the mirror in the bath to ensure that the underside paddle is positioned 180° from the top paddle.

### 21.3.8  Step 8

Position the TAV and loading system over the catheter tip of the delivery system, and advance until the TAV paddles align with the paddle attachment pockets, and then retract the tip guide tube to the belly region of the valve so that the paddles lay down into the pockets of the paddle attachment.

The paddles must be properly seated in the pockets of the paddle attachment before continuing (Fig. 21.9c, d). At this stage, a misload is an improperly loaded bioprosthesis, which can result in damage to the valve, delivery system, or both, and can negatively impact deployment and performance of the valve if not recognized. Due to a nitinol capsule within the delivery system, direct visual detection of misloads within the capsule is not possible; however, misloads can typically be identified through higher than normal force required to move the capsule forward, "pops" or sudden movement of TAV frame or delivery system, observing the delivery system move toward one side in the loading bath when advancing the capsule, or observing a bent, curved, or discolored capsule. In any event, a final inspection under fluoroscopy must be made prior to implantation to verify that the valve is properly loaded.

Paddles not properly seated increase loaded valve profile beyond inner capsule diameter specifications, require greater force to deploy or recapture, and can possibly contribute to delivery system failure or suboptimal deployment performance. To

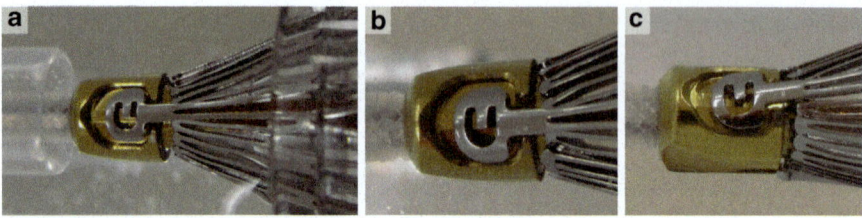

**Fig. 21.10** Paddle seating. (**a**) Correct: paddle and stem fully within pocket; (**b**) *top-down view*: paddles appear seated within the pocket, though adjacent crowns may be overlapping; (**c**) *oblique angle view*: overlapping crowns prevent the paddle stem from seating within the paddle pocket

prevent this, ensure that the top and bottom paddles are completely seated within the paddle pockets, as indicated by a spade-shaped outline around the paddle and "stem," and ensure that the outflow crowns are straight and evenly spaced and do not interfere with the paddle "stems" from seating within the pocket. View from multiple angles to verify position (Fig. 21.10).

### 21.3.9    Step 9

Rotate the handle to advance the capsule guide tube so that the flexible section covers the paddle attachment pockets; stop when the paddles are covered by the elastic tip of the capsule guide tube. Carefully watch for any movement of the valve when advancing the capsule, as this can indicate the paddles have come out the paddle attachment pockets. Use the mirror to visually inspect both paddles, and ensure that they are correctly seated in the pockets of the paddle attachment before advancing to the next step because advancing the capsule before the paddles are fully seated could damage the capsule and result in emboli.

### 21.3.10    Step 10

Continue advancing the capsule to further secure the paddles to the paddle attachment, stopping when the tips of the outflow crowns are in the elastic portion of the sheath guide tube and the capsule covers the top portion of the paddles. Carefully watch for any movement of the valve when advancing the capsule as this can indicate the paddles have come out the paddle attachment pockets. Ensure that both paddles and all outflow crowns are captured within the capsule and sheath guide tube before advancing to the next step (Fig. 21.11).

### 21.3.11    Step 11

Continue to advance the capsule forward, and stop when "tactile indicator" feedback is felt (approximately when the distal edge of the capsule covers the top of the

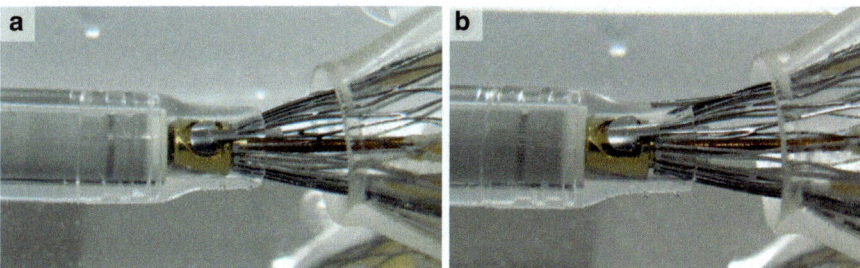

**Fig. 21.11** The paddle in the paddle attachment pockets. (**a**) Correct: crowns captured under the capsule guide tube. (**b**) Incorrect: crown outside capsule guide tube

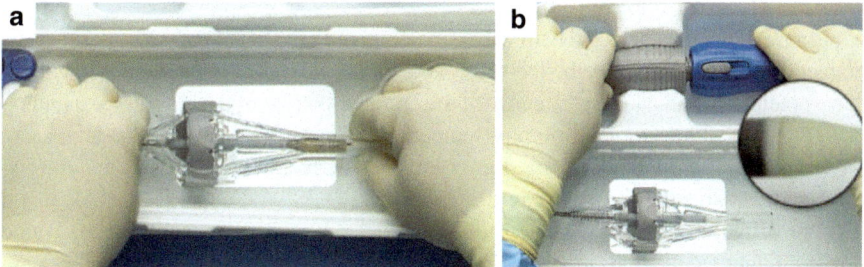

**Fig. 21.12** (**a**) Step 12. (**b**) Step 13: properly seated tip

commissure pads). Stop advancing the capsule at any point if excess force is noticed when closing the capsule or if the capsule angles toward the loading bath sides (Fig. 21.12a).

### 21.3.12 Step 12

Remove the backplate and the tip guide tube from the inflow cone, and gently agitate the loading tool while keeping it submerged in the bath to free any bubbles from the valve. Holding the capsule guide tube stationary, push the inflow cone in one uninterrupted movement toward the capsule until the entire inflow portion of the valve is compressed within the inflow cone. Ensure "on-axis" advancement of the inflow cone to ensure that all inflow crowns are captured evenly (Fig. 21.12b).

### 21.3.13 Step 13

Continue to advance the capsule over the TAV by rotating the deployment knob, and stop when the capsule edge is within 5 mm of the catheter tip. Remove the outflow cone, inflow cone, and capsule guide tube to provide better visualization of the distal edge of the capsule, and resume capsule closure until the distal edge of the capsule meets the shelf of the tip. This may require use of the overdrive feature to advance the capsule beyond its standard range of motion. Once the capsule meets the shelf of the tip, rotate the deployment knob in the opposite direction until it can move back and forth freely to relieve the force built up in the system.

### 21.3.14 Step 14

Visually and tactilely examine the capsule to verify that the valve was loaded properly. A misload can typically be identified by the presence of a bump or protrusion, especially around the paddle attachment area, discoloration in the capsule, and/or a kinked or bent capsule (Fig. 21.13).

In case of misload detected before the capsule reaches the top of the commissure pads, retract the capsule to unsheathe the valve, and reload (up to this point, the TAV will not have potentially damaged the integrity of the crimped portion of the capsule), expanding the TAV in the third rinse bath at room temperature, if necessary, before reloading.

Instead, if the misload occurred after the capsule reaches the top of the commissure pads, unsheathe the valve, remove from the DCS, and expand the TAV using the third rinsing bath with sterile saline at room temperature, examining the frame for permanent deformation, frayed sutures, or valve damage. If no problems are found, the TAV an attempt to be loaded a second time can be made; however, the loader must replace the delivery system, and utilize new loading bath and bath water. Additionally, examine the compression loading system for scratches or permanent deformation, and replace if problems are found.

### 21.3.15 Step 15

Provided no misload is detected, remove the stylet and flush the remaining three flush ports for the guidewire, stability layer, and InLine sheath (Fig. 21.14). Leave the THV submerged until implantation.

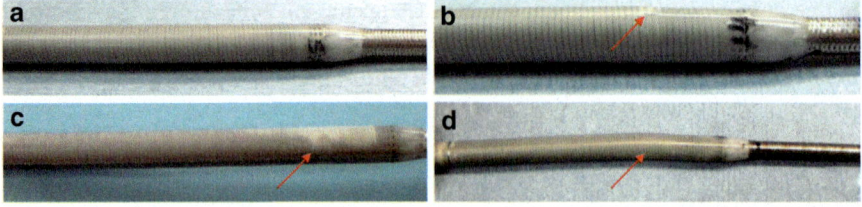

**Fig. 21.13** Loaded capsules. (**a**) Correctly loaded capsule; (**b**) misload, bump with white discoloration; (**c**) white discoloration running length of capsule; (**d**) capsule kinked or bent

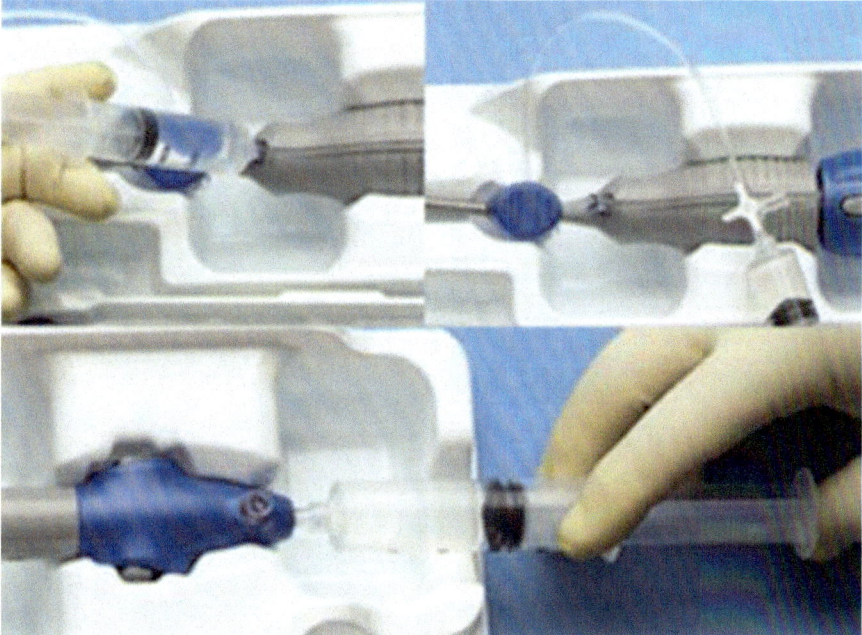

**Fig. 21.14**  Final flush

## 21.4    Pre-procedure

### 21.4.1  Fluoro Load Inspection

Prior to inserting the system in the patient, conduct a fluoroscopic inspection of the loaded delivery system to ensure it is properly loaded. In this case, the DCS will appear as a straight and smooth capsule, with the paddles seated symmetrically within the paddle attachment (Fig. 21.15a, b).

To ensure an accurate load assessment, using an anteroposterior imaging projection, hold the flush ports to the side (3:00/9:00), and rotate a few degrees in either direction until both paddles are visible simultaneously. Use high resolution cine (30 FPS) and magnification for best visibility. Rest capsule flat on patient or table for stability so radiopaque marker band appears as a straight line.

Focus inspection on the following areas to confirm characteristics of a good load (Fig. 21.15c):

1. Paddles: same height within the pockets and equidistant from paddle attachment
2. Outflow crowns: aligned straight and parallel to the distal end of the paddle attachment
3. Capsule: straight and free of any bends or curves with node bands appearing straight and uniform

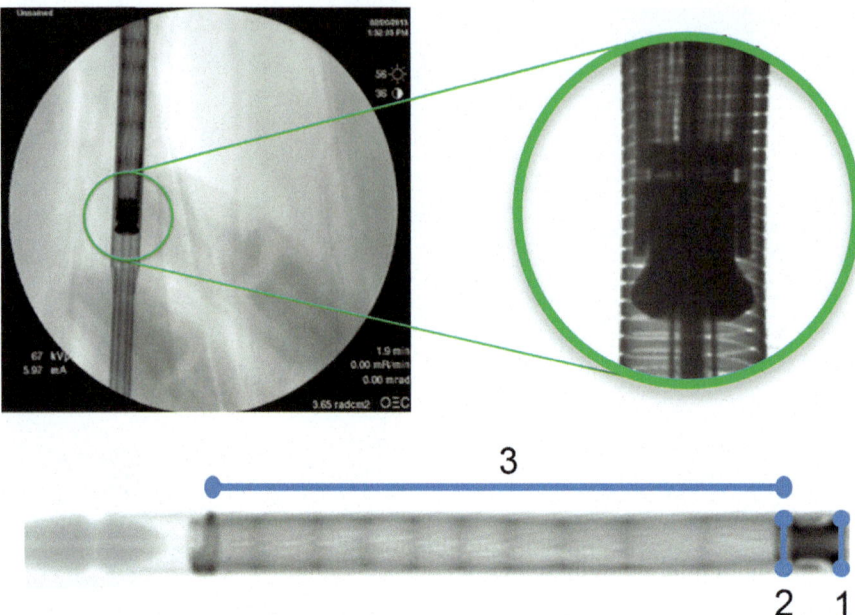

**Fig. 21.15** Fluoro load inspection: properly loaded valve. Focus inspection on the following areas to confirm characteristics of a good load: (1) paddles, same height within the pockets and equidistant from paddle attachment; (2) outflow crowns, aligned straight and parallel to the distal end of the paddle attachment; and (3) capsule, straight and free of any bends or curves, with node bands appearing straight and uniform

Misloads under fluoroscopic inspection will appear as any large gap between a paddle and pocket, asymmetrical position of paddles within pockets (i.e., one higher/lower than the other), outflow crowns not in a straight line parallel to paddle attachment edge, bent or angled capsule, misaligned node bands (not perpendicular to the capsule), and shadow or outline present, indicating a bent outflow strut.

If any indication of a misload is identified, the delivery system has to be replaced with a new system, and the valve can be reloaded if no damage is noticed upon inspection.

### 21.4.2 End Cap Safety Mechanism

The end cap is a component connecting the tip retrieval mechanism to the delivery system handle, held in place by two plastic tabs and slots. It can separate if the system experiences higher than expected deployment forces, similar to those generated by deploying a misloaded valve. If the end cap separates, the valve can be recaptured, but cannot be further deployed (Fig. 21.16).

**Fig. 21.16** End cap safety mechanism

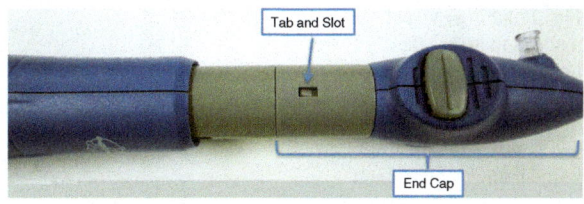

## 21.5 Procedure

After balloon valvuloplasty, the catheter is loaded onto the guidewire, with the flush ports pointing up. Under fluoroscopic guidance, the catheter is advanced over the guidewire to the aortic annulus, allowing the system to orient itself to the anatomy as it is advanced.

Before starting the deployment, the operator must find the coplanar image projection of the aortic cusps, and then adjust to see radiopaque marker as a straight line. If both cannot be achieved together, radiopaque marker alignment is preferred. Target implant depth is 3–5 mm, midway between node 0 (inflow edge of frame) and node 1 to just below node: due to minor valve frame length differences, the operator must assess valve position from frame inflow (node 0) and not the edge of the marker band (Fig. 21.17a, b).

Once the target implant depth is obtained, the second operator starts the deployment (consider controlled pacing (90–130 BPM) during deployment in patients with aortic regurgitation and/or large anatomies).

The first 1/3 of the bioprosthesis is deployed by rotating the actuator very slowly and in short increments in the direction of the marked arrows. Anticipate 1:1 capsule response after approximately two turns of the deployment knob. Valve position is assessed on fluoroscopy throughout deployment, and adjustment of position as necessary can be obtained until annular contact of the frame (Fig. 21.18a, b).

If satisfied with valve position at annular contact, the operator continues to deploy the valve until just before the "point of no recapture." Once blood pressure drops (because cardiac output is temporarily occluded by the deploying valve), the deployment must be quicker until blood pressure recovers, making sure not to advance past the point of no recapture. The tactile indicator provides feedback to indicate that the capsule is nearing the point of no recapture.

Before the point of no recapture, valve position and performance must be carefully evaluated, adjusting imaging projection to remove parallax in shell inflow to precisely determine valve position and assess hemodynamic angiography and echo.

If satisfied with valve position and performance, the valve can be fully deployed. To reduce potential for valve movement, it is advisable to release tension in the system just before final release by retracting the guidewire, slightly pushing on delivery system, and turning deployment knob very slowly to allow

**Fig. 21.17** (**a**) Visual markers to assess the implant depth. (**b**) Due to minor valve frame length differences, make sure to assess valve position from frame inflow (node 0) and not the edge of the marker band

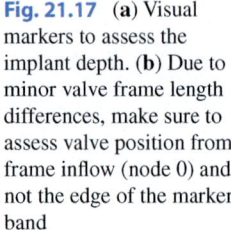
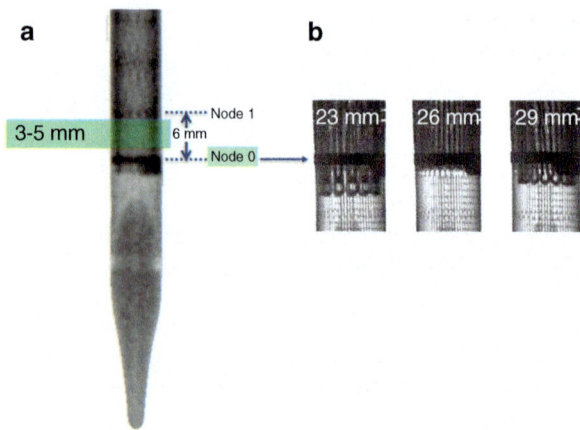

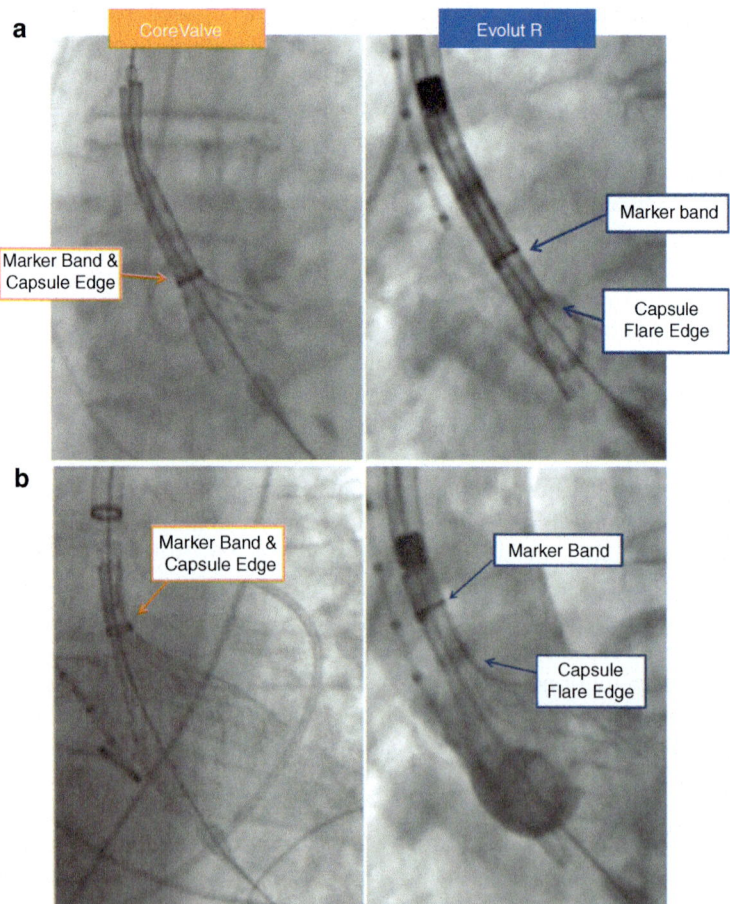

**Fig. 21.18** Deployment considerations: appreciate the visual landmark differences between Evolut® R and CoreValve when determining deployment depth. (**a**) Visual landmarks at 1/3 deployment, (**b**) visual landmarks at 2/3 deployment

the paddles to detach one at a time. Eventually the operator must confirm detachment of frame paddles under fluoroscopy, and center the nose cone before withdrawing the device.

Prior to withdrawing the system to the descending aorta, the operator must ensure that the catheter tip is coaxial with the inflow portion of the bioprosthesis, and release tension on the guidewire to center if not coaxial.

The system is withdrawn to the descending aorta, and the device is closed and locked using the "gray to blue" method (slide back the deployment knob trigger and retract the gray handrest to the blue deployment knob (gray to blue)). Prior to removing the device, verify that the catheter is locked by pulling on the deployment knob and tip retrieval mechanism to ensure they are locked in position. Then stabilize the InLine sheath, and withdraw the system until the capsule contacts the InLine sheath, verifying under fluoroscopy that the tip is not over- or under-captured prior to removal, and withdraw the catheter and EnVeo InLine sheath as a single unit. If experiencing excessive force, verify that the capsule tip is not over- or under-captured (Fig. 21.19).

When using the InLine sheath only, immediately replace with a separate 14 Fr vessel introducer sheath upon removal to maintain hemostasis. The introducer can be used for advancing a balloon, in case prosthesis post-dilatation is required [6].

### 21.5.1   Recapture

The valve can be partially or fully recaptured at any time prior to the point of no recapture by rotating the deployment knob in the opposite direction of the arrows.

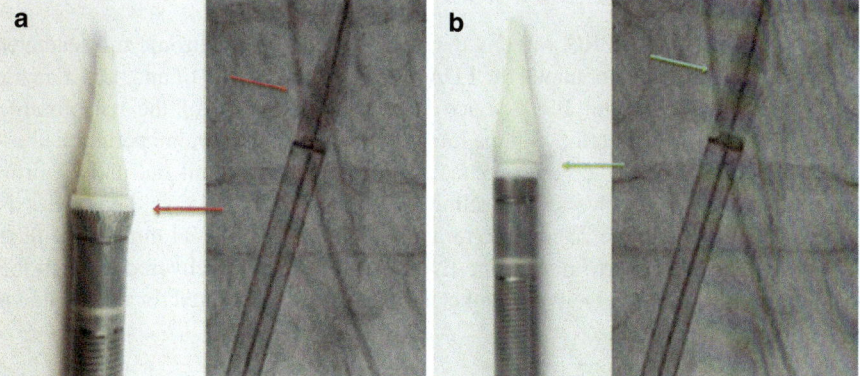

**Fig. 21.19** Look for what appears like a small gap between the capsule and nose cone under fluoroscopy, and use the deployment knob to advance or retract the capsule as necessary. (**a**) Properly captured tip. (**b**) Over-captured tip

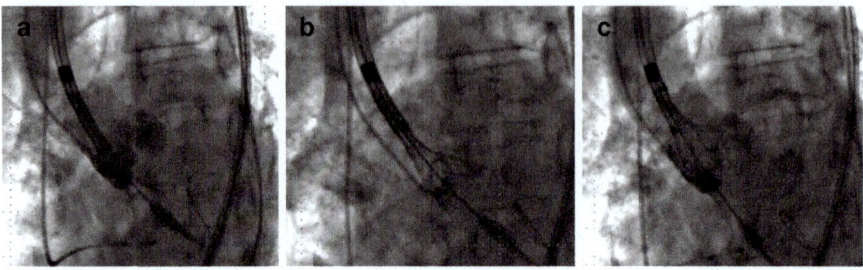

**Fig. 21.20** (**a**) Initial position. (**b**) Annular contact. (**c**) 2/3 deployment

Decision to recapture is typically made at two points in the procedure: 1/3 deployment (upon annular contact) and just before reaching the point of no recapture. Prior to the point of no recapture, the valve can be recaptured three times: the first two attempts to reposition and redeploy the valve. A third attempt must be a complete recapture for retrieval from the patient (Fig. 21.20).

If the valve is too low, recapture and reposition when frame is no longer in contact with the native leaflets. Remember that the valve will occlude cardiac output between 2/3 and 1/3 recapture. In case of too high valve positioning or pop-out, ensure that the inflow portion of the valve is above the native leaflets as it is recaptured, and fully recapture the bioprosthesis before readvancing through the native valve. Recapture/resheathing should be viewed as a safety net for suboptimal valve implantation; if the valve is deployed at an acceptable depth with good hemodynamic results, it may not be necessary to recapture or resheathe. (Table 21.2) summarizes all procedural steps.

## 21.6    The Evolut PRO

The CoreValve Evolut PRO valve is the latest generation Medtronic transcatheter aortic valve. The device obtained the FDA approval in March 2017 and the CE mark in July 2017. The Evolut PRO device follows the platform of the recapturable CoreValve Evolut R System, with the integration of an outer porcine pericardial tissue wrap that adds surface area contact between the valve and the native aortic annulus to further advance valve sealing performance (Fig. 21.21). The device is currently available in the 23 mm, 26 mm and 29 mm sizes (the 34 mm size will be also available in the next future). The Evolut PRO system is delivered through the 16F equivalent EnVeo R Delivery Catheter System and is indicated for vessels down to 5.5 mm.

**Table 21.2** Procedure step

Sizing
- Follow IFU sizing matrix utilizing MSCT measurements

Vascular access
- Choose appropriate access approach and sheath selection (e.g., InLine sheath, 18 Fr introducer sheath)
- Ensure access vessel is sufficiently dilated before inserting InLine sheath

Guidewire placement
- Place a 6 Fr straight pigtail catheter in the NCC
- Advance a second pigtail catheter into the ventricle to assess pre-implant hemodynamics
- Shape guidewire with a curve (or use pre-shaped wire like Medtronic Confida™ guidewire) and position at apex of left ventricle
- Maintain strict fluoroscopic surveillance of guidewire throughout procedure

Load inspection
- Inspect the loaded Evolut R TAV using fluoroscopy to ensure proper loading

BAV
- If using InLine sheath, use 14 Fr introducer for BAV
- Balloon size based on current recommendations

Device insertion
- Ensure InLine sheath is flush with the capsule during device insertion
- Ensure flush ports point up and hold loosely to allow system to orient to anatomy as inserted within patient

Imaging projection and alignment
- Adjust imaging projection to achieve a coplanar view of aortic cusps
- Adjust view to remove parallax in radiopaque marker band
- Use radiopaque marker alignment if coplanar view and marker band alignment cannot be achieved together
- Allow system to align itself within the native annulus and maintain contact with the top of the aortic arch for maximum stability

Deployment
- Start deployment at a target implantation depth of 3–5 mm
- Anticipate a 1:1 catheter response after 1 to 2 turns
- Consider controlled pacing (90–130 bpm)
- Slowly deploy first 1/3 and reposition as necessary until annular contact
- Assess valve position/PVL using angiography and echo between tactile indicator and point of no recapture
- Release tension prior to valve release by retracting the guidewire, pushing on the delivery system, and slowly turning the deployment knob

Recapture/Resheathe
- Recapture up to three times, as appropriate, when the valve is deployed in a suboptimal position
- Fully recapture and retrieve delivery system if recaptured a third time

EnVeo R DCS retrieval
- Center the nose cone before withdrawing the delivery system
- Close capsule and lock system by moving the gray front grip to the deployment knob, and confirm nosecone is flush against capsule
- Withdraw capsule until flush against the InLine sheath, and check for over-capture prior to withdrawing
- When using the InLine sheath, immediately close or replace with a 14 Fr vessel introducer sheath upon removal

Post assessment
- Wait 10 min to assess the hemodynamics, using echo-, angio-, and hemodynamics
- Intervene on any moderate and above PVL
- Follow post-dilatation balloon sizing guidance as applicable

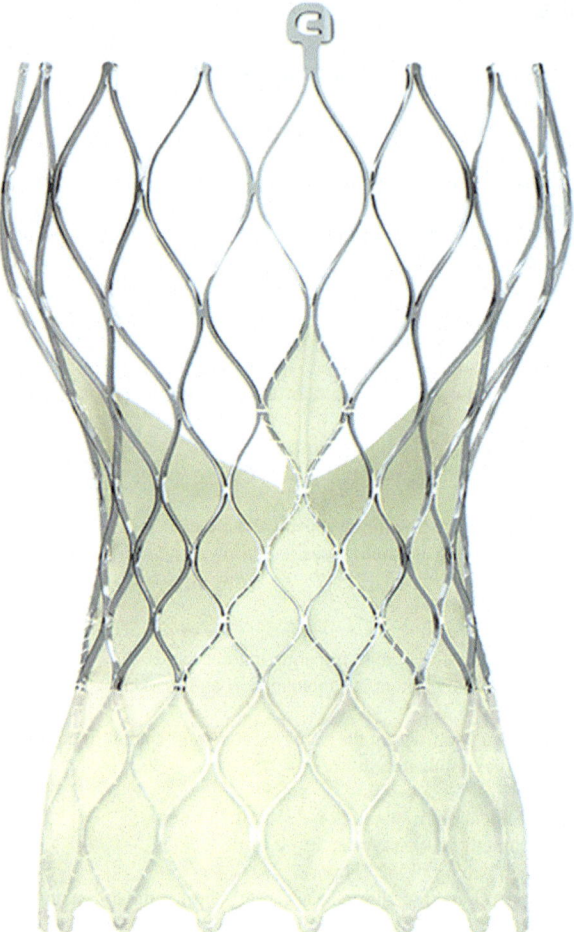

**Fig. 21.21** Evolut PRO transcatheter heart valve

## References

1. Grube E, Laborde JC, Zickmann B, et al. First report on a human percutaneous transluminal implantation of a self-expanding valve prosthesis for interventional treatment of aortic valve stenosis. Catheter Cardiovasc Interv. 2005;66:465–46.
2. Barbanti M, Webb JG, Gilard M, Capodanno D, Tamburino C. Transcatheter aortic valve implantation in 2017: state of the art. EuroIntervention. 2017;13:AA11–AA21.
3. Barbanti M, Binder RK, Freeman M, Wood DA, Leipsic J, Cheung A, Ye J, Tan J, Toggweiler S, Yang TH, Dvir D, Maryniak K, Lauck S, Webb JG. Impact of low-profile sheaths on vascular complications during transfemoral transcatheter aortic valve replacement. EuroIntervention. 2013;9:929–35.
4. Barbanti M, Buccheri S, Rodés-Cabau J, et al. Transcatheter aortic valve replacement with new-generation devices: A systematic review and meta-analysis. Int J Cardiol. 2017;245:83–9.
5. CoreValve Evolut® R System Valve Loading Procedure. Medtronic® Inc. 2014.
6. Barbanti M, Petronio AS, Capodanno D, et al. Impact of balloon post-dilation on clinical outcomes after transcatheter aortic valve replacement with the self-expanding CoreValve prosthesis. JACC Cardiovasc Interv. 2014;7:1014–21.

# Transcatheter Aortic Valve Implantation: Boston Lotus

# 22

Lennart van Gils and Nicolas M. Van Mieghem

## 22.1   Description of the Valve and Delivery System

The Lotus valve system (Boston Scientific, Marlborough, MA, USA) consists of a trileaflet bovine pericardial valve supported on a braided nitinol frame (Fig. 22.1). A central radiopaque marker facilitates positioning of the prosthesis within the aortic root. The frame is covered with an Adaptive Seal at the inflow segment that adapts to aortic root irregularities and minimizes paravalvular leak (Fig. 22.2). This transcatheter heart valve is currently available in three sizes—23, 25, and 27 mm (Fig. 22.3)—covering a range of annulus diameters from 19 to 27 mm. In fully deployed state, all sizes have a frame height of 19 mm. The 23 mm model can be delivered through an 18 Fr sheath (small), while the 25 and 27 mm valves require a 20 Fr (large) sheath. Lotus is typically inserted with a transfemoral approach, though direct aortic and trans-axillary alternative access is possible. Implantation of a Lotus valve requires the following components:

- A support guidewire: either a manually curved Super/Extra Stiff 0.035″ guidewire (260 cm for 23 mm and 275 for 25 and 27 mm) or a pre-shaped Safari[2] guidewire with an extra-small, small, or large curve (Fig. 22.4).
- Lotus introducer—small for 23 mm and large for 25 and 27 mm (Fig. 22.5).
- Lotus valve delivery system, with pre-mounted Lotus valve—103 cm for 23 and 113 cm for 25 and 27 mm (Fig. 22.6). The pre-shaped angulated delivery system should help negotiate the thoracic aorta.
- Prostar or double Perclose ProGlide (Abbott Vascular, Abbot Park, Illinois, USA) suture-based closure for transfemoral access (Fig. 22.7).

L. van Gils, M.D. • N.M. Van Mieghem, M.D., Ph.D. (✉)
Department of Interventional Cardiology, Thoraxcenter, Erasmus Medical Center, Room Bd 171 's Gravendijkwal 230, 3015 CE Rotterdam, Netherlands
e-mail: n.vanmieghem@erasmusmc.nl

© Springer International Publishing AG 2018
C. Tamburino et al. (eds.), *Percutaneous Treatment of Left Side Cardiac Valves*,
https://doi.org/10.1007/978-3-319-59620-4_22

**Fig. 22.1** The Lotus valve
(Courtesy of Boston
Scientific Corporation)

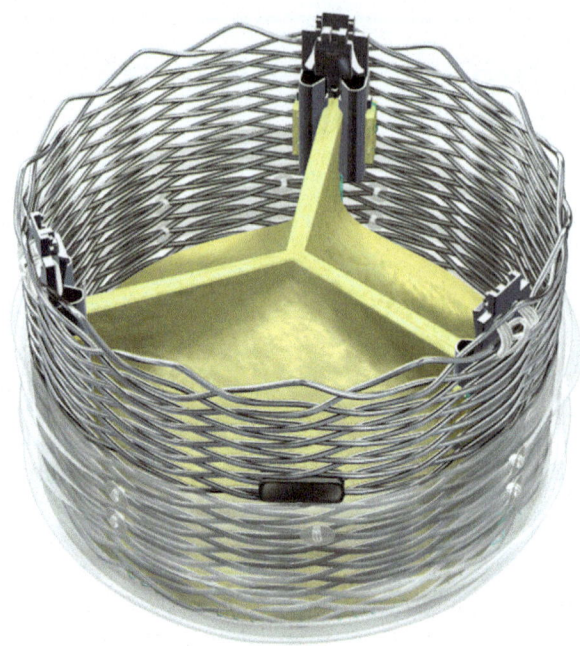

**Fig. 22.2** The Adaptive
Seal technology covers the
inflow segment of the
Lotus valve frame and
adapts to aortic root
irregularities and, hence,
minimizes paravalvular
leak (Courtesy of Boston
Scientific Corporation)

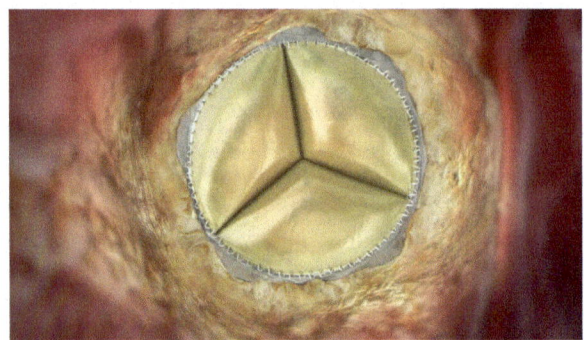

**Fig. 22.3** The three
available Lotus valve
sizes—23, 25, and
27 mm—accommodating
annulus diameters ranging
from 20 to 27 mm
(Courtesy of Boston
Scientific Corporation)

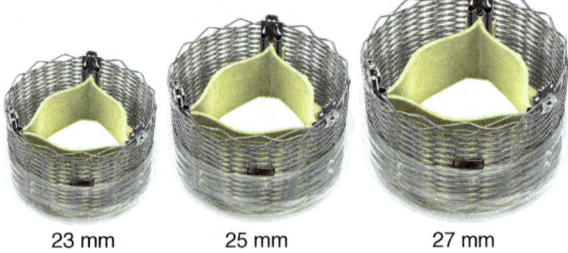

23 mm                25 mm                          27 mm

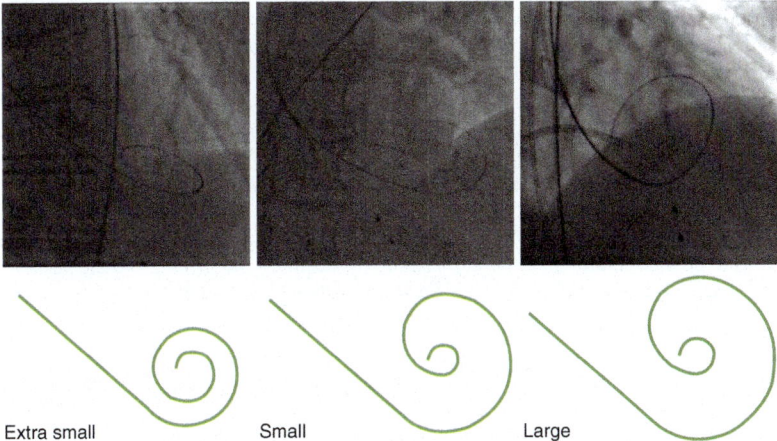

Extra small    Small    Large

**Fig. 22.4** The pre-curved Safari$^2$ wire comes in three curve sizes to facilitate stability for valve implantation in small and large ventricles

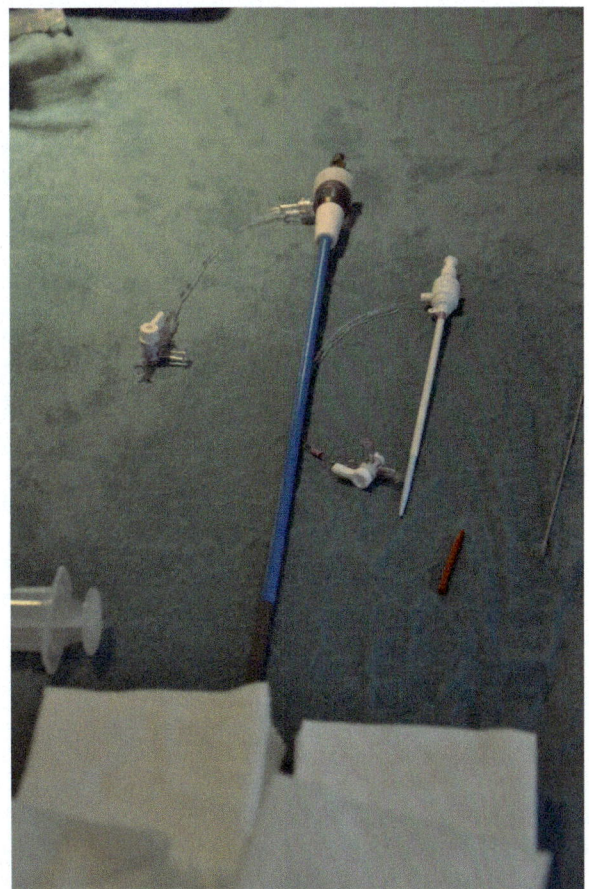

**Fig. 22.5** Lotus introducer (small). The light blue 18 Fr Lotus introducer accommodates transfemoral access for the small Lotus delivery system (23 mm valve)

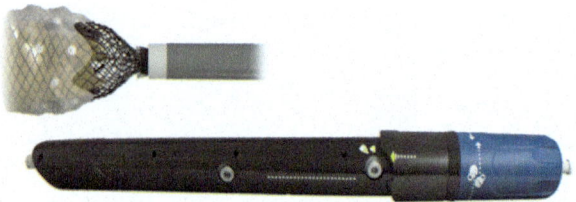

**Fig. 22.6** Lotus delivery system. Top, the pre-mounted Lotus valve; bottom, the intuitive delivery handle with the blue control knob for unsheathing/re-sheathing and locking and the black release cover for release of the valve (Courtesy of Boston Scientific Corporation)

**Fig. 22.7** Double Perclose ProGlide systems. ProGlide provides percutaneous suture-based closure of femoral access arteriotomies, ranging from 5 Fr to 21 Fr

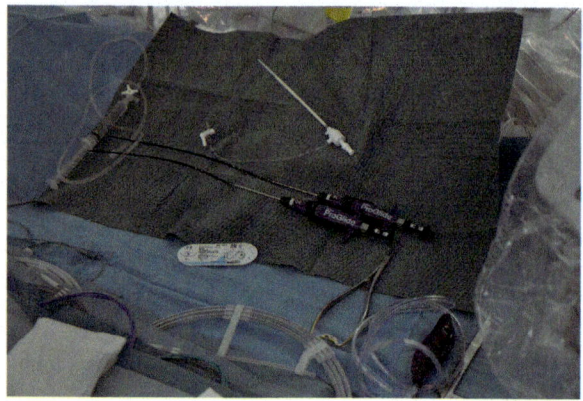

The bioprosthesis is coupled to the delivery system with three coupling fingers (Fig. 22.8). The three fingers hatch with the buckles at the top of the frame. Initially the frame expands during unsheathing. The unique feature of Lotus is the locking mechanism that follows after the frame is fully unsheathed but still elongated. The locking mechanism implies connecting the buckles (top of the frame) with the posts (level of valve leaflets), similar to fastening a seatbelt. The valve shortens and expands radially during the locking process (Fig. 22.9). After locking, the valve is fully deployed, and its position relative to the coronary ostia and presence of para-valvular aortic regurgitation can be assessed. Still, at this stage, the bioprosthesis can be repositioned or retrieved. The delivery handle of the delivery system is ergonomic and intuitive (Fig. 22.6). A large blue control knob regulates unsheathing and locking by rotating counterclockwise. Clockwise rotation will lead to re-sheathing. The release cover proximal to the blue control knob can be slid forward to release the valve from the catheter.

## 22.2 Prosthesis Loading

The loading procedure for the 23, 25, and 27 mm valves is identical. When removed from the package, the valve is sealed within a bottle stopcock at the distal end of the delivery system. The stopcock contains glutaraldehyde for valve conservation:

**Fig. 22.8** Three fingers connect the Lotus valve to the delivery system throughout the entire implantation process. The fingers are attached to the buckles on the frame and can be released when the result after complete locking is satisfactory (Courtesy of Boston Scientific Corporation)

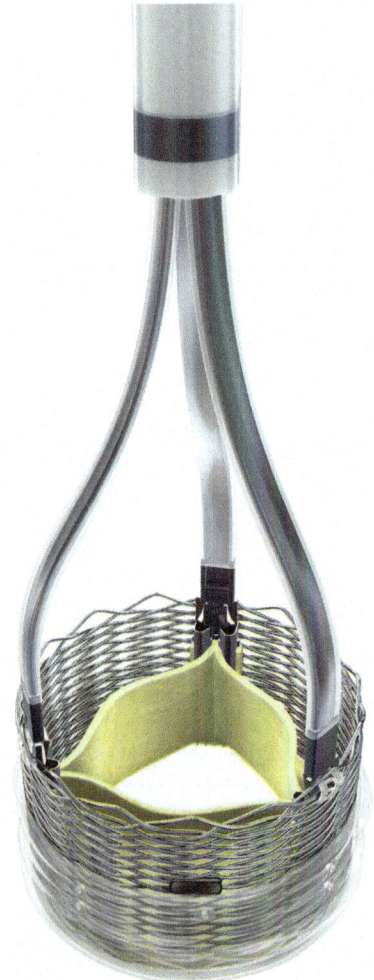

1. Remove the Luer cap from the bottle stopcock, and attach it to the waste bag to drain the glutaraldehyde solution.
2. Flush the guidewire port at the distal end of the delivery system.
3. Remove the valve from the stopcock (Fig. 22.10).
4. Visually inspect the valve for abnormalities (catheter tip and finger connection, collar and buckle interaction, sheathing aids, nosecone, valve leaflets), and flush the system (Fig. 22.11).
5. Lock the valve by turning the blue control knob counterclockwise, to ensure post and buckles engage without a gap and there is no twisting (Fig. 22.12).
6. Turn the blue control knob clockwise to ensure post and buckles disengage symmetrically.
7. Rinse the valve with agitation 2 × 60 s.
8. Insert a stylet in the nosecone and flush the system with saline.

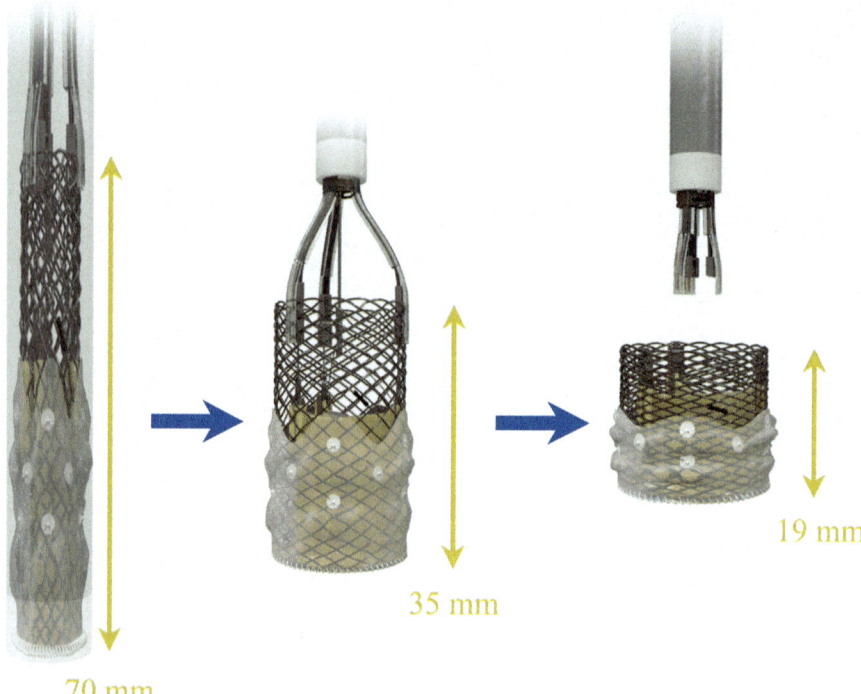

70 mm

35 mm

19 mm

**Fig. 22.9** When fully sheathed, the Lotus valve frame has a height of 70 mm. During unsheathing the height of the valve frame shrinks to 35 mm, while the diameter of the valve increases. During the locking process, the frame shrinks to a height of 19 mm and reaches its final configuration with maximal sealing of the annulus

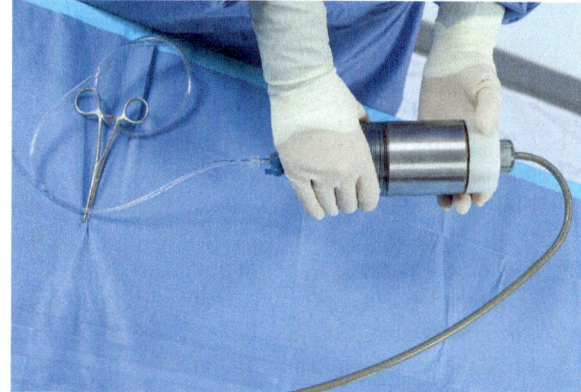

**Fig. 22.10** The pre-mounted Lotus valve is conserved in a bottle stopcock containing glutaraldehyde (Courtesy of Boston Scientific Corporation)

**Fig. 22.11** Before delivery, the valve is visually screened for abnormalities by checking the catheter tip and finger connection, collar and buckle interaction, sheathing aids, nosecone, and valve leaflets, followed by flushing of the system (Courtesy of Boston Scientific Corporation)

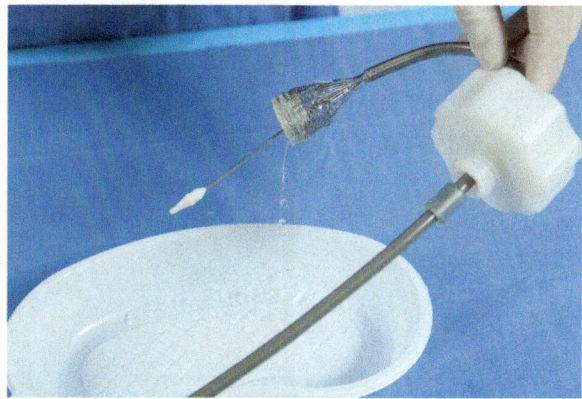

**Fig. 22.12** The blue control knob on the delivery handle facilitates unsheathing/locking of the Lotus valve (rotating counterclockwise) and re-sheathing (rotating clockwise). This mechanism is checked before valve delivery

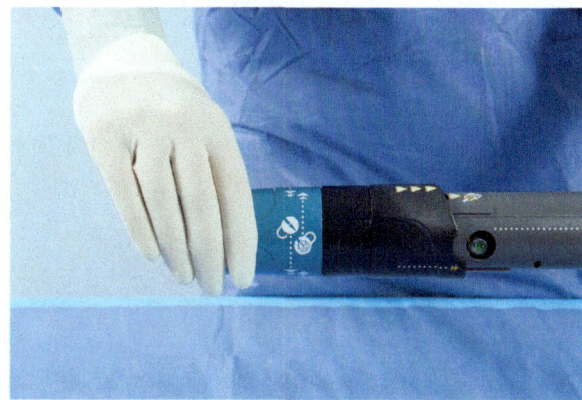

9. Remove air bubbles from the leaflets by agitating the valve.
10. Submerge the valve in saline, and wait until the valve can be delivered.
11. Once the valve can be delivered, gently start sheathing the valve by turning the blue control knob clockwise.
12. Remove the stylet and inspect the catheter tip. The delivery system is ready.

## 22.3   Typical Transfemoral Implantation Procedure

### 22.3.1  Obtaining Vascular Access

1. Obtain controlled access to the left and right common femoral arteries, preferably under fluoroscopy or ultrasound guidance (Fig. 22.13).
2. Obtain venous access for a temporary right ventricular pacing wire.
3. Position the temporary pacing wire in the apex of the right ventricle, and test the pacemaker.

**Fig. 22.13** Echo-guided puncture of the right common femoral artery. On an axial plane the location of the vessel can be accurately determined

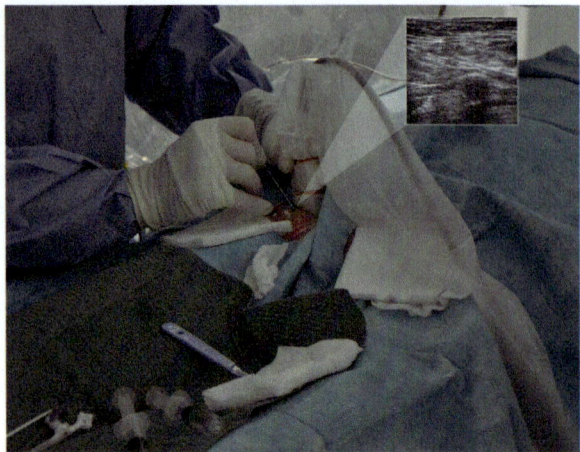

**Fig. 22.14** Angiogram of the aortic valve in a perpendicular plane with all cusps aligned (NCC-RCC-LCC). An optimal working projection contributes to an accurate valve implantation

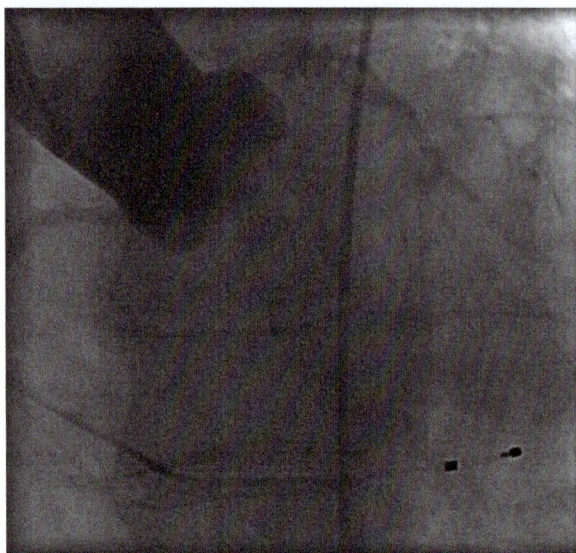

4. Insert a pigtail catheter through the left femoral artery, and position at the level of the noncoronary cusp; confirm a coaxial C-arm projection with a contrast injection to have all cusps in one plane (Fig. 22.14).
5. Preclosure with two 6 F Perclose ProGlide systems (or 1 Prostar) in the right femoral artery.
6. Insert the 18 F introducer (small) or 20 F (large), depending on the bioprosthesis size (Fig. 22.5).

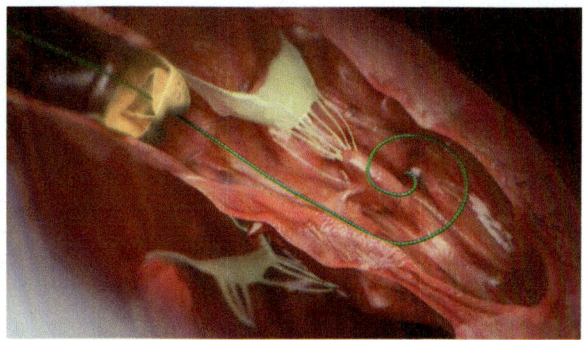

**Fig. 22.15** Animation of a Safari[2] wire positioned in the left ventricle (Courtesy of Boston Scientific Corporation)

7. Cross the aortic valve with a 0.035 straight tip wire, and advance a catheter in the left ventricle.
8. Confirm ventricular pressures and transaortic gradient.
9. Exchange for a Safari wire (Figs. 22.4 and 22.15). Ensure the pre-shaped curve of the Safari wire is positioned in the apex, and the soft part of the wire is entirely curled in the ventricle. This will provide enough safe migration space for the nosecone (see below).
10. Decide whether to perform balloon predilatation. In our practice, balloon predilatation is performed only exceptionally.

## 22.3.2 Valve Delivery

1. Hold the pre-shaped delivery system in an S-curve, and insert over the Safari wire into the body (Fig. 22.16a).
2. Advance the assembly gently, under fluoroscopic guidance, keeping guidewire control and checking proper orientation along the descending aorta (Fig. 22.16b). The radiopaque marker should be facing the right side of the delivery system on an AP fluoroscopic view before entering the aortic arch (Fig. 22.17).
3. Smoothly advance the system along the aortic arch (Figs. 22.16b and 22.17).
4. Cross the native aortic valve and ensure the nitinol braid is below the aortic annulus (Fig. 22.18a1).
5. Determine the final landing zone of the radiopaque marker.
6. Start unsheathing the valve by turning the blue control knob counterclockwise (Figs. 22.16c and 22.18a2/a3/a4).
7. Avoid excessive device migration into the left ventricle. The Lotus valve functions early during deployment; there should be no hemodynamic compromise.
8. As the valve deployment evolves, a waist will appear, and the radiopaque marker is displaced toward the ventricle.
9. The framework shortens from 70 to 35 mm upon unsheathing.

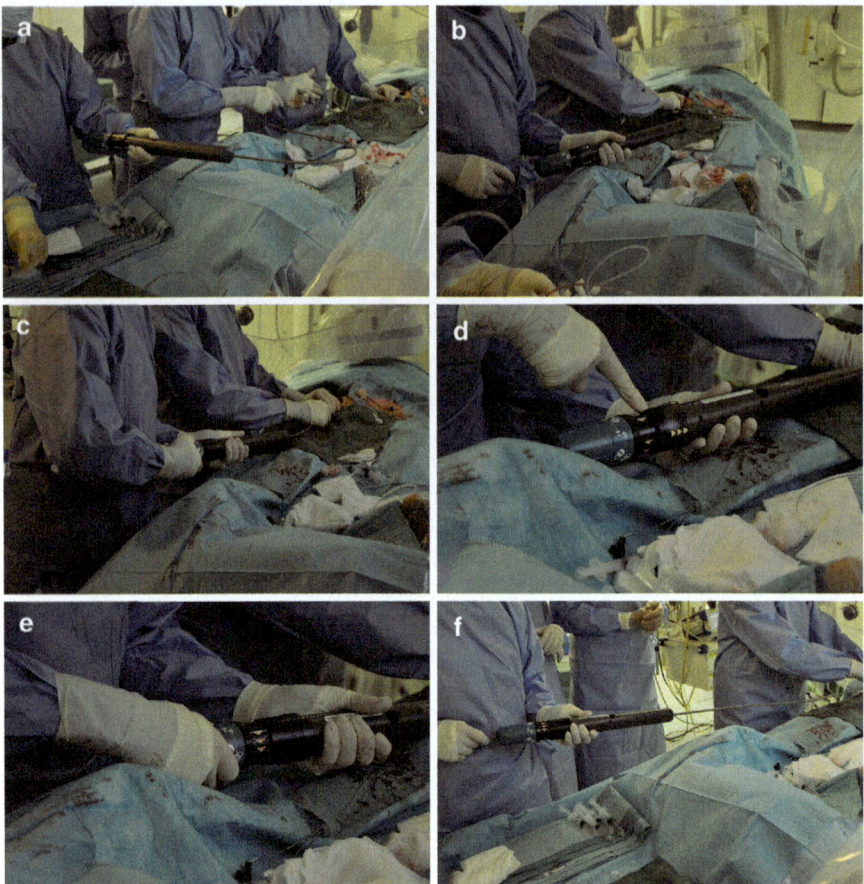

**Fig. 22.16** Stepwise Lotus valve implantation: (**a**) delivery system is held in the pre-shaped S-curve before introduction; (**b**) delivery system is smoothly advanced by pushing forward through the Lotus introducer; (**c**) when the tip of the delivery system is in the correct position (with the nitinol braid below the native annulus), the valve can be unsheathed and locked by turning the blue knob counterclockwise; (**d**) release cover is slid toward the patient and turned clockwise to release the valve; (**e**) blue control knob is turned counterclockwise to re-sheath the disconnected fingers and nosecone; (**f**) delivery system is pulled back gently through the introducer

### 22.3.3 Locking

The next step is locking the valve by connecting the buckles (cranial) and posts (caudal).

1. Before initiating the final locking process, confirm that the fluoroscopy projections show all three buckles and posts (Fig. 22.18b1).
2. Gently turn the blue control knob counterclockwise while confirming that the buckles and posts approach symmetrically. During this process, the frame height will shrink from 35 to 19 mm (Fig. 22.18b2).

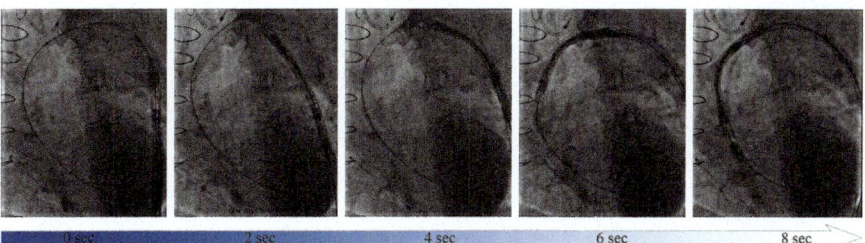

**Fig. 22.17** During crossing of the aortic arch (in approximately 8 s), the delivery system is carefully monitored to ensure that the radiopaque marker follows the outer curve of the arch

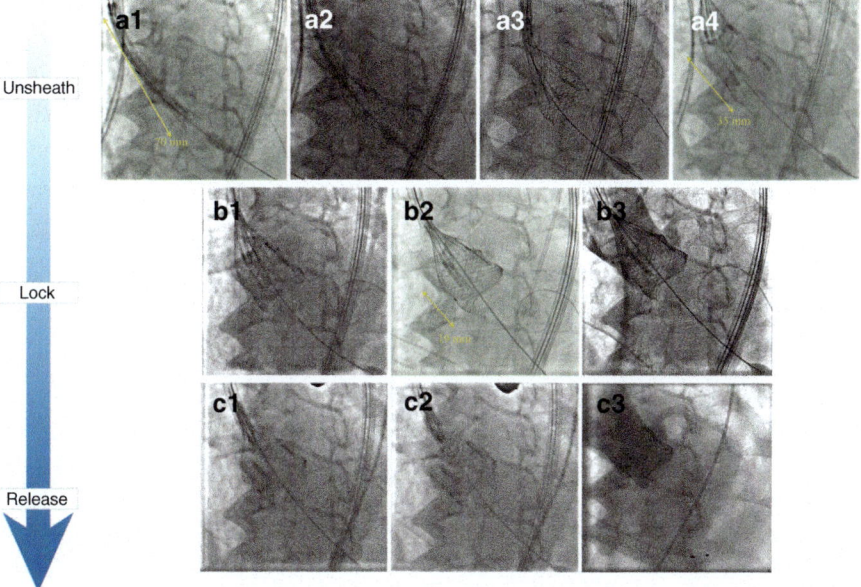

**Fig. 22.18** Unsheathing: (**a1**) fully sheathed Lotus valve (frame height 70 mm) with the distal tip of the nitinol frame below the native annulus; (**a2/3**) unsheathing of the valve. The valve functions early during deployment; (**a4**) fully unsheathed valve (frame height 35 mm). Locking: (**b1**) locking of the frame in a correct fluoroscopic image with all buckles and posts visible; (**b2**) fully locked frame (frame height shrinks to 19 mm); (**b3**) angiogram to confirm correct positioning after locking and absence of significant paravalvular regurgitation. At this stage, the valve is still fully repositionable and re-sheathable. Release: (**c1/2**) disconnecting the fingers from the frame buckles; (**c3**) final angiogram to evaluate position and paravalvular regurgitation

3. The valve is completely locked, resistance is felt, and a force limiter is tripped. An audible sound is heard.
4. Final valve positioning relies on the confirmation that the distal braid is below the annulus (this may allow for a high position) or by landing the radiopaque marker at its predetermined location.

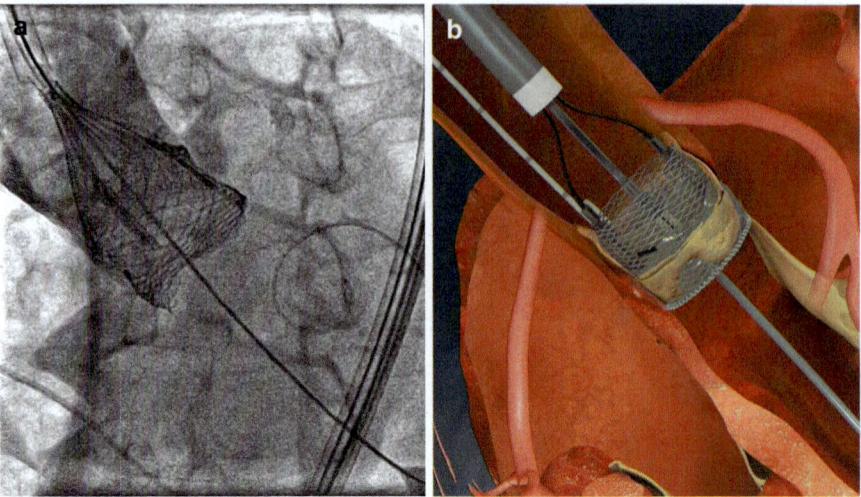

**Fig. 22.19** Fully locked Lotus valve before release on fluoroscopy (**a**) and reconstructed (**b**). The valve can be repositioned at this stage

5. After locking the valve, a contrast injection may help confirm valve positioning in terms of implantation depth, position relative to the coronary ostia, and paravalvular regurgitation (Figs. 22.19 and 22.18b3).

### 22.3.4 Release

1. Slide the release cover (located distal to the blue knob) in the direction of the patient (Fig. 22.16d).
2. Turn the release cover clockwise. The release pin moves upward. The valve is released (Fig. 22.18c1/2).
3. When the valve is completely released, start re-sheathing the fingers and nosecone by turning the blue control knob clockwise. Gently pull the nosecone back into the descending aorta and fully re-sheath.
4. The final position of the Lotus valve can be properly visualized by transthoracic or transesophageal echocardiography (Fig. 22.20) and on fluoroscopy (Fig. 22.21).

### 22.3.5 Repositioning

The repositionability/retrievability feature allows for precise valve delivery even in complex anatomies (e.g., horizontal aorta (Fig. 22.22)) and readjustment when paravalvular regurgitation is present (Figs. 22.23 and 22.24). The Lotus bioprosthesis is fully repositionable and retrievable until the valve is fully locked and the release pin is removed. Re-sheathing is done by turning the blue control knob clockwise.

**Fig. 22.20** Long-axis transesophageal echocardiographic view of the Lotus valve after final release

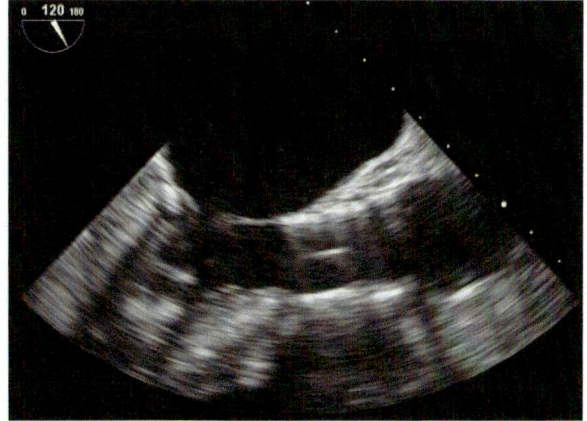

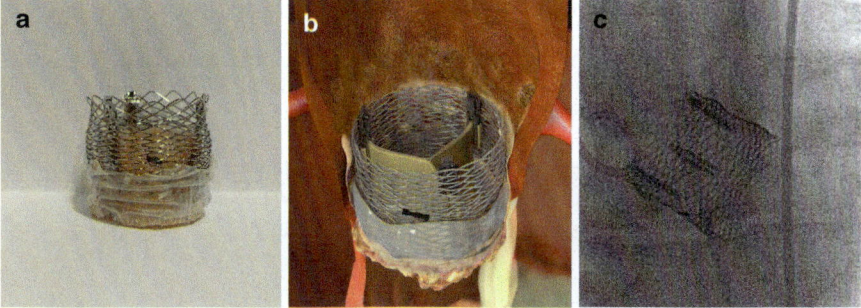

**Fig. 22.21**  The Lotus valve after final locking and release: (**a**) lotus valve with central radiopaque marker and Adaptive Seal; (**b**) reconstruction of a Lotus valve in the correct anatomical position; (**c**) fluoroscopic image of the Lotus valve

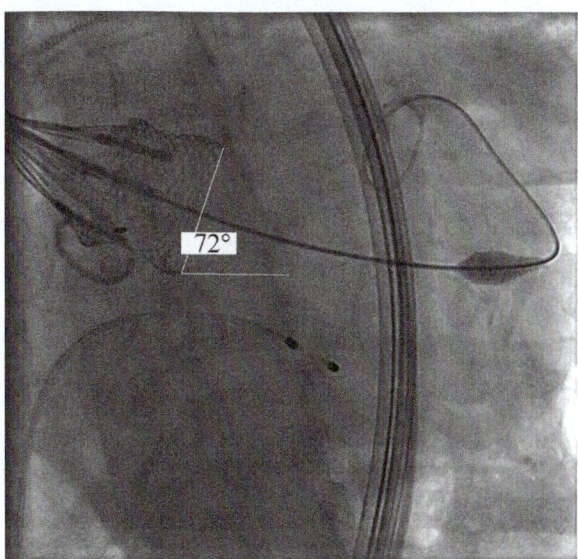

**Fig. 22.22**  Fluoroscopic image of a fully locked Lotus valve in an extremely horizontal aorta with an angle of 72°

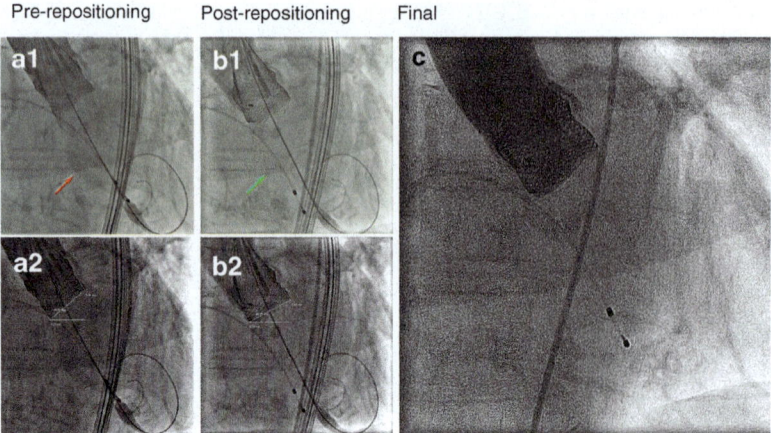

**Fig. 22.23** Repositioning of the Lotus valve on fluoroscopy: (**a1**) aortic angiogram pre-repositioning, moderate paravalvular aortic regurgitation; (**b1**) aortic angiogram post-repositioning, no aortic regurgitation. (**a2/b2**) Angle and depth measurements before and after implantation confirming a slight tilting of the frame between pre- and post-repositioning, with a similar depth of implantation; (**c**) final aortic angiogram with no aortic regurgitation

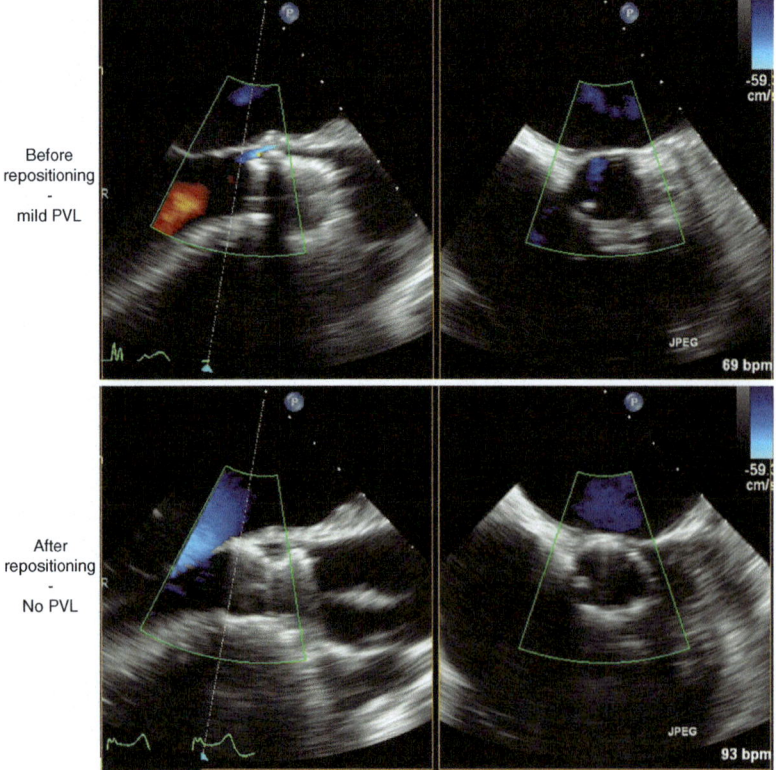

**Fig. 22.24** Repositioning of the Lotus valve on transesophageal echocardiography: there was a mild paravalvular leak (at 11 o'clock on short axis), which was resolved after repositioning

## 22.4   Procedure and Sizing Tips and Tricks

The Lotus delivery system requires a minimum arterial vessel diameter of 6 mm. The Lotus valve can be implanted in a wide range of native valve diameters (19–27 mm). Figure 22.25 illustrates the sizing matrix. The 23 mm Lotus fits annulus and LVOT diameters ranging from 20 to 23 mm, the 25 mm Lotus from 23 to 25 mm, and the 27 mm Lotus from 25 to 27 mm. The Adaptive Seal of the Lotus valve can help eliminate the incidence of paravalvular regurgitation. In our opinion, the left ventricular outflow tract dimensions are equally important for Lotus sizing. Excessive oversizing relative to the LVOT and overall depth of implantation may affect the occurrence of conduction disorders and need for pacemakers. It is important to bear in mind that the bioprosthesis will dominate the anatomy, suggesting a more circular final geometry. Coronary obstructions can be avoided by pre-procedure MSCT planning and by checking the Lotus position before release. The bioprosthesis can be repositioned when needed.

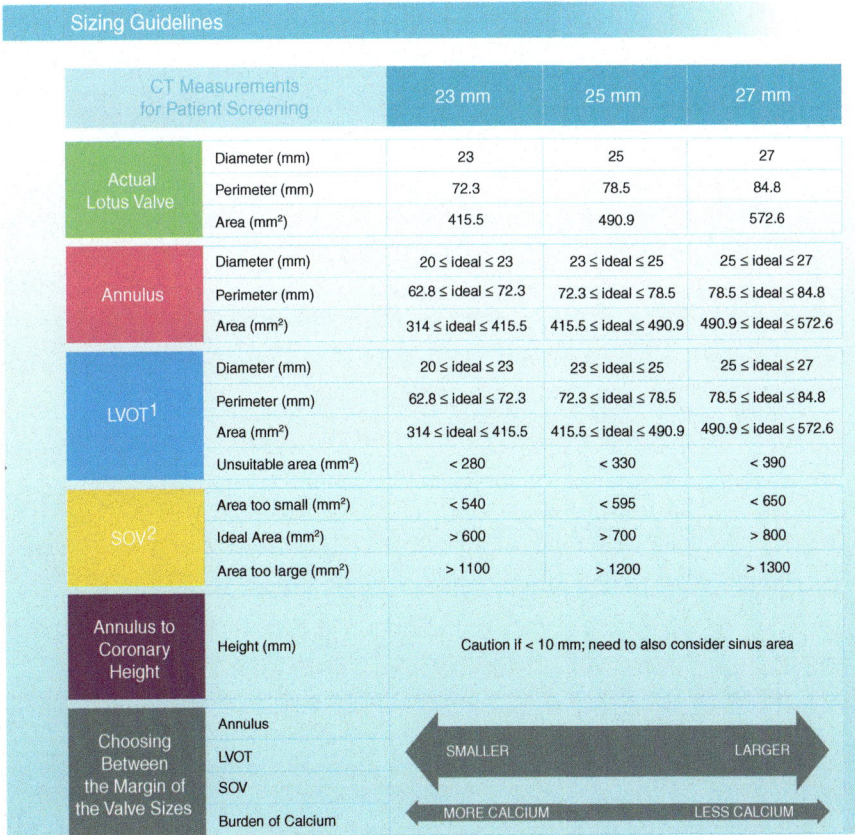

**Fig. 22.25**  Lotus valve sizing guidelines (Courtesy of Boston Scientific Corporation)

# Transcatheter Aortic Valve Implantation: Boston ACURATE and ACURATE-neo TF

# 23

Carmelo Sgroi, Claudia Ina Tamburino, and Gerlando Pilato

The Boston ACURATE platform is designed for all transcatheter aortic valve implantation (TAVI) access routes: transfemoral, transapical, and transaortic. These bioprostheses are based on a unique, self-seating, and self-sealing design that allows for optimal positioning of the valve.

## 23.1 The ACURATE TA and the ACURATE-neo™ Aortic Bioprostheses

### 23.1.1 Device Description

There are two types of aortic bioprostheses on the market: The first, the ACURATE, is currently implanted solely via transapical access. It was followed by the second-generation ACURATE-neo, which is implanted, instead, with a transfemoral approach. Both devices do not allow for re-sheathing, but repositioning is always possible.

The ACURATE TA™ transapical aortic bioprosthesis (Boston Scienti c, Marlborough, MA, USA) is composed of a radiopaque, Nitinol self-expandable support structure (stent), an integrated tri-leaflet biological tissue valve, and a polyethylene terephthalate (PET) fabric skirt. The biological valve is manufactured from three non-coronary porcine leaflets. The device has three stabilization arches for axial alignment, an upper crown for capping the aortic annulus, and a lower crown that is opened for full deployment over the native valve [1] (Fig. 23.1).

The ACURATE TA transapical delivery consists of a 33-Fr delivery catheter. This transapical delivery system is designed for a simple two-step deployment and stable positioning within the native annulus.

C. Sgroi (✉) • C.I. Tamburino • G. Pilato
Cardiac-Thoracic-Vascular Department, Ferrarotto Hospital, University of Catania, Catania, Italy
e-mail: carmelo_sgroi@hotmail.com

© Springer International Publishing AG 2018
C. Tamburino et al. (eds.), *Percutaneous Treatment of Left Side Cardiac Valves*,
https://doi.org/10.1007/978-3-319-59620-4_23

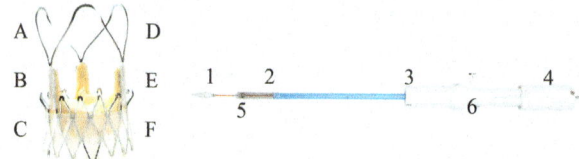

**Fig. 23.1** (*A*) STABILIZATION ARCHES for self-alignment of bioprosthesis; (*B*) UPPER CROWN for supra-annular anchoring and tactile feedback; (*C*) PET SKIRT allowing low incidence of paravalvular leak; (*D*) SELF-EXPANDING NITINOL for an anatomic conformability to the native annular shape; (*E*) WAIST to capture calcified leaflets; (*F*) LOWER CROWN allows minimal stent protrusion into the left ventricle and low risk of conduction system interference. (*1*) RADIOPAQUE TIP with sheathless, atraumatic insertion; (*2*) TRANSPARENT RADIOPAQUE HOUSING for greater visibility; (*3*) FLEXIBLE ISODIAMETRIC SHAFT to easily introduce through angled apical access; (*4*) ROTATION KNOB allows single operator deployment; (*5*) RADIOPAQUE MARKERS are a reference for correct bioprosthesis positioning; (*6*) SAFETY BUTTON allows controlled release, avoiding premature deployment of bioprosthesis

The transfemoral TAVI device (Boston Scienti c, Marlborough, MA, USA) consists of the ACURATE-neo™ aortic bioprosthesis and the ACURATE-TF™ transfemoral delivery system [2]. The ACURATE-neo™ aortic bioprosthesis is a second-generation transcatheter aortic valve composed of a porcine pericardial tissue valve sewn into a self-expanding Nitinol stent covered on the inside and outside, with an anti-leak porcine pericardial skirt. As for the first-generation ACURATE TA, the device has three stabilization arches for axial alignment and upper crown for capping the aortic annulus and a lower crown that is opened for full deployment over the native valve (Fig. 23.2). The design gives it a supra-annular position. The ACURATE-TF™ transfemoral delivery consists of a true 18-Fr flexible delivery catheter (Fig. 23.2). This transfemoral delivery system is designed for a simple two-step deployment and stable positioning within the native annulus.

## 23.1.2 Transfemoral Procedure (Figs. 23.3 and 23.4)

The implantation of the ACURATE-neo™ aortic bioprosthesis follows an intuitive controlled procedure. After the insertion of an 18–19-Fr transfemoral introducer sheath (Gore, SoloPath, or 19-Fr Cook), the ACURATE-TF™ flexible delivery catheter is advanced up to the aortic root. The native aortic valve is then crossed, and the prosthesis loader is usually placed 4–6 mm below the aortic annulus (Fig. 23.3a). The upper crown is opened to capture the native aortic leaflets, deflecting them downward away from the coronary ostia (Fig. 23.3b). With the pigtail catheter placed in the non-coronary or right cusp, an aortography confirms the accurate position. The stabilization arches are released to contact the aortic root (Fig. 23.3b), followed by self-deployment of the lower crown, obtained by rotating the second knob of the delivery catheter handle (Fig. 23.3c).

Importantly, unlike other self-expanding devices, the ACURATE-neo™ is initially released from the aorta rather than from the left ventricle outflow tract, with subsequent deployment of the sub-annular portion. This enables stability during

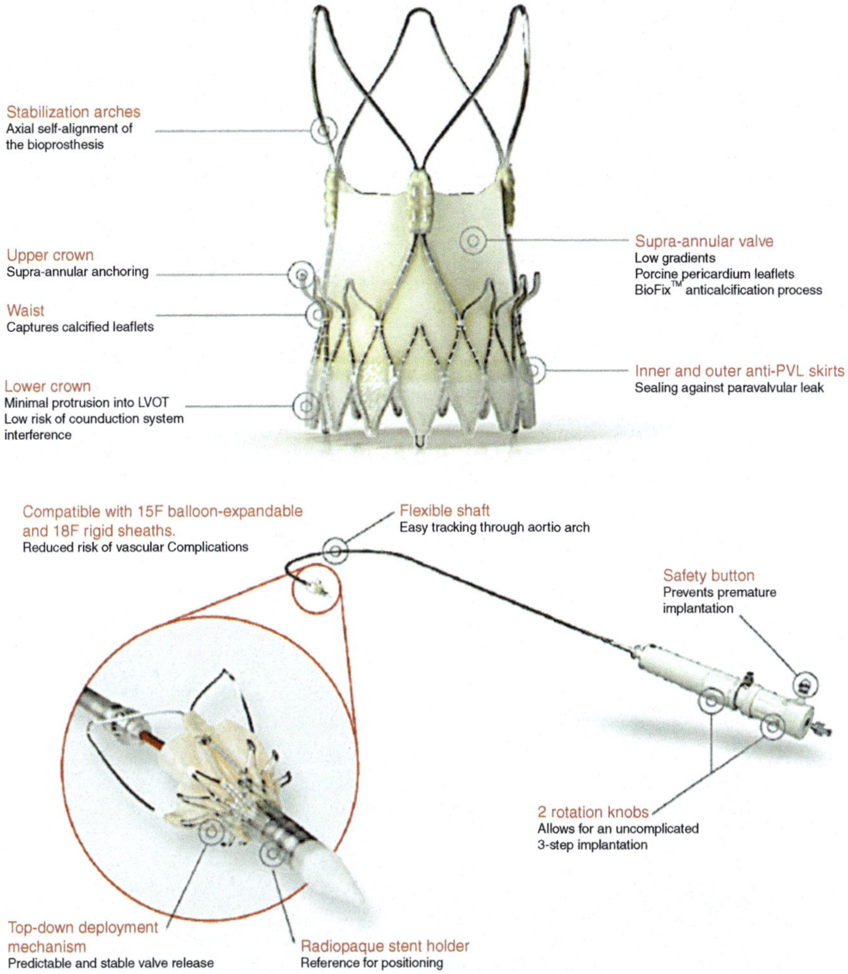

**Fig. 23.2** (**a**) The ACURATE-neo™ aortic bioprosthesis. The ACURATE-neo™ device has three stabilizer arches for axial alignment and a porcine pericardial tissue valve sewn into a self-expanding Nitinol stent. The upper crown and waist capture aortic leaflets centrally toward the aortic annulus, thereby minimizing coronary ostia obstruction. The lower crown is covered with an inner and outer anti-leak porcine pericardial skirt. The ACURATE-TF delivery system. True 18-Fr outer diameter delivery catheter. Knob 1: opens upper crown and sta- bilization arches. Knob 2: opens lower crown for valve self-deployment. Adapted from Symetis with permission ©Symetis 2016

valve positioning, as well as minimizes hemodynamic compromise during deployment. Indeed, the V shape of the device with the upper crown and stabilizers opened (Fig. 23.3b) avoids obstruction of antegrade blood flow during the positioning and self-deployment steps, thereby protecting against uncontrolled device movements and/or embolization. During the release steps of the device, it is important to keep the system tensioned toward the ventricle. If the operator is not satisfied with the position of the prosthesis (too low) before releasing the anchors, it is

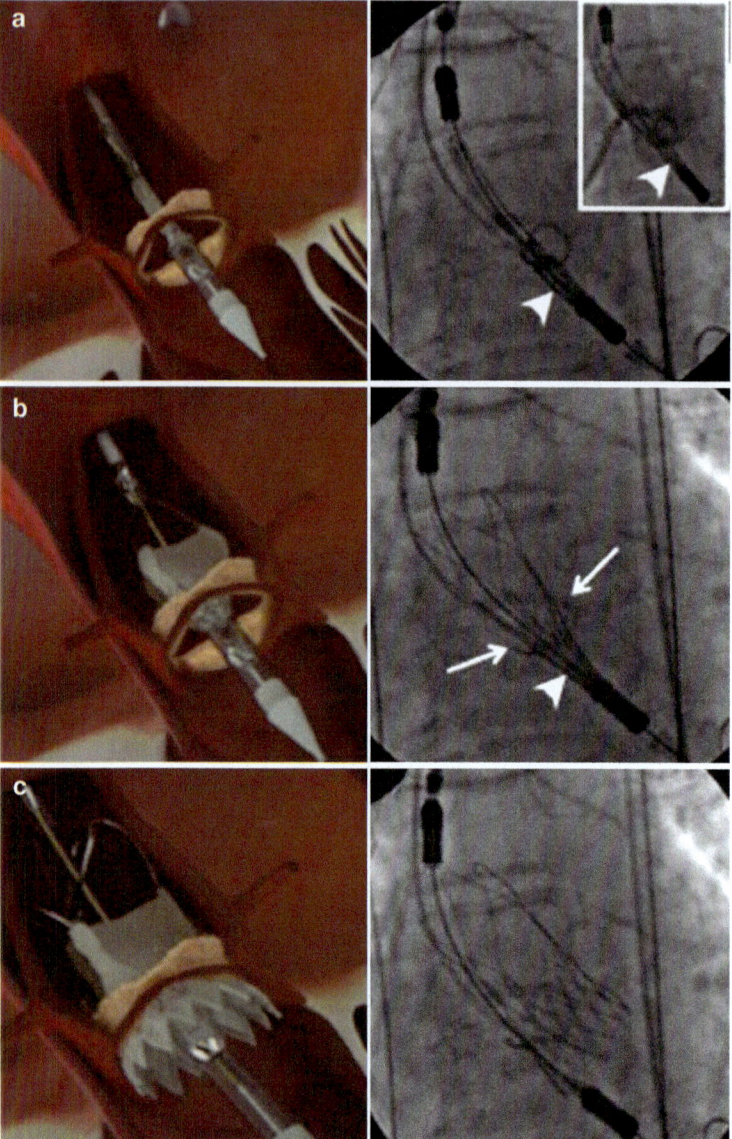

**Fig. 23.3** Transcatheter ACURATE-neo™ aortic valve implantation procedure. (**a**) Fluoroscopic alignment is obtained by placing the radiopaque marker (*arrowhead*) of the stent at the level of the aortic annulus (*white line*), with an implantation depth between 4 and 6 mm below the annulus. (**b**) Subsequently, opening of the stabilizer arches placed in the ascending aorta for axial self-alignment. The upper crown (*arrows*) captures the leaflets of the native aortic valve caudal away from the left main. Importantly, the ACURATE-neo™ is initially released from the aortic side, rather than from the left ventricular outflow tract, thereby obtaining stability during valve positioning/deployment, as well as minimizing hemodynamic compromise during deployment. Indeed, the V shape of the device with the upper crown and stabilizers opened protects against uncontrolled movements of the valve, as well as the obstruction of antegrade blood flow. (**c**) Fluoroscopic aspect of the implanted ACURATE-neo™ aortic bioprosthesis. Left panel schematic images are adapted from Symetis with permission Symetis 2016

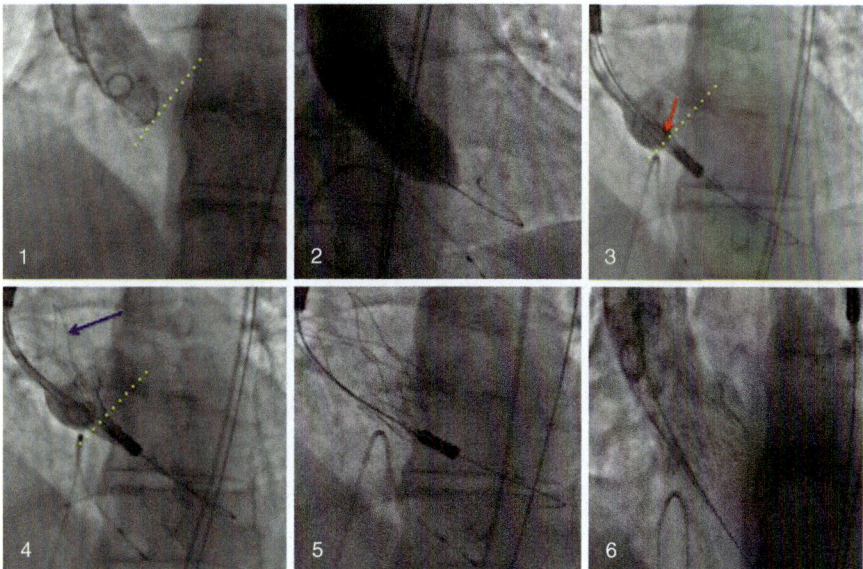

**Fig. 23.4** Transcatheter ACURATE-neo™ aortic valve implantation procedure: (*1*) aortogram showing the alignment of the coronary cusps for correct positioning of the valve (the *yellow line* indicates the virtual ring plane); (*2*) preimplantation valvuloplasty; (*3*) device placed inside the aortic valve. The *red arrow* indicates the radiopaque marker, which must be positioned in the annulus before starting the release of the device; (*4*) release of the stabilization arches (*blue arrow*); (*5*) release of the lower crown; (*6*) final post-TAVI control aortogram

advisable to pull the delivery system out of the ventricle and repeat the maneuver of crossing the native aortic valve. This needs to be done to avoid deploying the bioprosthesis with the tensioned system toward the aorta. There are two ways to ensure that the right tension is being applied on the system: (1) before and after releasing the anchoring, with left lateral fluoroscopic view, the system is positioned against the aortic lateral wall; (2) when the device is released completely, the nosecone of the delivery catheter releases tension, tending to migrate slightly inside the ventricle.

### 23.1.3 Transapical Procedure (Figs. 23.5 and 23.6)

The access side is prepared for a transapical procedure in a standard fashion, and the balloon aortic valvuloplasty is then performed. The crimped ACURATE TA is inserted through the left ventricle and is advanced to cross the native valve. Two radiopaque markers aid correct positioning. The knob of the delivery is then rotated for a commissural alignment. The partial release begins with the rotation of the knob until there is an intermediate stop created by the safety button on the delivery system. The stabilization arches and the upper crown are released. The upper crown engages the cusps of the native leaflets. The final release begins with the removal of the safety button and with the complete rotation of the knob. The valve detaches from the delivery system, leaving the lower crown fully expanded.

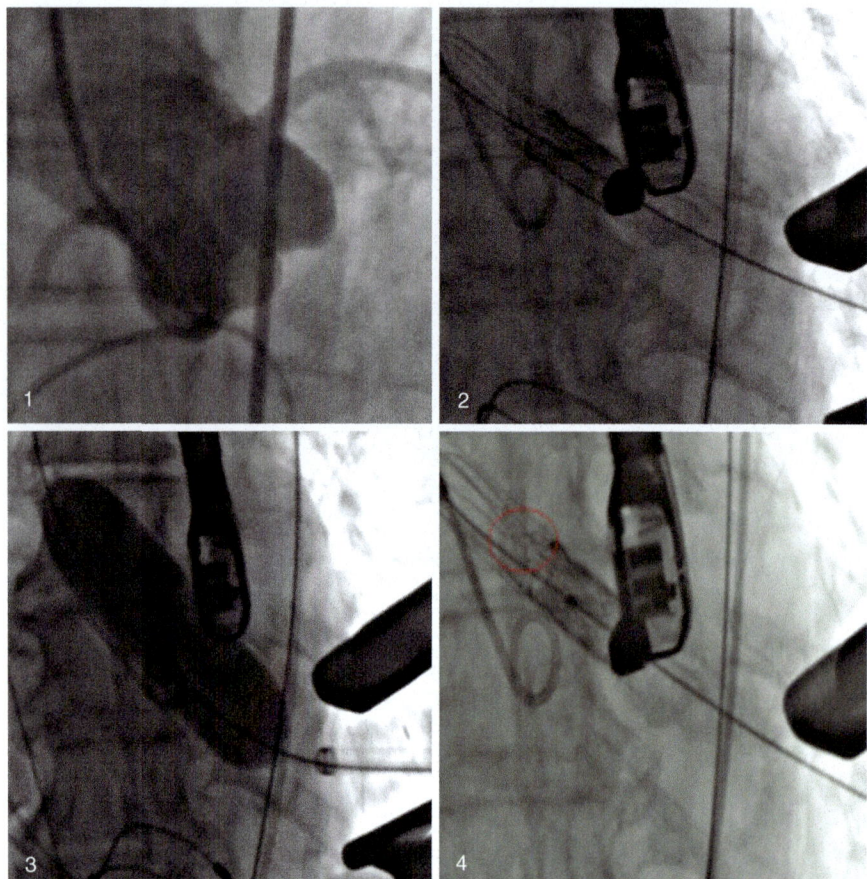

**Fig. 23.5** Transapical implantation of the Symetis device: (*1*) angiographic alignment, (*2*) pre-dilatation, (*3*) insertion, (*4*) commissural alignment

## 23.1.4 Patient Selection

ACURATE and ACURATE-neo are available in three sizes: S, M, and L. In choosing the right bioprosthesis, a preliminary multislice computed tomography scan is recommended. It provides an accurate and reproducible assessment of the valve annulus (maximum and minimum diameter, perimeter), sinuses of Valsalva, and minimum diameter of the vascular accesses. It also allows the operator to determine the angle of the aortic annulus in order to choose the most suitable vascular access (transfemoral or direct aortic) (Table 23.1).

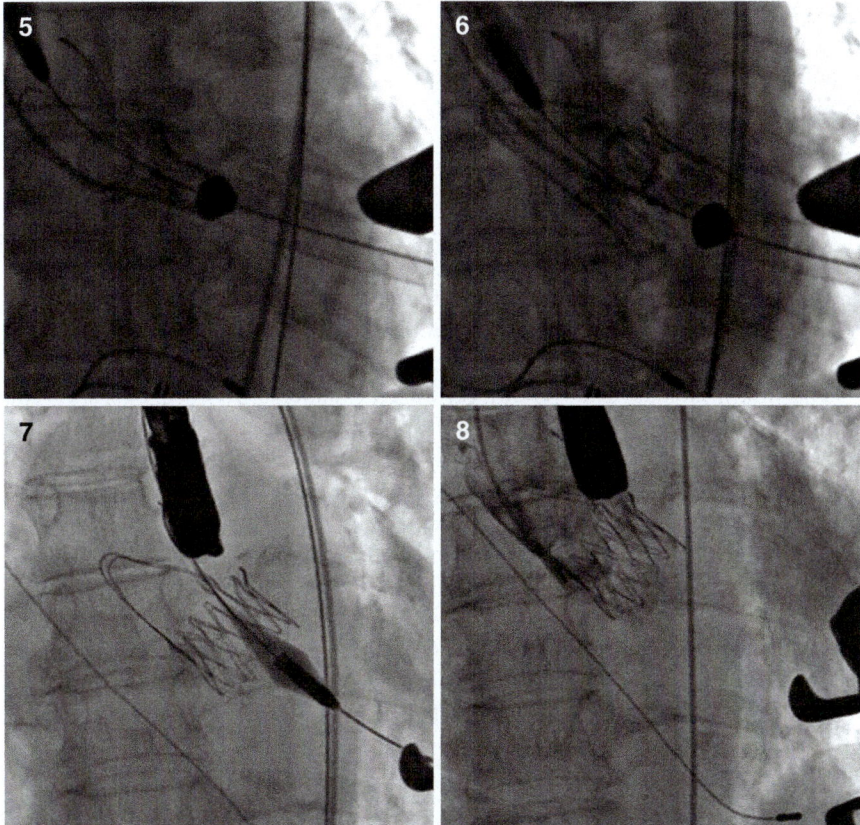

**Fig. 23.6** Transapical implantation of the Symetis device: (5) partial release, (6) full release, (7) retrieval of delivery system, (8) final angiography

**Table 23.1** The self-expandable ACURATE and ACURATE-neo THVs are available in three sizes, small "*S*," medium "*M*," and large "*L*," to fit into aortic annuluses between 21 and 27 mm

| Annulus size | S | M | L |
|---|---|---|---|
| Annulus size diameter (mm) | $21 \leq \emptyset < 23$ | $23 \leq \emptyset < 25$ | $25 \leq \emptyset < 27$ |
| Annulus size perimeter (mm) | 66–72 | 72–79 | 79–85 |
| Annulus size area (mm²) | 346–415 | 415–491 | 491–573 |

Specifically, ACURATE S is indicated for an annulus with a perimeter measuring 66–72 mm; ACURATE M is indicated for an annulus with a perimeter measuring 72–79 mm; and ACURATE L is indicated for an annulus with a perimeter measuring 79–85 mm.

According to the technical data sheet, the minimum distance required for the height of the coronaries is 8 mm. An 18-Fr introducer (compatible with the device) requires a minimum artery diameter of 6 mm. Self-expanding introducers can be used as well and require a minimum diameter of 5.5 mm.

## 23.1.5 Clinical Outcomes

The first-in-human use of the devices was in January 2012, in three patients. These patients have returned for a 12-month follow-up in good health and with good functioning of the device, without significant residual stenosis or paravalvular leakage.

The first-in-human trial (TF20) enrolled 20 patients between February and August 2012. In the TF20 trial, patients had a mean age of 84.8 ± 4.5 years and presented with a logistic EuroSCORE of 26.5 ± 8.0 (STS score 7.0 ± 5.2). The intended implantation could be performed in all patients. The procedural success was very high, at 95% ($n = 19$); only one patient had to be treated with a valve in valve due to too low initial placement. One patient had a grade 2 paravalvular leak, while all other patients had zero or trace leaks. The effective orifice area improved from 0.7 to 1.8 cm$^2$. The pacemaker rate was low, at 10% ($n = 2$). At 30 days, there was one stroke and one re-intervention (due to a ventricular septal defect at day 17). Importantly, there was no myocardial infarction and no death at 30 days of follow-up. In addition, there was a significant improvement in NYHA class in all patients.

The second study was carried out to obtain the CE Mark and enrolled 89 patients from January 2012 to October 2013. The mean age of the patients was 83.7 years ±4.4, with a logistic EuroSCORE of 26.6 ± 7.7 (STS score 7.5 ± 8.2). The device was successfully implanted in 94.4% of patients. The pacemaker implantation rate was 9%. Mortality at 30 days was 3.4%. There were two cases of stroke (2.2%), four cases of moderate post-TAVI aortic regurgitation (4.9%), and no case of aortic regurgitation worse than moderate. There were no cases of myocardial infarction.

The data at 30 days of the Symetis ACURATE *Neo*™ Valve Implantation Using Transfemoral Access (SAVI TF) Registry were presented at the 2016 EuroPCR. A total of 1000 patients were enrolled from October 2015 to April 2016 at 25 European centers. The mean age of the patients was 81.1 years ±5.2, with a logistic EuroSCORE of 18.1 ± 12.5 (STS score 6 ± 5.6). The pacemaker implantation rate was 8.2%. Mortality at 30 days was 1.3%. There were 19 (1.9%) cases of stroke, 39 (4%) cases of moderate post-TAVI aortic regurgitation, and no case of aortic regurgitation worse than moderate. There were no cases of myocardial infarction.

A Symetis S was implanted in 26.2% of cases, Symetis M in 43%, and Symetis L in 30.8% (Table 23.2).

**Table 23.2** Symetis SAVI
TF Registry presented by
Prof. Moellmann at EuroPCR
2016, LBCT, May 17, 2016

| Patients | 1000 |
|---|---|
| Permanent pacemaker | 8.2% |
| Paravalvular leak at 7 days | 4.1% |
| All-cause mortality | 1.3% |

# References

1. Kempfert J, Möllmann H, Walther T. Symetis ACURATE TA valve. EuroIntervention. 2012;8:Q102–Q10.
2. Barbanti M, Webb JG, Gilard M, Capodanno D, Tamburino C. Transcatheter aortic valve implantation in 2017: state of the art. EuroIntervention. 2017;13:AA11–21.

# Transcatheter Aortic Valve Implantation: Abbott Portico

# 24

Carmelo Sgroi, Claudia Ina Tamburino, and Martina Patanè

## 24.1 Device Description

The Portico (Abbott Vascular) valve (Fig. 24.1a) is a self-expanding transcatheter aortic prosthesis that was clinically evaluated in the Portico CE trial. In this prospective, multicenter study, safety, and performance of the Portico system (23 and 25 mm valves delivered through 18 Fr transfemoral resheathable delivery system) were tested on 100 patients with severe symptomatic aortic stenosis, 50 for each valve size. The results through 12 months showed that the Portico system produces clinically significant and sustained improvements in patient outcomes. Additionally, this study establishes an excellent safety profile at 30 days with the Portico system in terms of mortality, permanent pacemaker rate, moderate/severe paravalvular leak (PVL), major stroke rate, and major vascular complications. The good hemodynamic results were sustained up to 12 months, with the mean aortic gradient constantly stable at about 9.9 mmHg and valve area at 1.6 cm². The functional NYHA class remained improved and remained stable at follow-up [1].

In January 2016, results at 30 days from the "Multicentre Clinical Study Evaluating a Novel Self-Expanding and Resheathable Transcatheter Aortic Valve System" were presented, confirming the data previously obtained by the Portico CE trial.

The Portico valve (Fig. 24.1a) is a self-expanding stent, made of super-elastic nitinol, with shape memory, and a preset finish temperature, set below body temperature, to ensure that the valve fully opens to the annulus diameter on deployment, and has sufficient radial force to seal and anchor.

C. Sgroi (✉) • C.I. Tamburino • M. Patanè
Ferrarotto Hospital, University of Catania, Catania, Italy
e-mail: carmelo_sgroi@hotmail.com

© Springer International Publishing AG 2018
C. Tamburino et al. (eds.), *Percutaneous Treatment of Left Side Cardiac Valves*,
https://doi.org/10.1007/978-3-319-59620-4_24

431

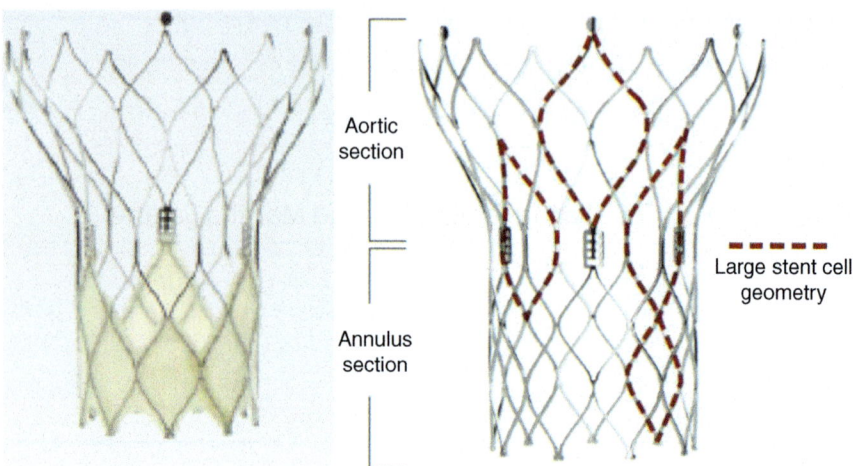

**Fig. 24.1** Portico (St. Jude Medical) valve; *left*, overview of the prosthesis; *right*, details of the nitinol prosthesis

This stent design and its proprietary manufacturing process also optimize the stent's radial forces. The two components of stent radial force—radial resistive force (RRF) and chronic outward force (COF)—are both augmented for performance. The RRF is optimized to allow for room temperature loading of the Portico valve and resheathability at body temperature. Additionally, the COF is enhanced to ensure optimal valve anchoring and apposition within the native annulus [2].

The stent design has two primary sections: (1) annulus, with a higher cell density that provides support for the valve and has higher radial force for optimal anchoring, apposition, and sealing, and (2) aortic, with lower cell density and lower stent radial force, which ensures optimal valve alignment and conformability within the ascending aorta [2].

The stent has an open cell design (Fig. 24.1b), which reduces the overall metal content and allows the valve to conform around calcific nodules in the annulus anatomy. In addition, this allows for coronary access post implant with a 15.8 F catheter [2]. The Portico valve has also been implanted via the transapical approach.

The Portico valve is designed to be fully resheathable and repositionable at the implant site and retrievable, if needed. All options are available until the valve is fully deployed. Short valve height allows for sealing without the valve extending deep into the left ventricular outflow tract (LVOT)—to help mitigate conduction system disturbances while maintaining access to the coronary ostia (Fig. 24.2). More precisely, the Portico valve is designed to be implanted at the annular level, extending no more than 5 mm into the LVOT, hence, as mentioned, potentially minimizing conduction defects. Also, large stent cells (Fig. 24.1b) in the annulus section of the stent allow for conformability and provide annular sealing to help minimize PVL and facilitate engagement of the coronary ostia postimplantation. Moreover, the contoured leaflet design allows for optimal leaflet coaptation in round and elliptical annulus configurations.

| Portico valve size (mm) | Leaflet/cuff height (mm) | Total height (mm) |
|---|---|---|
| 23 | 26 | 50 |
| 25 | 28 | 53 |
| 27 | 28 | 49 |
| 29 | 29 | 50 |

**Fig. 24.2** Portico valve technical dimensions

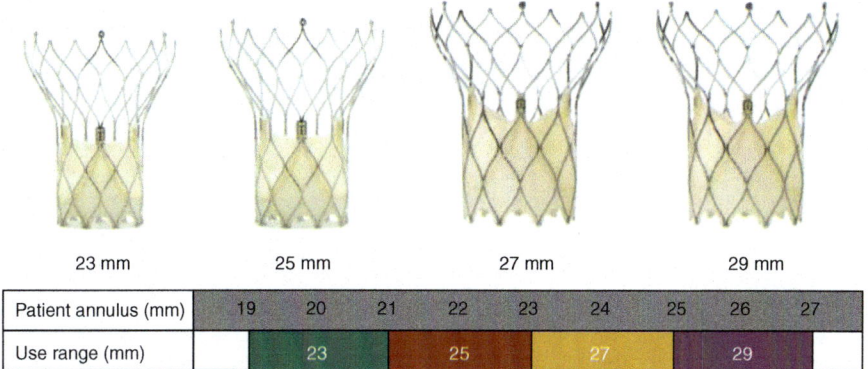

| Patient annulus (mm) | 19 | 20 | 21 | 22 | 23 | 24 | 25 | 26 | 27 |
|---|---|---|---|---|---|---|---|---|---|
| Use range (mm) | | 23 | | 25 | | 27 | | 29 | |

**Fig. 24.3** Portico valve size chart

The bovine leaflets and porcine pericardial sealing cuff are equipped with Linx™ anticalcification treatment, which is also performed in the Trifecta™, Epic™, and Epic Supra surgical valve designs. This treatment reduces free aldehydes [3, 4], extracts lipids [5], minimizes uptake of cholesterol, and stabilizes leaflet collagen [6]. Of note, there is no clinical data currently available that evaluates the long-term impact of anticalcification tissue treatment in humans.

The prosthesis comes in four different sizes, allowing treatment of the annulus ranging from 19 to 27 mm (Fig. 24.3).

## 24.2  Packaging

The valve is supplied sterile and non-pyrogenic, packaged in a formaldehyde storage solution, and supplied on a disposable holder. The transfemoral three-component system includes the valve, the loading system, and the delivery system (Fig. 24.4); no specialized accessories or ancillary products are required. The valve requires rinsing for a total time of 20 s (twice: 10 s each time in two different bowls).

**Fig. 24.4** Portico valve (**a**) loading system: (*1*) loading tube; (*2*) loading funnel; (*3*) base insert; (*4*) loading base; (*5*) leaflet testers; (**b**) delivery system

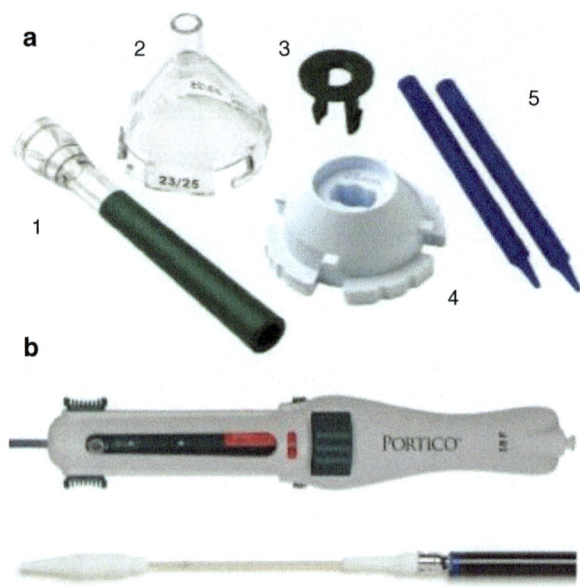

The 24 Fr delivery system used for the transapical approach is composed of a tapered nose cone, a capsule containing the compressed valve, and a handle with a thumbwheel that allows the release or resheathing of the valve while rotating clockwise or counterclockwise, respectively. The inner shaft contains a radiopaque marker that provides a reference point and contributes, as does the curved shape of the capsule, to a better valve alignment in the aortic annulus.

## 24.3    Patient Selection and Sizing

The Portico TAVI system is currently available as a 23, 25, 27, and 29 mm device, covering annulus diameters ranging from 19 to 27 mm (Fig. 24.3).

Careful evaluation of the aortic root and vascular access site is mandatory for patient selection and prosthesis size choice. Multislice computed tomography (MSCT) is the gold standard for evaluating anatomy before a TAVI procedure.

The Portico 23 and 25 mm valves are loaded on an 18 Fr delivery system, while the Portico 27 and 29 mm valves are loaded on a 19 Fr delivery system. Minimum access diameter is therefore 6 mm for the two smaller sizes and 6.5 mm for the two bigger sizes. Key measurements for a correct valve size include annulus diameter, area and perimeter, sinus of Valsalva width and height, and ascending aorta diameter (Fig. 24.5). Also, a minimum to maximum annulus axis ratio measurement of ≥0.7 is recommended, since the Portico valve is an annular-functioning valve, and thus severe eccentric annulus anatomy could affect its function.

Refer to Table 24.1 for further patient selection characteristics.

| Portico valve size | Annulus range (mm) | Ascending aorta diameter (mm) | Area (mm²)* | Perimeter (mm)* |
|---|---|---|---|---|
| 23 mm | 19–21 | 26–36 | 277–346 | 60–66 |
| 25 mm | 21–23 | 28–38 | 338–415 | 66–73 |
| 27 mm | 23–25 | 30–40 | 405–491 | 72–79 |
| 29 mm | 25–27 | 32–42 | 479–573 | 79–85 |

**Fig. 24.5** Portico valve sizing specific according to instructions for use labeling. (*Asterisk*) Recommendation based on circular or elliptical geometry (≥0.73 ratio)

**Table 24.1** Patient selection guide

| Characteristic | Selection criteria | |
|---|---|---|
| | Required per IFU | Off label per IFU |
| Vasc access diameter for 18 F delivery system | ≥6 mm | <6 mm |
| Vasc access diameter for 19 F delivery system | ≥6.5 mm | <6.5 mm |
| | Recommended | Not recommended |
| Atrial or ventricular thrombus | Not present | Present |
| Aortic and vascular conditions | Normal | Stenosis, tortuosity, severe calcification |
| Mitral regurgitation | ≤Grade 3 | >Grade 3 |
| Annulus eccentricity | Minor/major axis ratio ≥ 0.73 | Minor/major axis ratio < 0.73 |
| LV ejection fraction | ≥20% | <20% |
| Sinus of Valsalva width | ≥27 (23 and 25 mm valves) | <27 mm (23 and 25 mm valves) |
| | ≥29 mm (27 mm valve) | <29 mm (27 mm valve) |
| | ≥31 mm (29 mm valve) | <31 mm (29 mm valve) |
| Sinus of Valsalva height | ≥15 mm | <15 mm |
| Sub-aortic stenosis | Not present | Present |
| Annulus to brachiocephalic (TAo) | ≥80 mm | <80 mm |
| LV depth—apex to annulus (TA) | ≥4.5 cm | <4.5 cm |
| Coronary artery disease | Not clinically significant | Untreated; clinically significant |
| | Recommended | Moderate-high risk |
| LV hypertrophy | Normal to mild (0.6–1.8 cm) | Severe (≥1.8 cm) |
| Aortic arch angulation | Large radius turn | High angulation or sharp bend |
| Annulus to aorta angle (TF, TA, left sub) | ≤70 ° | >70 ° |
| Annulus to aorta angle (right SC) | ≤30 ° | >30 ° |

## 24.4 Preparation and Loading Procedure (Courtesy of St. Jude Medical)

### 24.4.1 Handling

1. Review the temperature indicator on the valve packaging to ensure it has remained within the required temperature range.
2. Examine the valve and container carefully, and do not use if there is any sign of leaking, damage, or deterioration.
3. Open the container by breaking the plastic seal and removing the screw top lid. Leave the valve and holder in the jar and solution until ready to use (Fig. 24.6a).
4. Carefully grasp the valve holder and remove the valve from the jar (Fig. 24.6b).
5. Remove the valve from the valve holder by carefully compressing the valve stent circumferentially (Fig. 24.6c).

### 24.4.2 Rinsing

1. Within the sterile field, prepare two sterile basins each with 500 mL of sterile isotonic saline at room temperature.
2. Holding the aortic (non-leaflet) end of the valve, fully immerse the valve in the sterile isotonic saline solution in the first basin (Fig. 24.7a).
3. Continually rinse the valve for 10 s, using a gentle back-and-forth motion.

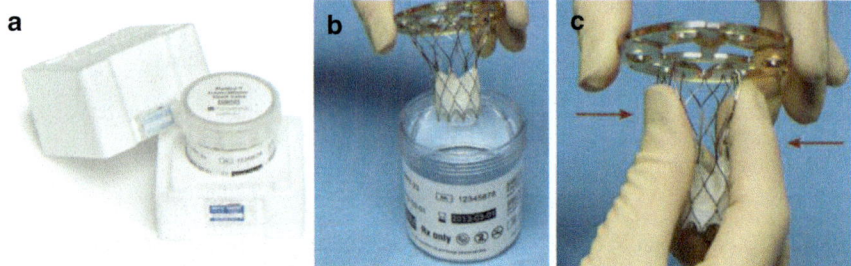

**Fig. 24.6** Preparation and loading procedure. Handling (courtesy of St. Jude Medical)

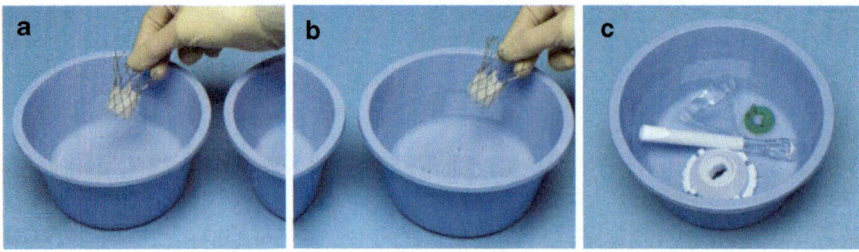

**Fig. 24.7** Preparation and loading procedure. Rising (courtesy of St. Jude Medical)

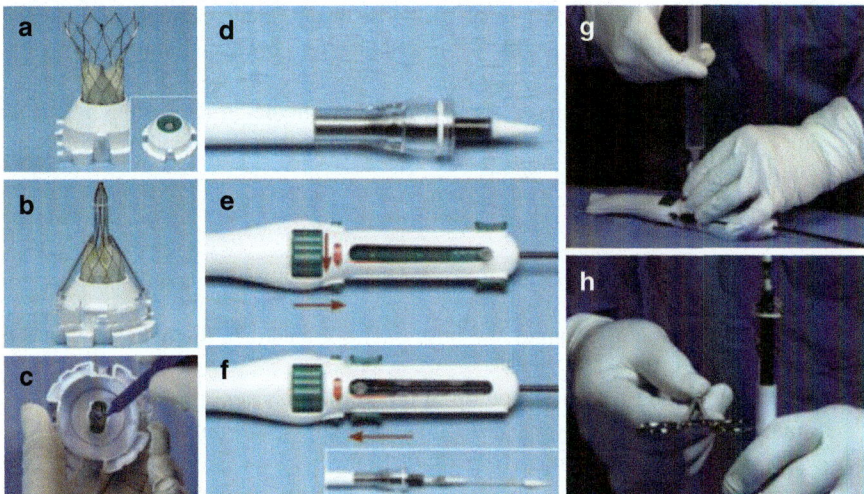

**Fig. 24.8** Preparation and loading procedure. Preparing (courtesy of St. Jude Medical)

4. Repeat steps (2) and (3) in the second basin (Fig. 24.7b).
5. After rinsing, leave the valve immersed in the second basin. Do not allow the tissue to dry.
6. Within the sterile field, prepare a separate sterile basin with 500 mL of sterile isotonic saline at room temperature, and immerse the loading base, base insert, loading funnel, and loading tube (Fig. 24.7c).

### 24.4.3 Preparing

1. Confirm valve size to be implanted. For the 23 mm valve, place the green base insert into the loading base.
2. Place the annulus end of the valve onto the loading base on top of the green insert (Fig. 24.8a).
3. Wet the loading funnel with sterile saline and place over the aortic end of the valve (Fig. 24.8b).
4. Gently push the loading funnel down over the valve, rotating the loading funnel slightly until it locks into the loading base.
5. Look through the underside of the loading base to ensure there is an opening through the leaflets. If necessary, use the leaflet tester to gently push the leaflets toward the stent frame (Fig. 24.8c).
6. Wet a 4″ × 4″ gauze with sterile saline and wipe the shaft of the delivery system.
7. Slide the loading tube over the protective sheath, advancing to just below the distal tip of the protective sheath (Fig. 24.8d).
8. Advance the locking buttons to the forward position and slide the 80% release lever to the right (Fig. 24.8e).

9. Fully retract the sliding mechanism to expose the retainer receptacle (Fig. 24.8f).
10. Fill a 20 cc syringe with sterile saline and attach to the sheath flush port with a stopcock (Fig. 24.8g).
11. Holding the distal tip of the delivery system upright, de-air the system by injecting 15–20 cc of saline into the sheath flush port and tapping the loading tube to dislodge air bubbles (Fig. 24.8h).

### 24.4.4 Loading

1. Compress the loading funnel and base to slightly actuate the aortic end of the valve (Fig. 24.9a).
2. Carefully thread the radiopaque tip of the delivery system through the loading funnel and base assembly, ensuring that the tip passes through the center of the valve to avoid leaflet damage (Fig. 24.9b).
3. Engage the three retainer tabs onto the retainer receptacle by releasing compression (inset).
4. Retract the locking buttons, and turn the deployment/resheath wheel opposite the direction of the arrow on the handle to encapsulate the retainer tabs within the protective sheath.
5. Advance the loading tube and align the black indicator line on the loading tool with the distal end of the protective sheath (Fig. 24.9c).
6. Turn the deployment/resheath wheel opposite the direction of the arrow until the funnel is fully seated in the loading tube.
7. Unlock and remove the loading base from the loading funnel (Fig. 24.9d).
8. Gently inject saline into the loading funnel to cover the valve, and tap the delivery system radiopaque tip to remove air bubbles from the inner shaft.

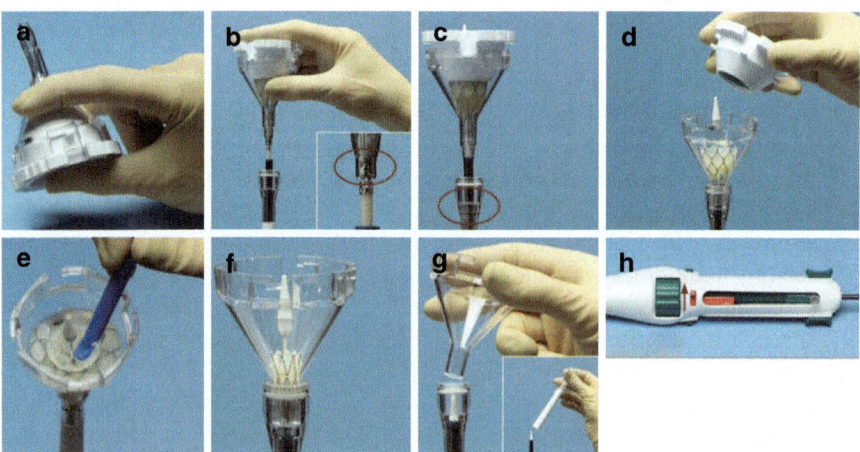

**Fig. 24.9** Preparation and loading procedure. Loading (courtesy of St. Jude Medical)

9. Slide the leaflet tester from top to bottom of each leaflet to remove any remaining air bubbles, and ensure no leaflet tissue is trapped between stent struts (Fig. 24.9e).
10. Fully encapsulate the valve in the sheath using the deployment/resheath wheel (Fig. 24.9f).
11. Massage the delivery system shaft from the proximal end to the distal end to close any gap between the sheath and the radiopaque tip.
12. Pour saline out of the loading funnel, and slide the loading funnel and loading tube off the distal end of the delivery system (Fig. 24.9g).
13. Slide the delivery system 80% release lever to the LEFT (opposite direction of the arrow on the delivery system handle) (Fig. 24.9h).
14. Flush the lumen with sterile isotonic saline.

## 24.5  Procedural and Deployment Characteristics

The Portico valve is currently available as a 23, 25, 27, and 29 mm device, accommodating annulus diameters ranging from 19 to 27 mm. The Portico valve can be delivered by transfemoral, transaxillary, transaortic, or transapical access. For retrograde access, a standard 18 Fr introducer is recommended for the 23 mm and the 25 mm valve prosthesis, and a 19 Fr introducer is recommended for the larger size valve prosthesis. A minimum vascular access diameter of 6 mm is required for the 18 Fr delivery system and of 6.5 mm for the 19 Fr delivery system. For the anterograde approach, a 24 Fr sheathless dedicated delivery system is needed.

The procedure is performed in a standard fashion. Once the preferred vascular approach and closure are chosen, an 18 or 19 Fr introducer (according to valve prosthesis size) is advanced, the aortic valve is crossed, and a stiff guidewire is accommodated into the left ventricle apex. The use of an extra-stiff wire is not recommended. Balloon aortic valvuloplasty with rapid ventricular pacing is suggested before valve implantation (size according to native valve annulus diameter). A pigtail previously inserted from the contralateral side and positioned at the inferior bottom of the non-coronary cusp serves as a landmark and for performing a small aortogram. At this point, the deployment projection should be assessed (having the three cusps aligned). The valve is then advanced with the delivery system through the annulus, and the inner member marker band (Fig. 24.10) must be aligned with the native aortic valve annulus plane, and, if needed, the releasing projection should be changed in order to align the annulus end of the frame to a straight line (Fig. 24.12a).

Deployment of the valve can then start by turning the deployment wheel clockwise on the handle of the delivery system. The valve is gradually released, with no rush, as the valve is fully functioning at initial deployment, and no rapid ventricular pacing is needed (Figs. 24.11 and 24.12).

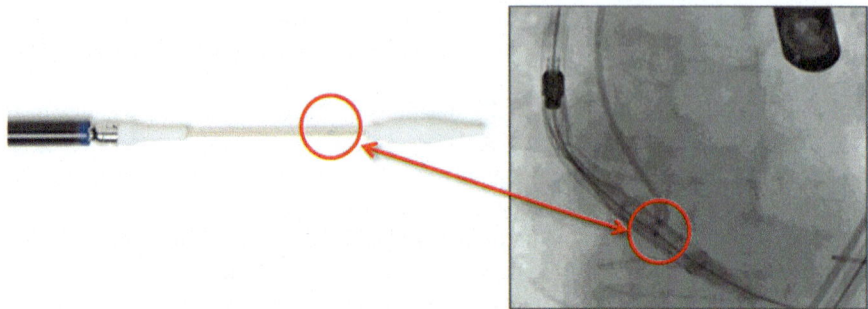

**Fig. 24.10** Inner marker band must be aligned to native valve annulus plan (courtesy of St. Jude Medical)

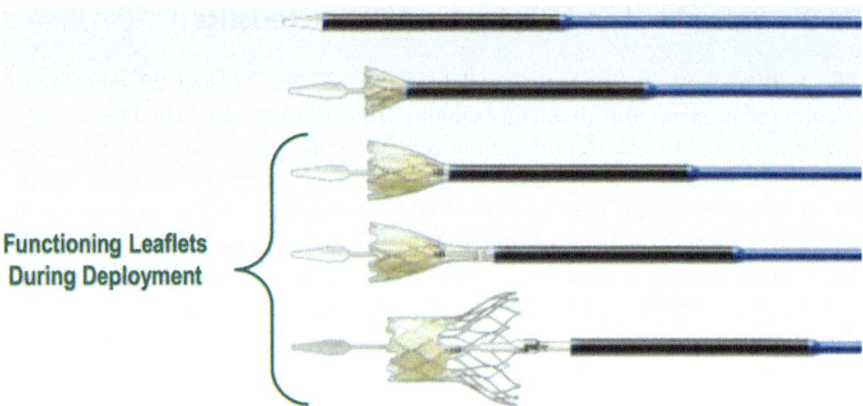

**Functioning Leaflets During Deployment**

**Fig. 24.11** Portico valve deployment steps. The valve is fully functioning at initial deployment ensuring a hemodynamic stability and giving time to operator to calmly assess placement before full release (courtesy of St. Jude Medical)

Target placement is 3 mm, keeping in mind that half stent cell height is 7 mm for the 23 and 25 mm valves and 8 mm for the 27 mm and the 29 mm valves (acceptable ranges are 1–9 mm for 23 mm and 25 mm valves and 1–10 for 27 mm and 29 mm valves). In heavy calcification a deeper implantation is recommended, with a target of 5 mm in the LVOT, since in the bench test a lower implantation showed a more uniform expansion and better apposition of the prosthesis (Fig. 24.13). It is important to maintain a neutral delivery system throughout tracking and deployment and to wait for the valve to respond to wheel turns before making any adjustment to the catheter position. If the position is correct, deployment should be continued until the safety release lever is engaged (a red lever on the handle of the delivery system) (Fig. 24.4b), which corresponds to 80% release of the prosthesis (Fig. 24.12c). This is the point of no return. In fact, until this point the valve can be easily be resheathed if the position is not satisfactory. The degree of resheathing can be tailored depending on need. If the valve is a bit too high, partial resheathing

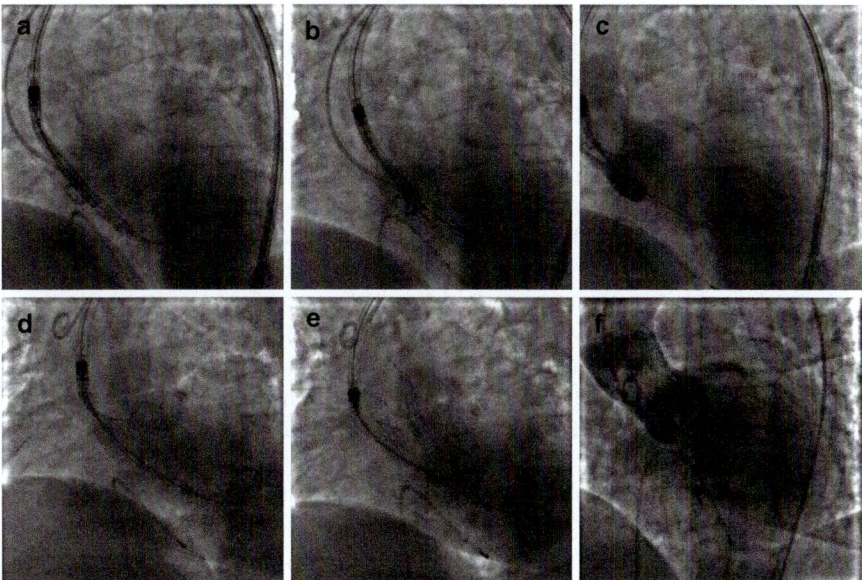

**Fig. 24.12** Implanting procedure (referred to the text for step-by-step explanation)

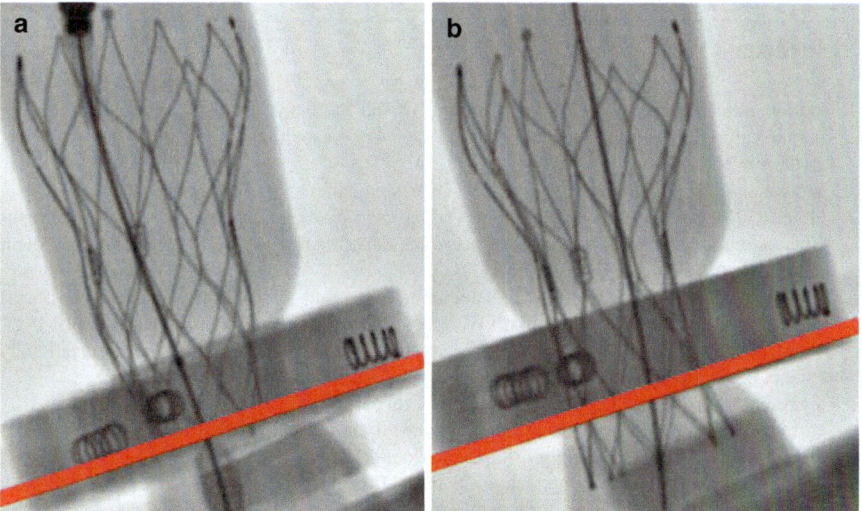

**Fig. 24.13** Bench testing simulating heavy calcification on native annulus. (**a**) A higher implantation may create under-expansion and malapposition, (**b**) a deeper deployment (~5 mm) creates a more uniform expansion and better apposition (courtesy of St. Jude Medical)

will allow repositioning, while if the prosthesis valve has migrated in the ascending aorta, complete resheathing is needed to recross the native valve. This is also the case if the implantation is too deep. Due to the fact that nitinol can lose its radial force after resheathing, it is recommended to change the prosthesis with a new one if there are more than two resheathings. If satisfied with the valve position, the release lever can be pushed, and the valve can be fully deployed (Fig. 24.12d, e). Before final release of the prosthesis, an aortogram should be done to reapprove the position. After complete deployment of the valve, attention must be paid to the three valve anchor tabs attached to the delivery system (Fig. 24.12e). They all have to be released prior to withdrawing the catheter in order to prevent valve embolization. It is recommended that their release is confirmed in at least two differing views. If one of the tabs seems to be still attached to the system, a slight rotation of the system (45–90 °) should be performed, and the guidewire should be gently pulled back in order to change the angulation with the delivery system. After complete deployment of the valve, the delivery system should be gently pulled back in the descending aorta. In order to prevent valve embolization due to nosecone interference with the prosthesis, the guidewire should be slightly pulled so the nosecone is in the middle of the valve instead of the side. After retreating the system on the descending aorta, the delivery system must be closed by pulling the handle away from the sliding mechanism instead of advancing the sliding mechanism.

After deployment, valve function should be assessed using standard methods (Fig. 24.12f), and if post-dilatation is needed, it can be done. In this case, a rapid ventricular pacing is recommended in order to minimize the risk of embolization of the valve [7].

## References

1. Manoharan G. Portico CE Trial Assessment of the St. Jude Medical Portico Transcatheter Aortic Valve Implant and the Transfemoral Delivery System. EuroPCR 2014. Paris. 20–23, 2014. $N = 100$.
2. Vietmeier K, Principal R&D Engineer, St. Jude Medical.
3. Frater RWM, Seifter E, Liao K, et al. In: Gabbay S, Wheatley D, editors. Advances in antical-cific and antidegenerative treatment of heart valve bioprostheses, vol. 8. 1st ed. Austin: Silent Partners Inc.; 1997. p. 105–13.
4. Kelly SJ, Ogle MF, Carlyle WC, et al. Biocompatibility and calcification of bioprosthetic heart valves. Society for Biomaterials, Sixth World Biomaterials Congress Transaction, 2000;13534.
5. Vyavahare N, Hirsch D, Lerner E, et al. Prevention of bioprosthetic heart valve calcification by ethanol preincubation: efficacy and mechanisms. Circulation. 1997;95(2):479–88.
6. Vyavahare N, Hirsch D, Lerner E, et al. Prevention of calcification of glutaraldehyde-crosslinked porcine aortic cusps by ethanol preincubation: mechanistic studies of protein structure and water-biomaterial relationships. J Biomed Mater Res. 1998;40(4):577–85.
7. Barbanti M, Petronio AS, Capodanno D, et al. Impact of balloon post-dilation on clinical outcomes after transcatheter aortic valve replacement with the self-expanding CoreValve prosthesis. JACC Cardiovasc Interv. 2014;7:1014–21.

# Transcatheter Aortic Valve Implantation: Other Devices

# 25

Martina Patanè, Ketty la Spina, and Alessio La Manna

Supported by favorable data from first-generation devices, TAVI has undergone rapid technological advancements. The focus on these innovations was on limiting complications found with early TAVI devices such as paravalvular regurgitation, conduction disturbances, valve malpositioning, and the impossibility of repositioning and retrieving the prosthesis. Innovations were achieved both on device designs and on delivery system technologies. Some second-generation devices have already received the CE Mark (Sapien 3, Edwards Lifesciences; CoreValve Evolut R, Medtronic; Portico™, St. Jude Medical, St. Paul, MN, USA; ACURATE neo™, Symetis, Ecublens, Switzerland; Lotus™, Boston Scientific, Marlborough, MA, USA), while other devices are in early clinical evaluation but have yet to receive the CE Mark.

Current second-generation devices have already been deeply discussed in preceding chapters. In this chapter, we provide a brief overview of non-CE Mark second-generation devices.

## 25.1 BIOVALVE (Biotronik AG, Bülach, Switzerland)

BIOVALVE (Biotronik AG, Bülach, Switzerland) (Fig. 25.1) is a resheathable porcine pericardial valve consisting of a skirt and three leaflets mounted on a nitinol stent and is delivered through an 18 Fr delivery system (Fig. 25.2). The prosthesis

M. Patanè (✉)
Division of Cardiology, Centro Cuore Morgagni, Pedara, Italy
e-mail: martipatane@gmail.com

K. la Spina • A. La Manna
Division of Cardiology, Ferrarotto Hospital, University of Catania, Catania, Italy

© Springer International Publishing AG 2018
C. Tamburino et al. (eds.), *Percutaneous Treatment of Left Side Cardiac Valves*,
https://doi.org/10.1007/978-3-319-59620-4_25

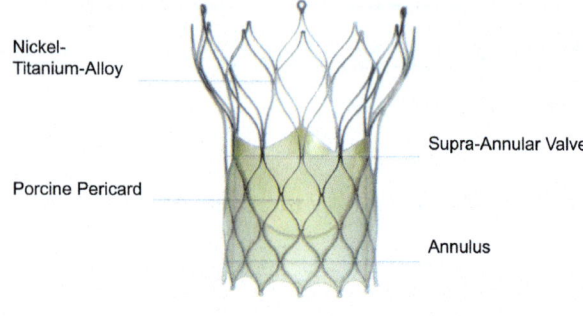

**Fig. 25.1** BIOVALVE prosthesis (courtesy of Biotronik AG, Bülach, Switzerland)

Nickel-Titanium-Alloy

Porcine Pericard

Supra-Annular Valve

Annulus

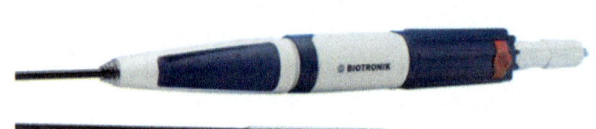

**Fig. 25.2** BIOVALVE delivery system (courtesy of Biotronik AG, Bülach, Switzerland)

**Table 25.1** BIOVALVE M (29 mm) characteristics

| | |
|---|---|
| Annulus diameter | 23–26 mm |
| Inflow diameter | 29 mm |
| Outflow diameter | 42 mm |
| Height without eyelets | 49 mm |
| Cells over circumference | 12 |
| Cells over length | 3 |
| Height of cell/rhombus | 12 mm |
| Valve position | Supra-annular |

has a supra-annular valve design to allow a large effective orifice area. The length of the rhombi that constitute the nitinol frame varies over the length of the stent. Different rhombi lengths correlate with different radial forces. The inflow end has the shortest cells and, thus, the highest radial force, allowing a correct anchoring of the prosthesis in the initial phase of the release. The outflow end has the longest cells and the least amount of radial force in order to provide flexibility in the stent to follow the ascending aorta curve. The larger cell size in the outflow tract also allows unrestricted access to the coronary arteries.

The prosthesis is currently available in size M (29 mm) accommodating annulus diameters from 23 to 26 mm (Table 25.1). Additional sizes are under development.

The BIOVALVE can be implanted through a transfemoral approach with a dedicated 18 Fr 360° flexible delivery system. The implantation is controlled by an ergonomic handle, which provides 1:1 response between handle and valve deployment. Target implantation depth is 6 mm below the annulus. A safety release button ensures a controlled deployment up to the resheathing limit (80% of full release). At this point, the valve is fully functioning, and positioning can be calmly assessed. If not satisfactory, the valve can be resheathed, repositioned, and redeployed. Final release starts by pressing the safety buttons and fully releasing the valve.

Feasibility and safety of this second-generation device were assessed in the BIOVALVE-I study [1]. In this first-in-human study, 13 patients were enrolled. Thirty-day early safety for VARC-2 was observed in two patients (15.4%), and device success was obtained in nine patients (69.2%). One patient (7.7%) had at least moderate aortic regurgitation, and three (23.1%) patients received a permanent pacemaker (PM) implantation.

## 25.2    CENTERA Valve

The CENTERA valve (Edwards Lifesciences) (Fig. 25.3) is a self-expanding, repositionable valve composed of a nitinol frame, a trileaflet bovine pericardial tissue valve (at annular level), and a polyethylene terephthalate skirt. The stent frame is shorter than other self-expanding valves (~20 mm), and the ventricular edge is flared and covered with a polyethylene terephthalate skirt. This, on

**Fig. 25.3** CENTERA valve (courtesy of Edwards Lifesciences)

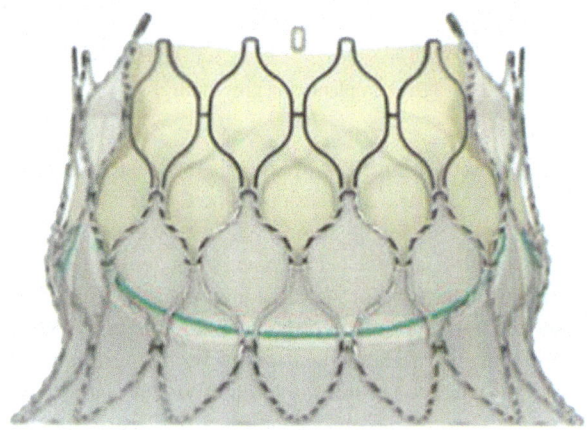

| CENTERA Valve Size | 23 mm | 26 mm | 29 mm |
|---|---|---|---|
| Native Valve Annulus Size (CT) Area Derived Diameter | 18-21 mm | 21-24 mm | 24-26 mm |

**Fig. 25.4** CENTERA valve size

**Fig. 25.5** CENTERA valve motorized delivery system (courtesy of Edwards Lifesciences)

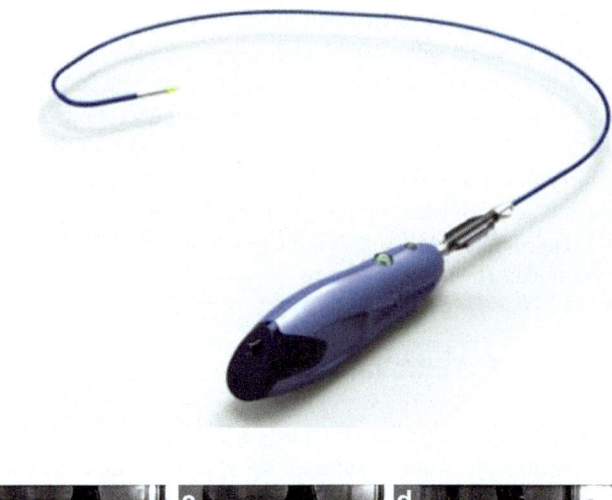

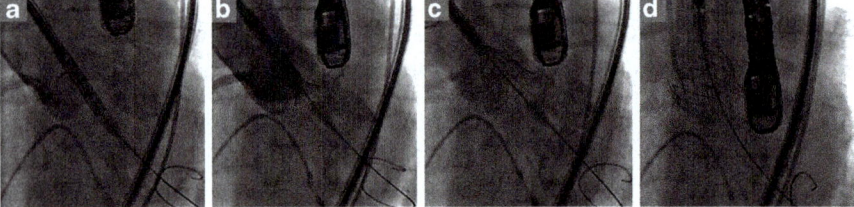

**Fig. 25.6** CENTERA implantation procedure

the one hand, minimizes prosthesis protrusion in the ventricular side and, on the other, reduces paravalvular leak. The CENTERA valve is available as a 23, 26, and 29 mm valve, covering annular sizes between 18 and 26 mm (Fig. 25.4). Thanks to its low profile, the CENTERA valve is deployed through a 14 Fr delivery system with a transfemoral or subclavian approach (Fig. 25.5). This delivery system consists of a delivery catheter and a detachable, motorized handle that allows accurate valve placement and repositioning by a single operator. The handle has two buttons, allowing for either valve deployment (large button) or valve loading (small button). The catheter incorporates a deflection mechanism to assist in traversing the aortic arch and facilitate coaxial positioning with the native valve. TAVI with the CENTERA system is implanted with a standard technique. After crossing the valve with the delivery system, deployment should be started, in a coaxial view, with the motorized handle. The ventricular edge of the prosthesis should be positioned around 2–4 mm below the annulus (Fig. 25.6a). Once the operator is satisfied with the prosthesis position, full position should be achieved by continuing to press the deployment button on the handle (Fig. 25.6b). Otherwise, the recapture button should be pressed to retract and reposition the prosthesis. It is important to note that the valve can be recaptured and repositioned prior to 70% of its deployment. Operators should also bear in mind that this prosthesis obstructs left ventricle outflow tract at 50% of its deployment, so rapid ventricular pacing is recommended during the final deployment stage. After checking final position of the prosthesis (Fig. 25.6c), detachment of the valve from the delivery system should be achieved by using the valve release mechanism located at the bottom of the handle.

A next-generation CENTERA system, fully repositionable and with an enhanced delivery system articulation, is currently under development.

In human clinical experience [2], the procedure has been found to be feasible and safe. Device success was obtained in all 15 patients (100%), paravalvular leak at 30 days was none/trivial in 3 patients (23%), mild in 9 (69%), and moderate in 1 (8%). A permanent PM was implanted in four patients (27%). Survival was 87% at 30 days and 80% at 1-year follow-up.

## 25.3   JenaValve

The JenaValve (JenaValve Technology GmbH, Munich, Germany) (Fig. 25.7) is a native porcine aortic valve mounted on a self-expanding nitinol support, with a porcine pericardial skirt to prevent paravalvular leak. JenaValve features a unique clip fixing mechanism of the native aortic valve leaflet that offers secure anchorage of the prosthesis even in the absence of calcifications. Thanks to this characteristic and to the promising results, the JenaValve is the only TAVI system worldwide for aortic regurgitation with the CE Mark. The JenaValve covers annuli ranging from 21 to

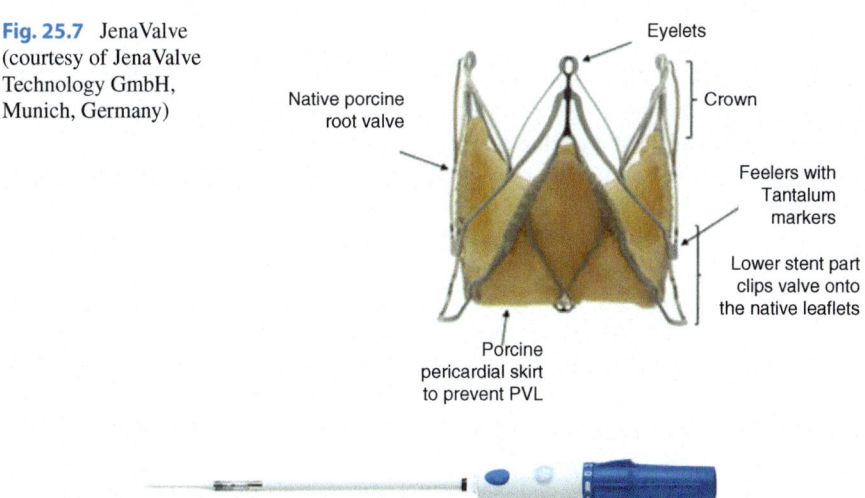

**Fig. 25.7** JenaValve (courtesy of JenaValve Technology GmbH, Munich, Germany)

Native porcine root valve

Eyelets

Crown

Feelers with Tantalum markers

Lower stent part clips valve onto the native leaflets

Porcine pericardial skirt to prevent PVL

**Fig. 25.8** JenaValve transapical delivery system (courtesy of JenaValve Technology GmbH, Munich, Germany)

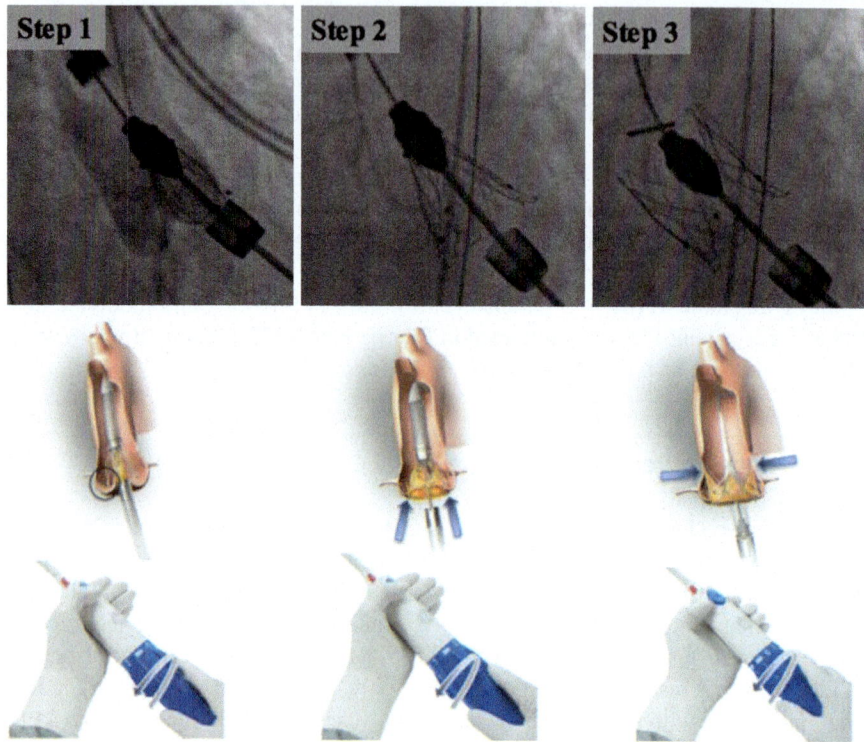

**Fig. 25.9** JenaValve three-step implantation

27 mm. Three sizes are available (23, 25, and 27 mm). The JenaValve is implanted through a sheathless 32 Fr delivery system with a transapical approach (Fig. 25.8).

After punction of the left ventricle apex, a soft guidewire is advanced into the descending aorta and exchanged with a stiff wire. At this point, if necessary, a balloon aortic valvuloplasty (BAV) should be performed. After eventual BAV, the 32 Fr delivery system is advanced over the wire through the native valve. At this point, valve deployment should start with the easy three-step implantation: (step 1) release of position feelers, (step 2) clipping of aortic cusps, and (step 3) full deployment (Fig. 25.9).

The post-market registry (JUPITER [3]) recently showed promising 1-year results. A total of 180 patients were enrolled. Procedure success was 95% ($n = 171$); conversion to surgical aortic valve replacement (SAVR) was necessary in five patients (2.8%). All-cause mortality at 30 days was 11.1%, all-cause mortality after 30 days was 13.1%, and combined efficacy at 1 year was 80.8%. At 1-year follow-up, paravalvular leak was none/trace in 49 patients (82.4%), mild in 12 patients (19.0%), and moderate in 2 patients (3.2%).

**Fig. 25.10** JenaValve Pericardial TAVI System

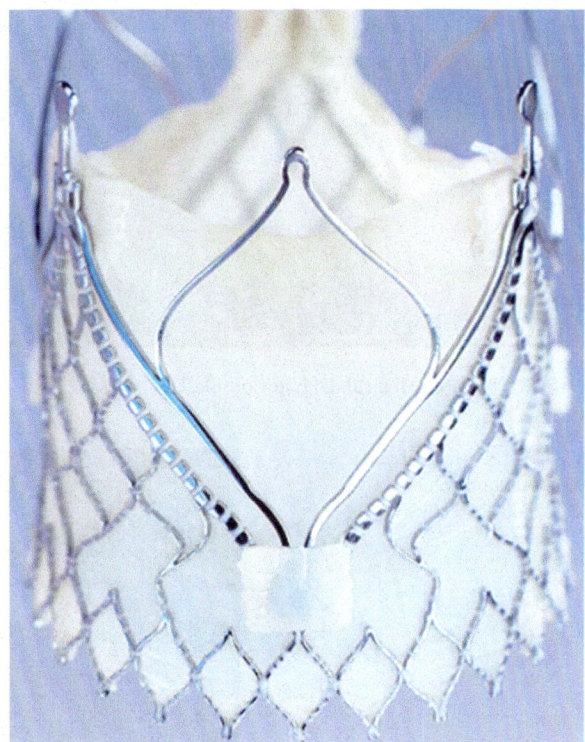

The next-generation JenaValve Pericardial TAVI System (Fig. 25.10) is currently under clinical evaluation with both transapical (22 Fr) and transfemoral (19 Fr) delivery systems.

## 25.4 Valve Medical

Recently an ultralow profile (12 Fr) TAVI system is under evaluation: the Valve Medical. This newer valve device is of a modular design (Fig. 25.11). In fact, the frame and the valve are separate and are assembled in the ascending aorta during TAVI implantation. The stent is made of a nitinol self-expanding frame module inserted in an optimal annular location. The valve is made of a single piece of pericardium fixed on a mandrel, with fewer stiches than other TAVI devices, which should improve manufacturability and durability. The valve is not crimped but folded, and all sizes are delivered by the same ultralow profile 12 Fr delivery

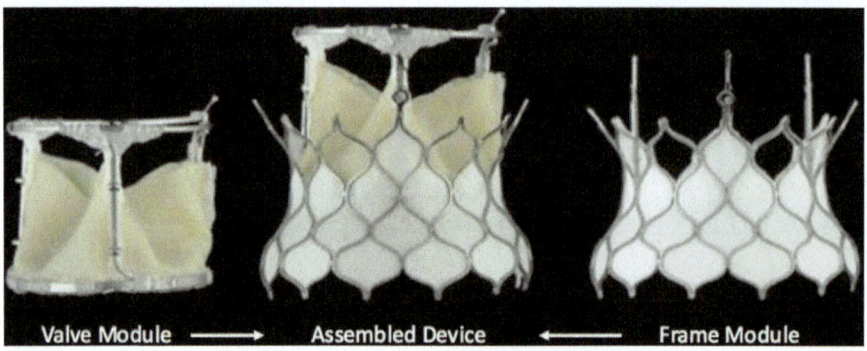

**Fig. 25.11** Valve Medical. Ultralow profile TAVI system

**Fig. 25.12** Medical valve
temporary parachute
descending aorta valve

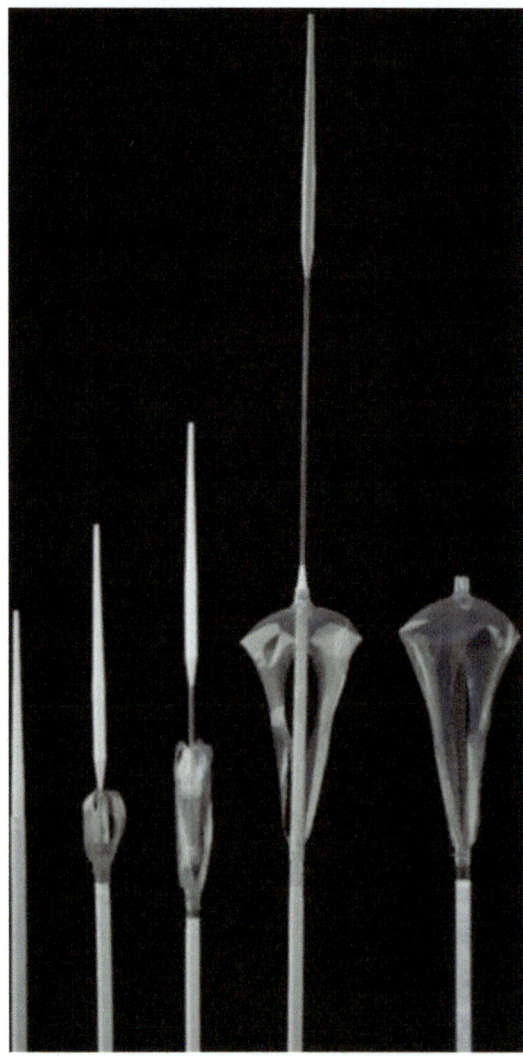

**Fig. 25.13** TRISKELE
UCL-TAV

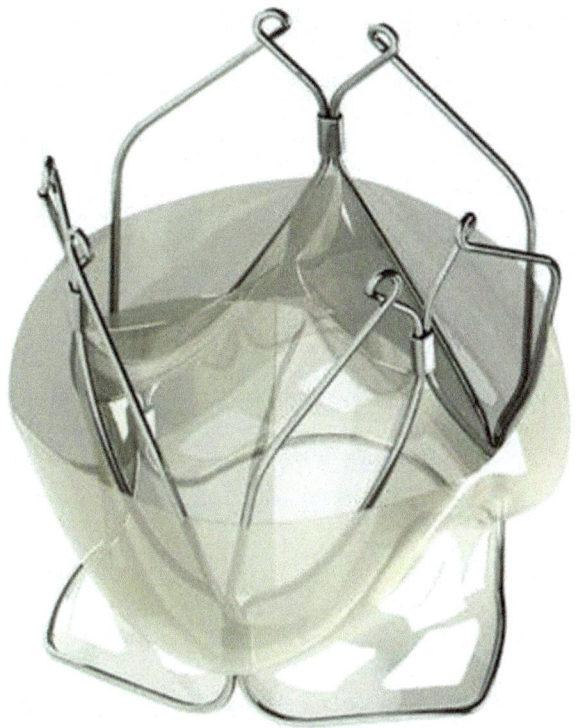

catheter. The valve is meant to be implanted with a transfemoral approach. During implantation, a temporary mono-leaflet, polymeric valve is inserted in the descending aorta for safety reasons (Fig. 25.12). The stent frame is then advanced through the native valve, and after its releasing, the valve module is opened in the ascending aorta and docked to the frame.

## 25.5 TRISKELE UCL-TAV

Recently, a new-generation TAVI was developed by the University College London: the TRISKELE UCL-TAV (Fig. 25.13). This novel device is made of a self-expandable nitinol stent and a trileaflet valve made of a novel polymer nanocomposite. The polymer is also used to create a sealing skirt, reducing paravalvular regurgitation. This polymer has enhanced physiochemical properties and resistance to calcification and thrombosis, with superior in vivo biostability. It has demonstrated superior mechanical properties compared with porcine and bovine pericardial tissues [4]. The TRISKELE UCL-TAV is currently under preclinical evaluation.

# References

1. Treede H, Lubos E, Conradi L, Deuschl F, Asch FM, Weissman NJ, Schofer N, Schirmer J, Koschyk D, Blankenberg S, Reichenspurner H, Schaefer U. Thirty-day VARC-2 and performance data of a new self-expanding transcatheter aortic heart valve. EuroIntervention. 2015;11(7):785–92; [Epub ahead of print].
2. Binder RK, Schäfer U, Kuck KH, Wood DA, Moss R, Leipsic J, Toggweiler S, Freeman M, Ostry AJ, Frerker C, Willson AB, Webb JG. Transcatheter aortic valve replacement with a new self-expanding transcatheter heart valve and motorized delivery system. JACC Cardiovasc Interv. 2013;6:301–7.
3. Silaschi M, Treede H, Rastan AJ, Baumbach H, Beyersdorf F, Kappert U, Eichinger W, Rüter F, de Kroon TL, Lange R, Ensminger S, Wendler O. The JUPITER registry: 1-year results of transapical aortic valve implantation using a second-generation transcatheter heart valve in patients with aortic stenosis. Eur J Cardiothorac Surg. 2016;50(5):874–81; [Epub ahead of print].
4. Rahmani B, Burriesci G, Mullen M, Seifalian A, Tzamtzis S, Yap J. A new generation transcatheter heart valve with a novel nanocomposite material and fully retrievable design. J Am Coll Cardiol Intv. 2013;60(17):B34.

# Complications Post-TAVI

# 26

Chekrallah Chamandi and Josep Rodés-Cabau

Transcatheter aortic valve replacement (TAVR) has become the standard of care for inoperable patients with symptomatic severe aortic stenosis [1] and a good alternative to surgical aortic valve replacement for patients at high surgical risk [2]. Worldwide, two types of transcatheter heart valves (THVs) have been most used to date: the balloon-expandable Edwards valve (Cribier-Edwards, Edwards SAPIEN, SAPIEN XT, and SAPIEN 3; Edwards Lifesciences, Irvine, CA) and the self-expandable CoreValve system (CoreValve, Evolut, Evolut R; Medtronic, Minneapolis, MN). In the past few years, other transcatheter valves have also received CE mark approval and are now commonly used (e.g., Direct Flow, Lotus Valve, Portico, JenaValve, Symetis). Despite significant progress in the technology of transcatheter valves over the last decade, several complications remain associated with this less-invasive procedure. This chapter seeks to review the major significant complications following TAVR. Methods of prevention and treatment of those hurdles will also be appraised.

## 26.1 Paravalvular Leak

Paravalvular leak (PVL) is a complication of aortic valve prostheses and is seen more frequently after TAVR than after SAVR (Table 26.1) [3–14]. The incidence of moderate or severe PVL after TAVR has been reported to be 12–21%, which is approximately sixfold higher than that after SAVR [15]. Residual moderate-to-severe AR is clinically relevant and has been associated with an increased risk of all-cause mortality.

C. Chamandi, M.D. • J. Rodés-Cabau, M.D. (✉)
Quebec Heart and Lung Institute, Laval University, Quebec City, QC, Canada
e-mail: Josep.Rodes@criucpq.ulaval.ca

© Springer International Publishing AG 2018
C. Tamburino et al. (eds.), *Percutaneous Treatment of Left Side Cardiac Valves*,
https://doi.org/10.1007/978-3-319-59620-4_26

**Table 26.1** Incidence of AR after TAVR in major registries and randomized trials

| Study | No patients | Type of THV | Moderate-severe AR (%) |
|---|---|---|---|
| PARTNER cohort B (3) | 179 | 100% Edwards SAPIEN | 13.2 |
| PARTNER cohort A (4) | 348 | 100% Edwards SAPIEN | 10.6 |
| SOURCE Registry (5) | 1038 | 100% Edwards SAPIEN | 1.9 |
| FRANCE 2 (6) | 3195 | 70% Edwards SAPIEN, 30% CoreValve | 16.5 |
| Canadian Registry (7) | 339 | 18% Cribier-Edwards, 82% Edwards SAPIEN | 10 |
| GARY (8) | 3876 | 53% Edwards SAPIEN, 42% CoreValve, 5% other | 6.2 |
| UK-TAVI Registry (9) | 870 | 48% Edwards SAPIEN, 52% CoreValve | 13.6 |
| PRAGMATIC Plus Registry (10) | 793 | 43% Edwards SAPIEN, 57% CoreValve | 1.9 |
| TAVI Sentinel Pilot Registry (11) | 4571 | 57% Edwards SAPIEN, 43% CoreValve | 9 |
| STS/ACC TVT Registry (12) | 7710 | 100% Edwards SAPIEN | 8.5 |
| ADVANCE Registry (13) | 1015 | 100% CoreValve | 15.6 |
| CHOICE trial (14) | 241 | 50% Edwards SAPIEN, 50% CoreValve | 3.7 |

*ACC* American College of Cardiology, *AR* aortic regurgitation, *GARY* German Aortic Valve Registry, *PARTNER* Placement of AoRTic TraNscathetER Valve trial, *STS* Society of Thoracic Surgeons, *TAVR* transcatheter aortic valve replacement, *THV* transcatheter heart valve

According to the Valve Academic Research Consortium (VARC)-2 criteria [16], the criteria for severe PVLs include a regurgitant volume $\geq 60$ mL, a regurgitant fraction $\geq 50\%$, an effective regurgitant orifice area $\geq 0.3$ cm$^2$, and a holosystolic diastolic flow reversal in the descending aorta and a circumferential extent of PVL $> 30\%$. On the other hand, mild PVL is determined by a regurgitant volume of $<30$ mL, a regurgitant fraction of $<30\%$, an effective regurgitant orifice area of $<0.1$ cm$^2$, and the absence of diastolic flow reversal in the descending aorta and a circumferential extent of the PVL less than 10%. The rates of mild, moderate, and severe PVL following TAVR range from 7.8 to 40.8%, 5 to 37.9%, and 0.5 to 13.6%, respectively [17]. Indeed, in a weighted meta-analysis of 12,926 patients from 45 studies, the pooled incidence rate of moderate or severe PVL was 11.7% [18]. This large variation in PVL rate might be explained by the lack of standardization across medical institutions in the procedure and differences in valve types and sizes, combined with the various imaging modalities used and the numerous challenges in grading PVL.

Several observational studies have shown a higher rate of moderate–severe PVL associated with the CoreValve system compared with the balloon-expandable Edwards valve [9, 19]. These observations were confirmed by the CHOICE randomized controlled trial, which compared the valve performance and clinical outcomes associated with the Edwards SAPIEN XT valve vs. the CoreValve system. The main results showed a lower number of patients in the balloon-expandable group with more than mild AR compared with the self-expandable valve cohort (4.1% vs. 18.3%; RR, 0.23; $p < 0.001$) [14].

The progression of PVL over time is still a matter of debate. Data from the PARTNER trial reported that PVL had increased by $\geq 1$ grade in 22.4% of 80 patients, remained the same in 46.2%, and amended by $\geq 1$ grade in 31.5% of patients [4]. On the other hand, studies reporting the PVL incidence over several time points found diminishing rates of moderate or severe PVL with the self-expanding CoreValve system. In the cohort of patients deemed at extreme risk for surgery in the CoreValve US trial, the frequency of moderate or severe paravalvular AR was lower at 12 months post-TAVR (4.2%) than at hospital discharge (10.7%; $p < 0.004$ for paired analysis) [20]. Similarly, in the high-risk population of the CoreValve US trial, 76.2% of patients with moderate or severe PVL at discharge had mild or no regurgitation at 1 year [21]. This finding could be attributed not only to the use of computed tomography assessment for valve size selection, higher placement of the valve within the annulus, and sustained expansion of the nitinol frame and geometric remodeling of the annular–bioprosthesis interface but also to the death of patients with higher-grade PVL [2, 4, 21]. In addition, 2 years after TAVR with a self-expandable CoreValve, the proportion of patients with moderate-to-severe PVL remained stable [22].

### 26.1.1 Impact of PVL on Mortality

Two large meta-analyses showed that moderate or severe AR post-TAVR is associated with 2.12- and 2.27-fold of overall 1-year mortality, respectively [15, 18]. In the Italian registry [23], data on 663 patients who underwent TAVR with a self-expandable CoreValve system showed that PVL $\geq 2$ was not associated with early 30-day mortality. Nonetheless, multivariable analysis indicated a hazard ratio (HR) of 3.79 for late mortality beyond 30 days ($p = 0.003$). In the FRANCE-2 registry, post-procedural AR $\geq$ grade 2 was a strong independent predictor of 1-year mortality for both balloon-expandable (HR = 2.50; $p < 0.001$) and self-expandable (HR = 2.11; $p < 0.001$) THV. Post-procedural AR $\geq$ grade 2 was well endured in individuals with AR $\geq$ grade 2 at baseline (1-year mortality = 7%) but was associated with high mortality in many other subgroups: renal failure (43%), AR < grade 2 at baseline (31%), low transaortic gradient (35%), or non-femoral delivery (45%) [24]. Moreover, Miyazaki et al. [25] recently found that moderate-to-severe PVL was associated with increased 2-year estimated mortality in the cohort of patients with a baseline ejection fraction of <40%, while there was no difference in the group of patients with a baseline ejection fraction $\geq$40%. Therefore, operators should probably be even more careful to avoid PVL in the subgroup of patients with reduced baseline left ventricular function. In the extreme risk cohort of the CoreValve US trial, 1-year mortality was associated with total severe AR at the time of discharge [20]. The same trial randomized high-risk patients to TAVR versus SAVR. The rates of moderate or severe PVL were higher following TAVR but did not appear to have an adverse effect on overall survival [21]. Interestingly, results from the cohort A of the PARTNER trial demonstrated that with balloon-expandable THV, even mild PVL was associated with a worse survival at 2 years and at 5 years [4, 26]. The explanation for the relationship between mild PVL and mortality still needs to be clarified. In a study by Jerez-Valero et al. looking at 1735 patients undergoing TAVR with a balloon-expandable transcatheter heart valve (THV) or a self-expandable valve, it was shown that the acuteness of AR impacts the clinical outcomes [27]. Indeed, acute moderate-to-severe AR was independently associated with increased risk of mortality, compared with none/trace/mild AR (adjusted HR: 2.37; $p < 0.001$) and chronic moderate-to-severe AR (adjusted HR: 2.24; $p < 0.015$). There were no significant differences in survival rates between patients with chronic moderate-to-severe and none/trace/mild AR ($p > 0.50$).

## 26.1.2 Mechanisms and Predictors of PVL

TAVR is a less-invasive procedure and requires preprocedural imaging to analyze the degree of calcification and the dimensions of the aortic valve and the aortic root. The procedure involves the implantation under fluoroscopy and echocardiography of a circular bioprosthesis in a usually oval-shaped native aortic annulus. The three main mechanisms of PVL are incomplete apposition of the THV against the native annulus due to significant calcification [28–30], undersizing of the valve [31, 32], and malpositioning of the device [33]. Table 26.2 summarizes the numerous predictors of PVL identified in the literature according to valve type.

A recent study showed that a point-of-care hemostatic test, the CT-ADP, was predictive of the presence or absence of paravalvular aortic regurgitation after TAVR. The test was also predictive of the rate of death 1 year after the procedure [34].

**Table 26.2** Predictors of PVL after TAVR according to valve type

| | |
|---|---|
| Edwards | Older age |
| | Male gender |
| | NYHA IV |
| | Annular size—larger aortic annulus |
| | Transfemoral approach |
| | Calcification of the aortic valve |
| | Area cover index[a] |
| | Low cover index[b] |
| | Operator's experience |
| CoreValve | Peripheral vascular disease |
| | History of heart failure |
| | Chronic renal insufficiency |
| | Prosthesis mismatch |
| | Low implantation |
| | Larger aortic annulus |
| | Increased angle of LVOT to ascending aorta |

*LVOT* left ventricular outflow tract
[a]Area cover index: (1-annulus area/prosthesis nominal area)
[b]Cover index: (100 × [prosthesis diameter − TEE annulus diameter/prosthesis diameter])

### 26.1.3 Role of Imaging to Prevent PVL

Multidetector computed tomography (MDCT) plays an important role in the workup of patients who are candidates for TAVR, as well as in the evaluation of patients with PVL (Figs. 26.1 and 26.2). The 3D image reconstruction of the aortic annulus allows multiplanar measurements of annular diameter, area, and perimeter. Willson et al. showed that in 109 patients who underwent MDCT assessment pre-TAVR with a balloon-expandable device, MDCT-derived 3D measurements were predictive of PVL following TAVR [35]. Transcatheter bioprostheses that were oversized relative to the MDCT mean annular diameter by at least 1 mm and annular area by at least 10% had a reduced risk of moderate or severe PVL. Yet, device oversizing is associated with a greater risk of coronary occlusion, annular rupture, and bradyrhythmias. In a study by Mylotte et al., adherence to MDCT-based oversizing was associated with a reduced incidence of PVL, while adherence to a bidimensional transesophageal echocardiogram (TEE)-based sizing was not [36]. Indeed, in a retrospective analysis of 157 patients who underwent CoreValve implantation, THV oversizing was 20.1% when the measurements were made on TEE, while oversizing was only 10.4% when computed tomography diameters were retrospectively used. Thus, the MDCT analysis posited that up to 50% of patients had received an inappropriate CoreValve size. When MDCT-based sizing criteria were met, there was a 21% decrease in the incidence of PVL (14% vs. 35%; $p < 0.003$). In a recent study by Jilaihawi et al. including 256 patients, it was shown that cross-sectional 3D echocardiographic sizing of the aortic annulus dimension provides discrimination of post-TAVR paravalvular aortic

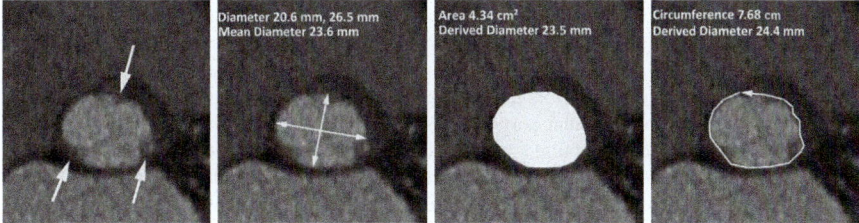

**Fig. 26.1** Determination of aortic annulus dimensions in CT. After an appropriate plane that exactly contains the three lowest insertion points of the coronary cusps has been created, three different methods of determining aortic annulus size have been proposed. The long and short diameter can be measured to calculate the mean diameter. The area can be measured, and the diameter can be deducted under the assumption that this area changes to a circle when a valve is implanted. Finally, it can be assumed that the circumference will stay constant during the implantation and the diameter can be derived from the circumference, again assuming that the annulus will achieve a perfectly circular shape. The more eccentric the aortic annulus, the more these three measurements will differ from one another, with the circumference-based method yielding the largest results. Taken from SCCT expert consensus document on computed tomography imaging before transcatheter aortic valve implantation (TAVI)/transcatheter aortic valve replacement (TAVR) Stephan Achenbach, MD, FSCCTa,*, Victoria Delgado, MDb, Jorg Hausleiter, MDc, Paul Schoenhagen, MDd, James K. Min, FSCCTe, Jonathon A. Leipsic, MD, FSCCT. Journal of Cardiovascular Computed Tomography (2012) 6, 366–380

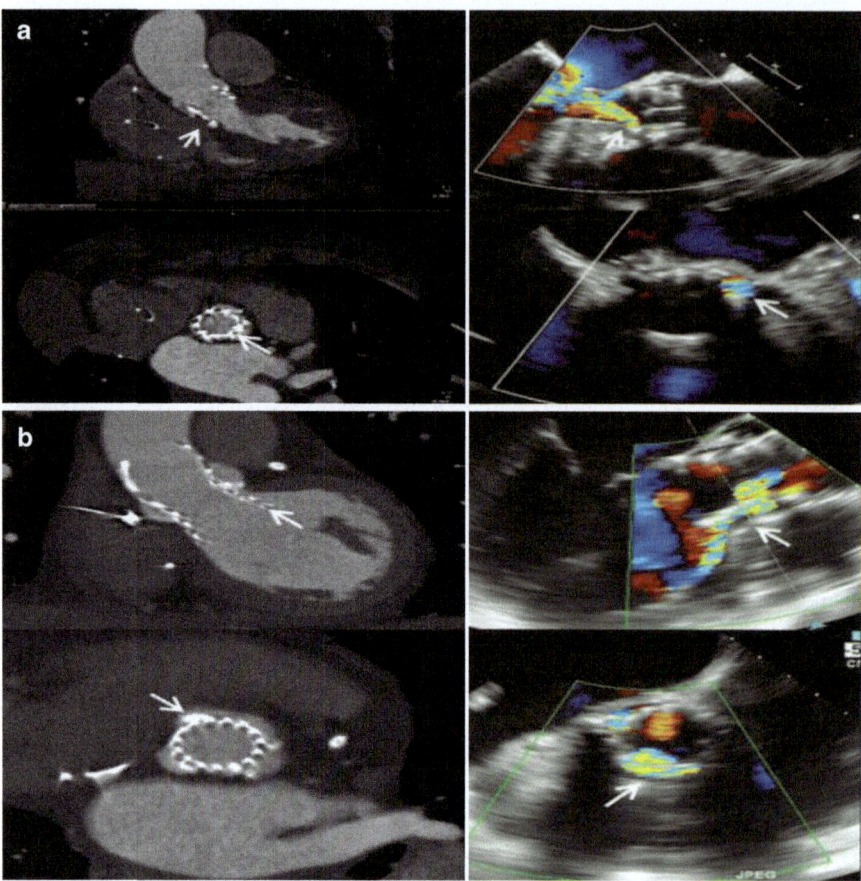

**Fig. 26.2** Pathophysiological factors determining paravalvular aortic regurgitation. (**a**) Example of a patient with mild paravalvular aortic regurgitation at the level of the hinge point, with the membranous interventricular septum (*arrow*). Multidetector-row computed tomography shows a bulky calcification at this level (*arrow*). The short-axis view shows mild paravalvular aortic regurgitation at the level of the left coronary cusp. Note on the multidetector-row computed tomography the presence of calcifications at this level surrounding the prosthetic frame (*arrow*). (**b**) Deep implantation of a self-expandable transcatheter aortic valve, causing significant paravalvular aortic regurgitation (*arrow*). Multidetector-row computed tomography allows accurate assessment of the deployment of the valve. In addition, there is a paravalvular regurgitant jet originating at the level of the right coronary cusp. Multidetector-row computed tomography shows the presence of a bulky calcified right coronary cusp pushed away following valve deployment (*arrow*). Taken from open issues in transcatheter aortic valve implantation. Part 2: procedural issues and outcomes after transcatheter aortic valve implantation. Jeroen J. Bax, Victoria Delgado, Vinayak Bapat, Helmut Baumgartner, Jean P. Collet, Raimund Erbel, Christian Hamm, Arie P. Kappetein, Jonathon Leipsic, Martin B. Leon, Philip MacCarthy, Nicolo Piazza, Philippe Pibarot, William C. Roberts, Josep Rodés-Cabau, Patrick W. Serruys, Martyn Thomas, Alec Vahanian, John Webb, Jose Luis Zamorano, and Stephan Windecke. European Heart Journal (2014) 35, 2639–2654 doi:10.1093/eurheartj/ehu257

regurgitation that is significantly superior to that of 2D-TEE [37]. Therefore, if MDCT data are unavailable for TAVR sizing, cross-sectional data from 3D-TEE should be obtained. In another study, individuals with severe symptomatic aortic stenosis who had both contrast MDCT and 3D-TEE for annulus assessment before balloon-expandable TAVR were assessed [38]. This study used a new method for analyzing 3D-TEE image-generated annulus measurements that closely approximated those of MDCT. Moreover, the two 3D modalities predicted mild or greater PVL with similar accuracy. In conclusion, it seems clear that at present, a 3D imaging modality, either MDCT or 3D-TEE, should be used for THV sizing.

### 26.1.4 Treatment of PVL

There is no clear algorithm for the management of PVL after TAVR. Careful positioning of the THV is important to avoid PVL. Real-time echocardiogram, 3D angiographic reconstruction with rotational aortogram, and careful selection of the best coplanar fluoroscopic view can facilitate the appropriate positioning of the THV and may theoretically lead to less frequent PVL.

When the transcatheter valve is implanted in a very calcified aortic valve with bulky calcifications that prevent complete expansion of the frame, balloon post-dilatation can reduce paravalvular AR, ensuring full expansion of the frame and improving the sealing of the aortic annulus, though there is still risk of annulus rupture [39]. In a single-center trial, Daneault et al. reported that post-dilatation was performed in 41% of cases to reduce PVL in patients with greater than mild PVL after balloon-expandable TAVR [39]. Factors associated with a higher risk for balloon post-dilatation were a larger annulus, smaller cover index, transfemoral approach, and a larger transcatheter valve size. Of note, there was a tendency toward a higher incidence of cerebrovascular events in the post-dilatation group. However, there were no significant disparities in major aortic injury, THV embolization, rupture of the membranous septum, trauma to the conduction system, and permanent pacemaker implantation rates between groups.

In another study on post-dilatation, by Nombela-Franco et al., post-dilatation was performed in 28% of patients [40]. Post-dilatation reduced PVL by at least one grade in 71% of patients, with residual AR of <2 in about half of the patients. Transfemoral approach and degree of valve calcification were identified as predictors of the need for post-dilatation. Post-dilatation was also linked to a higher incidence of cerebrovascular events at 1 month (11.9% vs. 2.0%; $p = 0.006$). The influence of post-dilatation on mortality after TAVR has yet to be determined.

In patients with too shallow or too deep implantation of the transcatheter valve, transcatheter valve in valve can be an effective technique for reducing a significant PVL. This technique can also be used in patients with moderate-to-severe transvalvular AR. In a cohort of 2554 patients included in the PARTNER trial, a valve-in-valve procedure was performed in 63 patients (2.5%) [41]. In 36.1% of these patients, valve in valve was done because of severe PVL, and in half of the cases, it was performed because of severe central aortic regurgitation due to malpositioning of the THV or leaflet dysfunction. Patients who required a second valve had higher 1-year mortality (HR: 1.86; $p = 0.041$) compared with those with single valve implantation.

A multicenter international registry sought to evaluate the outcomes of percutaneous closure of post-TAVR PVL [42]. In this study, transcatheter implantations of a closure device were performed in 24 patients (Fig. 26.3). The most frequently used device (80% of the cases) was the Amplatzer Vascular Plug (St. Jude Medical, St. Paul, MN, USA), and 89% of the procedures were technically successful (defined as the successful deployment of a device, with immediate reduction of PVR to a final grade $\leq 2$ as assessed by echocardiography). The 1-, 6-, and 12-month survival rates were 83.3%, 66.7%, and 61.5%, respectively. The majority of the deaths were attributable to a noncardiac etiology.

## 26.1.5 New TAVR Systems

There are several new TAVR systems with enhanced anti-PVL properties that have been associated with very low rates of PVL following the procedure, much lower than those reported with the older-generation transcatheter valves (Fig. 26.4).

The SAPIEN 3 system (Edwards Lifesciences) incorporates an optimized cobalt chromium alloy frame (which allows for an extremely low-crimped profile, with high radial strength), pericardial leaflets, and an outer sealing skirt surrounding the bottom of the valve with the objective of reducing PVL. Several studies have shown lower rates of $\geq$ mild PVLs compared with those observed with the older-generation balloon-expandable valve [50, 51]. Recently, the 1-year follow-up results of the PARTNER II SAPIEN 3 High Risk Cohort showed that no or trace PVL was present in 68.1% of patients, mild PVL was seen in 29.1%, moderate PVL was present in 2.7%, and no patient had severe PVL [43]. A recent meta-analysis found that the S3 valve was associated with significantly less moderate-to-severe PVR compared with the XT valve (1.6% vs. 6.9%, respectively, OR: 0.28, 95% CI 0.15–0.51, $p < 0.0001$) [52].

The Medtronic Evolut R valve offers the option of fully recapturing and repositioning the valve to obtain optimal valve positioning. These new features, combined

$\longrightarrow$

**Fig. 26.3** Treatment of significant paravalvular aortic regurgitation after transcatheter aortic valve implantation. Implantation of an AMPLATZER Vascular Plug III closure device to seal a severe paravalvular aortic regurgitation as observed in the parasternal short-axis view, with a circumferential extent 0.20% (**a**). The device is inserted between the native aortic root and the prosthetic frame (*arrows*) (**b**), resulting in significant reduction of the paravalvular regurgitant jet (**c**). Taken from open issues in transcatheter aortic valve implantation. Part 2: procedural issues and outcomes after transcatheter aortic valve implantation. Jeroen J. Bax, Victoria Delgado, Vinayak Bapat, Helmut Baumgartner, Jean P. Collet, Raimund Erbel, Christian Hamm, Arie P. Kappetein, Jonathon Leipsic, Martin B. Leon, Philip MacCarthy, Nicolo Piazza, Philippe Pibarot, William C. Roberts, Josep Rodés-Cabau, PatrickW. Serruys, Martyn Thomas, Alec Vahanian, JohnWebb, Jose Luis Zamorano, and StephanWindecke. European Heart Journal (2014) 35, 2639–2654 doi:10.1093/eurheartj/ehu257

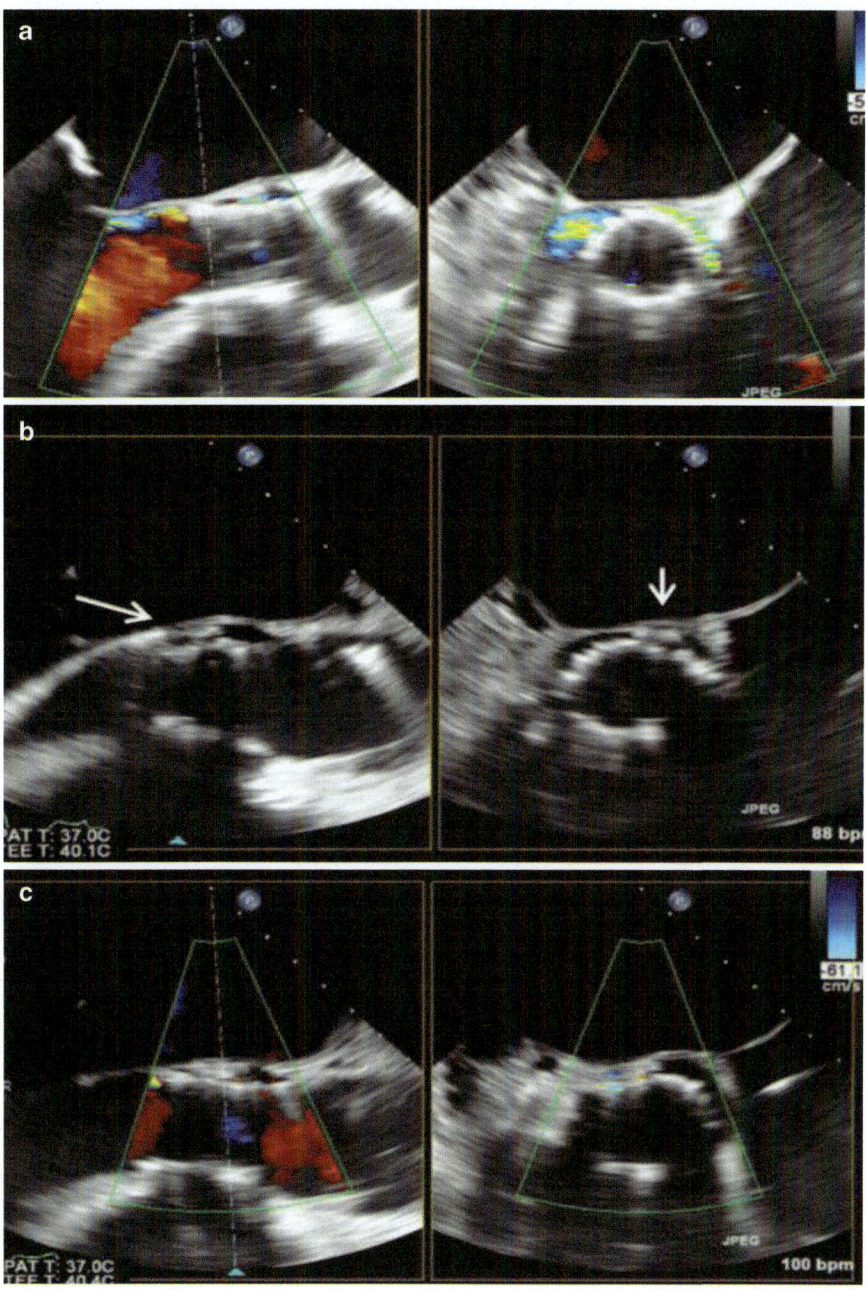

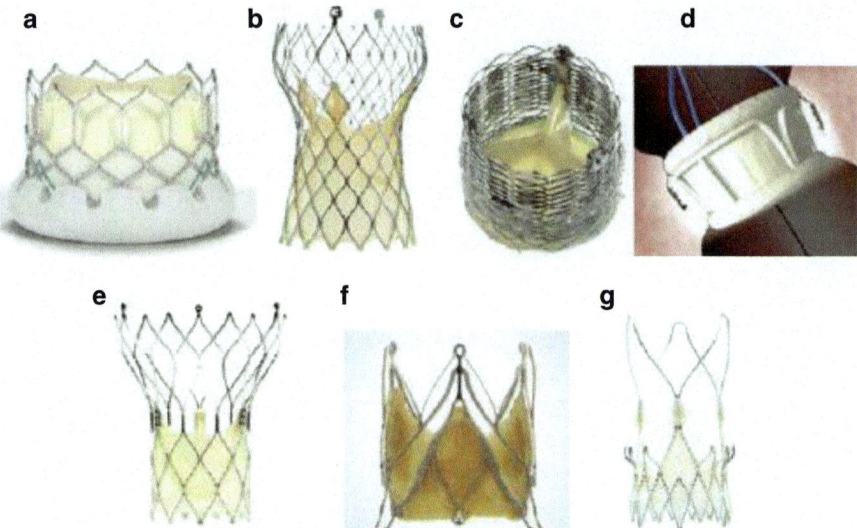

**Fig. 26.4** Newer-generation valves. (**a**) SAPIEN 3, (**b**) Evolut R, (**c**) Lotus Valve, and (**d**) Direct Flow valve, (**e**) Portico, (**f**) JenaValve, (**g**) Symetis ACURATE. Taken from Expert Rev. Cardiovasc Ther. 2015 Nov;13(11):1251–62. doi: 10.1586/14779072.2015.1096778. Reducing periprocedural complications in transcatheter aortic valve replacement: review of paravalvular leaks, stroke and vascular complications. Paradis JM, Altisent OA, Rodés-Cabau J

with an extended sealing skirt, were designed to reduce PVL. Thirty-day results showed a moderate-to-severe PVL rate of 3.4% [44].

The Lotus Valve (Boston Scientific) is a second-generation self-expanding valve with a bovine pericardial tissue valve incorporated in a nitinol stent. This stent frame minimizes the risk of paravalvular AR with its new-age sealing system (urethane membrane), which adapts to the irregular surface of the ring (Fig. 26.4). Results of the REPRISE II trial indicated that 86.4% of patients had no paravalvular regurgitation at 1 year and 2.3% had only a trace of regurgitation. No patient had moderate or severe paravalvular regurgitation at 1 year [45].

The Direct Flow valve (Direct Flow Medical) consists of a nonmetallic percutaneous bovine pericardial valve with an expandable Dacron polyester double-ring design containing noncompliant angioplasty balloon technology (Fig. 26.4). The upper (aortic) and lower (ventricular) ring balloons, interconnected by a tubular bridging system, can be pressurized independently through position-fill lumens. A multicenter registry including 100 patients showed a rate of mild or moderate PVL of 28% and 1%, respectively, with no cases of severe PVL at 30 days [46]. At 1 year, PVL was none or trace in 79% of the patients. Total aortic regurgitation was none or trace in 68% and mild or less in 100% of the patients [53].

The Portico self-expandable valve (St. Jude) is an annular functioning, trileaflet bovine pericardial valve, mounted on a self-expanding nitinol frame. The skirt is made from porcine pericardium and works synergistically with the widely spaced conformable nitinol frame to seal the native annulus and mitigate PVL. It is fully re-sheathable. To date, there have been no reports of severe aortic valve regurgitation at 30 days based on site-reported echocardiographic analysis [47, 54].

The JenaValve™ (JenaValve Technology GmbH) is a second-generation THV, designed to ease correct positioning and to reduce the incidence of paravalvular regurgitation and complete heart block. It enables calcium-independent annular fixation by engaging the native aortic cusps through an active clipping mechanism for fixation, with tactile feedback during implantation. Allowing for anatomically aligned positioning, without the need for rapid ventricular pacing during implantation, it is also fully repositionable during the first step of implantation. Data at 1 year showed a rate of significant PVL of 3.5% [48].

The ACURATE platform (Symetis) is based on a self-seating and self-sealing design that allows for optimal positioning of the THV, which could potentially reduce PVL. Initial experience with this new device showed a rate of mild PVL of 25.1%, none/trace PVL of 72.6%, and relevant (≥2) PVL of 2.3% [49].

## 26.2    Conduction Disturbances

The occurrence of conduction disturbances and the need for permanent pacemaker implantation (PPI) after TAVR remain a concern. The close proximity of the conduction system to the aortic annulus can lead to a mechanical interaction between the stent frame of the transcatheter valve prosthesis and the left bundle branch, which in turn can translate into the occurrence of a left bundle branch block (LBBB) and eventually into a high-grade or complete atrioventricular block (AVB).

The rate of new-onset LBBB post-TAVI is ~27% (ranging from 4 to 57%) [55], and the rate of PPI is ~17% (from 2 to 51%) [56]. Wide variations have been reported across studies and according to valve type, and rates of new PPI are also reportedly higher with certain newer-generation transcatheter valve systems (Tables 26.3 and 26.4). Overall, the incidence of both new-onset LBBB and PPI is higher following use of the self-expanding CoreValve system (~48% and 28%, respectively) compared with the balloon-expandable Edwards SAPIEN/SAPIEN XT valve (~14% and 6%, respectively) [55, 56, 64]. Indeed, the increased risk of PPI associated with the CoreValve prosthesis compared with the Edwards SAPIEN/SAPIEN XT valve was confirmed in a randomized trial (37.6% vs. 17.3%, $p < 0.001$) [14]. A slow but significant reduction in the rate of conduction abnormalities and need for PPI associated with both transcatheter valve types has been observed over time [55, 65]. This may be related to improvements in delivery systems, increased experience with, and knowledge of, the factors associated with conduction disturbances post-TAVI, in addition to the implementation of more restrictive indications for PPI [65].

However, early results show a lack of reduction or even an increase in the rate of conduction system disturbances associated with these so-called

**Table 26.3** PPM incidence in major registries (according to valve type)

| Edwards | Author's name | No. | 30-day mortality (no.) | Incidence of PPM (%) |
|---|---|---|---|---|
| Belgium[1] | Bosmans et al. | 187 | 6 | 5 |
| France[2] | Eltchaninof et al. | 166 | 20 | 5.4 |
| France II[3] | Gilard et al. | 2107 | 195 | 11.5 |
| PARTNER EU[4] | Lefevre et al. | 130 | 13 | 2.3 |
| Source XT[5] | Wendler et al. | 2688 | 216 | 9.5 |
| PARTNER I A[6] | Smith et al. | 348 | 12 | 3.8 |
| PARTNER I B[7] | Leon et al. | 179 | 9 | 3.4 |
| PARNER II B[8] | Webb et al. | 276 | 14 | 5.9 |
| PARTNER II B (XT)[8] | Webb et al. | 284 | 10 | 6.8 |
| PARTNER II – IR[9] | Leon et al. | 1011 | 62 | 8.5 |
| Spain[10] | Sabaté et al. | 809 | 78 | 4.8 |
| Multicenter[11] | Wendler et al. | 120 | 5 | 12.5 |
| French[12] | Watanabe et al. | 170 | 14 | 4.8 |
| Suisse TAVI[13] | Binde et al. | 445 | 20 | 11 |
| *CoreValve* | | | | |
| Belgium[1] | Bosmans et al. | 141 | 3 | 22 |
| France[2] | Eltchaninof et al. | 78 | 11 | 25.6 |
| France II[3] | Gilard et al. | 1043 | 91 | 24.2 |
| CoreValve Pivotal[14] | Buellesfeld et al. | 126 | 19 | 26.2 |
| Italy[15] | Barbanti et al. | 1326 | 56 | 24 |
| Australia[16] | Meredith et al. | 506 | 21 | 28.4 |
| Spain[10] | Sabaté et al. | 610 | 44 | 17 |
| French[12] | Watanabe et al. | 150 | 15 | 19.3 |
| US CoreValve (high risk)[17] | Adams et al. | 390 | 13 | 19.8 |
| US CoreValve (extreme risk)[18] | Popma et al. | 489 | 41 | 21.6 |
| ADVANCE trial[19] | Linke et al. | 1015 | 45 | 26.4 |
| *New-generation valves* | | | | |
| SAPIEN S3 | Herrmann et al. [43] | 583 | 15 | 13.3 |
| Evolut R | Manoharan et al. [44] | 60 | 0 | 11.7 |
| Lotus | Meredith et al. [45] | 120 | 5 | 28.6 |
| Direct flow | Schofer et al. [46] | 100 | 1 | 17 |
| Portico | Manoharan [47] | 100 | 3 | 9.8 |
| JenaValve | Silaschi et al. [48] | 180 | 20 | 14.4 |
| Symetis | Kempfert el al [49] | 250 | 17 | 10 |

**Table 26.4** Incidence of new LBBB in major studies

| Study | Valve type (%) | Sample size (no.) | Age (mean) | New LBBB (%) |
|---|---|---|---|---|
| Carrabba et al. [57] | MCRS (100) | 92 | 81 | 37 |
| Schymik et al. [58] | ESV (81) MCRS (19) | 634 | 82 | 31.1 |
| Urena et al. [59] | ESV (100) | 668 | 79 | 11.8 |
| Houthuizen et al. [60] | ESV (53) MCRS (47) | 476 | 81 | 28.7 |
| Nazif et al. [61] | ESV (100) | 1151 | 84 | 10.5 |
| Franzoni et al. [62] | ESV (63) MCRS (37) | 238 | 79 | 26.5 |
| Testa et al. [63] | MCRS (100) | 818 | 82 | 22.5 |

new-generation valves [66]. Specifically, an increased rate of PPI has been reported with the use of the third-generation balloon-expandable Edwards valve compared with previous generations of the Edwards valve. This finding has been attributed to the incorporation of an external fabric cuff in the inferior part of the valve intended to minimize paravalvular leak. A higher (more aortic) valve depth implantation of this new-generation valve might help in preventing the higher risk of PPI [67].

Clinical predictors of an increased risk of new-onset LBBB include, in addition to valve prosthesis type, depth of implantation, presence of preexisting conduction abnormalities (longer baseline QRS duration), and TAVI within the native aortic valve (as opposed to valve-in-valve procedures). Also, baseline characteristics such as male gender, absence of prior valve surgery, the presence of porcelain aorta, and preexisting conduction abnormalities (mainly preexisting right bundle branch block, left anterior hemiblock, and first-degree AV block) have been identified as independent predictors of the need for PPI post-TAVI [55]. Similarly, intraprocedural AV block, implantation depth, use of the CoreValve system, and balloon predilatation are independently associated with an increased likelihood of PPI [55, 56, 64].

The main reason for pacemaker implantation following TAVI is the occurrence of a high-grade or complete AVB followed by sick sinus syndrome and severe symptomatic bradycardia. However, new-onset persistent LBBB following TAVI has been considered by some centers to be an indication for prophylactic pacemaker implantation, and this may partially explain the differences between centers/studies regarding the pacemaker implantation rate.

The onset of conduction disturbances after TAVR can vary, with the majority of cases being periprocedural or occurring within the first week of the procedure [68]. Delayed high-degree AVB (up to 8 days) is rarer and is reported to occur more frequently in men and in patients with conduction disorders in the ECG-recorded post-TAVR. Thus, most authors suggest continuous electrocardiographic monitoring for at least 48 h is needed in such patients [55, 68].

Data on the clinical impact of new conduction disturbances post-TAVR remain controversial. A recent meta-analysis by Regueiro et al. showed that new-onset LBBB is significantly associated with higher risk of cardiac death (RR of 1.39; 95% CI, 1.04–1.86; $p = 0.03$) and need for PPI at 1-year follow-up (RR, 2.18; 95% CI, 1.28–3.70; $p < 0.01$), while periprocedural PPI seemed not to be associated with an increased risk of death (global or cardiac) within a year of TAVR [69].

## 26.3 Vascular Complications

Preventing vascular complications is a major issue in TAVR. The use of large-diameter catheters and the high-risk profile of the TAVR population are the two main reasons for the high rate of vascular complications. In a meta-analysis of 3519 patients, the pooled incidence rate of major vascular complications was 11.9% [70]. Rates can vary considerably depending on the access route, valve type and size, and definitions used to report vascular complications. In the TF cohort of the PARTNER trial, the 30-day major and minor vascular complication rates were of 15.3% and 11.9%, respectively [71]. The most frequent vascular complications were vascular dissection (62.8%), vascular perforation (31.3%), access site hematoma (22.9%), and retroperitoneal bleeding (9.5%).

In the FRANCE-2 registry, the overall rate of major vascular complications was 4.7%, as defined by the VARC-1 criteria. More complications were reported in the CoreValve group compared with the Edwards THV patients (4.5% vs. 2.7%, respectively) [6]. No significant difference was found when comparing patients who received a CoreValve to those who had an Edwards THV (9.3% vs. 12.3%; HR: 0.735; $p = 0.34$) in the PRAGMATIC PLUS initiative, after a propensity score matching for sheath size [10]. Two large meta-analyses found that the overall rates of major vascular complications were higher in the transarterial (mainly trans-femoral) compared with the transapical approach [72, 73]. Nonetheless, interpretation of the data on vascular complications is difficult since the studies published before the VARC era used different and arbitrary definitions. The implementation of the VARC-2 criteria may have resulted in a higher rate of reported major VC after TAVI compared with VARC-1 criteria, mainly by the inclusion of major bleeding events [74].

The occurrence of major vascular complications has been linked to a higher 1-month and 1-year all-cause and cardiovascular mortality in numerous studies [5, 10, 71, 74]. On the other hand, the occurrence of minor vascular complications has no impact on mortality.

## 26.3.1 Predictors of Vascular Complications

The main determinants of vascular complications after transfemoral TAVR are small vessel diameter, severe atherosclerotic disease, bulky calcification, and tortuosity of the iliofemoral axis [75]. By multivariable analysis in 127 patients undergoing transfemoral TAVR, the independent predictors of VARC-1 major vascular complications were sheath-to-femoral artery ratio (SFAR) (HR: 186.2; $p = 0.006$), early center experience (HR: 3.66; $p = 0.023$), and femoral artery calcium score (HR: 3.44; $p = 0.026$). Neither the type of device nor the diameter of the introducer sheath predicted major vascular complications [76].

Peripheral vascular disease and a sheath external diameter greater than the minimal artery diameter have been shown to be other predictors of vascular complications in an analysis of 137 TAVR patients [77]. In the multivariable analysis of the PRAGMATIC initiative, determinants of major vascular complications included sheath size and female gender [78]. In the PARTNER trial, female gender was also recognized as a strong, independent predictor of major vascular complications (HR: 2.31; $p = 0.03$) [71]. Table 26.5 summarizes main predictors of major vascular complications after TAVR.

**Table 26.5** Predictors of vascular complications in TAVR

| Peripheral vascular disease |
| --- |
| Female gender |
| Early center experience |
| Sheath external diameter |
| SFAR > 1.05 |
| SFAAR > 1.35 |
| Sheath size > 20 Fr |

*SFAAR* sheath-to-femoral artery area ratio, *SFAR* sheath-to-femoral artery ratio

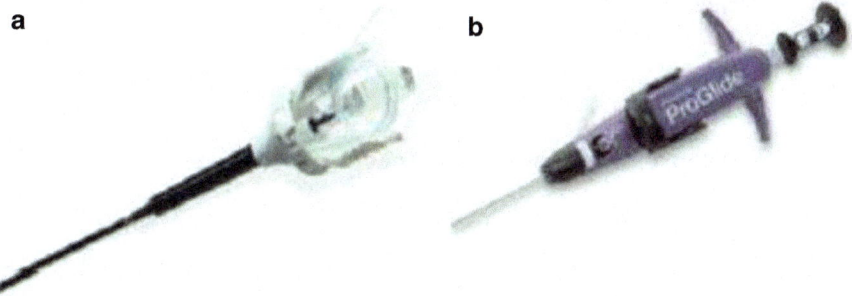

**Fig. 26.5** (**a**) Prostar XL Percutaneous Vascular System (Abbott Vascular, Abbott Park, IL, USA) and (**b**) Perclose ProGlide Suture-Mediated Closure System (Abbott Vascular, Abbott Park, IL, USA). Taken from Expert Rev. Cardiovasc Ther. 2015 Nov;13(11):1251–62. doi: 10.1586/14779072.2015.1096778. Reducing periprocedural complications in transcatheter aortic valve replacement: review of paravalvular leaks, stroke and vascular complications. Paradis JM, Altisent OA, Rodés-Cabau J

## 26.3.2 Reducing the Risk of Vascular Complications

Since the introduction of percutaneous closure devices, this technique has been employed in the vast majority of centers for transfemoral access, replacing the conventional surgical cutdown. The results of percutaneous closure have been similar to those of surgical cutdown, and it has the advantage of facilitating recovery and discharge. The fully percutaneous technique is, however, associated with a learning curve process and improved results, and progressively lowering rates of vascular complications are expected with increasing experience [77, 78].

The most commonly used vascular closure devices are the Prostar XL percutaneous vascular surgical system (Abbott Vascular, Abbott Park, IL, USA) and the Perclose ProGlide suture-mediated closure system (Abbott Vascular) (Fig. 26.5). The CLOsure device iN TRansfemoral aOrtic vaLve implantation (CONTROL) multicenter study recently found that after propensity score matching, the rate of major vascular complications was higher in the group of patients undergoing percutaneous TAVR with the Prostar device compared with those undergoing TAVR with the Perclose ProGlide system (7.4% vs. 1.9%; $p = 0.001$). Nevertheless, the rate of in-hospital mortality was similar with both the devices (4.9% vs. 3.5%; $p = 0.2$) [79].

In addition to improving the valve platform characteristics, some of the newer-generation valve systems have incorporated lower profile delivery systems that have translated into a significant reduction in vascular complications. This is the case of the SAPIEN 3 valve and the Commander delivery catheter (Edwards Lifesciences), which can be advanced through a 14 Fr expandable sheath [43, 52], and the last generation of the CoreValve system (Evolut R; Medtronic, Minnesota, MN, USA), which can be introduced through a 14 Fr sheath (true 18 Fr outer diameter) [44].

## 26.4 Stroke

### 26.4.1 Incidence of Cerebrovascular Events

The occurrence of cerebrovascular events (CVE) is associated with significant morbidity and mortality and remains one of the most worrisome complications associated with TAVR, especially with the tendency toward treating lower surgical risk patients as in the recently published PARTNER-2 (Placement of AoRTic TraNscathetER-2) trial [80].

However, recent studies [80–82] have suggested a decrease in CVE over time, down to rates of 2.5–3% compared with earlier TAVR appraisals [83].

In a large meta-analysis of 64 studies involving 72,318 patients, the overall rate of CVE was 3.3% (range 1–11%) at 30 days, with no significant differences between single and multicenter studies, or according to CVE adjudication availability [84]. In the high-risk cohort of the randomized PARTNER trial, in which TAVR was compared with SAVR, the rates of stroke and transient ischemic attack were higher after TAVR at both 1 month (5.5% TAVR vs. 2.4% SAVR; $p = 0.04$) and 1 year (8.3% TAVR vs. 4.3% SAVR; $p = 0.04$) [2]. However, this early risk diminished over time, with similar stroke incidences at 2 years (11.2% TAVR vs. 6.5% SAVR; $p = 0.05$) [11] and 5 years (15.9% TAVR vs. 14.7% SAVR; $p = 0.35$) [26].

No significant difference in stroke rate was found between TAVR and SAVR in the randomized US CoreValve trial, at 1 month and 1 year [20].

On the other hand, clinically silent cerebral embolism has been associated with more lingering neurological impairment, most importantly a decline in neurocognitive function, and deterioration of dementia [85]. Mechanistic studies using diffusion-weighted cerebral MRI have found new cerebral lesions in 68–91% of patients after TAVR irrespective of the valve type and approach (transfemoral or transapical) [86, 87]. These lesions were usually multiple and dispersed in both hemispheres in a pattern suggesting cerebral embolization. Despite the high frequency of new cerebral lesions on MRI in these series, the long-term clinical significance of these cerebral lesions remains unknown.

The definition of stroke varied across the studies, and, usually, there was no independent adjudication of the event. In an effort to make TAVR studies more rigorous and to avoid a clinical data conundrum that may render comprehensive evaluation of the data very complex and the comparison of inter-study results challenging, VARC proposed standardized definitions for numerous end points, including stroke [16]. According to VARC-2, a stroke can be defined as an acute episode of a focal or global neurological deficit with at least one of the following: change in the level of consciousness, hemiplegia, hemiparesis, numbness or sensory loss affecting one side of the body, dysphasia or aphasia, hemianopia, amaurosis fugax, or other neurological signs or symptoms consistent with stroke. Also, the duration of a focal or global neurological deficit should be >24 or <24 h if there is available neuroimaging evidence of a new hemorrhage or infarct or if the neurological deficit results in death. A stroke can also be categorized as ischemic if it is an acute episode of focal cerebral, spinal or retinal dysfunction caused by infarction of the central nervous system tissue, or hemorrhagic if it is an acute episode of focal or global cerebral or spinal dysfunction caused by intraparenchymal, intraventricular, or subarachnoid hemorrhage. A stroke can be classified as undetermined if there is insufficient information to allow categorization as ischemic or hemorrhagic. Finally, a stroke can be called disabling if the modified Rankin score is 2 or more at 90 days and there is an increase in at least one modified Rankin score category from an individual's pre-stroke baseline.

## 26.4.2 Risk Factors and Predictors of Neurological Events

Numerous variables have been described as potential predictors of CVE after TAVR. It is known that most of the procedural cerebral embolic events during TAVR occur during balloon valvuloplasty, manipulation of catheters across the aortic valve, and THV deployment [88]. However, it has been shown that about 50% of the CVE may occur more than 24 h after TAVR [89]. Those neurological events likely have a thrombogenic origin and may reflect the highly comorbid profile of TAVR candidates.

In a large meta-analysis of 64 studies, Auffret et al. showed that men were at lower risk for CVE (RR, 0.82; $p = 0.02$), while chronic kidney disease (RR, 1.29; $p = 0.03$), new-onset atrial fibrillation post-TAVR (RR, 1.85; $p = 0.005$), and procedures performed within the first half of a center's experience (RR, 1.55; $p = 0.003$) were associated with an increased risk. Balloon post-dilation tended to be associated with a higher risk of CVE (RR, 1.43; $p = 0.07$). Valve type (balloon expandable vs. self-expandable, $p = 0.26$) and approach (transfemoral vs. non-transfemoral, $p = 0.81$) did not predict CVE [84].

Likewise, another meta-analysis of 25 multicenter registries and 33 single-center studies failed to show a significant difference in stroke rates between valve type and approach [90].

In a subanalysis of the PARTNER trial, having a smaller aortic valve area was correlated with an increased risk of early stroke, probably because tight stenotic valves have more calcification that could embolize during TAVR [89]. On the other hand, being a non-TF candidate, having a history of stroke or transient ischemic attack, and more advanced functional disability were recognized as the risk factors for late neurological events. In this subanalysis, preoperative rhythm was not associated with post-TAVR neurologic events. Table 26.6 summarizes the main mechanisms of cerebrovascular events following TAVR.

| Table 26.6 Mechanisms of CVE following TAVR | *Procedural* |
| --- | --- |
| | Manipulation of the catheter, wire, and THV within the aorta and across the aortic valve |
| | Balloon aortic valvuloplasty |
| | Balloon post-dilatation |
| | Valve embolization, need for second valve |
| | Air embolism |
| | Thromboembolism |
| | Hypotension |
| | Hypertension following TAVR |
| | *Non-procedural* |
| | Female gender |
| | Chronic kidney disease |
| | Atrial fibrillation |
| | Diabetes |
| | Prior stroke |
| | Atherosclerosis burden |

### 26.4.3 Impact of Cerebrovascular Events on Mortality After TAVR

In the previously mentioned meta-analysis by Eggebrecht et al. [83], stroke following TAVR was associated with a 3.5-fold increased mortality within the first 30 days. CVE was also found to be associated with higher rates of mortality in the Italian registry (CoreValve system) and in the PARTNER trial (Edwards THV) [23, 89]. In the multicenter study by Nombela-Franco et al. [91], the influence of cerebrovascular events on mortality was determined by the severity of the neurological event. Indeed, only the events leaving permanent sequelae were associated with lower survival at 30 days and 1 year.

### 26.4.4 Prevention of Stroke

Several cerebral protection devices have been developed with the objective of reducing CVE that occur primarily during or immediately after TAVR [92]. These protection devices work by filtering or deflecting the debris away from the cerebral circulation while allowing ongoing cerebral perfusion.

The Embrella Embolic Deflector (EED) device (Edwards Lifesciences, Irvine, CA, USA) (Fig. 26.6) is a percutaneous 6 Fr compatible embolic protection device made of an oval-shaped nitinol frame with a porous polyurethane membrane covering, which is attached to a 110-cm-long nitinol shaft. Once deployed, the petals extend and cover the ostium of the innominate artery as well as the origin of the left common carotid artery. In the feasibility and exploratory efficacy PROTAVI-C study [93], EED was deployed in 41 patients. It did not prevent the incidence of cerebral microemboli during TAVR or new transient ischemic lesions on magnetic resonance imaging. However, compared with the control group, there was a reduction in cerebral lesion volume when EED was used.

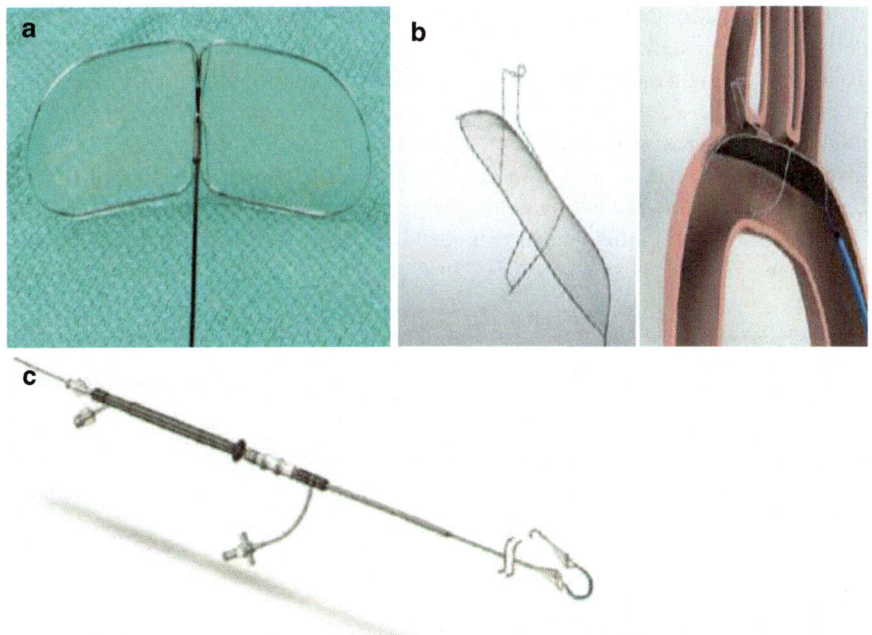

**Fig. 26.6** Examples of embolic protection devices. (**a**) Embrella™ embolic deflector device. (**b**) TriGuard™ cerebral protection device. (**c**) Claret Montage ™ dual filter embolic protection device. Taken from Expert Rev. Cardiovasc Ther. 2015 Nov;13(11):1251–62. doi: 10.1586/14779072.2015.1096778. Reducing periprocedural complications in transcatheter aortic valve replacement: review of paravalvular leaks, stroke and vascular complications. Paradis JM, Altisent OA, Rodés-Cabau J

The TriGuard HDH embolic deflection device (Keystone Heart Ltd., Caesarea, IL, USA) (Fig. 26.6) is a temporary, biocompatible filter made of fine nitinol wires, which is delivered via a 9 Fr transfemoral introducer sheath placed in the aortic arch and secured in position by an atraumatic stabilizer in the ostium of the innominate artery. All three major cerebral arteries in the aortic arch (innominate, left common carotid, and subclavian arteries) are covered by the filter portion, which maintains blood flow to the cerebral vessels through 130 mm pores while deflecting larger emboli to the descending aorta. An antithrombotic coating is present to reduce the formation of thrombus at the surface of the device. In the recently published DEFLECT III study [94], 85 patients undergoing TAVR were randomized to TriGuard protection or to no protection. TriGuard was associated with a lower rate of new ischemic brain lesions (11.5% vs. 26.9%), fewer new neurologic deficits detected by the National Institutes of Health Stroke Scale (3.1% vs. 15.4%; $p = 0.16$), improved Montreal Cognitive Assessment scores, better performance on a delayed memory task ($p = 0.028$) at discharge, and a greater than twofold increase in recovery of normal cognitive function (Montreal Cognitive Assessment score > 26) at 30 days. More data are expected from the ongoing REFLECT randomized trial.

The Claret Montage embolic protection device is a 6 Fr compatible catheter delivered over a standard coronary guidewire and delivers two filters (Fig. 26.6). To protect the right carotid artery, the first filter is deployed in the brachiocephalic trunk. Then, the second filter is positioned in the left common carotid artery. Of a total of 40 patients who underwent TAVR with the use of this device, 75% had macroscopic material captured in the device filter baskets, consisting of thrombotic material and tissue fragments compatible with aortic valve leaflet [95]. These findings substantiate the urgent need to decrease cerebrovascular embolization during TAVR.

## 26.5 Coronary Occlusion

Symptomatic coronary obstruction following TAVR is also a rare (<1%) but life-threatening complication, most often caused by the displacement of the calcified native cusp over the coronary ostium, mainly of the LCA (Fig. 26.7). It has been shown to occur more frequently in women, in patients receiving a balloon-expandable

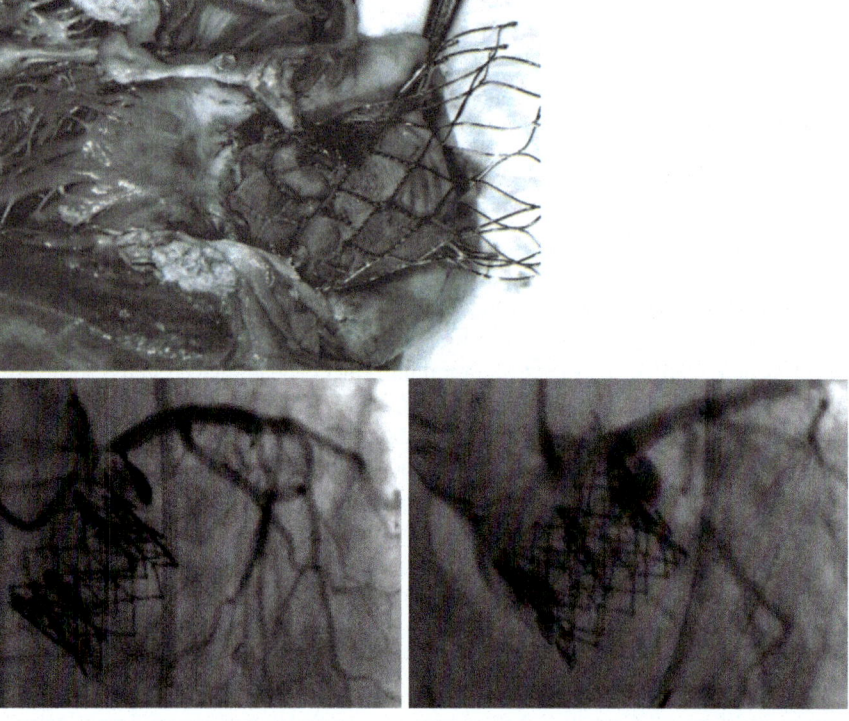

**Fig. 26.7** Autopsy showing a self-expandable valve (Portico) occluding the ostium of the right coronary artery. (*Left*) LM obstruction after deployment of a second balloon-expandable valve (SAPIEN), successfully treated with angioplasty and stent implantation (*Right*). Images acquired at our institute

valve, and in those with a previous surgical bioprosthesis. Lower-lying coronary ostium (<12 mm) and shallow sinus of Valsalva (<30 mm) were associated anatomic factors [96].

Because acute and late mortality remains very high (8.3%) despite successful treatment, it is essential to try to anticipate and prevent the occurrence of this complication. Therefore, pre-interventional imaging with computed tomography and/or transesophageal echography should be used to gather information on this issue, since some potential problems can be anticipated and thus prevented. In these cases, a type of valve with a lower risk of coronary obstructions should be used, or conventional surgical valve replacement considered the potentially better option.

The vast majority of patients will present with rapid hemodynamic deterioration and persistent severe hypotension, significant ST changes, or procedural ventricular arrhythmias. Hemodynamic support and percutaneous treatment are successful in most cases as long as the revascularization efforts are effective within a few minutes. In difficult cases, it may be helpful to initiate a temporary extracorporeal circulation and convert to open-heart surgery.

## 26.6 Annular Rupture and Free Wall Perforation

Aortic annular rupture is a rare, life-threatening complication of TAVR that occurs at a rate of 1.1% [97]. It has been shown that moderate or severe LVOT/subannular calcification and significantly oversized prostheses (≥20% area oversizing) are the most important risk factors associated with aortic root rupture. Smaller annular size or sinotubular junction, bulky calcification, implantation of a balloon-expandable device, and aggressive balloon pre- or post-dilation should also be considered as potential predictors [98] (Fig. 26.8).

The rupture can occur at the annular level, sinus of Valsalva, LVOT, or sinotubular junction. While uncontained aortic root rupture is associated with very high morbidity and mortality (48%), it seems that contained periaortic rupture/hematoma has better prognoses [98, 99].

This complication is very hard to predict. Preprocedural CT analysis is crucial in detecting unfavorable anatomy (LVOT calcifications), and aggressive oversizing with regard to the LVOT diameter should be avoided, especially in fragile elderly patients. Emergent conversion to an open-heart surgery, pericardial drainage, and comfort care are the existing management options.

Cardiac tamponade has been described as occurring in 0.2–4.3% of cases, with a higher probability in retrograde transvascular techniques than with transapical access [100]. The major mechanisms leading to this complication include annular or aortic root rupture, perforation of the right ventricle (RV) caused by the temporary pacing lead, and perforation of the LV by a guidewire. Once diagnosed, perforations from the venous (i.e., RV) side can often be treated effectively by pericardiocentesis with reinfusion of the blood into the femoral vein, while arterial perforations (i.e., LV perforations or annular rupture) frequently require immediate surgical interventions.

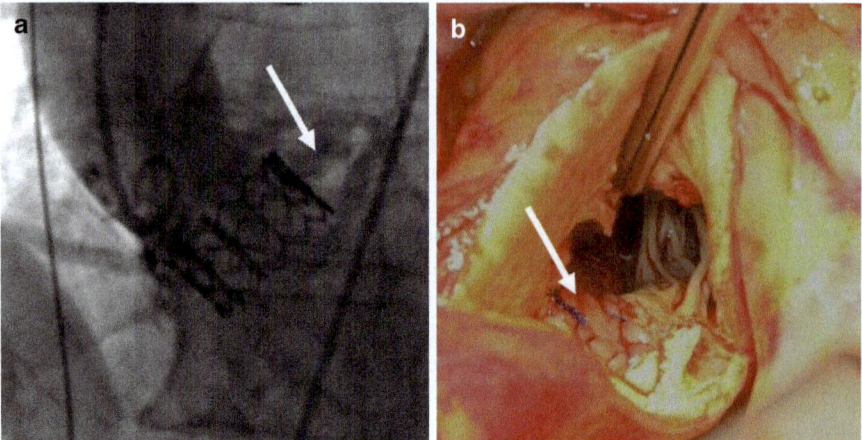

**Fig. 26.8** Annular rupture: (**a**) After implantation of a balloon-expandable prosthesis, final angiography shows a rupture of the aortic root, with leakage of contrast agent into the pericardium (*white arrow*). (**b**) Operative site of a ruptured annulus that has been successfully repaired with a patch (*white arrow*). Taken from Complications of transcatheter aortic valve implantation (TAVI): how to avoid and treat them. Möllmann H, Kim WK, Kempfert J, Walther T, Hamm C. Heart. 2015 Jun;101(11):900–8. doi: 10.1136/heartjnl-2013-304708

## 26.7 Long-Term Valve-Related Complications: Thrombosis and Degeneration

Though THV thrombosis is a rare complication (1.2%), little is known about its real incidence, clinical implications, and predisposing factors. Results among studies vary according to valve type, clinical/imaging diagnostic criteria, timing of follow-up, and antithrombotic/anticoagulation regimen. It is known that a majority of patients present with worsening dyspnea and increased THV gradients. It has been shown that most cases of THV thrombosis occur within a year of TAVI (median time of onset of 6 months) and a preponderance following balloon-expandable valve implantation [101]. Latib et al. reported an incidence of THV thrombosis of 0.61% in a multicenter retrospective registry of >4000 patients, based mainly on TTE. All cases were detected within 2 years of TAVR (median of 180 days) [102]. No association with valve type or other predisposing factors was noted.

In a large multicenter study, involving 10 centers and 2418 patients, Del Trigo et al. found that the overall incidence of VHD, defined as an absolute increase in mean transprosthetic gradient ≥10 mmHg (on TTE) between discharge and last follow-up, was 4.5% [103]; 2.8% occurred within the first year. Independent associated factors were lack of anticoagulation therapy, a valve-in-valve procedure, use of an ≤23 mm transcatheter valve, and a greater BMI. No difference with valve type was noted.

However, recent reports have found that conventional TTE follow-up post-TAVR is inferior for the detection of THV thrombosis compared to contrast-enhanced

**Table 26.7** Current guidelines for antithrombotic therapy post-TAVR

American Heart Association/American College of Cardiology/Society of Thoracic Surgeons
1. Aspirin should be used indefinitely
2. Concomitant clopidogrel for 3–6 months
3. If vitamin K antagonist is indicated, no concomitant clopidogrel

European Society of Cardiology
1. Aspirin or clopidogrel indefinitely
2. Combination of aspirin and clopidogrel early after TAVI
3. If vitamin K antagonist is indicated, no antiplatelet therapy

multidetector computed tomography (MDCT). Indeed, it has the ability to detect THV thrombosis in asymptomatic patients with no evidence of THV obstruction on TTE and can potentially lead to increased risk of stroke, THV obstruction with heart failure, or reduced long-term THV durability [104, 105].

Similarly, Hansson et al. employed MDCT in addition to TTE and TEE, in 460 consecutive patients undergoing TAVR with the Edwards SAPIEN XT or SAPIEN 3 valves, at 1- to 3-month follow-up. The incidence of overall thrombosis was 7%, of which only 18% were clinically overt obstructive THV thrombosis. On multivariable analysis, larger THV (29 mm) and no post-TAVR warfarin treatment independently predicted THV thrombosis [106]. Twenty-five percent of patients were on aspirin alone.

The most commonly used treatment regimen for THV thrombosis is anticoagulation, which has proven to be efficacious in more than 80% of patients [102, 106]. In other cases, percutaneous TAVR in TAVR or open-heart surgery can be considered. However, a significant concern regards the antithrombotic regimen that should be used post-TAVR, its duration, and whether anticoagulation is indicated or not (Table 26.7) [107, 108]. Currently, dual antiplatelet therapy (ASA + clopidogrel) is recommended and used in most centers, but the duration of clopidogrel varies widely. Future studies, such as the ongoing ARTE (Aspirin Versus Aspirin + Clopidogrel Following Transcatheter Aortic Valve Implantation) pilot trial (NCT01559298) should provide key data to inform future large-scale, clinical trials. On the other hand, data on the protective effect of anticoagulant therapy is expected to be provided with ongoing randomized trials, such as the GALILEO trial (NCT02556203) and the POPular-TAVI trial (NCT02247128).

### Conclusions

In this chapter, the most common complications following TAVR have been briefly reviewed. Despite major advances in TAVR, PVLs, stroke, conduction disturbances, and vascular complications are still significant complications associated with this less-invasive procedure. The presence of moderate-to-severe PVL following TAVR is definitely associated with decreased survival. New or emerging THV devices may reduce this hurdle by allowing controlled deployment, repositioning, or even retrieval of the valve and by better annular sealing. Post-procedural stroke is also associated with worse survival post-TAVR and is still one of the most feared complications by both the patient and operator. The use of newer, smaller, less-traumatic catheters, improved technique, increased operator's experience, and the use of embolic protection devices could eventually contribute to lowering the risk of cerebrovascular events associated with TAVR. Conduction disturbances and the need for PPI are the most frequent complications of TAVR, and its occurrence has seemingly increased with some of the newer-generation transcatheter valves. Finally, for vascular complications, thorough assessment of the iliofemoral arteries with MDCT, careful patient selection, improved experience, and the use of alternate access routes (transapical, transaortic, subclavian, carotid, transcaval) can sometimes be necessary to avoid major vascular complications. Moreover, lower sheath profile, fully percutaneous access, and echocardiographic-guided access also represent technological advances that can potentially reduce the occurrence of vascular complications in the setting of TAVR.

As the use of TAVR expands to include lower-risk populations, it is mandatory to develop new technologies that will reduce the rate of complications following TAVR and will therefore ensure a favorable risk–benefit ratio for both the existing and the new, less-comorbid patient populations.

# References

1. Leon MB, Smith CR, Mack M, et al. Transcatheter aortic-valve implantation for aortic stenosis in patients who cannot undergo surgery. N Engl J Med. 2010;363:1597–607.
2. Smith CR, Leon MB, Mack MJ, et al. Transcatheter versus surgical aortic-valve replacement in high-risk patients. N Engl J Med. 2011;364:2187–98.
3. Makkar RR, Fontana GP, Jilaihawi H, et al. Transcatheter aortic-valve replacement for inoperable severe aortic stenosis. N Engl J Med. 2012;366:1696–704.
4. Kodali SK, Williams MR, Smith CR, et al. Two-year outcomes after transcatheter or surgical aortic-valve replacement. N Engl J Med. 2012;366:1686–95.
5. Thomas M, Schymik G, Walther T, et al. One-year outcomes of cohort 1 in the Edwards SAPIEN Aortic Bioprosthesis European Outcome (SOURCE) registry: the European registry of transcatheter aortic valve implantation using the Edwards SAPIEN valve. Circulation. 2011;124:425–33.
6. Gilard M, Eltchaninoff H, Iung B, et al. Registry of transcatheter aortic-valve implantation in high-risk patients. N Engl J Med. 2012;366:1705–15.
7. Rodes-Cabau J, Webb JG, Cheung A, et al. Long-term outcomes after transcatheter aortic valve implantation: insights on prognostic factors and valve durability from the Canadian multicenter experience. J Am Coll Cardiol. 2012;60:1864–75.
8. Hamm CW, Mollmann H, Holzhey D, et al. The German Aortic Valve Registry (GARY): in-hospital outcome. Eur Heart J. 2014;35:1588–98.
9. Moat NE, Ludman P, de Belder MA, et al. Long-term outcomes after transcatheter aortic valve implantation in high-risk patients with severe aortic stenosis: the UK TAVI (United Kingdom Transcatheter Aortic Valve Implantation) Registry. J Am Coll Cardiol. 2011;58:2130–8.
10. Chieffo A, Buchanan GL, Van Mieghem NM, et al. Transcatheter aortic valve implantation with the Edwards SAPIEN versus the Medtronic CoreValve Revalving system devices: a multicenter collaborative study: the PRAGMATIC Plus Initiative (Pooled-RotterdAm-Milano-Toulouse In Collaboration). J Am Coll Cardiol. 2013;61:830–6.

11. Di Mario C, Eltchaninoff H, Moat N, et al. The 2011–12 pilot European Sentinel Registry of Transcatheter Aortic Valve Implantation: in-hospital results in 4571 patients. Euro-Intervention. 2013;8:1362–71.

12. Mack MJ, Brennan JM, Brindis R, et al. Outcomes following transcatheter aortic valve replacement in the United States. JAMA. 2013;310:2069–77.

13. Linke A, Wenaweser P, Gerckens U, et al. Treatment of aortic stenosis with a self-expanding transcatheter valve: the International Multi-centre ADVANCE Study. Eur Heart J. 2014;35(38):2672–84. doi:10.1093/eurheartj/ehu162.

14. Abdel-Wahab M, Mehilli J, Frerker C, et al. Comparison of balloon-expandable vs self-expandable valves in patients undergoing transcatheter aortic valve replacement: the CHOICE randomized clinical trial. JAMA. 2014;311:1503–14.

15. Takagi H, Umemoto T, for the ALICE (All-Literature Investigation of Cardiovascular Evidence) Group. Impact of paravalvular aortic regurgitation after transcatheter aortic valve implantation on survival. Int J Cardiol. 2016;221:46–51.

16. Kappetein AP, Head SJ, Généreux P, et al. Updated standardized endpoint definitions for transcatheter aortic valve implantation: the valve academic research consortium-2 consensus document. J Am Coll Cardiol. 2012;60:1438–54.

17. Lerakis S, Hayek SS, Douglas PS. Paravalvular aortic leak after transcatheter aortic valve replacement: current knowledge. Circulation. 2013;127:397–407.

18. Athappan G, Patvardhan E, Tuzcu EM, et al. Incidence, predictors, and outcomes of aortic regurgitation after transcatheter aortic valve replacement: meta-analysis and systematic review of literature. J Am Coll Cardiol. 2013;61(15):1585–9.

19. Nombela-Franco L, Ruel M, Radhakrishnan S, et al. Comparison of hemodynamic performance of self-expandable CoreValve versus balloon-expandable Edwards SAPIEN aortic valves inserted by catheter for aortic stenosis. Am J Cardiol. 2013;111(7):1026–33.

20. Popma J, Adams D, Reardon M, et al. Transcatheter aortic valve replacement using a self-expanding bioprosthesis in patients with severe aortic stenosis at extreme risk for surgery. J Am Coll Cardiol. 2014;63:1972–81.

21. Adams DH, Popma JJ, Reardon MJ, et al. Transcatheter aortic-valve replacement with a self-expanding prosthesis. N Engl J Med. 2014;370:1790–8.

22. Reardon MJ, Adams DH, Kleiman NS, et al. 2-Year outcomes in patients undergoing surgical or self-expanding transcatheter aortic valve replacement. J Am Coll Cardiol. 2015;66:113–21.

23. Tamburino C, Capodanno D, Ramondo A, et al. Incidence and predictors of early and late mortality after transcatheter aortic valve implantation in 663 patients with severe aortic stenosis. Circulation. 2011;123:299–308.

24. van Belle E, Juthier F, Susen S, et al. Postprocedural aortic regurgitation in balloon-expandable and self-expandable transcatheter aortic valve replacement procedures: analysis of predictors and impact on long-term mortality: insights from the FRANCE2 Registry. Circulation. 2014;129:1415–27.

25. Miyazaki S, Agricola E, Panoulas VF, et al. Influence of baseline ejection fraction on the prognostic value of paravalvular leak after transcatheter aortic valve implantation. Int J Cardiol. 2015;190:277–81.

26. Mack MJ, Leon MB, Smith CR, et al. 5-Year outcomes of transcatheter aortic valve replacement or surgical aortic valve replacement for high surgical risk patients with aortic stenosis (PARTNER 1): a randomised controlled trial. Lancet. 2015;1:8.

27. Jerez-Valero M, Urena M, Webb JG, et al. Clinical impact of aortic regurgitation after transcatheter aortic valve replacement: insights into the degree and acuteness of presentation. JACC Cardiovasc Interv. 2014;7:1022–32.

28. Koos R, Mahnken AH, Dohmen G, et al. Association of aortic valve calcification severity with the degree of aortic regurgitation after transcatheter aortic valve implantation. Int J Cardiol. 2011;150:142–5.

29. Colli A, D'Amico R, Kempfert J, et al. Transesophageal echocardiographic scoring for transcatheter aortic valve implantation: impact of aortic cusp calcification on postoperative aortic regurgitation. J Thorac Cardiovasc Surg. 2011;142:1229–35.

30. Yared K, Garcia-Camarero T, Fernandez-Friera L, et al. Impact of aortic regurgitation after transcatheter aortic valve implantation: results from the REVIVAL trial. JACC Cardiovasc Imaging. 2012;5:469–77.
31. Détaint D, Lepage L, Himbert D, et al. Determinants of significant paravalvular regurgitation after transcatheter aortic valve: implantation impact of device and annulus discongruence. JACC Cardiovasc Interv. 2009;2:821–7.
32. Schultz CJ, Tzikas A, Moelker A, et al. Correlates on MSCT of paravalvular aortic regurgitation after transcatheter aortic valve implantation using the Medtronic CoreValve prosthesis. Catheter Cardiovasc Interv. 2011;78:446–55.
33. Généreux P, Head SJ, Hahn R, et al. Paravalvular leak after transcatheter aorticvalve replacement: the new Achilles' heel? A comprehensive review of the literature. J Am Coll Cardiol. 2013;61:1125–36.
34. Van Belle E, Rauch A, Vincent F, et al. Von Willebrand factor multimers during transcatheter aortic-valve replacement. N Engl J Med. 2016;375(4):335–44. doi:10.1056/NEJMoa1505643.
35. Willson AB, Webb JG, Labounty TM, et al. 3-dimensional aortic annular assessment by multidetector computed tomography predicts moderate or severe paravalvular regurgitation after transcatheter aortic valve replacement: a multicenter retrospective analysis. J Am Coll Cardiol. 2012;59:1287–94.
36. Mylotte D, Dorfmeister M, Elhmidi Y, et al. Erroneous measurement of the aortic annular diameter using 2-dimensional echocardiography resulting in inappropriate CoreValve size selection: a retrospective comparison with multislice computed tomography. JACC Cardiovasc Interv. 2014;7:652–61.
37. Jilaihawi H, Doctor N, et al. Aortic annular sizing for transcatheteraortic valve replacement using cross-sectional 3-dimensional transesophageal echocardiography. J Am Coll Cardiol. 2013;61:908–16.
38. Khalique OK, Kodali SK, Paradis JM, et al. Aortic annular sizing using a novel 3-dimensional echocardiographic method use and comparison with cardiac computed tomography. Circ Cardiovasc Imaging. 2014;7:155–63.
39. Sinning JM, Werner N, Nickenig G, Grube E. Challenges in transcatheter valve treatment: aortic regurgitation after transcatheter aortic valve implantation. EuroIntervention. 2013;9(Suppl):S72–6.
40. Nombela-Franco L, Rodes-Cabau J, DeLarochelliere R, et al. Predictive factors, efficacy, and safety of balloon post-dilation after transcatheter aortic valve implantation with a balloon-expandable valve. JACC Cardiovasc Interv. 2012;5:499–512.
41. Makkar RR, Jilaihawi H, Chakravarty T, et al. Determinants and outcomes of acute transcatheter valve-in-valve therapy or embolization: a study of multiple valve implants in the U.S. PARTNER trial (Placement of AoRTic TraNscathetER Valve Trial Edwards SAPIEN Transcatheter Heart Valve). J Am Coll Cardiol. 2013;62:418–30.
42. Saia F, Martinez C, Gafoor S, et al. Long-term outcomes of percutaneous paravalvular regurgitation closure after transcatheter aortic valve replacement: a multicenter experience. JACC Cardiovasc Interv. 2015;8:681–8.
43. Herrmann HC, Thourani VH, Kodali SK, et al. One-year clinical outcomes with SAPIEN 3 transcatheter aortic valve replacement in high-risk and inoperable patients with severe aortic stenosis. Circulation. 2016;134(2):130–40. doi:10.1161/CIRCULATIONAHA.116.022797.
44. Manoharan G, Walton AS, Brecker SJ, et al. Treatment of symptomatic severe aortic stenosis with a novel resheathable supra-annular self-expanding transcatheter aortic valve system. JACC Cardiovasc Interv. 2015;8(10):1359–67.
45. Meredith IT, Walters DL, Dumonteil N, et al. 1-Year outcomes with the fully repositionable and retrievable lotus transcatheter aortic replacement valve in 120 high-risk surgical patients with severe aortic stenosis: results of the REPRISE II study. JACC Cardiovasc Interv. 2016;9(4):376–84.
46. Schofer J, Colombo A, Klugmann S, et al. Prospective multicenter evaluation of the direct flow medical transcatheter aortic valve. J Am Coll Cardiol. 2014;63(8):763–8.

47. Manoharan G, Linke A, Möllmann H, et al. Multicentre clinical study evaluating a novel resheathable annular functioning self-expanding transcatheter aortic valve system: safety and performance results at 30 days with the Portico system. EuroIntervention. 2016;12:768–74.
48. Silaschi M, Treede H, Rastan AJ, et al. The JUPITER registry: 1-year results of transapical aortic valve implantation using a second-generation transcatheter heart valve in patients with aortic stenosis. Eur J Cardiothorac Surg. 2016;50(5):874–81.
49. Kempfert J, Holzhey D, Hofmann S, et al. First registry results from the newly approved ACURATE TA™ TAVI system. Eur J Cardiothorac Surg. 2015;48(1):137–41.
50. Webb J, Gerosa G, Lefèvre T, et al. Multicenter evaluation of a next-generation balloon-expandable transcatheter aortic valve. J Am Coll Cardiol. 2014;64:2235–43. doi:10.1016/j.jacc.2014.09.026.
51. Herrmann HC. New transcatheter aortic valve prosthesis sets a new standard. J Am Coll Cardiol. 2014;64:2244–5. doi:10.1016/j.jacc.2014.08.042.
52. Ando T, Briasoulis A, Holmes AA, Taub CC, Takagi H, Afonso L. Sapien 3 versus Sapien XT prosthetic valves in transcatheter aortic valve implantation: a meta-analysis. Int J Cardiol. 2016;220:472–8. doi:10.1016/j.ijcard.2016.06.159.
53. Lefèvre T, Colombo A, Tchétché D, et al. Prospective multicenter evaluation of the direct flow medical transcatheter aortic valve system: 12-month outcomes of the evaluation of the direct flow medical percutaneous aortic valve 18F system for the treatment of patients with severe aortic stenosis (DISCOVER) study. JACC Cardiovasc Interv. 2016;9(1):68–75.
54. Sondergaard L, Worthley S, Rodes J, Maisano F. Safety and performance of the Portico valve in patients with severe aortic stenosis and excessive surgical risk: a first report of 30-day results from the PORTICO I study. Published in Abstracts EuroPCR 2016, May 2016.
55. Bax JJ, Delgado V, Bapat V, et al. Open issues in transcatheter aortic valve implantation. Part 2: procedural issues and outcomes after transcatheter aortic valve implantation. Eur Heart J. 2014;35:2639–54.
56. Siontis GC, Jüni P, Pilgrim T, et al. Predictors of permanent pacemaker implantation in patients with severe aortic stenosis undergoing TAVR: a meta-analysis. J Am Coll Cardiol. 2014;64:129–40.
57. Carrabba N, Valenti R, Migliorini A, et al. Impact on left ventricular function and remodeling and on 1-year outcome in patients with left bundle branch block after transcatheter aortic valve implantation. Am J Cardiol. 2015;116:125–31.
58. Schymik G, Tzamalis P, Bramlage P, et al. Clinical impact of a new left bundle branch block following TAVI implantation: 1-year results of the TAVIK cohort. Clin Res Cardiol. 2015;104:351–62.
59. Urena M, Webb JG, Cheema A, et al. Impact of new-onset persistent left bundle branch block on late clinical outcomes in patients undergoing transcatheter aortic valve implantation with a balloon-expandable valve. JACC Cardiovasc Interv. 2014;7:128–36.
60. Houthuizen P, van der Boon RM, Urena M, et al. Occurrence, fate and consequences of ventricular conduction abnormalities after transcatheter aortic valve implantation. EuroIntervention. 2014;9:1142–50.
61. Nazif TM, Williams MR, Hahn RT, et al. Clinical implications of new-onset left bundle branch block after transcatheter aortic valve replacement: analysis of the PARTNER experience. Eur Heart J. 2014;35:1599–607.
62. Franzoni I, Latib A, Maisano F, et al. Comparison of incidence and predictors of left bundle branch block after transcatheter aortic valve implantation using the CoreValve versus the Edwards valve. Am J Cardiol. 2013;112:554–9.
63. Testa L, Latib A, De Marco F, et al. Clinical impact of persistent left bundle-branch block after transcatheter aortic valve implantation with CoreValve Revalving System. Circulation. 2013;127:1300–7.
64. Van der Boon RM, Nuis RJ, Van Mieghem NM, et al. New conduction abnormalities after TAVI—frequency and causes. Nat Rev Cardiol. 2012;9:454–63.

65. Petronio AS, Sinning JM, Van Mieghem N, et al. Optimal implantation depth and adherence to guidelines on permanent pacing to improve the results of transcatheter aortic valve replacement with the Medtronic CoreValve system: the CoreValve prospective, international, post-Market ADVANCE-II Study. JACC Cardiovasc Interv. 2015;8:837–46.

66. Urena M, Rodés-Cabau J. Managing heart block after transcatheter aortic valve implantation: from monitoring to device selection and pacemaker indications. EuroIntervention. 2015;11(suppl W):W101–5. doi:10.4244/EIJV11SWA30.

67. Tarantini G, Mojoli M, Purita P, Napodano M, D'Onofrio A, Frigo A, Covolo E, Facchin M, Isabella G, Gerosa G, Iliceto S. Unravelling the (arte)fact of increased pacemaker rate with the Edwards SAPIEN 3 valve. EuroIntervention. 2015;11:343–50. doi:10.4244/EIJY14M11_06.

68. Toggweiler S, Stortecky S, Holy E, et al. The electrocardiogram after transcatheter aortic valve replacement determines the risk for post-procedural high-degree AV block and the need for telemetry monitoring. JACC Cardiovasc Interv. 2016;9(12):1269–76.

69. Regueiro A, Abdul-Jawad Altisent O, Del Trigo M, et al. Impact of new-onset left bundle branch block and periprocedural permanent pacemaker implantation on clinical outcomes in patients undergoing transcatheter aortic valve replacement: a systematic review and meta-analysis. Circ Cardiovasc Interv. 2016;9(5):e003635.

70. Genereux P, Head SJ, Van Mieghem NM, et al. Clinical outcomes after transcatheter aortic valve replacement using valve academic research consortium definitions: a weighted meta-analysis of 3,519 patients from 16 studies. J Am Coll Cardiol. 2012;59:2317–26.

71. Genereux P, Webb JG, Svensson LG, et al. Vascular complications after transcatheter aortic valve replacement: insights from the PARTNER (Placement of AoRTic TraNscathetER Valve) trial. J Am Coll Cardiol. 2012;60:1043–52.

72. Khatri PJ, Webb JG, Rodes-Cabau J, et al. Adverse effects associated with transcatheter aortic valve implantation: a meta-analysis of contemporary studies. Ann Internal Med. 2013;158:35–46.

73. Panchal HB, Ladia V, Amin P, et al. A meta-analysis of mortality and major adverse cardiovascular and cerebrovascular events in patients undergoing transfemoral versus transapical transcatheter aortic valve implantation using edwards valve for severe aortic stenosis. Am J Cardiol. 2014;114(12):1882–90.

74. Steinvil A, Leshem-Rubinow E, et al. Vascular complications after transcatheter aortic valve implantation and their association with mortality reevaluated by the valve academic research consortium definitions. Am J Cardiol. 2015;115(1):100–6.

75. Genereux P, Head SJ, Wood DA, et al. Transcatheter aortic valve implantation: 10-year anniversary. Part II: clinical implications. Eur Heart J. 2012;33:2399–402.

76. Hayashida K, Lefèvre T, Chevalier B, et al. Transfemoral aortic valve implantation new criteria to predict vascular complications. JACC Cardiovasc Interv. 2011;4:851–8.

77. Toggweiler S, Gurvitch R, Leipsic J, et al. Percutaneous aortic valve replacement: vascular outcomes with a fully percutaneous procedure. J Am Coll Cardiol. 2012;59:113–8.

78. Van Mieghem NM, Tchetche D, Chieffo A, et al. Incidence, predictors, and implications of access site complications with transfemoral transcatheter aortic valve implantation. Am J Cardiol. 2012;110:1361–7.

79. Barbash IM, Barbanti M, Webb J, et al. Comparison of vascular closure devices for access site closure after transfemoral aortic valve implantation. Eur Heart J. 2015;36(47):3370–9.

80. Leon MB, Smith CR, Mack MJ, et al. Transcatheter or surgical aortic-valve replacement in intermediate-risk patients. N Engl J Med. 2016;374:1609–20.

81. Holmes DR, Brennan JM, Rumsfeld JS, et al. Clinical outcomes at 1 year following transcatheter aortic valve replacement. JAMA. 2015;313:1019–28.

82. Walther T, Hamm CW, Schuler G, et al. Perioperative results and complications in 15,964 transcatheter aortic valve replacements: prospective data from the GARY registry. J Am Coll Cardiol. 2015;65:2173–80.

83. Eggebrecht H, Schmermund A, Voigtlander T, Kahlert P, Erbel R, Mehta RH. Risk of stroke after transcatheter aortic valve implantation (TAVI): a meta-analysis of 10,037 published patients. EuroIntervention. 2012;8:129–38.

84. Auffret V, Regueiro A, Del Trigo M, et al. Predictors of early cerebrovascular events in patients with aortic stenosis undergoing transcatheter aortic valve replacement. J Am Coll Cardiol. 2016;68(7):673–84.
85. Bendszus M, Stoll G. Silent cerebral ischaemia: hidden fingerprints of invasive medical procedures. Lancet Neurol. 2006;5:364–72.
86. Fairbairn TA, Mather AN, Bijsterveld P, Worthy G, Currie S, Goddard AJ, Blackman DJ, Plein S, Greenwood JP. Diffusion-weighted MRI determined cerebral embolic infarction following transcatheter aortic valve implantation: assessment of predictive risk factors and the relationship to subsequent health status. Heart. 2012;98:18–23.
87. Rodes-Cabau J, Dumont E, Boone RH, Larose E, Bagur R, Gurvitch R, Bedard F, Doyle D, De Larochelliere R, Jayasuria C, Villeneuve J, Marrero A, Cote M, Pibarot P, Webb JG. Cerebral embolism following transcatheter aortic valve implantation: comparison of transfemoral and transapical approaches. J Am Coll Cardiol. 2011;57:18–28.
88. Drews T, Pasic M, Buz S, et al. Transcranial Doppler sound detection of cerebral microembolism during transapical aortic valve implantation. Thorac Cardiovasc Surg. 2011;59:237–42.
89. Miller DC, Blackstone EH, Mack MJ, et al. Transcatheter (TAVR) versus surgical (AVR) aortic valve replacement: occurrence, hazard, risk factors, and consequences of neurologic events in the PARTNER trial. J Thorac Cardiovasc Surg. 2012;143:832–843.e13.
90. Athappan G, Gajulapalli RD, Sengodan P, et al. Influence of transcatheter aortic valve replacement strategy and valve design on stroke after transcatheter aortic valve replacement: a meta-analysis and systematic review of literature. J Am Coll Cardiol. 2014;63:2101–10.
91. Nombela-Franco L, Webb JG, de Jaegere PP, et al. Timing, predictive factors, and prognostic value of cerebrovascular events in a large cohort of patients undergoing transcatheter aortic valve implantation. Circulation. 2012;126:3041–53.
92. Freeman M, Barbanti M, Wood DA, et al. Cerebral events and protection during transcatheter aortic valve replacement. Catheter Cardiovasc Interv. 2014;84:885–96.
93. Rodes-Cabau J, Kahlert P, Neumann F-J, et al. Feasibility and exploratory efficacy evaluation of the Embrella Embolic Deflector system for the prevention of cerebral emboli in patients undergoing transcatheter aortic valve replacement: the PROTAVI-C pilot study. JACC Cardiovasc Interv. 2014;7:1146–55.
94. Lansky AJ, Schofer J, Tchetche D, et al. A prospective randomized evaluation of the TriGuard™ HDH embolic DEFLECTion device during transcatheter aortic valve implantation: results from the DEFLECT III trial. Eur Heart J. 2015;36:2070–8.
95. Van Mieghem NM, Schipper MEI, Ladich E, et al. Histopathology of embolic debris captured during transcatheter aortic valve replacement. Circulation. 2013;127:2194–201.
96. Ribeiro HB, Webb JG, Makkar RR, et al. Predictive factors, management, and clinical outcomes of coronary obstruction following transcatheter aortic valve implantation: insights from a large multicenter registry. J Am Coll Cardiol. 2013;62:1552–62.
97. Généreux P, Head SJ, Van Mieghem NM, Kodali S, Kirtane AJ, Xu K, Smith C, Serruys PW, Kappetein AP, Leon MB. Clinical outcomes after transcatheter aortic valve replacement using valve academic research consortium definitions: a weighted meta-analysis of 3,519 patients from 16 studies. J Am Coll Cardiol. 2012;59:2317–26.
98. Barbanti M, Yang T-H, Rodes-Cabau J, et al. Anatomical and procedural features associated with aortic root rupture during balloon-expandable transcatheter aortic valve replacement. Circulation. 2013;128:244–53.
99. Pasic M, Unbehaun A, Dreysse S, Buz S, Drews T, Kukucka M, D'Ancona G, Seifert B, Hetzer R. Rupture of the device landing zone during transcatheter aortic valve implantation: a life-threatening but treatable complication. Circ Cardiovasc Interv. 2012;5:424–32.
100. Rezq A, Basavarajaiah S, Latib A, et al. Incidence, management, and outcomes of cardiac tamponade during transcatheter aortic valve implantation: a single-center study. JACC Cardiovasc Intervent. 2012;5:1264–72.
101. Córdoba-Soriano JG, Puri R, Amat-Santos I, et al. Valve thrombosis following transcatheter aortic valve implantation: a systematic review. Rev Esp Cardiol (Engl Ed). 2015;68(3):198–204.

102. Latib A, Naganuma T, Abdel-Wahab M, et al. Treatment and clinical outcomes of transcatheter heart valve thrombosis. Circ Cardiovasc Interv. 2015;8.
103. Del Trigo M, Muñoz-Garcia AJ, Wijeysundera HC, et al. Incidence, timing, and predictors of valve hemodynamic deterioration after transcatheter aortic valve replacement: multicenter registry. J Am Coll Cardiol. 2016;67:644–55.
104. Leetmaa T, Hansson NC, Leipsic J, et al. Early aortic transcatheter heart valve thrombosis: diagnostic value of contrast-enhanced multidetector computed tomography. Circ Cardiovasc Interv. 2015;8.
105. Pache G, Schoechlin S, Blanke P, et al. Early hypo-attenuated leaflet thickening in balloon-expandable transcatheter aortic heart valves. Eur Heart J. 2016;37(28):2263–71.
106. Hansson NC, Grove EL, Andersen HR, et al. Transcatheter aortic heart valve thrombosis: incidence, predisposing factors, and clinical implications. J Am Coll Cardiol. 2016;68(19):2059–69. pii: S0735-1097(16)34936-1
107. Holmes DR Jr, Mack MJ, Kaul S, et al. 2012 ACCF/AATS/SCAI/STS expert consensus document on transcatheter aortic valve replacement: developed in collabration with the American Heart Association, American Society of Echocardiography, European Association for CardioThoracic Surgery, Heart Failure Society of America, Mended Hearts, Society of Cardiovascular Anesthesiologists, Society of Cardiovascular Computed Tomography, and Society for Cardiovascular Magnetic Resonance. J Thorac Cardiovasc Surg. 2012;144:e29–84.
108. Vahanian A, Alfieri O, Andreotti F, et al. Guidelines on the management of valvular heart disease (version 2012): the Joint Task Force on the Management of Valvular Heart Disease of the European Society of Cardiology (ESC) and the European Association for Cardio-Thoracic Surgery (EACTS). Eur J Cardiothorac Surg. 2012;42:S1–S44.

# TAVI Postprocedural Management

# 27

Piera Capranzano and Corrado Tamburino

## 27.1 Antithrombotic Therapy

### 27.1.1 Background and Rationale

Despite recent progresses in technology and operator experience and high procedural success rates, the transcatheter aortic valve implantation (TAVI) is associated with a non-negligible risk of thrombotic events, especially ischemic stroke. This risk of stroke is particularly high in the periprocedural period, but it steadily maintains during follow-up [1, 2]. Multiple factors can contribute to stroke in TAVI patients, including the following: introduction and manipulation of large valve systems in calcified arteries; exposition of tissue factor or arterial embolization of thrombogenic and inflammatory material subsequent to the important tissue injury caused by the positioning and implantation of the prosthesis valve when crushing the native valve; thrombi generated in areas of turbulent flow or blood stasis created by the new device overlying the native valve, especially in the case of small valve areas; tissue injury of the aortic wall triggering the thrombus formation; thromboembolism from bioprosthetic leaflets; peripheral vascular disease; and atrial fibrillation. This latter arrhythmia, in particular, is an important contributing factor, as it is present before the procedure in a relevant proportion (about 30%) of patients undergoing TAVI. In addition, it can develop newly after TAVI during follow-up in about 20% of patients who were on sinus rhythm at the time of the procedure [3]. Of importance, the advanced age and large burden of comorbidities typical of TAVI patients lead to a frequently high CHA2DS2-VASC score associated with a high annual risk of stroke.

P. Capranzano, M.D. (✉) • C. Tamburino, M.D., Ph.D.
Cardiovascular Department, Ferrarotto Hospital, University of Catania, Catania, Italy
e-mail: pcapranzano@gmail.com

© Springer International Publishing AG 2018
C. Tamburino et al. (eds.), *Percutaneous Treatment of Left Side Cardiac Valves*,
https://doi.org/10.1007/978-3-319-59620-4_27

Few cases of leaflet thrombosis in transcatheter bioprosthetic aortic valves have been reported [4]. In particular, symptomatic transcatheter aortic valve thrombosis is rare, occurring within the first 2 years after TAVI in <1% of cases [4]. Echocardiographic findings of leaflet thrombosis cases include a markedly elevated mean aortic valve pressure gradient, presence of thickened leaflets or thrombotic apposition of leaflets in 77%, and a thrombotic mass on the leaflets in the remaining 23% of patients [4]. The most common clinical presentation is exertional dyspnea (65%), while 31% of patients have no worsening symptoms, and the valve thrombosis is detected on routine follow-up echocardiography [4]. Of note, in most patients (88%), anticoagulation therapy results in a significant decrease in the aortic valve pressure gradient within 2 months [4]. However, due to absent or mild clinical manifestations, the frequency of valve thrombosis may be underestimated if early echocardiographic assessment is not systematically done. This was highlighted in a recent study in which subclinical reduced leaflet motion, likely due to thrombosis, was not uncommon in three different small cohorts [5]. Therapeutic anticoagulation with warfarin was associated with significantly lower rates of reduced leaflet motion than was dual antiplatelet therapy (DAPT) [5]. In a recent study, among 405 consecutive patients undergoing TAVI with the Edwards SAPIEN XT or SAPIEN 3, the contrast-enhanced multidetector computed tomography (MDCT) showed hypo-attenuated leaflet thickening, indicating valve thrombosis in 28 (7%) patients [6]. A total of 23 (5.7%) patients had subclinical valve thrombosis, while 5 (1.2%) patients experienced clinically overt obstructive thrombosis. The risk of valve thrombosis in patients not receiving warfarin was higher compared with patients receiving warfarin, 10.7% vs. 1.8% [6]. Treatment with warfarin effectively reverted thrombosis and normalized valve function in 85% of patients as documented by follow-up transesophageal echocardiography and MDCT [6]. However, the clinical impact of subclinical reduced leaflet motion remains undetermined.

The risks of stroke and valve thrombosis in TAVI patients established the rationale for antithrombotic therapy, antiplatelet (single or DAPT), and/or anticoagulant. The possible predominant pathogenetic role of thrombin over platelets in the cerebrovascular events occurring after TAVI, non-infrequent new-onset atrial fibrillation, and possible bioprosthesis thrombosis suggests the greater potential usefulness of anticoagulant with respect to antiplatelet therapy, even in patients with no specific concomitant indications for anticoagulation. However, in selecting antithrombotic therapy, it should be considered that patients undergoing TAVI are at high risk of bleeding. Bleedings are frequent complications of TAVI during the periprocedural phase occurring in about 15–30% of patients [2, 7]. Also late major bleedings, in which the antithrombotic therapy plays a role, are common and are known to have a negative prognostic impact [7]. For this reason, in patients undergoing TAVI, it is crucial to identify the antithrombotic regimen that can be effective but also safe. Indeed the risk of bleeding related to the use of specific antithrombotic drugs may not counterbalance the risk of stroke or that of prosthesis valve thrombosis. However, the optimal antithrombotic therapy for TAVI patients is still a matter of debate, and though little evidence is available, it is currently under investigation in several studies.

### 27.1.1.1 Current Evidence and Practical Recommendations

During the procedure, the most used antithrombotic strategy is unfractionated heparin (UFH) administered as an initial intravenous bolus of 5000 IU plus eventual additional bolus to achieve an activated clotting time $\geq$ 250 s for the entire procedure. Reversal of UFH with protamine at the end of the procedure is usually considered standard local institutional practice. This common antithrombotic strategy during the TAVI procedure is corroborated by a recent randomized study (BRAVO-3) assessing UFH vs. bivalirudin in 802 patients undergoing transfemoral TAVI [8]. Compared with UFH, bivalirudin did not significantly reduce rates of major bleeding at 48 h or net adverse cardiovascular events at 30 days, though the non-inferiority for the latter end point was met [8]. Thus, considering the cost of heparin and the lack of an antidote for bivalirudin, according to the results of the BRAVO-3 trial, UFH should remain the standard of care.

Evidence on the antithrombotic treatment after TAVI is scant, and thus the optimal regimen has yet to be established. Empirically, in patients without a specific indication for oral anticoagulation, antiplatelet drugs are commonly used after TAVI. In particular, the general consensus is to prescribe DAPT with aspirin and clopidogrel for 3–6 months and aspirin in single chronic therapy thereafter. However, the use of DAPT has not been evidence based. Four studies have compared aspirin in monotherapy versus DAPT after TAVI, concluding that aspirin alone tended to reduce major bleeding, with no increase in ischemic stroke [9–12]. These studies were small, including 672 patients overall, and only 2 were randomized, not allowing for definite conclusions on the superior net clinical benefit of single therapy versus DAPT after TAVI. However, the consistency and biological plausibility of overall safety results suggest that a therapy with a single antiplatelet may be a viable strategy for patients with a relative higher risk of bleeding. Considering that most cases of ischemic stroke occur during the first 30 days after TAVI, a reasonable antithrombotic regimen could consist in prescribing DAPT for at least one month and, thereafter, continuing with aspirin only. The latter strategy was adopted in the PARTNER 2A trial [13], where the absolute increase of ischemic stroke between 30 days and 1 year was lower (about half) than that of life-threatening or disabling bleeding. These findings would appear to argue against the use of prolonged regimens of DAPT after TAVI. The ongoing ARTE (aspirin vs. aspirin + clopidogrel following TAVI pilot trial) and POPular-TAVI (antiplatelet therapy for patients undergoing TAVI) studies will help to define the role of DAPT compared with aspirin in monotherapy after TAVI.

Finally, it is still unknown whether anticoagulation would be better for TAVI patients with no specific indication compared with the antiplatelet therapy. This issue has being addressed in two large randomized studies. The GALILEO (Global multicenter, open-label, randomized, event-driven, active-controlled study comparing a rivAroxaban-based antithrombotic strategy with an antipLatelet-based strategy after transcatheter aortIc vaLve rEplacement to Optimize clinical outcomes) trial randomized TAVI patients with no atrial fibrillation or other indications for oral anticoagulation to rivaroxaban 10 mg daily for long-term plus aspirin 75–100 mg for the first 3 months or to aspirin 75–100 mg for long-term plus clopidogrel for the first 3 months). The ATLANTIS (Anti-Thrombotic Strategy to Lower All Cardiovascular and Neurologic Ischemic and Hemorrhagic Events after Trans-Aortic Valve

Implantation for Aortic Stenosis) trial compared apixaban 5 mg bid (2.5 mg bid in specific subgroups) with antiplatelet therapy or warfarin in patients without oral anticoagulation indications. Until the results of these studies are available, oral anti-coagulation cannot be routinely used in TAVI patients without other concomitant specific indications (e.g., atrial fibrillation, venous thromboembolism). However, a strict monitoring at follow-up is needed to detect new-onset atrial fibrillation and a subclinical valve prosthesis dysfunction likely due to thrombosis, which would require oral anticoagulation alone.

## 27.1.2 In-Hospital Care

### 27.1.2.1 ICU Care

After the procedure, a short period of observation (about 48 h) is needed in an intensive care unit (ICU). Careful monitoring of vital signs and an accurate clinical examination are absolutely necessary to detect, early on, the onset of complications and to diagnose or rule out any states of heart failure or neurological impairment (Table 27.1). For example, the sudden onset of hypotension and signs of peripheral

**Table 27.1** Postprocedural management

| | |
|---|---|
| After procedure (until discharge) | Vital signs (temperature, heart rate, systolic blood pressure, and respiratory rate) |
| | Cardiovascular and neurological evaluation |
| | Laboratory work: CBC, creatinine, blood urea nitrogen, CK, CK-MB, liver enzymes, clotting parameters, electrolytes |
| | Pulse-oximetry oxygen saturation |
| | Monitoring of central venous pressure and input/output: fluid infusion for AK1 or dehydration |
| | Check of vascular accesses and color Doppler in case of suspicion of hematoma |
| | 12-lead ECG |
| | Removal of temporary pacemaker within 24 h and implantation of permanent pacemaker, if necessary (complete atrioventricular block) |
| | Holter ECG |
| | TTE |
| | Prophylactic antibiotic therapy |
| 30 days after hospital discharge | Brief physical examination, including vital signs |
| | Cardiac health status, including NYHA functional status CBC, creatinine, blood urea nitrogen |
| | TTE |
| | 12-lead ECG |
| | Quality of life measure |
| | Endocarditis prophylaxis |
| | Documentation of adverse events |
| 3 months; 6, 12, 18, and 24 months; and yearly after 24 months | Brief physical examination, including vital signs |
| | Cardiac health status, including NYHA functional status |
| | CBC, creatinine, blood urea nitrogen |
| | TTE |
| | 12-lead ECG |
| | Quality of life measure (at 12-month follow-up only) |
| | Endocarditis prophylaxis |
| | DoD documentation of adverse events |

hypoperfusion can point toward a diagnosis of cardiogenic shock secondary to valve malfunction, ventricular dysfunction, cardiac tamponade, retroperitoneal hematoma, arrhythmia, or myocardial infarction; signs of neurological impairment, such as aphasia, hyposthenia, confusion, or memory deficit, point instead to a suspicion of brain ischemia, which must be carefully investigated by complete neurological examination and a brain computed tomography scan.

Special attention must also be paid to (Table 27.1):

- Laboratory tests
- Renal function and fluid balance
- Vascular access
- Rhythm control
- Transthoracic echocardiogram (TTE)

**Laboratory Tests**

A routine check of laboratory examinations is recommended immediately after the procedure and every 24 h. The blood count is useful for the early detection of anemia secondary to occult bleeding, leukocytosis due to infection, and thrombocytopenia. Thrombocytopenia is a rare side effect linked to the use of thienopyridines, UFH, and low molecular weight heparin (LMWH). The use of a thienopyridine can be associated with the onset of thrombotic thrombocytopenic purpura, a condition marked by intravascular clotting, thrombocytopenia, and bleeding. In this case, platelet transfusion is contraindicated, except for cases of major bleeding, while plasmapheresis and fresh plasma administration are useful [14].

If there is a suspicion of thrombocytopenia secondary to the administration of heparin (either UFH or LMWH), early detection of the form that arises as a result of an immune-type mechanism is necessary; this is known as heparin-induced thrombocytopenia (HIT) and is less common than the nonimmune-mediated form yet more serious because it is associated with a high risk of thromboembolic events. In this case, administration of the drug must be stopped, and non-heparin anticoagulants must be used [15].

Blood urea nitrogen and creatinine values should be monitored to assess kidney function and diagnose acute kidney injury (AKI), while careful monitoring of serum electrolytes should be performed frequently over the first 48 h or in the presence of polyuria for the early detection of a state of depletion and for adequate correction.

Other laboratory examinations include the specific cardiac enzymes CK, CK-MB, and troponin-I necessary to diagnose acute myocardial ischemia, which may be caused, after TAVI, by embolization of calcific debris, displacement of native aortic leaflets, or large bulky calcium deposits over coronary artery ostia. In this case, an angiogram should be done to rule out coronary artery obstruction. Liver enzymes and clotting parameters should be monitored frequently.

**Renal Function and Fluid Balance**

In TAVI procedures, AKI is defined as an absolute reduction in kidney function occurring within 72 h after the procedure as follows: (1) stage 1, increase in serum creatinine to 150–200% (1.5—2.0 × increase compared with baseline) or increase of $\geq0.3$ mg/dL ($\geq26.4$ mmol/L); (2) stage 2, increase in serum creatinine to 200–300% (2.0–3.0 × increase compared with baseline); and (3) stage 3, increase in serum creatinine to 300% (>3 × increase compared with baseline) or serum creatinine of $\geq4.0$ mg/dL ($\geq354$ mmol/L) with an acute increase of at least 0.5 mg/dL (44 mmol/L). The TAVI procedure is associated with varying degrees of postprocedural AKI, ranging from 12 to 57% [16]. Preventive intravenous hydration with isotonic saline solution is known to decrease the risk of AKI. Some authors have shown benefits of the use of $N$-acetyl-cysteine administered 24 h before the procedure along with adequate hydration in patients with existing kidney failure [17, 18]. The recent PROTECT-TAVI (PROphylactic effecT of furosEmide-induCed diuresis with matched isotonic intravenous hydraTion in Transcatheter Aortic Valve Implantation) study has assessed the impact on AKI prevention after TAVI of the RenalGuard System (PLC Medical Systems, Milford, Massachusetts), a device that delivers intravenous fluids matched to the urine output [19]. In 112 patients undergoing TAVI, matched isotonic intravenous hydration by the RenalGuard System continued for 4 h after the procedure was associated with lower AKI rates compared with standard saline solution hydration continued for 6 h after the procedure ($n = 3$ [5.4%] vs. $n = 14$ [25.0%], respectively, $p = 0.014$], with most cases (94%) being stage 1.

Careful monitoring of the fluid balance and central venous pressure is necessary to diagnose depleted intravascular volume states, provide adequate hydration, and reduce the risk of AKI. Therefore, a Foley catheter should be retained at least for the first 24 h after the procedure to facilitate input/output monitoring. It has been observed that after TAVI, a significant number of patients with normal kidney function develop AKI. It is believed that this condition is almost certainly secondary to depleted intravascular volume developing immediately after an intense polyuric phase. It has been hypothesized that polyuria is caused by a sudden and significant rise in cardiac output after valve implantation followed by kidney hyperperfusion [20]. Therapy must be mainly aimed at correcting oliguria secondary to hypovolemia, with an adequate supply of fluids. Diuretic therapy can be useful in patients in whom oliguria persists, even though normovolemia, hemodynamics, and kidney perfusion pressure have been restored.

### Vascular Access

Major vascular complications are frequent in transfemoral TAVI (about 9%), and many of these are linked to the use of heparin, atheromatosis, calcification, and vascular bed tortuosity in these elderly patients and the use of large-gauge introducers [13]. These complications include hematomas, pseudoaneurysm, arteriovenous fistulas, dissections, retroperitoneal bleeding (in the case of transfemoral access), stenosis, and distal embolization. The introducer insertion site and distal pulses should be checked every 15 min during the first hour after the procedure and then every hour, to detect any signs of bleeding, hematomas, ecchymosis, pulsatile masses, murmurs, weak pulses, or signs of ischemic damage in the limbs. Patients must also be immobilized for 12 h after arterial hemostasis. Small hematomas and mild murmurs are frequent and do not require any diagnostic investigation or medical treatment. Clinical evidence of a large and progressively growing mass should lead to suspicion of a hematoma or pseudoaneurysm and hence be assessed by color Doppler ultrasound, especially if it is associated with a sudden development of anemia. Color Doppler ultrasound also allows for the diagnosis of arteriovenous fistulas, which can cause groin pain or new-onset murmurs. Groin hematomas are usually stable and spontaneously vanish without any need for specific treatment. Pseudoaneurysms and arteriovenous fistulas require, as a first therapeutic strategy, ultrasound-guided compression repair (UGCR): the hematoma and the arterial breach should be identified; gradual compression should be applied until the flow from the artery to the hematoma stops; it should then be compressed until an echo-reflecting clot forms inside the hematoma, and then a sturdy compressive medication applied for at least 24–48 h (Fig. 27.1); if the procedure is ineffective, surgical hemostasis is needed [21].

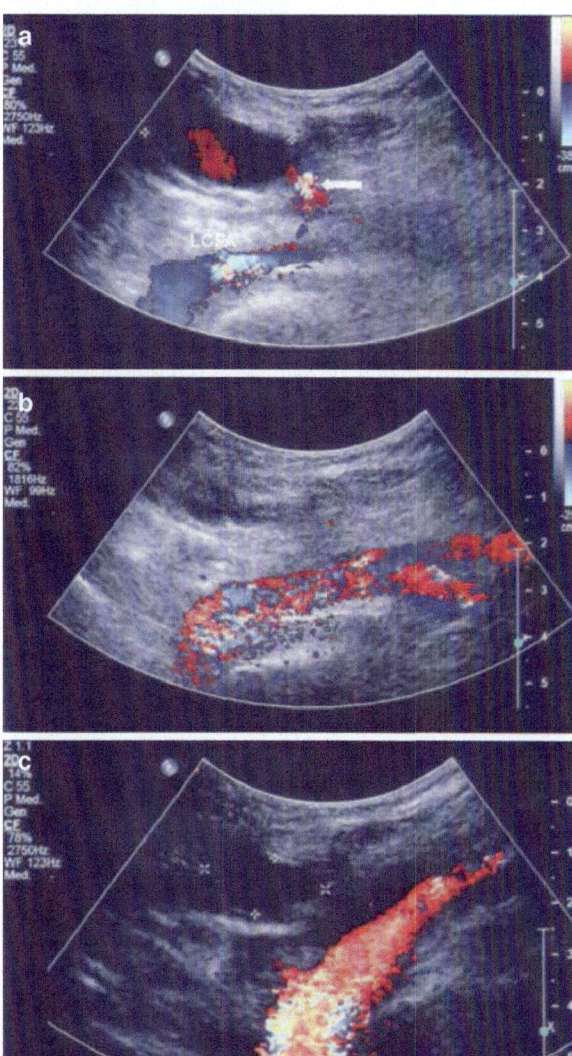

**Fig. 27.1** Doppler ultrasound showing the evolution of a femoral artery pseudoaneurysm (FAP) after ultrasound-guided compression repair (UGCR) in a patient undergoing transfemoral implantation of aortic device. The first image (**a**) shows FAP and blood effusion (*white arrow*) through the left common femoral artery (LCFA) 4 h after the procedure; the second (**b**) shows the lack of communicating tract from LCPA after UGCR; the third (**c**) is a predischarge check showing complete solution of the FAP

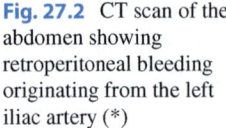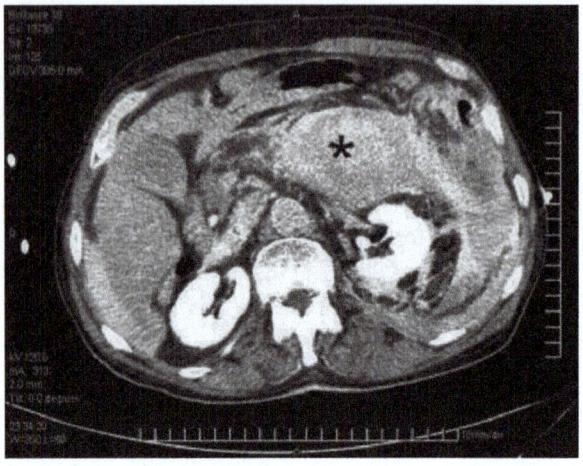

**Fig. 27.2** CT scan of the abdomen showing retroperitoneal bleeding originating from the left iliac artery (*)

The diagnosis of retroperitoneal hematoma is more challenging. It is a dangerous complication caused by a high arterial access site, above the inguinal ligament, from which blood exudate flows freely into the retroperitoneum, causing abdominal or back pain without any evidence of groin hematoma. The signs also include bleeding with no apparent origin and no pain, inexplicable hypotension, and recurrent episodes of vagal crisis. Retroperitoneal hematoma is diagnosed by tomography, which should be performed urgently (Fig. 27.2). Most of these cases of bleeding require surgery. The gradual or sudden development of anemia following these vascular complications requires, in many cases, transfusion with concentrated red blood cells.

Dissection or iliofemoral stenosis cases are generally treated by percutaneous angioplasty with balloon and stent implantation, while in the case of peripheral embolization, embolectomy or surgery is necessary.

### Rhythm Control

Arrhythmias can occur after TAVI, so continuous ECG monitoring by telemetry is necessary. Atrioventricular or intraventricular conduction disorders are among the most frequent arrhythmic complications in TAVI. Atrial fibrillation secondary to alterations in the electrolyte balance can occasionally characterize the postprocedural course.

It is known that aortic valvuloplasty is marked by the intraprocedural onset of total left bundle branch block (LBBB) or atrioventricular block (AVB) of various degrees. In the great majority of cases, conduction disorders spontaneously resolve [22, 23]. TAVI has a higher incidence of conduction disorders.

Self-expanding valves are marked by the onset of total AVB in about 10–30% of cases [24] versus about 5–7% for balloon-expandable valves [25]. Most of the total AVB and all LBBB cases are intraprocedural; however, there is a small percentage of patients who can develop symptomatic late total AVB between postprocedure day 5 and day 30 (Figs. 27.3 and 27.4).

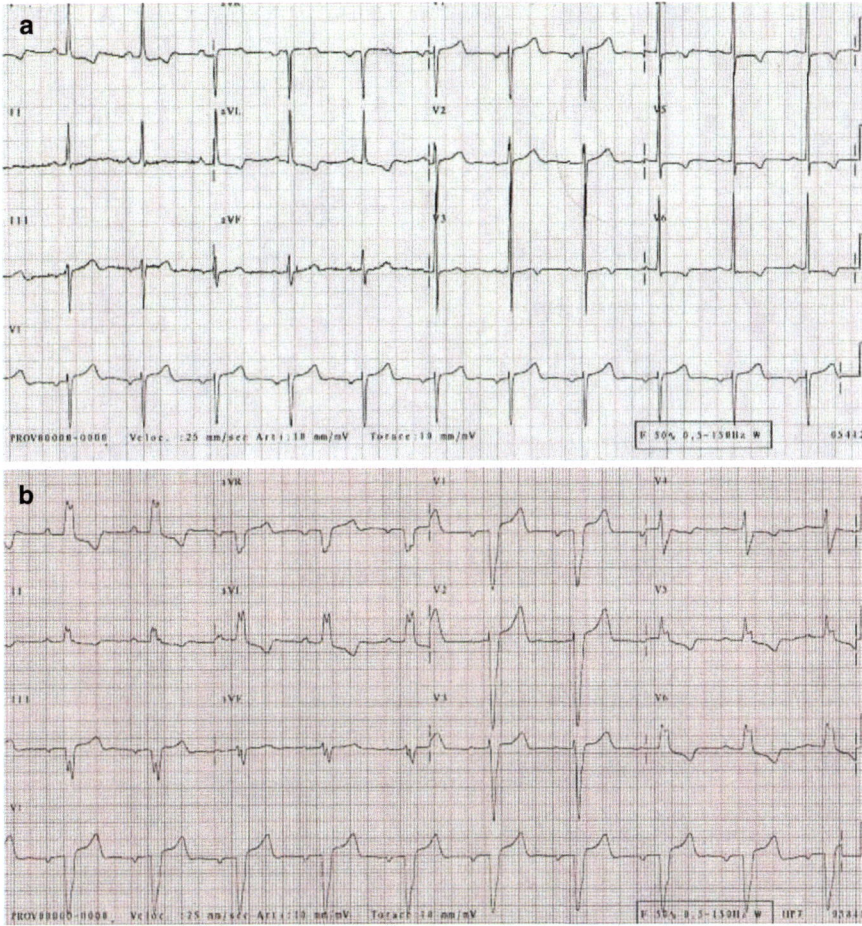

**Fig. 27.3** (a) Baseline ECG recording from a patient prior to transfemoral CoreValve implantation. (b) A 12-lead ECG recording from the same patient immediately after transfemoral implantation of a CoreValve prosthesis. The patient developed a new left bundle branch block

The predictors of total AVB have not yet been fully defined. Of the risk factors involved in cardiac surgery, the following can be considered: pre-existing bundle branch block (especially of the right branch), preprocedural aortic regurgitation, prior myocardial infarction, pulmonary hypertension, and electrolyte imbalances [26, 27]. Some authors have suggested, based on the close anatomical relations existing between the atrioventricular conduction system and the aortic valve apparatus, that the expansion of the device may cause mechanical trauma in the conduction system, especially in patients with calcified annulus, worsening pre-existing conduction defects or generating of new ones. One study showed that the mean distance from the proximal (or ventricular) end of the frame of the CoreValve prosthesis to the lower

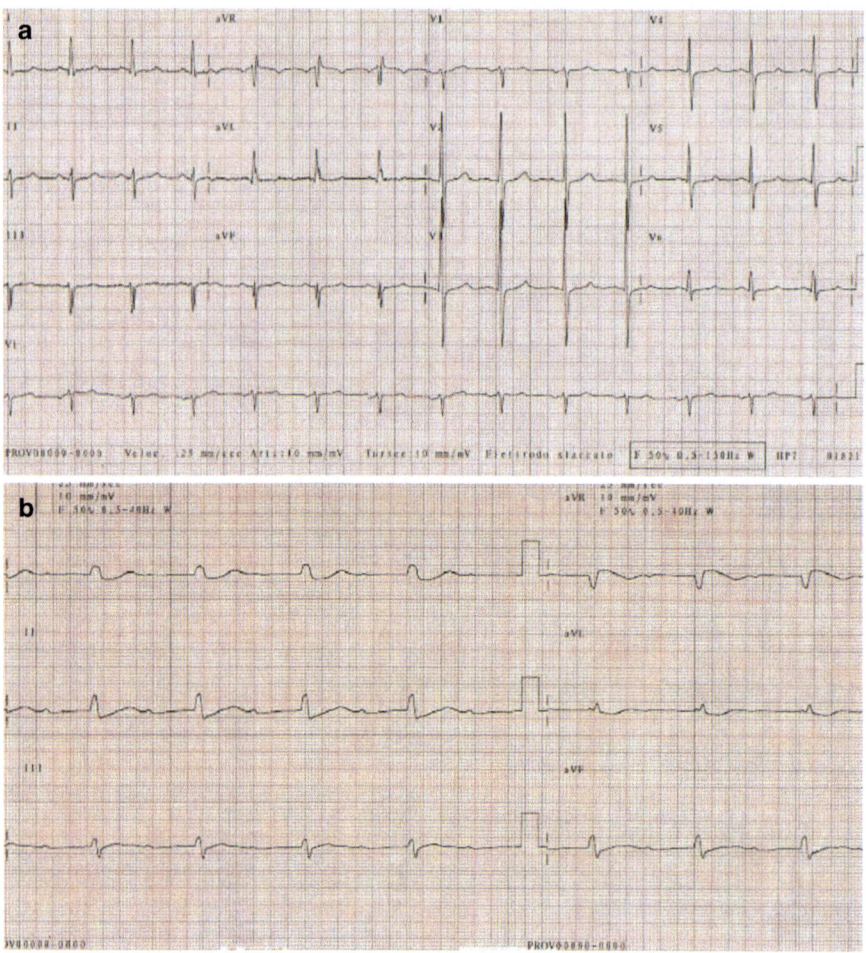

**Fig. 27.4** (**a**) Baseline ECG recording from a patient prior to transfemoral CoreValve implantation. (**b**) A 12-lead ECG obtained 1 day after implantation of the CoreValve device: identification of a symptomatic, third-degree atrioventricular block led to the implantation of a permanent pacemaker

edge of the noncoronary cusp is significantly greater in patients with new-onset LBBB than in patients without new-onset LBBB. Therefore, there exists the possibility of the aortic prosthesis overlapping the left bundle branch with mechanical compression.

Furthermore, the low implantation of the device has been identified as an independent predictor of post-TAVI pacemaker implantation [28]. Therefore, better device placement inside the left ventricular outflow tract may limit the risk of developing conduction disorders and, hence, the need for pacemaker implantation [24, 29]. Other studies have suggested that potential predictors of permanent pacing requirement consist of left axis deviation at baseline and LBBB with left axis deviation, the presence of severe septal hypertrophy, and baseline thickness of the native noncoronary cusp [30]. However, it seems that the presence of right bundle branch block before the procedure is the most powerful predictor of permanent pacemaker [24, 28].

In the case of intraprocedural total AVB, a pacemaker must be implanted within 24 h, both because it seldom resolves spontaneously and because it is recommended to remove the temporary pacemaker as soon as possible due to the risk of displacement of the lead inside the right ventricle and hence of perforation and cardiac tamponade. If arrhythmias do not occur in the first 24 h, the temporary pacemaker should be removed, and rhythm control by telemetry and a periodic ECG is recommended over the next 5 days. In the case of an advanced-degree conduction disorder (AVB II type 2 or third degree) within 48 h of the procedure, permanent pacing, usually dual chamber, is needed. A recent study of patients implanted with a CoreValve device recommends a higher threshold of attention for patients with severe septal hypertrophy, who have had periprocedural AVB or in whom a 29 mm device has been implanted [31].

Other conduction defects observed within the first 48 h after TAVI include LBBB, first-degree AVB, right bundle branch block (RBBB), and atrial fibrillation. Of these, LBBB is definitely the most common and does not require any specific treatment, solely regular ECG control at follow-up. Holter ECG monitoring, 24 h before and 48 h after the procedure, can help predict or detect any major arrhythmias. Ventricular arrhythmias or fibrillation seldom appear after these procedures, though they may occur in the presence of ventricular dysfunction, concurrent coronary artery disease, or electrolyte imbalances (e.g., potassium depletion).

### Transthoracic Echocardiogram

TTE should be done immediately after TAVI and after 24 h and then, as long as there is no clinical worsening, before discharge. The TTE allows assessment of the mean transaortic gradient and effective aortic orifice area, the presence and degree of aortic and mitral regurgitation, left ventricular contractility, estimated pulmonary artery pressure, the position of the temporary pacemaker lead in the right ventricle, and pericardial effusion. The assessment of aortic regurgitation is important. Mild paravalvular leaks secondary to device expansion have no hemodynamic relevance and usually disappear after a few weeks (Fig. 27.5). Multiple or major paravalvular leaks are less common, but they must be detected early, as they may cause heart

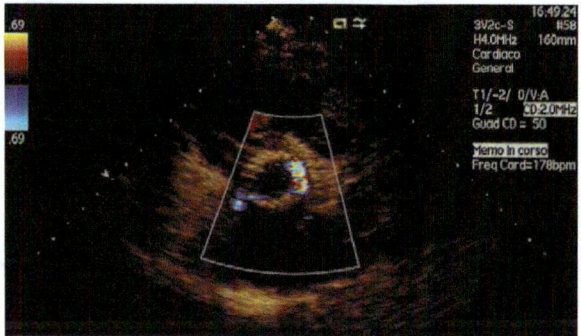

**Fig. 27.5** Echocardiographic parasternal short-axis view, showing mild periprosthetic leak after transfemoral implantation of CoreValve device

failure due to volume overload in the left ventricle, especially in the case of reduced contractility. The detection of a high pressure gradient or a diastolic pressure below 50 mmHg can help with recognition of this complication. Aortic regurgitation after TAVI is nearly always paravalvular and can be explained by inadequate sizing of the valve due to inadequate annulus size measurement before TAVI or lack of sufficient ranges of frame sizes, insufficient expansion of the frame due to severe calcification of leaflets and aortic root, leaflet malcoaptation, and malposition of the valve [32]. In the last case, usually, for the CoreValve Revalving System, the valve is in too low a position; the leaks come above the prosthesis skirt, which guarantees the sealing of the valve to the annulus; and there are always two jets in symmetrical and opposite locations [33].

In the case of pericardial effusion, it is important to determine whether it is secondary to left ventricle perforation by the stiff guidewire used during the procedure or to right ventricle perforation by the temporary pacemaker (Fig. 27.6). The former complication is a dramatic event leading to cardiac tamponade. The latter, which occurs after the procedure in most cases, is less serious yet more difficult to diagnose. In general, it is marked by the onset of unexpected bradycardia and hypotension. Pericardial effusion can also be secondary to bleeding of the access site (apex of the left ventricle) used during transapical implantation. After diagnosing the presence of pericardial effusion, fluids must be administered, concentrated red blood cells should be transfused, heparin should be reversed if the patient is decoagulated, and subxiphoid pericardiocentesis with the positioning of an 8 Fr pigtail should be done within a short period of time. If complete hemostasis is not achieved following pericardiocentesis, surgical draining and suture are needed. The systolic pulmonary artery pressure can be a good indirect hemodynamic parameter and is an index of the degree of impairment of left cardiac function and, hence, of the overload on the right ventricle.

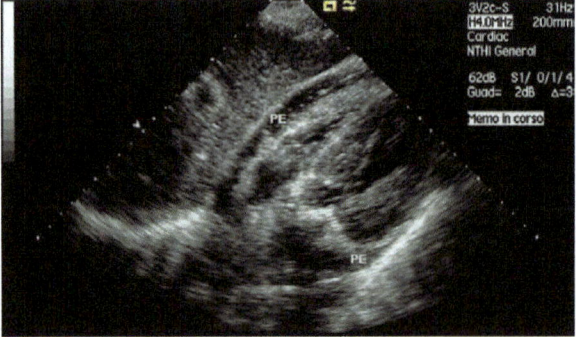

**Fig. 27.6** Echocardiographic subcostal view showing the presence of pericardial effusion secondary to puncture of the right ventricle by the temporary pacemaker in a patient undergoing transfemoral implantation of aortic valve device. Effusion became evident 4 h after the procedure and pericardiocentesis was successfully performed. *PE* pericardial effusion

### 27.1.2.2 General Preventive Measures

Prevention of endocarditis includes antibiotic prophylaxis, especially against staphylococci, for 3 days after the procedure, accurate skin disinfection and overall care, and early removal of the venous accesses and Foley catheter. In the case of signs of infection like leukocytosis or fever, the causes should be thoroughly investigated by means of diagnostic examinations such as urine culture to exclude an infection of the urinary tract, chest X-ray to detect any pulmonary infections, blood cultures, and microbiology examinations of the central catheters. If deemed necessary, targeted antibiotic therapy should be started while taking into due account the possible risk of sepsis. Hematological parameters should be monitored for evidence of disseminated intravascular coagulation.

Finally, early patient mobilization should be achieved in order to avoid complications like muscular atrophy, constipation, bed ulcers, and thrombophlebitis and to reduce the length of hospital stay. In some cases, admission to centers specializing in cardiac rehabilitation may be recommended for an earlier recovery of motor functions.

### 27.1.2.3 Before Hospital Discharge

Before discharge, an accurate assessment of the cardiac and extracardiac status is needed and comprises a clinical examination, ECG, TTE, and blood examinations. The vascular accesses, in the case of transfemoral/trans-subclavian, and the scar, in the case of transapical TAVI, must be accurately examined. Holter ECG monitoring can be indicated after TAVI in patients at high risk of developing conduction disorders.

A progressive reduction in the length of hospital stay has been associated with increasing experience in post-TAVI management [34]. Early discharge (within 72 h) after transfemoral TAVI has shown to be feasible and does not seem to jeopardize the early safety of the procedure when performed in a subset of patients selected by clinical judgment [34].

### 27.1.2.4 Medium-Term Management (Out of Hospital)

As there is no standard management after TAVI, standard management protocols already used in cardiac surgery can be applied (Table 27.1) [35].

The clinical and ECG follow-up should be scheduled, at least in the early phase, by the cardiology centers where the procedure is performed. The first cardiology visit should be scheduled 4 weeks after discharge if there is no period of cardiac rehabilitation. The next visits should be scheduled at 3, 6, and 12 months from the procedure and then every 6 months, except for cases in which the visit is urgently needed due to a worsening in the patient's clinical conditions.

The first visit must comprise a thorough clinical examination, an assessment of the NYHA functional class and quality of life, an ECG, a check of laboratory examinations, and a TTE to assess ventricular function, valve structure and function, any signs of device displacement or interference with adjacent anatomical structures, the presence of thrombi or vegetation on the device structures, and signs of pericardial effusion. If there is a suspicion of valve malfunction or in the case of poor transthoracic acoustic window, a transesophageal echocardiogram (TEE) should be performed, as it allows better definition of the anatomical structures.

Blood examinations, including plasma lactic dehydrogenase (LDH), haptoglobin, and reticulocyte count, should be monitored for the risk of hemolysis. In the case of a suspicion of hemolytic anemia, TEE should be performed to rule out paraprosthetic leaks [36].

As stated above, the risk of intravalvular thrombosis and thromboembolism in the biological valve can be considered low, but it increases in the presence of depressed ventricular function, valve deterioration, or device distortion due to poor positioning [35]. In any event, in these cases, the clinical suspicion must be confirmed by TTE, TEE, or cinefluoroscopy [37]. Occlusive prosthetic thrombosis should be treated surgically, though in critical and high-risk patients, thrombolysis can be a therapeutic alternative [35, 36].

Thromboembolism can have multifactorial causes: thrombi, vegetation on the device, or abnormal flow conditions created by a degenerated prosthesis or other sources. Only after a thorough diagnostic pathway is it possible to start appropriate treatment. In the case of nonocclusive prosthetic thrombosis and thromboembolic events, anticoagulation therapy should be started.

The risk of endocarditis is higher in the first 3–6 months after device implantation, although it is constantly present [35]. Some cases of endocarditis after TAVI have been reported [38–40] (Fig. 27.7). Therefore, antibiotic prophylaxis should be

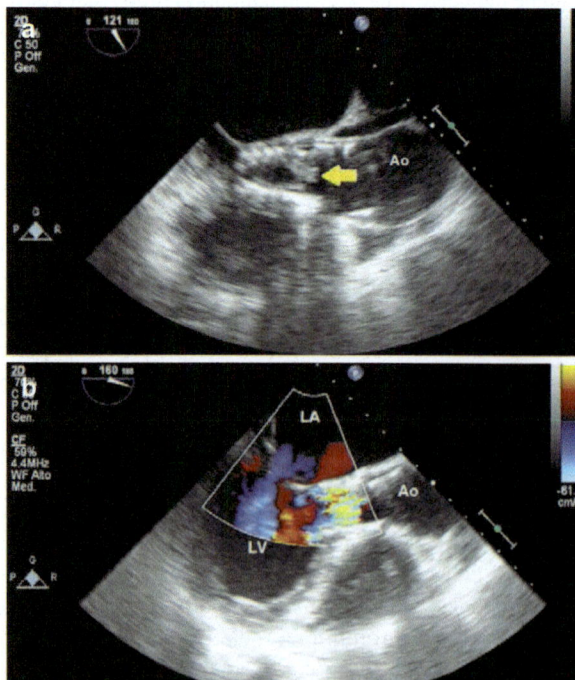

**Fig. 27.7** (**a**) A large vegetation arising from the prosthetic leaflets of a CoreValve is revealed by TEE (*yellow arrow*). (**b**) Severe intraprosthestic regurgitation is detected in the same patient by color-flow Doppler imaging. *Ao* aorta, *LA* left atrium, *LV* left ventricle

provided in all conditions at risk, such as dental, endoscopic, and surgical procedures. Antibiotic therapy to prevent endocarditis must be specific to the type of procedure the patient is undergoing, according to standard protocols. If there is a clinical suspicion of endocarditis, the patient must be admitted to a hospital and undergo serial blood cultures and TTE to confirm the diagnostic hypothesis.

The treatment of endocarditis on valve implants requires a multidisciplinary approach involving the cardiologist, cardiac surgeon, and infectious disease physician. If an early diagnosis is reached and there is no indication for surgical treatment, targeted IV antibiotic therapy for at least 4–6 weeks is sufficient.

Surgery is only necessary if appropriate medical therapy is not enough to cure the disease (persistent bacteremia, hemodynamic impairment, embolism) [35].

# References

1. Barbanti M, Gulino S, Tamburino C, et al. Antithrombotic therapy following transcatheter aortic valve implantation: what challenge do we face? Expert Rev Cardiovasc Ther. 2016;14:381–9.
2. Rodés-Cabau J, Dauerman HL, Cohen MG, et al. Antithrombotic treatment in transcatheter aortic valve implantation: insights for cerebrovascular and bleeding events. J Am Coll Cardiol. 2013;62:2349–59.
3. Sannino A, Gargiulo G, Schiattarella GG, et al. A meta-analysis of the impact of pre-existing and new-onset atrial fibrillation on clinical outcomes in patients undergoing transcatheter aortic valve implantation. EuroIntervention. 2015;12(8):e1047–56. pii: 20150323-05.12
4. Latib A, Naganuma T, Abdel-Wahab M, et al. Treatment and clinical outcomes of transcatheter heart valve thrombosis. Circ Cardiovasc Interv. 2015;8(4).
5. Makkar RR, Fontana G, Jilaihawi H, et al. Possible subclinical leaflet thrombosis in bioprosthetic aortic valves. N Engl J Med. 2015;373:2015–24.
6. Hansson NC, Grove EL, Andersen HR, et al. Transcatheter aortic heart valve thrombosis: incidence, predisposing factors, and clinical implications. J Am Coll Cardiol. 2016;68(19):2059–2069. pii: S0735-1097(16)34936-1. doi:10.1016/j.jacc.2016.08.010.
7. Généreux P, Cohen DJ, Mack M, et al. Incidence, predictors, and prognostic impact of late bleeding complications after transcatheter aortic valve replacement. J Am Coll Cardiol. 2014;64:2605–15.
8. Dangas GD, Lefèvre T, Kupatt C, et al. Bivalirudin versus heparin anticoagulation in transcatheter aortic valve replacement: the randomized BRAVO-3 trial. J Am Coll Cardiol. 2015;66:2860–8.
9. Ussia GP, Scarabelli M, Mulè M, et al. Dual antiplatelet therapy vs aspirin alone in patients undergoing transcatheter aortic valve implantation. Am J Cardiol. 2011;108:1772–6.
10. Stabile E, Pucciarelli A, Cota L, et al. SAT-TAVI (single antiplatelet therapy for TAVI) study: a pilot randomized study comparing double to single antiplatelet therapy for transcatheter aortic valve implantation. Int J Cardiol. 2014;174:624–7.
11. Poliacikova P, Cockburn J, de Belder A, et al. Antiplatelet and antithrombotic treatment after transcatheter aortic valve implantation—comparison of regimes. J Invasive Cardiol. 2013;25:544–8.
12. Durand E, Blanchard D, Chassaing S, et al. Comparison of two antiplatelet therapy strategies in patients undergoing transcatheter aortic valve implantation. Am J Cardiol. 2014;113:355–60.
13. Leon MB, Smith CR, Mack MJ, et al. Transcatheter or surgical aortic-valve replacement in intermediate-risk patients. N Engl J Med. 2016;374:1609–20.
14. Bennett CL, Kim B, Zakarija A, et al. Two mechanistic pathways for thienopyridine-associated thrombotic thrombocytopenic purpura: a report from the SERF-TTP research group and the RADAR project. J Am Coll Cardiol. 2007;50:1138–43.

15. Shantsila E, Lip GYH, Chong BH. Heparin-induced thrombocytopenia. Chest. 2009;135: 1651–64.
16. Généreux P, Kodali SK, Green P, et al. Incidence and effect of acute kidney injury after transcatheter aortic valve replacement using the new valve academic research consortium criteria. Am J Cardiol. 2013;111:100–15.
17. Briguori C, Colombo A, Violante A, et al. Standard vs double dose of N-acetylcysteine to prevent contrast agent associated nephrotoxicity. Eur Heart J. 2004;25:206–11.
18. Birck R, Kzossok S, Markowetz F, et al. Acetylcysteine for prevention of contrast nephropathy: meta-analysis. Lancet. 2003;362:598–603.
19. Barbanti M, Gulino S, Capranzano P, et al. Acute kidney injury with the RenalGuard System in patients undergoing transcatheter aortic valve replacement: The PROTECT-TAVI Trial (PROphylactic effecT of furosEmide-induCed diuresis with matched isotonic intravenous hydraTion in Transcatheter Aortic Valve Implantation). JACC Cardiovasc Interv. 2015;8: 1595–604.
20. Ussia GP, Scarabelli M, Mulè M, et al. Postprocedural management of patients after transcatheter aortic valve implantation procedure with self-expanding bioprosthesis. Catheter Cardiovasc Interv. 2010;76:757–66.
21. Schaub F, Theiss W, Busch R, et al. Management of 219 consecutive cases of post-catheterization pseudoaneurysm. J Am Coll Cardiol. 1997;30:670–5.
22. NHLBI balloon valvuloplasty registry participants. Percutaneous balloon aortic valvuloplasty. Acute and 30-day follow-up results in 67 patients from the NHLBI balloon valvuloplasty registry. Circulation. 1991;84:2383–97.
23. Otto CM, Mickel MC, Kennedy JW, et al. Three-year outcome after balloon aortic valvuloplasty. Insights into prognosis of valvular aortic stenosis. Circulation. 1994;89:642–50.
24. Piazza N, Onuma Y, Jesserun E, et al. Early and persistent intraventricular conduction abnormalities and requirements for pacemaking after percutaneous replacement of the aortic valve. JACC Cardiovasc Interv. 2008;1:310–6.
25. Sinhal A, Altwegg L, Pasupati S, et al. Atrioventricular block after transcatheter balloon expandable aortic valve implantation. JACC Cardiovasc Interv. 2008;1:305–9.
26. Limongelli G, Ducceschi V, D'Andrea A, et al. Risk factors for pacemaker implantation following aortic valve replacement: a single centre experience. Heart. 2003;89:901–4.
27. Koplan BA, Stevenson WG, Epstein LM, et al. Development and validation of a simple risk score to predict the need for permanent pacing after cardiac valve surgery. J Am Coll Cardiol. 2003;41:795–801.
28. Fraccaro C, Buja G, Tarantini G, et al. Incidence, predictors, and outcome of conduction disorders after transcatheter self-expandable aortic valve implantation. Am J Cardiol. 2011;107: 747–54.
29. Calvi V, Puzzangara E, Pruiti GP, et al. Early conduction disorders following percutaneous aortic valve replacement. Pacing Clin Electrophysiol. 2009;32:126–30.
30. Jilaihawi H, Chin D, Vasa-Nicotera M, et al. Predictors for permanent pacemaker requirement after transcatheter aortic valve implantation with the CoreValve bioprosthesis. Am Heart J. 2009;157:860–6.
31. Khawaya MZ, Rajani R, Cook A, et al. Permanent pacemaker insertion after CoreValve transcatheter aortic valve implantation: incidence and contributing factors (the UK CoreValve collaborative). Circulation. 2011;123:951–60.
32. De Jaegere PP, Piazza N, Galema TW, et al. Early echocardiographic evaluation following percutaneous implantation with the self-expanding CoreValve revalving system aortic valve bioprosthesis. EuroIntervention. 2008;4:351–7.
33. Piazza N, Schultz C, De Jaegere PP, et al. Implantation of two self-expanding aortic bioprosthetic valves during the same procedure insights into valve-in-valve implantation ("Russian doll concept"). Catheter Cardiovasc Interv. 2009;73:530–9.
34. Barbanti M, Capranzano P, Ohno Y, et al. Early discharge after transfemoral transcatheter aortic valve implantation. Heart. 2015;101:1485–90.

35. Butchart EG, Gohlke-Bärwolf C, Antunes MJ, et al. Working groups on valvular heart disease, thrombosis, cardiac rehabilitation, exercise physiology and European Society of Cardiology. Recommendations for the management of patients after heart valve surgery. Eur Heart J. 2005;26:2463–71.
36. Vahanian A, Baumgartner H, Bax J, et al. Guidelines on the management of valvular heart disease: the Task Force on the management of valvular heart disease of the European Society of Cardiology. Eur Heart J. 2007;28:230–68.
37. Montorsi P, De Bernardi F, Muratori M, et al. Role of cine fluoroscopy, transthoracic and TEE in patients with suspected prosthetic valve thrombosis. Am J Cardiol. 2000;85:58–64.
38. Webb JG, Altwegg L, Boone RH, et al. Transcatheter aortic valve implantation: impact on clinical and valve-related outcomes. Circulation. 2009;119:3009–16.
39. Gotzmann M, Mügge A. Fatal prosthetic valve endocarditis of the CoreValve ReValving System. Clin Res Cardiol. 2011;100:715–7.
40. Carnero-Alcázar M, Maroto Castellanos LC, Camicer JC, et al. Transapical aortic valve prosthetic endocarditis. Interact Cardiovasc Thorac Surg. 2010;11:252–3.

# Transcatheter Therapy for Aortic Stenosis: A Review of the Literature

# 28

Davide Capodanno and Simona Gulino

## 28.1 Early Proof of Concept Cases

"Even if the development of transcatheter aortic valve implantation (TAVI) can be considered a success story today, it is nothing short of a miracle, as the project appeared particularly challenging - not to say totally unrealistic - at its origin in the early 1990s." These are the words that Cribier used to define the history of TAVI as a genuine odyssey, which, however, over the years has been increasingly recognized as a revolutionary technique in aortic valve stenosis (AS).

The start of all this can be dated back to the early 1980s, when the limits of balloon aortic valvuloplasty (BAV) emerged [1, 2]. The routine observation that high-pressure balloon inflation could open all calcified aortic valves in a circular fashion led to the idea that a balloon-expandable stent with a high radial force might be expanded within the native valve to prevent restenosis and a valvular structure might be inserted within the stent to mimic native valve function. This combination of stent frame and valvular structure opened the way to the replacement of the aortic valve by using mini-invasive catheterization techniques. In the years that followed, several studies in animals investigated the feasibility of the technique. Henning Anderson developed a transluminal catheter technique to implant an artificial aortic valve in pigs, in 1992, using a balloon-expandable stent [3]. Philipp Bonhoeffer performed the first human percutaneous valve implantation in a 12-year-old boy with stenosis and insufficiency of a prosthetic conduit from the right ventricle to the pulmonary artery with a bovine jugular valve in 2000 [4]. However, it took up to

D. Capodanno (✉)
Ferrarotto Hospital, University of Catania, Via Citelli 6, 95124 Catania, Italy
e-mail: dcapodanno@gmail.com

S. Gulino
Division of Cardiology – Ferrarotto Hospital, University of CataniaCatania, Italy

© Springer International Publishing AG 2018
C. Tamburino et al. (eds.), *Percutaneous Treatment of Left Side Cardiac Valves*,
https://doi.org/10.1007/978-3-319-59620-4_28

501

2002 for TAVI to make its debut on the medical scene, when Alain Cribier performed the first human TAVI using a balloon-expandable valve through a transseptal approach in a 57-year-old-male with severe AS, cardiogenic shock, and a left ventricular ejection fraction of 12% [5]. The first self-expanding valve was implanted in a human in 2004, using a bovine pericardial trileaflet nitinol stent in a 73-year-old woman with severe, symptomatic AS using a retrograde approach through the common iliac artery. The first case history, by Cribier in 2004, proved the feasibility of this novel technique using balloon-expandable devices [6]; success was achieved in five of six patients, with a decrease in transaortic gradient and an increase in valve area. In this initial experience, the antegrade approach was used and, as already stated, abandoned for the retrograde and transapical approach. These two approaches were investigated by a French team, which studied 36 patients [7]; 27 were treated with success (75%), 23 with the retrograde approach, and 4 with the transapical technique. The incidence of major adverse cardiac and cerebrovascular events (MACCEs) at 30 days and at 6 months was 26% (six deaths) and 37% (ten deaths), respectively. A series of implants with the retrograde approach performed by Webb et al. [8] showed an initial success rate of 78%, which rose to 96% after the first 25 cases, thus proving the importance of the learning curve [9]. Thirty-day mortality was 12% as opposed to the expected 28%. At follow-up there was no evidence of valve deterioration, embolization, or intraprosthetic failure. Periprosthetic regurgitation was observed at 1 month in three cases, while in most patients there was a slight leak, with no significant hemodynamic consequences.

Commercial TAVI was approved in Europe in 2007, followed by the USA in 2011.

## 28.2    Landmark Single-Arm Multicenter National Registries

### 28.2.1 Investigator-Driven Registry

After the enthusiasm that greeted the first case studies, acceptance and expansion of TAVI were significant. In line with statements from the European Association of Cardiothoracic Surgery (EACTS) and the European Society of Cardiology (ESC) [10], several hundred patients were included in national registries conducted with the two models of valves and using the different approaches (Table 28.1). These registries contributed to a better appraisal of patient screening, improvements in technical modalities, and better prevention and management of complications. The immediate and long-term results kept improving with experience and advancing technologies; the procedural success rate progressively reached more than 95%. Excellent hemodynamic results, comparing favorably with the results of surgical aortic valve replacement (SAVR), lasting functional improvement, and improved survival were consistently observed. Complications were also shown to decrease with experience, reaching an acceptable level in this high-risk population, and were similar for both valve models, with the exception of a more frequent incidence of conduction disturbances with the CoreValve. Overall, the results of TAVI became more predictable.

**Table 28.1**  TAVI survival of the main national registry

| National registry | Authors (year) | Patients, n | Procedural success | 30 days survival | 1 year survival | 2 years survival | 3 years survival | 4 years survival | 5 years survival | 6 years survival |
|---|---|---|---|---|---|---|---|---|---|---|
| FRANCE registry | Eltchaninoff et al. (2010) | 244 | 98.3% | 87.3% | | | | | | |
| FRANCE 2 registry | Gilard et al. (2012) | 3195 | 96.9% | 90.3% | 76.0% | | | | | |
| Italian registry | Tamburino et al. (2011) | 663 | 98% | 94.6% | 85.0% | | | | | |
| | Ussia et al. (2012) | 181 | | | 76.4% | 69.7% | 65.2% | | | |
| | Barbanti et al. (2015) | 353 | | | 79% | 71% | 62% | 52% | 42% | |
| German registry | Zahn et al. (2010) | 697 | 98.4% | 87.6% | | | | | | |
| Gary registry | Walther et al. (2015) | 15,964 | | | | | | | | |
| UK registry | Moat et al. (2011) | 877 | | 92.9% | 78.6% | 73.7%, | | | | |
| | Duncan et al. (2015) | 850 | | | | | | | 45.5% | |
| | Ludman et al. (2015) | 3980 | | 93.7% | 81.7% | | 61.2% | | | 37.3% |
| STS/ACC TVT registry | Mack et al. (2013) | 7710 | 92% | 92.4% | | | | | | |
| | Holmes et al. (2015) | 12,182 | | 93% | 76.3% | | | | | |
| Canadian registry | Rodés-Cabau et al. (2010) | 339 | 93.3% | 10.4% | | | | | | |
| | Rodés-Cabau et al. (2012) | | | | | | | 45% | | |
| SOURCE registry | Thomas et al. (2010) | 2344 | | 93.7% TF 89.7% TA | | | | | | |
| | Thomas et al. (2011) | | | | 76.1% | | | | | |
| SOURCE XT registry | Schymik et al. (2015) | 2688 | | 93.7% | 80.6% | | | | | |
| ADVANCE | Linke et al. (2014) | 1015 | 96.5% | 4.5% | 21.2% | | | | | |

First results were available in 2010, when early safety and efficacy of TAVI were evaluated in the national **FRANCE Registry** [11]. Two hundred and forty-four high-surgical-risk patients (logistic EuroSCORE $\geq$20%, STS $\geq$ 10%, or contraindication to AVR) underwent TAVI with both Edwards SAPIEN and CoreValve prosthesis (68 and 32% of patients, respectively). The preferred approach was transarterial (transfemoral, 66%; subclavian, 5%); a transapical approach was used in 29% of patients. Device success rate was 98.3%, and 30-day mortality was 12.7%. Severe complications included stroke (3.6%), tamponade (2%), acute coronary occlusion (1.2%), and vascular complications (7.3%). A pacemaker was required in 11.8%. In 2012, the French results were updated in the **FRANCE 2 registry**, with a greater number of patients and with follow-up data at 1 year [12]. The reported procedural success rate was 96.9% in a total of 3195 patients undergoing TAVI with Edwards SAPIEN (66.9%) and Medtronic CoreValve (33.1%) devices. Approaches were either transarterial (transfemoral, 74.6%; subclavian, 5.8%; and other, 1.8%) or transapical (17.8%). Mortality rates at 30 days and 1 year were 9.7% and 24.0%, respectively. At 1 year, the incidence of stroke was 4.1%, and the incidence of periprosthetic aortic regurgitation was 64.5%. In a multivariate model, a higher logistic risk score, NYHA class III or IV symptoms, the use of a transapical TAVI approach, and a higher amount of periprosthetic regurgitation were significantly associated with reduced survival.

In 2010, the **German Registry** reported its results [13]. A total of 697 patients were included in the analysis, 666 (95.6%) of whom received a percutaneous implant, 26 (3.7%) a transapical implant, and 5 (0.7%) a transaortic implant. Both CoreValve (84.4%) and Edwards SAPIEN prostheses (15.6%) were used. Procedural success was achieved in 98.4% of cases; the inhospital mortality rate was 8.2%, and the 30-day mortality rate was 12.4%. Any residual aortic regurgitation was observed in 72.4% of patients, with a significant aortic insufficiency ($\geq$ Grade III) in only 16 patients (2.3%). Complications included pericardial tamponade in 1.8% and stroke in 2.8% of patients. Permanent pacemaker implantation after TAVI became necessary in 39.3% of patients. Recently, TAVI complication rates were evaluated based on prospective data from the German Aortic Valve Registry (**GARY**) [14]. From 2011 to 2013, a total of 15,964 TAVI procedures were registered. Overall inhospital mortality was 5.2%, while severe vital complications occurred in 5.0% of the population. Technical complications of the procedures occurred in 4.7% of patients and decreased significantly from 2011 to 2013.

In 2011, the **Italian Registry** investigated the incidence and predictors of early mortality at 30 days and late mortality between 30 days and 1 year after TAVI with the self-expanding CoreValve prosthesis [15]. In a total of 663 consecutive patients, the authors reported a procedural success of 98%. The cumulative incidences of mortality were 5.4% and 15% at 30 days and at 1 year, respectively. Predictors of late mortality between 30 days and 1 year were correlated with patient baseline conditions. In particular, a previous ischemic stroke or pulmonary edema was associated with a risk of late mortality of five and two times greater. In 2012, the 3-year results of the Italian CoreValve Registry were available on 181 patients [16]. The 5-year outcomes on 353 patients were available in 2015 [17], reporting an all-cause mortality at 1, 2, 3, 4, and 5 years of 21%, 29%, 38%, 48%, and 55.0%, respectively. Cardiovascular mortality was 10%, 14%, 19%, 23%, and 28.0%, respectively. The overall neurological event rate at 5 years was 7.5%, of which more than two-thirds occurred early after the procedure. During follow-up, there were 241 rehospitalizations for cardiovascular reasons in 164 (46%) patients. Among all rehospitalizations, acute heart failure was the most frequently reported (42.7%), followed by the need for permanent pacemaker implantation (17.4%). Late prosthesis failure occurred in five cases (1.4%); among these, redo TAVI was successfully carried out in two patients (0.6%) presenting with symptomatic prosthesis restenosis. The remaining three cases of prosthesis failure did not undergo further invasive interventions. Ten patients (2.8%) showed late mild stenosis. Valve thrombosis or late valve embolization was not reported.

Initial data from the **UK TAVI Registry** (United Kingdom Aortic Transcatheter Implantation) reported 30-day, 1-year, and 2-year survival rates after TAVI as 92.9%, 78.6%, and 73.7%, respectively, in 877 patients who underwent TAVI between January 1, 2007 and December 31, 2009 [18]. Both devices (Medtronic CoreValve = 452; Edwards SAPIEN = 410) and both the transfemoral and non-transfemoral approach (TF = 599, non-TF = 271) were used. In 2015, the authors analyzed long-term outcomes after TAVI and found 3- and 5-year survival rates of 61.2% and 45.5%, respectively [19]. They found that long-term survival after TAVI is largely determined by intrinsic patient factors. Other than stroke, procedural variables, including paravalvular aortic leak, did not appear to be independent predictors of long-term survival. A significant increase in deaths in the subgroup undergoing the non-transfemoral approach (18.5% vs. 22.7% at 1 year and 22.5% vs. 36.7% in 2 years) was also registered. The authors also assessed trends in the performance of TAVI in the UK from the first case in 2007 to the end of 2012, analyzing changes in case mix, complications, outcomes to 6 years, and predictors of mortality [20]. Overall 30-day mortality was 6.3%. One-year survival was 81.7%, falling to 37.3% at 6 years. Discharge by day 5 rose from 16.7% in 2007 and 2008 to 28% in 2012. The only multivariate pre-procedural predictor of 30-day mortality was Logistic EuroSCORE ≥40. During long-term follow-up, multivariate predictors of mortality were pre-procedural atrial fibrillation, chronic obstructive pulmonary disease, creatinine >200 μmol/L, diabetes mellitus, and coronary artery disease. The strongest independent procedural predictor of long-term mortality was periprocedural stroke. Non-femoral access and post-procedural aortic regurgitation were also significant predictors of adverse outcome.

A national registry (the Society of Thoracic Surgeons/American College of Cardiology Transcatheter Valve Therapy [**STS/ACC TVT] Registry**) was also initiated in the USA to report the initial commercial experience with TAVI [21]. A total of 7710 patients were included. The most common vascular access approach was transfemoral (4972 patients [64%]), followed by transapical (2197 patients [29%]) and other alternative approaches (536 patients [7%]). Device implantation success was achieved in 92% of cases. The overall inhospital mortality rate was 5.5%, and the stroke rate was 2.0%. Median hospital stay was 6 days (interquartile range [IQR], 4–10 days), with 4613 (63%) discharged home. Among patients with available follow-up at 30 days ($n$ = 3133), the incidence of mortality was 7.6% (non-cardiovascular cause, 52%); a stroke had occurred in 2.8% and re-intervention in 0.5%. In 2015, the data were updated, including 1-year outcomes, in a total of 12,182 patients [22]. Thirty-day mortality was 7.0%. In the first year after TAVI, patients were alive and out of the hospital for a median of 353 days (IQR, 312–359 days); 24.4% ($n$ = 2074) of survivors were rehospitalized once, and 12.5% ($n$ = 1525) were rehospitalized twice. At 1 year, the overall mortality rate was 23.7% ($n$ = 2450), the stroke rate was 4.1% ($n$ = 455), and the rate of the composite outcome of mortality and stroke was 26.0%. Temporal trends between 2012 and 2013 versus 2014 were also compared in an interim analysis [23], showing a change in procedure performance, with an increased use of moderate sedation, and increase in femoral access using percutaneous techniques. Vascular complication rates decreased (from 5.6% to 4.2%), while site-reported stroke rates remained stable at 2.2%.

The Canadian multicenter experience reported by Rodés-Cabau J. et al., published in 2010, reported the results achieved with the use of the Edwards valve between January 2005 and June 2009 through the transfemoral and transapical approaches in six Canadian centers [24]. Out of a total of 345 procedures (TF, 168; TA, 177) performed on 339 patients, procedural success was 93.3%, and 30-day mortality was 10.4% (TF, 9.5%; TA, 11.3%). At a median follow-up of 8 months, the mortality rate was 22.1%. In 2012, the same group evaluated the long-term outcomes after TAVI with special focus on the causes and predictors of late mortality and valve durability [25]. At a mean follow-up of 42 ± 15 months 188 patients (55.5%) had died. The causes of late death (152 patients) were noncardiac (59.2%), cardiac (23.0%), and unknown (17.8%). The predictors of late mortality were chronic obstructive pulmonary disease (HR, 2.18; 95% CI, 1.53–3.11), chronic kidney disease (HR, 1.08 for each decrease of 10 ml/min in estimated glomerular filtration rate; 95% CI, 1.01–1.19), chronic atrial fibrillation (HR, 1.44; 95% CI, 1.02–2.03), and frailty (HR, 1.52; 95% CI, 1.07–2.17). A mild nonclinically significant decrease in valve area was found at 2-year follow-up ($p$ < 0.01), but no further reduction in valve area was observed up to 4-year follow-up. No changes in residual aortic regurgitation and no cases of structural valve failure were observed during the follow-up period.

### 28.2.2 Post-marketing Registries

The **SOURCE Registry** (SAPIEN Aortic Bioprothesis European Outcome) [26] described outcomes in a consecutive group of patients treated during the first year of commercialization of the Edward SAPIEN prosthesis. It included 2344 patients divided into two cohorts: the first cohort consisted of 1038 patients enrolled in 32 centers during the commercial launch of the Edwards-SAPIEN THV device (Edwards Lifesciences); cohort 2 consisted of patients who received TAVI in the years following the marketing of the device. Data submitted for cohort 1 showed a 30-day mortality of 6.3% in transfemoral patients and 10.3% in transapical patients. The 1-year outcomes for cohort 1 of the SOURCE Registry were published in 2011 [27]; the Kaplan-Meier survival rates for the entire cohort were 76.1% (72.1% for the transapical approach and 81.1% for the femoral approach).

The SOURCE XT Registry (Edwards SAPIEN XT Aortic Bioprosthesis Multi-Region Outcome Registry) assessed the use and clinical outcomes with the SAPIEN XT valve in the real-world setting (2688 patients at 99 sites) [28]. Survival was 93.7% at 30 days and 80.6% at 1 year. At 30-day follow-up, the stroke rate was 3.6%, the rate of major vascular complications was 6.5%, the rate of life-threatening bleeding was 5.5%, and the rate of new pacemakers was 9.5%. A moderate/severe paravalvular leak was seen in 5.5% of patients. Multivariable analysis identified non-transfemoral approach, renal insufficiency, liver disease, moderate/severe tricuspid regurgitation, porcelain aorta, and atrial fibrillation as predictors of 1-year mortality.

During EuroPCR 2016, data concerning the SOURCE 3 post-approval registry were presented [29]. It is currently the largest registry of the SAPIEN 3 THV, involving a total of 1950 patients. The reported 30-day mortality was 1.9% and 4.0% in transfemoral TAVI and non-transfemoral TAVI, respectively, (the lowest mortality rate reported in the SOURCE data). Lower profile delivery system resulted in increased potential for transfemoral access. SAPIEN 3 provided excellent hemodynamic results, with very low rates of clinically significant PVL (3.1%).

In 2014, the results of the **ADVANCE** study were published [30]. This study evaluated outcomes following implantation of a self-expanding transcatheter aortic valve system in a fully monitored, multicenter "real-world" patient population in highly experienced centers. A total of 1015 patients were enrolled, showing the safety and effectiveness of the CoreValve System, with low mortality and stroke. At 30 days, the MACCE rate was 8.0%, and all-cause mortality and cardiovascular mortality were 4.5 and 3.4%, respectively. The rate of stroke was 3.0%. The life-threatening or disabling bleeding rate was 4.0% (2.8–6.3%). The 12-month rates of MACCE, all-cause mortality, cardiovascular mortality, and stroke were 21.2%, 17.9%, 11.7%, and 4.5%, respectively. The 12-month rates of all-cause mortality were 11.1, 16.5, and 23.6% among patients with a logistic EuroSCORE $\leq$ 10%, EuroSCORE 10–20%, and EuroSCORE $\geq$20%, respectively.

In the same year, the results of the CoreValve Extreme-Risk Registry were published [31]. This study sought to evaluate the safety and efficacy of the CoreValve prosthesis for the treatment of severe aortic stenosis in patients at extreme risk for surgery. The primary end point was a composite of all-cause mortality or major stroke at 12 months, which was compared with a prespecified objective performance goal (OPG). Forty-one sites in the USA recruited a total of 506 patients, of whom 489 underwent TAVI. The rate of all-cause mortality or major stroke at 12 months was 26.0% (upper two-sided 95% confidence bound, 29.9%) versus 43.0% with the OPG ($p < 0.0001$). Individual 30-day and 12-month events included all-cause mortality (8.4% and 24.3%, respectively) and major stroke (2.3% and 4.3%, respectively). Procedural events at 30 days included life-threatening/disabling bleeding (12.7%), major vascular complications (8.2%), and need for permanent pacemaker placement (21.6%). The frequency of moderate or severe paravalvular aortic regurgitation was lower 12 months after self-expanding TAVI (4.2%) than at discharge (10.7%; $p = 0.004$ for paired analysis).

## 28.3 Active-Controlled Multicenter Registries

In 2009, Piazza et al. reported the first prospective study comparing TAVI with CoreValve prosthesis and SAVR, in 1122 patients (TAVI, 114; SAVR, 1008) [32]. The crude mortality rate was greater in the TAVI group (9.6% vs. 2.3%; OR 4.57), but this population had a higher-risk profile (age, NYHA class III–IV, high logistic EuroSCORE, comorbidities). The univariate and multivariate analyses showed that these clinical characteristics were significantly correlated with a higher 30-day mortality. The analysis adjusted for propensity scores showed that among patients with a sufficient degree of overlapping (propensity score > 0.625) potentially eligible for a randomized comparison between TAVI and SAVR, 3/39 (8%) patients undergoing TAVI and 22/957 (2.8%) patients undergoing SAVR (adjusted OR ranged from 0.35 to 3.17) died. In the group with insufficient overlapping (propensity score < 0.625), 8/75 (10.7%) TAVI patients and 1/51 (2%) patients undergoing surgery died, thereby showing a significant increase in the odds ratio (adjusted OR ranged from 5.88 to 25.7). This result was explained by the authors as the presence of confounding factors not previously measured (the presence of porcelain aorta, mediastinal irradiation, or patient frailty), which might have affected the comparison between the two procedures.

Data of the comparative study of TAVI versus SAVR reported by Tamburino et al. were available in 2012 [33]. The study included the enrollment of 618 consecutive (218 undergoing TAVI and 400 undergoing isolated SAVR). Inhospital MACCE was more frequent in the SAVR group (7.8% vs. 14.0%, $p = 0.022$). This was also confirmed in the statistical adjustments by covariates and/or propensity score, with estimates of risk ranging from 2.2 to 2.6 at 30 days, 2.3 to 2.5 at 6 months, and 2.0 to 2.2 at 12 months. At 12 months, there was a significant difference in MACCE (TAVI vs. SAVR, 14.7% vs. 15.5%, $p = 0.894$), but an increased risk of late deaths from all causes was reported in the TAVI group (12.4% vs. 6.0%, $p = 0.007$). No significant difference was seen, not even in the analyses done after statistical adjustment, with regard to death, stroke, and myocardial infarction at any point of the follow-up.

In 2013, Piazza et al. compared all-cause mortality in patients at intermediate surgical risk undergoing TAVI or SAVR, creating 405 propensity score matched pairs of TAVI and SAVR patients with STS scores between 3% and 8% [34]. Of matched TAVI patients, 99 (24%) patients STS scores of <3%, 255 (63%) had scores between 3% and 8%, and 51 (13%) had scores of >8%. Cumulative all-cause mortality at 30 days and 1 year was similar among propensity score matched TAVI and SAVR patients at intermediate surgical risk. Among patients with STS scores between 3% and 8%, 20 (7.8%) versus 18 (7.1%) patients had died at 30 days (HR, 1.12; 95% CI, 0.58–2.15; $p = 0.74$) and 42 (16.5%) versus 43 (16.9%) patients had died at 1 year HR, 0.90; 95% CI, 0.57–1.42; $p = 0.64$) after TAVI and SAVR, respectively.

Another study, by Wenaweser et al., assessing clinical outcomes among patients with estimated low or intermediate surgical risk undergoing TAVI was published in 2013 [35]. A total of 389 consecutive patients undergoing TAVI were categorized according to the STS score into low (STS < 3%; $n = 41$, 10.5%), intermediate (STS ≥ 3% and ≤8%, $n = 254$, 65.3%), and high-risk (STS > 8%; $n = 94$, 24.2%) groups for the purpose of the study. Compared with patients at calculated high risk, well-selected patients with STS-defined intermediate or low risk appeared to have favorable clinical outcomes. Indeed, significant differences were found between the groups for all-cause mortality at 30 days (2.4 vs. 3.9 vs. 14.9%, $P < 0.001$) and all-cause mortality at 1 year (10.1 vs. 16.1 vs. 34.5%, $P = 0.0003$). No differences were found with regard to cerebrovascular accidents and myocardial infarction during 1-year follow-up.

Finally, in 2015, the results of the Italian OBSERVANT (Observational Study of Effectiveness of SAVR–TAVI Procedures for Severe Aortic Stenosis Treatment) study were published [36]. This analysis aimed to describe 1-year clinical outcomes of a large series of propensity-matched patients who underwent SAVR and trans-femoral TAVI. The matched population had a total of 1300 patients (650 per group). The propensity score method generated a low-intermediate risk population (mean logistic EuroSCORE 1, 10.2 ± 9.2% vs. 9.5 ± 7.1%, SAVR vs. transfemoral TAVI; $p = 0.104$). The results suggested that SAVR and transfemoral TAVI have comparable mortality, MACCE, and rates of rehospitalization due to cardiac problems at 1 year. In fact, at 1 year, the rate of death from any cause was 13.6% in the surgical group and 13.8% in the transcatheter group (HR, 0.99; 95% CI, 0.72–1.35; $p = 0.936$). Similarly, there were no significant differences in the rates of MACCE, which were 17.6% in the surgical group and 18.2% in the transcatheter group (HR, 1.03; 95% CI, 0.78–1.36; $p = 0.831$).

In the SAPIEN 3 observational study [37], 1077 intermediate-risk patients were assigned to receive TAVI with the SAPIEN 3 valve. The study assessed all-cause mortality and incidence of strokes, re-intervention, and aortic valve regurgitation at 1 year after implantation. These data were compared with those for intermediate-risk patients treated with surgical valve replacement in the PARTNER 2A trial between December 23, 2011 and November 6, 2013, using a prespecified propensity score analysis to account for between-trial differences in baseline characteristics. At 1-year follow-up, TAVI with SAPIEN 3 in intermediate-risk patients with severe aortic stenosis was associated with low mortality (7.4%), disabling strokes (2%), and moderate or severe paravalvular regurgitation (2%). The propensity score analysis indicated a significant superiority (−9.2%, 95% CI −13.0 to −5.4; $p < 0.0001$) for the composite outcome of mortality, strokes, and moderate or severe aortic regurgitation with TAVI compared with surgery, suggesting that TAVI might be the preferred treatment alternative in intermediate-risk patients.

## 28.4  Randomized Trials

Over the past decade, approximately 15,000 patients have been randomized in clinical trials of TAVI (Table 28.2).

The **PARTNER** (Placement of Aortic Transcatheter Valves) study was the first prospective randomized comparative study between TAVI and traditional medical

**Table 28.2** Early and late outcomes of TAVI in randomized trial and main active-controlled multicenter registry

| Authors (year) | Patients, n | Device success | 30 days survival | 1 year survival | 2 years survival | 3 years survival | 5 years survival |
|---|---|---|---|---|---|---|---|
| *Randomized trial comparing TAVI vs. SAVR* | | | | | | | |
| PARTNER A | | | | | | | |
| Smith et al. (2011) | 699 | | 96.6% vs. 93.5% | 75.8% vs. 73.2% | | | |
| Kodali et al. (2012) | | | | | 66.1% vs. 65.0% | | |
| Makkar et al. (2015) | | | | | | | 32.2% vs. 37.6% |
| PARTNER B | | | | | | | |
| Leon et al. (2010) | 358 | | 95.0% vs. 97.2% | 69.3% vs. 49.3% | | | |
| Makkar et al. (2012) | | | | | 56.7% vs. 32.0% | | |
| Kapadia et al. (2015) | | | | | | | 29.2% vs. 6.4% |
| PARTNER 2 | | | | | | | |
| Leon et al. (2016) | 2032 | | 93.9% vs. 92.0% | 85.5% vs. 83.6% | 80.7% vs. 78.9% | | |
| COREVALVE US | | | | | | | |
| Adams et al. (2014) | 795 | | | 85.8% vs. 80.9% | | | |
| NOTION | | | | | | | |
| Thyregod et al. (2015) | 280 | | | 96.9% vs. 83.7% | | | |
| *Active-controlled multicenter registries comparing TAVI vs. SAVR* | | | | | | | |
| OBSERVANT | | | | | | | |
| Tamburino et al. (2015) | 1300 | | | 86.2% vs. 86.4% | | | |
| SAPIEN 3 | | | | | | | |
| Thourani et al. (2016) | 1710 | | 98.9% vs. 96.0% | 92.6% vs. 87.0% | | | |
| *Randomized trial comparing balloon-expandable vs. self-expandable valves* | | | | | | | |
| CHOICE | | | | | | | |
| Abdel-Wahab et al. (2014) | 121 | 95.9% vs. 77.5% | 95.9% vs. 94.9% | | | | |

and surgical therapy. The primary end point was all-cause mortality at 1 year. US and Canadian patients were enrolled and divided into two treatment arms:

- The first arm (cohort B), of about 350 patients, comparing optimized medical therapy and aortic valvuloplasty versus TAVI in patients with absolute contraindication to aortic valve surgery [38]
- The second arm (cohort A), of about 700 patients, analyzing equivalence in terms of non-inferiority between TAVI and aortic valve surgery and TAVI in high-risk surgical patients (STS score > 10%) [39]

The implanted device was the first-generation Edwards SAPIEN valve (Edwards Lifesciences, Inc., Irvine, CA, USA) via transfemoral and transapical approach. The results of cohort B showed that TAVI in patients with severe AS, considered inoperable, can improve survival compared with conventional treatment (medical therapy and/or percutaneous valvuloplasty). In the first 30 days of follow-up, stroke and major vascular events were higher, as expected, in the TAVI group, but statistically significant only for the major vascular events ($p < 0.001$). However, at 1 year, the incidence of death from any cause was 30.7% in the TAVI group, compared with 50.7% in the standard therapy group ($p < 0.001$). Repeat hospitalization was also much lower in the TAVI group ($p < 0.001$). Among survivors at 1 year, the most advanced NYHA classes were lower in the TAVI group. It was also seen that the quality of life, investigated using the Kansas City Cardiomyopathy Questionnaire (KCCQ) and the Medical Outcomes Study Short Form-12 (SF-12) Health Survey, registered a significant increase in scores at 12 months only in the TAVI group while improving significantly compared with the baseline in both populations at 1 and 6 months. These results were confirmed at 2-year follow-up [40]. At 5 years, 42 (86%) of 49 survivors in the TAVI group had NYHA class 1 or 2 symptoms compared with 3 of 5 (60%) in the standard treatment group [41]. Echocardiography after TAVI showed durable hemodynamic benefit, with no evidence of structural valve deterioration.

Data on cohort A led to the conclusion that TAVI in patients at high operative risk is not inferior to surgery (30-day mortality, 3.4% vs. 6.5%, $p = 0.07$; 1-year mortality, 24.2% vs. 26.8%; $p = 0.44$) [39]. At 2-year follow-up, the two treatments were similar with respect to mortality (33.9% vs. 35.0% $p = 0.78$), reduction in symptoms, and improved valve hemodynamics, but paravalvular regurgitation was more frequent after TAVI and was associated with increased late mortality [42]. In 2015, data on 5-year follow-up were published [43]: risk of death was 67.8% in the TAVI group compared with 62.4% in the SAVR group (HR, 1.04; 95% CI 0.86–1.24; $p = 0.76$). No structural valve deterioration requiring surgical valve replacement was recorded in either group. Moderate or severe aortic regurgitation occurred in 40 (14%) of 280 patients in the TAVI group and 2 (1%) of 228 in the SAVR group ($p < 0.0001$) and was associated with increased 5-year risk of mortality in the TAVI group (72.4% for moderate or severe aortic regurgitation vs. 56.6% for those with mild aortic regurgitation or less; $p = 0.003$).

The PARTNER 2 trial [44] investigated similar outcomes (primary end point: death from any cause or disabling stroke at 2 years) in a cohort of 2032 patients at intermediate risk undergoing either SAVR or TAVI with the following generation balloon-expandable SAPIEN XT valve (Edwards Lifesciences, Irvine, CA). Results have been recently published showing similar rates of death from any cause or disabling stroke. At 2 years, the Kaplan-Meier event rates were 19.3% in the TAVI group and 21.1% in the surgery group (HR in the TAVI group, 0.89; 95% CI, 0.73–1.09; $P = 0.25$). In the transfemoral-access cohort, TAVI resulted in a lower rate of death or disabling stroke than surgery (HR 0.79; 95% CI, 0.62–1.00; $P = 0.05$), while in the transthoracic-access cohort the outcomes were similar between the two groups. TAVI resulted in larger aortic valve areas than did surgery and also resulted in lower rates of acute kidney injury, severe bleeding, and new-onset atrial fibrillation. Surgery resulted in fewer major vascular complications and less paravalvular aortic regurgitation.

In November 2011, the results of the **STACCATO** trial [45] were published. It was designed as a prospective randomized study among A-TAVI and SAVR in elderly operable patients (age $\geq$ 70 or 75 years). The authors anticipated a surgical event rate, defined as a composite of 30-day all-cause mortality, major stroke, and/or renal failure of 13.5%, and an estimated event rate in the TAVI arm of 2.5%. The study began in November 2008, after the randomization of 70 patients (34 patients received A-TAVI and 36 SAVR) was prematurely discontinued, in May 2011, due to an excess of adverse events in the A-TAVI group, including an increased risk of major stroke and severe periprosthetic leakage.

The **NOTION** (Nordic Aortic Valve Intervention) trial compared TAVI with SAVR in an all-comers patient cohort [46]. A total of 280 patients $\geq$70 years old with severe aortic valve stenosis and no significant coronary artery disease were randomized 1:1 to TAVI using a self-expanding bioprosthesis versus SAVR. Mean age was 79.1 years, and 81.8% were considered low-risk patients. The primary outcome was the composite rate of death from any cause, stroke, or myocardial infarction (MI) at 1 year. In the intention-to-treat population, no significant difference in the primary end point was found (13.1% vs. 16.3%; $p = 0.43$ for superiority). The result did not change in the as-treated population. No difference in the rates of cardiovascular death or prosthesis re-intervention was found. Compared with SAVR-treated patients, TAVI-treated patients had more conduction abnormalities requiring pacemaker implantation, larger improvement in effective orifice area, more total aortic valve regurgitation, and higher NYHA functional class at 1 year. SAVR-treated patients had more major or life-threatening bleeding, cardiogenic shock, acute kidney injury (stage II or III), and new-onset or worsening atrial fibrillation at 30 days than did TAVI-treated patients.

The **CoreValve High-Risk Study** was a randomized trial comparing TAVI with a self-expanding transcatheter aortic valve bioprosthesis (CoreValve) with surgical aortic valve replacement in patients with severe aortic stenosis and an increased risk of death during surgery [47]. A total of 795 patients underwent randomization at 45 centers in the USA. In the as-treated analysis, the rate of death from any cause at 1 year was significantly lower in the TAVI group than in the surgical group (14.2% vs. 19.1%), with an absolute reduction in risk of 4.9 percentage points. The results were similar in the intention-to-treat analysis. In a hierarchical testing procedure, TAVI was non-inferior with respect to echocardiographic indexes of valve stenosis, functional status, and quality of life. Exploratory analyses suggested a reduction in the rate of major adverse cardiovascular and cerebrovascular events and no increase in the risk of stroke.

A randomized comparison of the balloon-expandable and the self-expandable device was available in 2014 with the **CHOICE** randomized clinical trial [48]. One hundred twenty-one patients were randomly assigned to receive a balloon-expandable valve (Edwards Sapien XT), and 120 were assigned to receive a self-expandable valve (Medtronic CoreValve). The use of a balloon-expandable valve resulted in a greater rate of device success than the use of a self-expandable valve (95.9% vs. 77.5%; RR, 1.24; 95% CI, 1.12–1.37; $p < 0.001$).This was attributed to a significantly lower frequency of residual more-than-mild aortic regurgitation (4.1% vs. 18.3%; RR, 0.23; 95% CI, 0.09–0.58; $p < 0.001$) and the less frequent need for implanting more than one valve (0.8% vs. 5.8%,$p = 0.03$) in the balloon-expandable valve group compared with the self-expandable valve group. Cardiovascular mortality at 30 days was similar in both groups (4.1% vs. 4.3%; RR, 0.97; 95% CI, 0.29–3.25; $p = 0.99$). The combined safety end point at 30 days, including all-cause mortality, major stroke, and other serious complications, occurred in 18.2% of those in the balloon-expandable valve group and in 23.1% of the self-expandable valve group (RR, 0.79; 95% CI, 0.48–1.30; $p = 0.42$). Placement of a new permanent pacemaker was less frequent in the balloon-expandable valve group (17.3% vs. 37.6%, $p = 0.001$).

Recently, the results of the **SURTAVI trial** [49] have been published, confirming the role of TAVI in patients at intermediate risk. This randomized trial compared TAVI (performed with the CoreValve or Evolut R transcatheter heart valve systems) with surgical aortic valve replacement in a total of 1660 patients at intermediate risk for surgery (Society of Thoracic Surgeons Predicted Risk of Mortality 4.5 ± 1.6%). At 24 months, the estimated incidence of the primary end point (composite of death from any cause or disabling stroke) was 12.6% in the TAVI group and 14.0% in the surgery group (95% credible interval [Bayesian analysis] for difference, −5.2– 2.3%; posterior probability of non-inferiority, >0.999). Surgery was associated with higher rates of acute kidney injury, atrial fibrillation, and transfusion requirements, whereas TAVI had higher rates of residual aortic regurgitation and need for pacemaker implantation. TAVI resulted in lower mean gradients and larger aortic valve areas than surgery.

## 28.5 Meta-analysis

The basic tenet of a meta-analysis is that there is a common truth behind all conceptually similar scientific studies but which has been measured with a certain error within individual studies.

Concerning TAVI, many meta-analyses have explored almost all fields of this procedure. The most recent meta-analysis investigating outcomes after TAVI or SAVR is that by Gargiulo et al. [50]. Data from this large meta-analysis included 5 randomized trials and 31 observational matched studies comparing mortality outcomes after TAVI or SAVR. A total of 16,638 patients were analyzed to compare clinical outcomes, including early (≤30-day) and midterm (≤1-year) mortality in adults with severe aortic stenosis undergoing either TAVI or SAVR (Fig. 28.1).

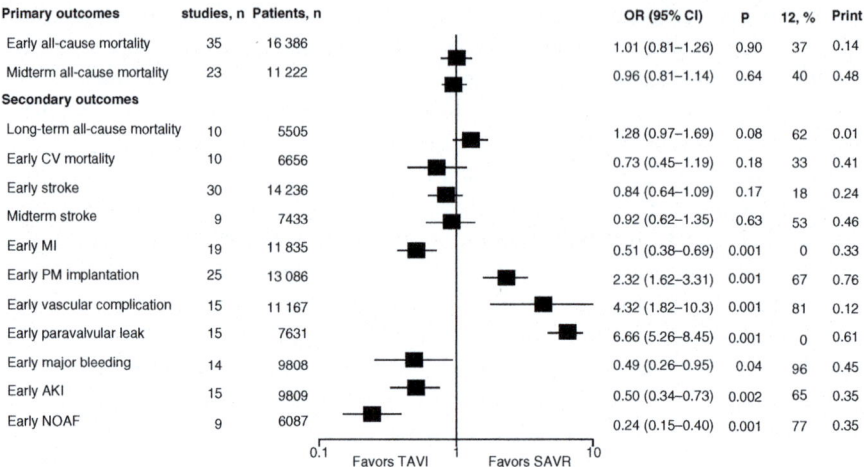

**Fig. 28.1** Forest plot for all outcomes of the meta-analysis by Gargiulo et al. [50]. Summary of Knapp–Hartung random-effects OR and 95% CI for all end points, including forest plots and details of studies and participants. *AKI* acute kidney injury, *CV* cardiovascular, *MI* myocardial infarction, *NOAF* new-onset atrial fibrillation, *OR* odds ratio, *P int* interaction P, *PM* pacemaker, *SAVR* surgical aortic valve replacement, *TAVI* transcatheter aortic valve implantation

Overall, there was no statistically significant difference in early and midterm all-cause mortality between TAVI and SAVR. Transfemoral TAVI provided mortality benefits over SAVR in trials. Analyses restricted to studies of patients at low to intermediate risk showed statistically nonsignificant reductions in early and midterm mortality with TAVI. Incidence of periprocedural myocardial infarction, major bleeding, acute kidney injury, and new-onset atrial fibrillation was lower with TAVI, but risk for pacemaker implantation, vascular complications, and paravalvular leak increased. Overall, there was a statistically nonsignificant increased risk in long-term (2- to 5-year) all-cause mortality with TAVI, while long-term mortality outcomes in patients at low to intermediate risk were inconclusive, with wide CIs.

## 28.6 Future Perspectives

Randomized studies with the goal of expanding TAVI indications and fill important knowledge gaps are increasing and ongoing (Fig. 28.2).

We are moving toward the expansion of clinical indications for intermediate and low-risk patients. The results of the **PARTNER 2A** randomized trial, the **SAPIEN 3i Propensity Score Analysis,** and, recently, the **SURTAVI trial** have just contributed to making TAVI a real alternative or preferred treatment option for patients at intermediate surgical risk.

Among the upcoming trial, the **UK TAVI** (ISRCTN57819173) is a multicenter randomized controlled trial, including 808 "all-comer" patients, to assess the clinical effectiveness and cost-utility of TAVI with any commercially available device, compared with conventional surgical aortic valve replacement in patients with

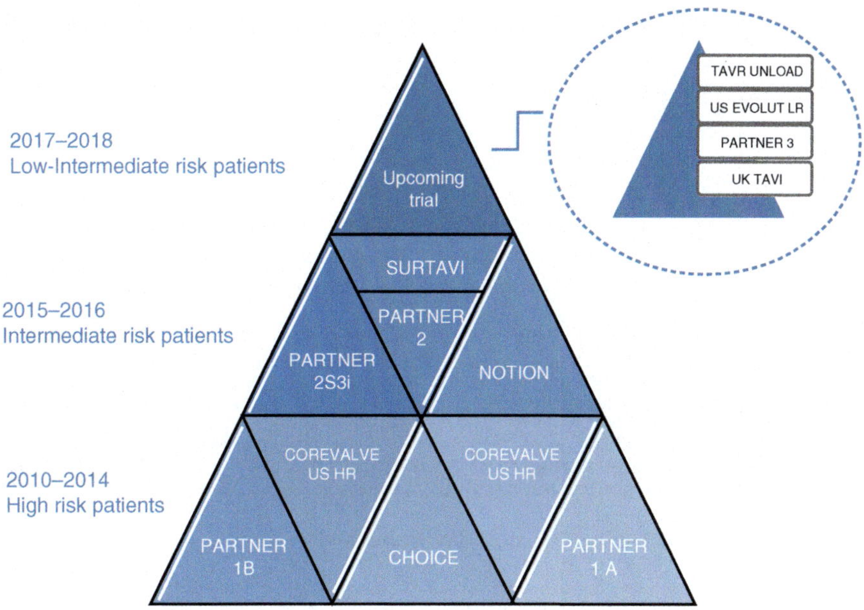

**Fig. 28.2** Overview of published and selected ongoing studies of transcatheter aortic valve implantation

severe symptomatic aortic stenosis who are at intermediate or high operative risk. The study started in August 2013 and will run until July 2016.

Two other non-inferiority trials using balloon-expandable (**PARTNER 3**, NCT02675114) and self-expanding prostheses (**Evolut R Low Risk**, NCT02701283) have recently initiated the recruitment of patients with heart team agreement on predicted perioperative mortality of <2% and <3%, respectively. PARTNER 3 will randomize transfemoral TAVI with the SAPIEN 3 valve (Edwards Lifesciences, Irvine, CA, USA) versus SAVR with a bioprosthetic valve, with a primary composite end point at 1 year, including all-cause mortality, all strokes, and rehospitalization. The Evolut R Low-Risk trial will randomize TAVI with the Evolut R and CoreValve prostheses versus SAVR with a bioprosthetic valve, with a primary composite end point at 2 years including all-cause mortality or disabling stroke. Results are expected in October 2018 and March 2018, respectively.

Moderate aortic stenosis patients with heart failure is another interesting field to be investigated. To address this, the **TAVR UNLOAD** (Transcatheter Aortic Valve Replacement to UNload the Left Ventricle in Patients with ADvanced Heart Failure, NCT02661451) is ongoing. A total of 600 patients with moderate aortic stenosis, symptomatic heart failure despite optimal medical therapy, and depressed left ventricular ejection fraction (>20% and <50%) will be randomized to TAVI with the SAPIEN 3 valve or optimal medical therapy alone. The two strategies will be investigated with respect to the hierarchical occurrence of all-cause mortality, disabling stroke, hospitalizations related to heart failure, or change in the KCCQ at 1 year.

Another expanding field of research regards new devices.

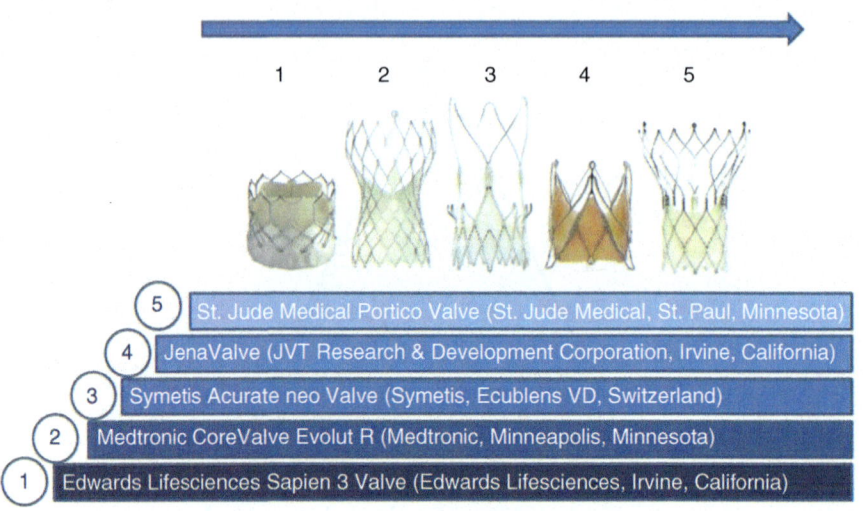

**Fig. 28.3** Overview of CE mark-approved TAVI systems

A great number of new TAVI devices, the so-called second-generation devices, have been investigated for a few years and incorporate features to address the limitations of the first-generation devices (i.e., lower profile, easier positioning, repositionability, and retrievability). Currently, nine TAVI systems are commercially available in Europe (Fig. 28.3).

TAVI with SAPIEN 3 in intermediate-risk patients with severe aortic stenosis has already been investigated, showing low rates of mortality, strokes, and regurgitation at 1 year [37].

Regarding the prosthesis (Medtronic, Minneapolis, Minnesota), the Evolut R CE Study found excellent procedural results, with a strong safety profile, exceptional outcomes, and strong hemodynamic performance, with the highest ever reported survival at 1 year (93.3%) [51]. Primary safety end points were mortality and stroke at 30 days. Primary clinical performance end points were device success for the VARC-2, and the percentage of patients with mild or less aortic regurgitation 24 h to 7 days post procedure. Repositioning was successful when required in all patients, with low rates of moderate or severe paravalvular aortic regurgitation and low permanent pacemaker implantation (11.7%).

The Symetis prosthesis obtained the CE mark at the end of 2011 and is currently commercially available in Europe. The first registry results were published in 2015 [52]. The registry was collected at 17 sites in Germany, Italy, Switzerland, and Argentina to treat 250 high-risk elderly patients. The procedural success rate was 98%, with two valve-in-valve procedures and three conversions to conventional surgery. The 30-day mortality rate was 6.8%. Post-implant echocardiography revealed a relevant paravalvular leak (moderate 2+) in 2.3% of patients, with all other patients showing either no/trace or a 1+ leak. The 30-day stroke rate was 2.8%. A new pacemaker implantation was required in 10.0% of patients.

The Lotus device is currently being assessed as part of the REPRISE (REpositionable Percutaneous Replacement of Stenotic Aortic Valve through

Implantation of Lotus™ Valve SystEm) clinical trial and of a global post-marketing study called RESPOND.

REPRISE I enrolled 11 symptomatic, high-surgical-risk patients undergoing TAVI with Lotus THV, supplying initial results to support proof of concept with this valve [53].

The REPRISE II [54] trial supported the granting of the CE mark. It presents the first report of 1-year outcomes of the 120 patients. All patients were successfully implanted with a Lotus valve, and 1-year clinical follow-up was available for 99.2% of patients. At 1 year of follow-up, the Lotus valve showed excellent valve hemodynamics, no moderate or severe paravalvular regurgitation, and significant and sustained improvement in NYHA functional class status, with good clinical outcomes. The all-cause mortality rate was 10.9%, disabling stroke rate 3.4%, and disabling bleeding rate 5.9%, with no repeat procedures for valve-related dysfunction. A total of 31.9% underwent new permanent pacemaker implantation at 1 year.

Three active-controlled randomized trials of TAVI devices are underway to generate efficacy data to support Food and Drug Administration clearance of transcatheter heart valves already approved for commercial use in Europe. All of these studies will target high- and extreme-risk patients with severe aortic stenosis:

1. PORTICO IDE ($N$ = 908, NCT02000115) is comparing the Portico™ (St. Jude Medical, St. Paul, MN, USA) valve and either SAPIEN or CoreValve systems.
2. SALUS (TranScatheter Aortic Valve RepLacement System Pivotal Trial The Safety and Effectiveness of the Direct Flow Medical Transcatheter Aortic Valve System) ($N$ = 649, NCT02163850) is comparing the Direct Flow Medical® (Direct Flow Medical, Santa Rosa, CA, USA) with the SAPIEN or CoreValve systems.
3. REPRISE III (Repositionable Percutaneous Replacement of Stenotic Aortic Valve Through Implantation of Lotus™ Valve System) ($N$ = 1032, NCT02202434) is a comparison of the Lotus™ (Boston Scientific, Marlborough, MA, USA) and CoreValve systems. A small investigator-initiated trial named REBOOT (REpositionable Versus BallOOn-expandable Prosthesis for Transcatheter Aortic Valve Implantation) ($N$ = 240, NCT02668484) is comparing the Lotus and SAPIEN 3 valves with respect to the incidence of new pacemaker implantation at 30 days. An industry-driven randomized trial of the ACURATE neo™ valve (Symetis, Ecublens, Switzerland) versus other TAVI systems is also planned.

Other new TAVI systems are in earlier phases of clinical testing as part of ongoing single-arm studies. These include:

- The Centera valve (Edwards Lifesciences), the safety and performance of which are the object of CENTERA-EU ($N$ = 200, NCT02458560)
- The JenaValve Pericardial TAVR System (JenaValve, Munich, Germany), which will be tested in two feasibility trials of high-risk patients with aortic stenosis ($N$ = 30, NCT02732691) or aortic regurgitation ($N$ = 30, NCT02732704) in Europe and the USA

# References

1. Letac B, Cribier A, Koning R, Bellefleur JP. Results of percutaneous transluminal valvulo-plasty in 218 adults with valvular aortic stenosis. Am J Cardiol. 1988;62(9):598–605.
2. Percutaneous balloon aortic valvuloplasty. Acute and 30-day follow-up results in 674 patients from the NHLBI Balloon Valvuloplasty Registry. Circulation. 1991;84(6):2383–97.
3. Andersen HR, Knudsen LL, Hasenkam JM. Transluminal implantation of artificial heart valves. Description of a new expandable aortic valve and initial results with implantation by catheter technique in closed chest pigs. Eur Heart J. 1992;13:704–8.
4. Bonhoeffer P, Boudjemline Y, Saliba Z, et al. Percutaneous replacement of pulmonary valve in a right-ventricle to pulmonary-artery prosthetic conduit with valve dysfunction. Lancet. 2000;356(9239):1403–5.
5. Cribier A, Eltchaninoff H, Bash A, et al. Percutaneous transcatheter implantation of an aortic valve prosthesis for calcific aortic stenosis: first human case description. Circulation. 2002;106: 3006–8.
6. Cribier A, Eltchaninoff H, Tron C, et al. Early experience with percutaneous transcatheter implantation of heart valve prosthesis for the treatment of end-stage inoperable patients with calcific aortic stenosis. J Am Coll Cardiol. 2004;43:698–70.
7. Cribier A, Eltchaninoff H, Tron C, et al. Treatment of calcific aortic stenosis with the percuta-neous heart valve: mid-term follow-up from the initial feasibility studies: the French experi-ence. J Am Coll Cardiol. 2006;47:1214–23.
8. Webb JG, Chandavimol M, Thompson CR, et al. Percutaneous aortic valve implantation retro-grade from the femoral artery. Circulation. 2006;113:842–50.
9. Grube E, Schuler G, Buellesfeld L, et al. Percutaneous aortic valve replacement for severe aor-tic stenosis in high-risk patients using the second- and current third-generation self-expanding corevalve prosthesis: device success and 30-day clinical outcome. J Am Coll Cardiol. 2007;50: 69–76.
10. Vahanian A, Alfieri O, Al-Attar N, et al. Transcatheter valve implantation for patients with aortic stenosis: a position statement from the European Association of Cardio-Thoracic Surgery (EACTS) and the European Society of Cardiology (ESC), in collaboration with the European Association of Percutaneous Cardiovascular Interventions (EAPCI). Eur Heart J. 2008;29(11):1463–70.
11. Eltchaninoff H, Prat A, Gilard M, et al. On behalf of the FRANCE Registry Investigators. Transcatheter aortic valve implantation: early results of the FRANCE (FRench Aortic National CoreValve and Edwards) registry. Eur Heart J. 2011;32:191–7.
12. Gilard M, Eltchaninoff H, Iung B, et al. Registry of transcatheter aortic valve implantation in high-risk patients. N Engl J Med. 2012;366(18):1705–15.
13. Zahn R, Gerckens U, Grube E, et al. On behalf of the German Transcatheter Aortic Valve Interventions—Registry Investigators. Transcatheter aortic valve implantation: first results from a multi-centre real-world registry. Eur Heart J. 2001;32:198–204.
14. Walther T, Hamm CW, Schuler G, et al., on behalf of the GARY Executive Board. Perioperative results and complications in 15,964 transcatheter aortic valve replacements. Prospective data from the GARY Registry. J Am Coll Cardiol. 2015;65(20):2173–80.
15. Tamburino C, Capodanno D, Mulè M, et al. Procedural success and 30-day clinical outcomes after percutaneous aortic valve replacement using current third-generation self-expanding CoreValve prothesis. J Invasive Cardiol. 2009;21:93–8.
16. Ussia GP, Barbanti M, Petronio AS, et al., on behalf of the CoreValve Italian Registry Investigators. Transcatheter aortic valve implantation: 3-year outcomes of self-expanding CoreValve prosthesis. Eur Heart J. 2012;33(8):969–76.
17. Barbanti M, Petronio AS, Ettori F, et al. 5-Year outcomes after transcatheter aortic valve implantation with CoreValve prosthesis. JACC Cardiovasc Interv. 2015;8(8):1084–91.
18. Moat NE, Ludman P, de Belder MA, et al. Long-term outcomes after transcatheter aortic valve implantation in high-risk patients with severe aortic stenosis: the U.K. TAVI (United Kingdom Transcatheter Aortic Valve Implantation) Registry. J Am Coll Cardiol. 2011;58:2130–8.

19. Duncan A, Ludman P, Banya W, et al. Long-term outcomes after transcatheter aortic valve replacement in high-risk patients with severe aortic stenosis. The U.K. Transcatheter Aortic Valve Implantation Registry. JACC Cardiovasc Interv. 2015:645–53.

20. Ludman PF, Moat N, de Belder MA, et al. Transcatheter aortic valve implantation in the United Kingdom: temporal trends, predictors of outcome, and 6-year follow-up: a report from the UK Transcatheter Aortic Valve Implantation (TAVI) Registry, 2007 to 2012. Circulation. 2015;131(13):1181–90.

21. Mack MJ, Brennan JM, Brindis R, et al., STS/ACC TVT Registry. Outcomes following transcatheter aortic valve replacement in the United States. JAMA. 2013;310(19):2069–77.

22. Holmes DR Jr, Brennan JM, Rumsfeld JS, et al. STS/ACC TVT Registry. Clinical outcomes at 1 year following transcatheter aortic valve replacement. JAMA. 2015;313(10):1019–28.

23. Holmes DR Jr, Nishimura RA, Grover FL, et al. STS/ACC TVT Registry. Annual Outcomes With Transcatheter Valve Therapy: From the STS/ACC TVT Registry. J Am Coll Cardiol. 2015 Dec 29;66(25):2813–23. .

24. Rode's-Cabau J, Webb JG, Cheung A, et al. Transcatheter aortic valve implantation for the treatment of severe symptomatic aortic stenosis in patients at very high or prohibitive surgical risk acute and late outcomes of the multicenter Canadian experience. J Am Coll Cardiol. 2010;55:1080–90.

25. Rodés-Cabau J, Webb JG, Cheung A, et al. Long-term outcomes after transcatheter aortic valve implantation; insights on prognostic factors and valve durability from the Canadian multicenter experience. J Am Coll Cardiol. 2012;60:1864–75.

26. Thomas M, Schymik G, Walther T, et al. Thirty-day results of the SAPIEN aortic Bioprosthesis European Outcome (SOURCE) Registry: a European registry of transcatheter aortic valve implantation using the Edwards SAPIEN valve. Circulation. 2010;122:62–9.

27. Thomas M, Schymik G, Walther T, et al. One-year outcomes of cohort 1 in the Edwards SAPIEN Aortic Bioprosthesis European Outcome (SOURCE) Registry: the European registry of transcatheter aortic valve implantation using the Edwards SAPIEN valve. Circulation. 2011;124:425–33.

28. Schymik G, Lefèvre T, Bartorelli AL, et al. European experience with the second-generation Edwards SAPIEN XT transcatheter heart valve in patients with severe aortic stenosis: 1-year outcomes from the SOURCE XT Registry. JACC Cardiovasc Interv. 2015;8(5):657–69.

29. SOURCE 3 post-approval registry - early outcomes in 1,946 TAVI patients with a third-generation balloon expandable transcatheter heart valve. Presented by O Wendler at EuroPCR 2016.

30. Linke A, Wenaweser P, Gerckens U, et al. Treatment of aortic stenosis with a self-expanding transcatheter valve: the International Multi-centre ADVANCE Study. Eur Heart J. 2014;35: 2672–84.

31. Popma JJ, Adams DH, Reardon MJ, et al. Transcatheter Aortic Valve Replacement Using a Self-Expanding Bioprosthesis in Patients with Severe Aortic Stenosis at Extreme Risk for Surgery. J Am Coll Cardiol. 2014, 1972;63(19):–81.

32. Piazza N, van Gameren M, Jüni P, et al. A comparison of patient characteristics and 30-day mortality outcomes after transcatheter aortic valve implantation and surgical aortic valve replacement for the treatment of aortic stenosis: a two-centre study. EuroIntervention. 2009;5:580–8.

33. Tamburino C, Barbanti M, Capodanno D, et al. Comparison of complications and outcomes to one year of transcatheter aortic valve implantation versus surgical aortic valve replacement in patients with severe aortic stenosis. Am J Cardiol. 2012;109(10):1487–93.

34. Piazza N, Kalesan B, van Mieghem N, et al. A 3-center comparison of 1-year mortality outcomes between transcatheter aortic valve implantation and surgical aortic valve replacement on the basis of propensity score matching among intermediate-risk surgical patients. JACC Cardiovasc Interv. 6(5, 2013):443–51.

35. Wenaweser P, Stortecky S, Schwander S, et al. Clinical outcomes of patients with estimated low or intermediate surgical risk undergoing transcatheter aortic valve implantation. Eur Heart J. 2013;34:1894–905.

36. Tamburino C, Barbanti M, D'Errigo P, et al. 1-Year outcomes after transfemoral transcatheter or surgical aortic valve replacement. Results from the Italian OBSERVANT Study. J Am Coll Cardiol. 2015;66(7):804–12.

37. Thourani VH, Kodali S, Makkar RR, et al. Transcatheter aortic valve replacement versus surgical valve replacement in intermediate-risk patients: a propensity score analysis. Lancet. 2016;387(10034):2218–25.
38. Leon MB, Smith CR, Mack M, et al. Transcatheter aortic-valve implantation for aortic stenosis in patients who cannot undergo surgery. N Engl J Med. 2010;363:1597–607.
39. Smith CR, Leon MB, Mack MJ, et al. Transcatheter versus surgical aortic-valve replacement in high-risk patients. N Engl J Med. 2011;364:2187–98.
40. Makkar RR, Fontana GP, Jilaihawi H, et al. Transcatheter aortic-valve replacement for inoperable severe aortic stenosis. N Engl J Med. 2012;366(18):1696–704.
41. Kapadia SR, Leon MB, Makkar RR, et al. 5-year outcomes of transcatheter aortic valve replacement compared with standard treatment for patients with inoperable aortic stenosis (PARTNER 1): a randomised controlled trial. Lancet. 2015;385(9986):2485–91.
42. Kodali SK, Williams MR, Smith CR, et al. Two-year outcomes after transcatheter or surgical aortic valve replacement. N Engl J Med. 2012;366:1686–95.
43. Mack MJ, Leon MB, Smith CR, et al. 5-year outcomes of transcatheter aortic valve replacement or surgical aortic valve replacement for high surgical risk patients with aortic stenosis (PARTNER 1): a randomised controlled trial. Lancet. 2015;385:2477–84.
44. Leon MB, Smith CR, Mack MJ, et al. Transcatheter or surgical aortic-valve replacement in intermediate-risk patients. N Engl J Med. 2016;374(17):1609–20.
45. Nielsen HH, Klaaborg KE, Nissen H, et al. A prospective, randomised trial of transapical transcatheter aortic valve implantation vs. surgical aortic valve replacement in operable elderly patients with aortic stenosis: the STACCATO trial. EuroIntervention. 2012;8:383–9.
46. Thyregod HG, Steinbruchel DA, Ihlemann N, et al. Transcatheter versus surgical aortic valve replacement in patients with severe aortic valve stenosis: 1-year results from the all-comers NOTION randomized clinical trial. J Am Coll Cardiol. 2015;65:2184–94.
47. Adams DH, Popma JJ, Reardon MJ, et al. Transcatheter aortic-valve replacement with a self-expanding prosthesis. N Engl J Med. 2014;370:1790–8.
48. Abdel-Wahab M, Mehilli J, Frerker C, et al. Comparison of balloon-expandable vs self-expandable valves in patients undergoing transcatheter aortic valve replacement. The CHOICE Randomized Clinical Trial. JAMA. 2014;311(15):1503–14.
49. Reardon MJ, Van Mieghem NM, Popma JJ, et al. Surgical or transcatheter aortic-valve replacement in intermediate-risk patients. N Engl J Med. 2017;376:1321–31.
50. Gargiulo G, Sannino A, Capodanno D, et al. Transcatheter aortic valve implantation versus surgical aortic valve replacement: a systematic review and meta-analysis. Ann Intern Med. 2016;165(5):334–44.
51. Manoharan G, Walton AS, Brecker SJ, et al. Treatment of symptomatic severe aortic stenosis with a novel resheathable supra-annular self-expanding transcatheter aortic valve system. JACC Cardiovasc Interv. 2015;8(10):1359–67.
52. Kempfert J, Holzhey D, Hofmann S, et al. First registry results from the newly approved ACURATE TA™ TAVI system. Eur J Cardiothorac Surg. 2015;48(1):137–41.
53. Meredith IT, Worthley SG, Whitbourn RJ, et al. Transfemoral aortic valve replacement with the repositionable Lotus Valve System in high surgical risk patients: the REPRISE I study. EuroIntervention. 2014;9(11):1264–70.
54. Meredith IT, Walters DL, Dumonteil N, et al. 1-year outcomes with the fully repositionable and retrievable lotus transcatheter aortic replacement valve in 120 high-risk surgical patients with severe aortic stenosis: results of the REPRISE II Study. JACC Cardiovasc Interv. 2016;9(4):376–84.

# Aortic Regurgitation

# 29

Piera Capranzano and Corrado Tamburino

## 29.1 Epidemiology

Aortic regurgitation (AR) is characterized by blood regurgitation from the aorta into the left ventricle (LV) due to the failure of the valve leaflets to adequately close during the diastolic phase of the cardiac cycle. AR is usually an acquired valve disease, while the congenital etiologies, mainly bicuspid morphology, are rarer. Acquired AR can be caused by primary disease of the aortic valve leaflets and/or abnormalities of the aortic root. The alterations of the aortic valve leaflets are more often of a calcific-degenerative nature, or a result of acute or chronic endocarditic valve processes, or due to myxomatous degeneration. There has been a progressive reduction in primary valve disease of rheumatic origin, which is now a rare event. Systemic arterial hypertension, aortic dissection, and connectivopathies such as Marfan's syndrome, Reiter's syndrome, Ehlers-Danlos syndrome, or rheumatoid arthritis alter the aortic root, leading to dilation and subsequent valve closure dysfunction [1]. Pure AR is far less common than aortic stenosis, affecting about 13% of patients with isolated, native left-sided valvular heart disease [2].

## 29.2 Pathophysiology

Valve failure can develop progressively (chronic AR), leaving the ventricle time to compensate for this defect, or acutely (acute AR) with no adaptation of the LV and often representing an emergency. The pathophysiological alterations resulting

P. Capranzano, M.D. (✉) • C. Tamburino, M.D., Ph.D.
Cardiovascular department, Ferrarotto Hospital, University of Catania, Catania, Italy
e-mail: pcapranzano@gmail.com

© Springer International Publishing AG 2018
C. Tamburino et al. (eds.), *Percutaneous Treatment of Left Side Cardiac Valves*,
https://doi.org/10.1007/978-3-319-59620-4_29

521

from AR are correlated to the degree of regurgitation and are different in chronic and acute AR. Chronic AR is a progressive condition involving several compensatory mechanisms [3]. In AR the overall systolic output volume comprises the antegrade output and the regurgitant volume, and the LV pumps the total volume into the aorta against high systemic impedance. The main compensatory mechanism is the rise in end-diastolic volume (increase in preload) caused by regurgitation. The LV manages to compensate volume overload by progressively dilating. In an initial phase, the rise in preload involves an increase in ventricular contractile efficiency, according to Starling's law. On the other hand, according to Laplace's law, LV dilation leads to an increase in systolic wall tension, which is addressed by the ventricle, with eccentric hypertrophy of the walls to normalize systolic stress. As a consequence, in AR, hypertrophy and dilation are combined. A valve defect can be well tolerated for a long time due to the compensatory mechanisms implemented.

As the pathology progressively evolves, due to the effects of chronic volume overload, hypertrophy can prove to be inadequate to dilation, thus leading to structural alterations of the ventricular myocardium. This brings about an increase in end-diastolic pressure and a reduction in systolic output, thus increasing left atrial and pulmonary vein and capillary pressure and eliciting the clinical manifestations of heart failure. The worsening in ventricular function is favored by the development of ischemic damage secondary to inadequate coronary artery perfusion due to reduced aortic diastolic pressure.

In acute AR, most frequently caused by acute infective endocarditis and aortic dissection, the inability of the LV to adapt to sudden volume overload leads to a rapid increase in ventricular diastolic pressure. This involves a sharp increase in atrial and pulmonary vein and capillary pressure, which elicits the clinical manifestations of acute heart failure, such as orthopnea and pulmonary edema [1, 3, 4].

## 29.3   Diagnosis

### 29.3.1 Noninvasive Diagnosis

In chronic AR patients, the symptoms due to reduced cardiac or coronary reserve, such as effort dyspnea and angina pectoris, have a late onset. Sudden onset of dyspnea at rest and low-flow symptoms characterize the clinical course of acute AR patients. Some of the objective signs typical of chronic AR are a wide and fast arterial pulse, increased differential pressure, decreasing aortic diastolic murmur, best audible in the third to fourth intercostal space on the left of the sternum in expiratory apnea, click and systolic ejection murmur, and end-diastolic murmur of mitral origin (the so-called Austin Flint murmur). In acute AR, the peripheral signs are missing, diastolic murmur is usually short, and there is a prevalence of the signs typical of low cardiac output and pulmonary venous congestion.

With regard to instrumental examinations, standard ECG can show the signs of left ventricular hypertrophy, left ventricular overload, or left bundle branch block

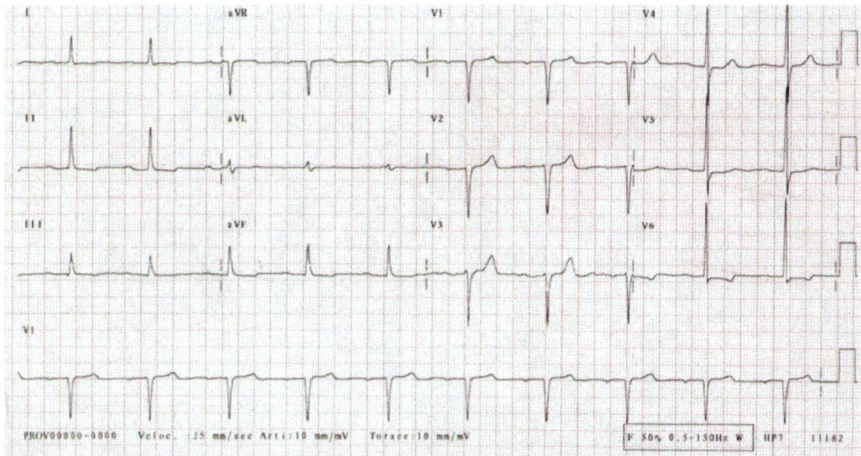

**Fig. 29.1** ECG picture of hypertrophy and left ventricular overload in patient with aortic regurgitation

(Fig. 29.1); these signs are not present in acute AR, in which sinus tachycardia and specific disorders in ventricular repolarization can occur.

Chest x-ray can show an increase in the volume of the LV and, at times, of the thoracic aorta, especially in the ascending tract. However, the key examination for noninvasive diagnosis of AR is transthoracic echocardiogram (TTE) with color Doppler ultrasound.

This method allows the following:

- Assessment of the anatomy and structural alterations of the aortic valve apparatus and the presence and severity of aortic root dilation
- Estimation of the presence and severity of AR
- Assessment of the structural adaptations and degree of LV impairment

TTE provides very accurate morphological and functional information on the aortic valve and root, identifying, for example, the presence of bicuspid aortic valve disease, the thickening and reduced mobility of the cusps in the degenerative or postrheumatic forms, thickened and redundant leaflets in myxomatosis, erosion and perforation of the cusps in forms secondary to endocarditis, and aortic ectasia in Marfan's syndrome. In addition, AR can also be secondary to degenerative processes affecting biological valve devices; in this case, TTE diagnosis uses the techniques applied for native valve disorders with small expedients [5].

M-mode examination can show high-frequency diastolic fluttering of the anterior mitral leaflet, inverse diastolic doming of the anterior mitral leaflet, and, in acute AR, early diastolic closing of the mitral valve.

The color Doppler technique shows blood regurgitation through the aortic valve during diastole and allows estimation of the severity, assessing the following parameters [6] (Fig. 29.2):

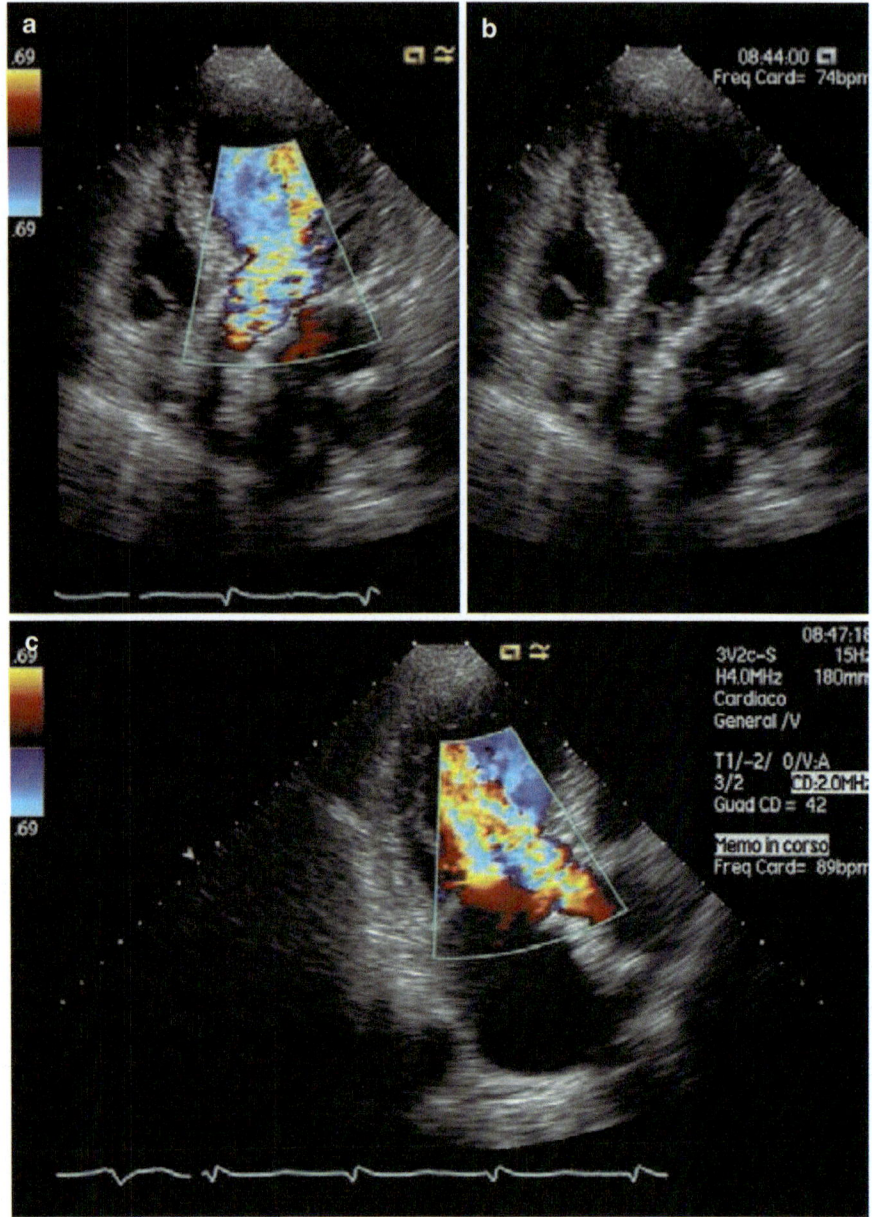

**Fig. 29.2** Color Doppler ECG in apical four-chamber view (**a** and **b**) and three-chamber view (**c**) showing severe aortic regurgitation

- Width and area of the regurgitant jet cross section
- Vena contracta
- Effective regurgitant orifice area (EROA) by the proximal isovelocity surface area (PISA) method

The width and cross-sectional area of the regurgitant jet must be measured in parasternal view, right below the aortic valve (within 1 cm of the valve). The relationship between the maximum width of the proximal jet and left ventricular outflow diameter, measured in parasternal long-axis view, or the relationship between the jet cross-sectional area and the LVOT, measured in parasternal short-axis view, makes it possible to estimate the severity of regurgitation [7]; AR is defined as severe if the relationship between the jet widths is ≥65% or the relationship between the jet areas is ≥60% [8] (Table 29.1).

Accurate measurement of the width and area of the regurgitant jet depends on the shape of the regurgitant orifice and jet direction; by occupying a small portion of the outflow tract, eccentric jets can lead to underestimation of the severity of the valvulopathy, while central jets, by contrast, can overestimate it. Measurement of the vena contracta, at the aortic valve, in parasternal long-axis view, makes it possible to distinguish between severe forms if it is >0.6 cm and mild forms if <0.3 cm [6, 9] (Table 29.1). In order to obtain accurate measurement of the vena contracta, the convergence flow, vena contracta, and jet should be clearly visible. The use of this parameter, though, is not indicated in the presence of multiple jets.

The PISA method is based on the principle of conservation of mass: according to this principle, the quantity of regurgitant flow through the aortic valve is obtained from the flow quantity of a proximal surface area with a known flow velocity. This method allows the quantitative estimation of the EROA and volume [10].

Imaging of the proximal flow convergence region by TTE is performed from the apical and parasternal views or the upper right sternal border. This method cannot be used in the case of multiple jets and is less accurate for eccentric jets. In addition, the presence of an aneurysm of the ascending aorta, which deforms the valve plane, can lead to an underestimation of the degree of AR. AR is defined as severe when the EROA is ≥0.30 cm² [6, 9, 11] (Table 29.1).

**Table 29.1** Criteria for the definition of aortic regurgitation severity

|  | Mild | Moderate | Severe |
|---|---|---|---|
| Doppler parameters |  |  |  |
| Jet width in LVOT-color flow Doppler | Small in central jets | Intermediate | Large in central jets |
| Jet deceleration rate (CW) (PHT, ms) | >500 | 500–200 | <200 |
| Diastolic flow reversal in descending aorta (PW) | Brief, early diastolic reversal | Intermediate | Holodiastolic reversal |
| Quantitative parameters |  |  |  |
| Jet width/LVOT width, % | <25 | 25–64 | ≥65 |
| Jet CSA/LVOT CSA, % | <5 | 5–59 | ≥60 |
| Vena contracta width, cm | <0.3 | 0.3–0.6 | ≥0.6 |
| RV, ml/beat | <30 | 30–59 | ≥60 |
| RF % | <30 | 30–49 | ≥50 |
| EROA, cm² | <0.10 | 0.10–0.29 | ≥0.30 |
| Structural parameters |  |  |  |
| LV size | Normal | Normal or dilatated | Usually dilatated |

*LVOT* left ventricular outflow tract, *CW* continuous wave Doppler, *PHT* pressure half-time, *PW* pulsed wave Doppler, *CSA* cross-sectional area, *RV* regurgitant volume, *RF* regurgitation fraction, *EROA* effective regurgitant orifice area, *LV* left ventricle

PW Doppler allows quantification of AR by calculating the regurgitant volume (RV) and regurgitant fraction (RF). Aortic RV is obtained by subtracting the systolic volume crossing the LVOT from the mitral inflow or pulmonary outflow volume. RF is obtained from the equation: RF = (aortic RV/LVOT systolic volume) × 100%.

The EROA can be calculated this way as well, since the flow volume is given by the product of the area by the time-velocity integral of the regurgitant jet at CW Doppler [12]. This method applies to multiple and eccentric jets, but cannot be used in the presence of MR that is worse than mild, except for those cases in which pulmonary output is used as reference. An RV ≥ 60 ml and EROA ≥0.30 cm$^2$ are consistent with severe AR [6, 9] (Table 29.1).

PW Doppler also allows the observation of a diastolic Doppler signal due to aortic diastolic flow reversal in either the ascending or descending aorta. With increasing AR, the duration and velocity of the reversal increase (Figs. 29.3 and 29.4).

CW color Doppler recording of the flow time-velocity curve of AR with an apical approach is marked by a rapid increase in velocity during isovolumetric relaxation, followed by a gradual slowdown during diastole and a sudden drop during

**Fig. 29.3** Transthoracic echocardiogram: color Doppler image of an aortic regurgitation jet recorded in the ascending aorta (Asc Ao)

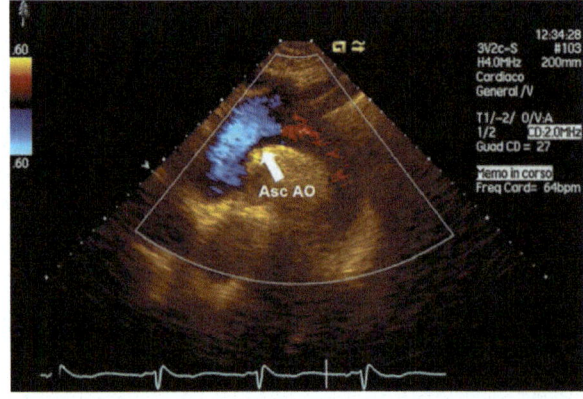

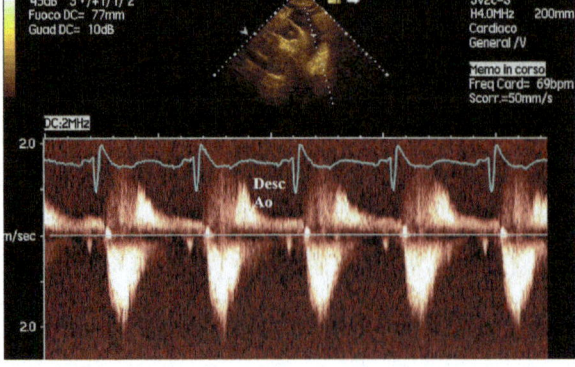

**Fig. 29.4** Transthoracic echocardiogram: PW Doppler of the flow in the descending aorta in patient with aortic regurgitation. The reverse diastolic flow can be seen during diastole. Descending aorta (Desc Ao)

**Fig. 29.5** Transthoracic echocardiogram: CW Doppler recording in a patient with aortic regurgitation showing how to measure the diastolic gradient of the regurgitant signal (AR) and the pressure half-time (PHT)

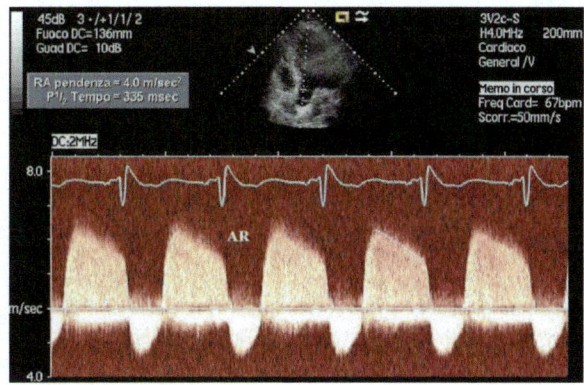

isovolumetric contraction. As the degree of severity of AR worsens, left ventricular diastolic pressure rises, and the pressure half-time (PHT) of the regurgitant flow and deceleration time of the mitral protodiastolic flow velocity become shorter [13]. A PHT > 500 ms is usually compatible with mild AR, whereas a value <200 ms is considered consistent with severe AR [6, 9] (Table 29.1) (Fig. 29.5). This technique has some limitations, though, as it is affected, for instance, by LV compliance, which, if reduced, leads to a shortening of PHT, due to the faster rise in LV pressure.

TEE is seldom used in the assessment of AR, but it may be needed if there is a poor acoustic window or if accurate assessment of aortic valve anatomy or Doppler scan is not possible.

Finally, in the overall assessment of a patient, an assessment of the LV is also needed for therapeutic and prognostic purposes; in particular, the increase in its end-systolic diameter to over 55 mm, without any other causes for volume overload, is an indication of severe ventricular function impairment.

The stress test in severe AR patients has not been validated. Cardiac MRI is recommended when the quality of the echocardiography images is not good or, together with multislice CT, for an assessment of the aorta when the echocardiography shows that it is dilated.

### 29.3.2 Invasive Diagnosis

The role of invasive diagnosis in AR is rather limited, since TTE and TEE provide an extensive and accurate analysis of the degree of regurgitation [9].

Cardiac catheterization may be useful in assessing differential pressure in the ascending aorta, but aortography with rapid injection of contrast in the aortic root (25–35 ml/s) is particularly successful in quantifying the degree of regurgitation (Fig. 29.6). In percutaneous treatment of pure aortic regurgitation, aortography is complementary to angio-CT and echocardiography to study the interaction of the device with the aortic apparatus and to achieve optimal implantation of the percutaneous device.

**Fig. 29.6** Aortogram in LAO view showing major regurgitation with contrast medium in the left ventricle (*asterisk*). *Ao* aorta, *LV* left ventricle

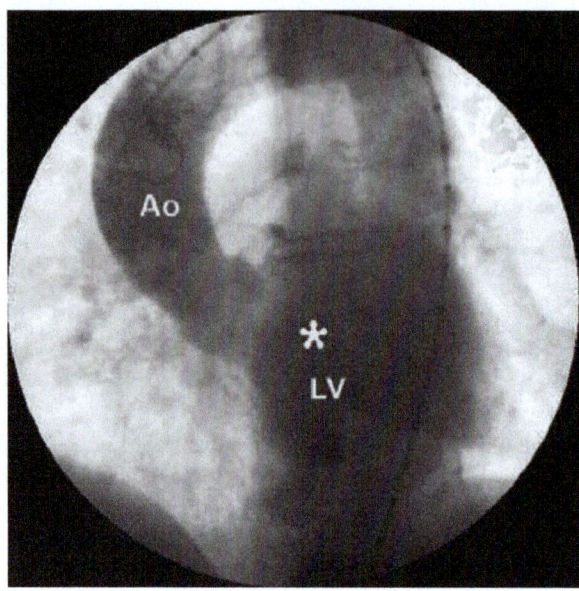

## 29.4    Timing of Interventions

Moderate or severe AR is generally associated with a favorable prognosis for many years. Among asymptomatic subjects with severe AR and normal left ventricle ejection fraction (LVEF), more than 45% of patients maintain this condition and normal ventricular function at 10 years [14–16], with a percentage of <6% a year developing left ventricular dysfunction [9]. The risk of sudden death in these patients is less than 0.5% a year. However, as for AS, once the patient becomes symptomatic, there is rapid and progressive worsening. Heart failure can occur along with episodes of pulmonary edema, or cases of sudden death, usually among previously symptomatic patients with major LV dilation. Presurgery data show that death in nonoperated patients usually occurs within 4 years of the onset of angina pectoris and within 2 years of the onset of heart failure [17]. Over the past 20 years, many surgical case histories have shown that a low LVEF is one of the most important determinants of mortality after valve replacement, especially when ventricular dysfunction is irreversible and does not improve after surgery [9].

It is more likely that left ventricular dysfunction is reversible if diagnosed early on, before the LVEF becomes so low that the ventricle dilates greatly and develops significant symptoms; therefore, surgical intervention is important before these alterations become irreversible [6].

When AR has an acute development, urgent surgery is clearly indicated due to hemodynamic instability. In the case of chronic AR, considering the excellent prognosis in the short and medium term, surgical repair must be delayed in patients with severe AR who are asymptomatic, have a good tolerance to effort, and have an LVEF >50% without marked LV dilation (i.e., end-diastolic diameter < 70 mm and end-systolic diameter < 50 mm). Similarly, without clear contraindications or associated pathologies, surgery is indicated in symptomatic patients with severe AR and asymptomatic patients with LVEF <50% and marked left ventricular dilation (end-diastolic diameter > 70 mm and end-systolic diameter > 50 mm). Since serious symptoms (NYHA class III or IV) and left ventricular dysfunction with LVEF <50% are independent risk factors for a worse postoperative survival, surgery must be performed in NYHA class II patients before they develop severe left ventricular dysfunction [18] (Table 29.2).

Finally, valve replacement must be performed regardless of the symptoms in cases of severe AR in patients who must undergo surgery for other contingent conditions (Table 29.2).

Indications for surgery in patients with severe AR secondary to aortic root dilation are similar to those for patients with primary valve disease. However, progressive expansion of the aortic root and/or a diameter > 50 mm in the case of Marfan's syndrome, greater than 50 mm (in the case of bicuspid valve with additional risk factors), and greater than 55 mm (in all other cases) with any other degree of regurgitation represent indications for surgery [18] (Table 29.2).

**Table 29.2** Indications for valve replacement in aortic regurgitation, adapted from the 2012 European Guidelines for the treatment of valve diseases

|  | Class of recommendation-level of evidence |
| --- | --- |
| *Severe AR* | |
| Symptomatic patients (dyspnea; NYHA classes II, III, and IV; or angina) | I-B |
| Asymptomatic patients with resting LVEF ≤50% | I-B |
| Patients undergoing CABG and surgery of the ascending aorta or on another valve | I-C |
| Asymptomatic patients with resting LVEF >50% with severe LV dilatation: | |
| End-diastolic dimension >70 mm | IIa-C |
| End-systolic dimension >50 (or 25 mm/m² BSA) | IIa-C |
| *Whatever the severity of AR* | |
| Patients who have aortic root disease with maximal aortic diameter | I-C |
| ≥50 mm for patients with Marfan's syndrome | IIa-C |
| ≥45 mm for patients with Marfan's syndrome with risk factors[a] | IIa-C |
| ≥50 mm for patients with bicuspid valves with risk factors[b] | |
| ≥55 mm for other patients | IIa-C |

*AR* aortic regurgitation, *NYHA* New York Heart Association, *CABG* coronary artery bypass grafting, *LV* left ventricle, *LVEF* left ventricular ejection fraction, *BSA* body surface area
[a]Family history of aortic dissection and/or aortic size increase >2 mm/year, severe AR or mitral regurgitation, desire for pregnancy
[b]Coarctation of the aorta, systemic hypertension, family history of dissection, or increase in aortic diameter > 2 mm/year

## 29.5    Percutaneous Therapy

Surgical valve replacement remains the treatment of choice in operable patients with native AR [18]. Transcatheter aortic valve replacement (TAVR) has become the standard of care for patients with aortic valve stenosis who have a prohibitive risk for surgical aortic valve replacement and an alternative to surgical aortic valve replacement in patients with aortic valve stenosis deemed at high surgical risk [18]. The role of TAVR for native severe AR treatment is rather marginal and currently consists of an "off-label" application in patients for whom cardiac surgery is an absolute contraindication; indeed the devices used are specifically designed for the treatment of aortic stenosis, to be implanted in heavily calcified and degenerated valves.

### 29.5.1  Patient Selection

As stated above, percutaneous treatment of native predominant AR has to be restricted only to patients with a prohibitive surgical risk based on the heart team assessment. Examples of comorbidities that heart teams considered significant enough to make the risk of surgery unacceptable include previous radiotherapy, hostile mediastinum, severe LV dysfunction, previous stroke, severe pulmonary hypertension, and severe pulmonary disease. Percutaneous devices specifically designed for native AR are in the development phase. On this background, from a clinical and anatomical perspective, patient selection is similar to that of aortic stenosis patients undergoing percutaneous replacement. Specifically, TAVR for AR can be attempted if the annulus is not at the upper limit for a specific device, and some technical issues have to be taken into account. However, it should be pointed out that TAVR in pure native AR represents an off-label indication for the majority of TAVR systems.

### 29.5.2  Procedure and Technical Aspects

The percutaneous technique is almost identical to the one used to treat AS, but some clarifications need to be made:

- Valvuloplasty before implantation is not performed.
- In AR of a native valve, there are generally no annulus calcifications (Fig. 29.6), while on the one hand, this reduces the incidence of complications due to the embolization of the calcium fragments during device expansion, and on the other, an important fluoroscopic landmarker to outline the annulus position and root anatomy is lost during valve release, which can be made more difficult, leading to major periprosthetic leaks. For an accurate positioning, some groups have advocated the use of two pigtail catheters for improved annular delineation (one catheter placed in the noncoronary sinus and the other in the left coronary sinus). Alternatively, transesophageal echocardiographic visualization can provide additional guidance but requires general anesthesia.

- Valve calcifications are an effective structure on which percutaneous biological devices can be anchored with a high radial force, reducing the risk of its migration and periprosthetic leaks to a minimum. For this reason, the use of rapid pacing is advisable for the deployment of the CoreValve/Evolut R for severe AR in order to decrease the regurgitant volume and systolic blood pressure, as well as the risk of prosthesis movement. It has been recommended that this be used at least from one-third frame deployment to two-thirds frame deployment. Indeed, this improves valve stability and reduces sudden movements and risk of valve dislocation during the one-third to two-thirds phases.
- Oversizing (significant more than 30% by area) of the device is advisable in AR without calcification to prevent dislocation and paravalvular regurgitation.

Due to all these technical challenges, valve deployment in an annulus without calcification and with a frequent concomitant dilation of the aortic root and/or the ascending aorta is more challenging and less predictable and can be complicated by supra-annular or ventricular dislocation of the prosthesis, the latter possibly occurring up to several hours after implantation.

The self-expanding Medtronic CoreValve (Medtronic, Minneapolis, Minnesota) has been used in the majority of cases due to its self-expanding frame with additional anchoring by means of support also against the ascending aorta [19]. Several newer-generation non-dedicated self-expanding transcatheter prostheses, such as the self-expandable and self-positioning ACURATE TA device (Symetis SA, Ecublens, Switzerland) and the self-expanding and repositionable Lotus Valve System (Boston Scientific, Marlborough, Massachusetts), have been investigated for the treatment of pure native AR [20, 21]. The risk of valve dislocation due to insufficient anchoring and annular rupture as a consequence of excessive oversizing have limited the use of these devices for native AR and prompted the development of dedicated devices enabling capture of aortic valve leaflets with specific clips to minimize the risk of valve embolization and paravalvular leaks. These more specific devices include the transapical, self-expanding JenaValve (JenaValve Technology, Munich, Germany) and J-Valve (JC Medical, Inc., Redwood City, California) [22, 23]. The JenaValve has three nitinol feelers, which facilitate "self-positioning" valve implantation. The three nitinol feelers and the frame of the prosthesis are integrated by an unmovable connection: each arm of the feelers is brought into the aortic sinuses, and the position of the prosthesis can be adjusted. The J-Valve has a self-expanding support frame connected movably with a three-prong clasper by three sutures; this movable connection allows adjusting the position of the prosthetic valve, while the clasper has already been placed in the aortic sinus. Thus, the claspers help in good positioning and also reinforce the anchoring of the prosthesis by clamping the native valve leaflets between it and the support frame.

In cases with a minimally calcified aortic annulus, the Helio transcatheter aortic anchoring device (Edwards Lifesciences) is another transfemoral system designed to enable annular fixation of a standard balloon-expandable SAPIEN XT transcatheter valve [24]. However, the Helio program has been interrupted.

## 29.5.3 Results

In 2013, the first and largest multicenter (14 centers) registry was published, including a total of 43 inoperable patients undergoing TAVR with the CoreValve prosthesis for the treatment of pure native AR [19]. The device success rate was 74.4%: eight patients required two transcatheter valves (18.6%), and nine patients (21%) had residual aortic regurgitation that was more than mild; one patient required conversion to open surgery [19]. The 30-day rate of major stroke was 4.7%. The all-cause mortality was 9.3% at 30 days and 21.4% at 12 months [19]. There was a strong correlation with absent valvular calcification [19]. Indeed, as stated above, absent aortic valve calcification may lead to reduced fixation of the lower part of the valve frame at the annulus during deployment, resulting in malpositioning. This may be exacerbated by enhanced movement of the prosthesis in the regurgitant jet. Dilation of the aortic root and ascending aorta, which is common in native AR, may also be a contributing factor. These limitations can be overcome by valve designs that are fully retrievable and repositionable, and valvular fixation can be improved even in the absence of calcifications.

The transapical TAVR with the use of the self-expandable and self-positioning ACURATE TA Symetis prosthesis in eight high-risk patients with pure severe AR was associated with no intraprocedural complications, with no stroke or deaths at 30 days, and with post-procedure AR grade I+ or lower in all eight patients [20].

The transapical, self-expanding JenaValve was associated with favorable clinical and hemodynamic results after 6 months in 31 patients [25]. Indeed, the implantation of the JenaValve was successful in 30 of 31 cases (97%); transcatheter heart valve dislodgement necessitated valve-in-valve implantation in one patient (3%) [25]. Post-procedural aortic regurgitation was none/trace in 28 of 31 (90.3%) and mild in 3 of 31 patients (9.7%) [25]. During follow-up, two patients underwent valvular reinterventions (surgical aortic valve replacement for endocarditis, valve-in-valve implantation for increasing paravalvular regurgitation) [25]. All-cause mortality was 13% at 30 days and 19% at 6 months [25]. A significant and persistent improvement in New York Heart Association class was observed [25].

In a recent report, six inoperable patients with native AR without significant valve calcification underwent successful transapical implantation of the J-Valve prosthesis [26]. During the follow-up period (from 31 days to 186 days), only one patient had trivial prosthetic valve regurgitation, and none of the patients had para-valvular leak of more than mild grade. There was no major postoperative complications or mortality [26].

## References

1. Braunwald E, Goldman L. Primary cardiology. 2nd ed. New York: Elsevier Science; 2003.
2. Iung B, Baron G, Butchart EG, et al. A prospective survey of patients with valvular heart disease in Europe: the euro heart survey on Valvular heart disease. Eur Heart J. 2003;24:1231–43.
3. Ti M, Sayeed MR, Stamou SC, et al. Pathophysiology of aortic valve disease. In: Cohn LH, editor. Cardiac surgery in the adult. New York: McGraw-Hill; 2008. p. 825–40.

4. Braunwald E, Fauci AS, Kasper DL, et al. Harrison's principles of internal medicine. 15th ed. New York: McGraw Hill; 2002.
5. Zoghbi WA, Chambers JB, Dumesnil JG, et al. Recommendations for evaluation of prosthetic valves with echocardiography and Doppler ultrasound. J Am Soc Echocardiogr. 2009;22: 975–1014.
6. Zoghbi WA, Eriquez-Sarano M, Foster E, et al. Recommendations for evaluation of the severity of native valvular regurgitation with two-dimensional and Doppler echocardiography. J Am Soc Echocardiogr. 2003;16:777–802.
7. Perry GJ, Helmcke F, Nanda NC, et al. Evaluation of aortic insufficiency by Doppler color flow mapping. J Am Coll Cardiol. 1987;9:952–9.
8. Bonow RO, Carabello BA, Chatteljee K, et al. ACC/AHA 2006 guidelines for the management of patients with valvular heart disease. J Am Coll Cardiol. 2006;48:1–148.
9. Vahanian A, Baumgartner H, Bax J, et al. Guidelines on the Management of Valvular Heart Disease: the task force on the management of Valvular heart disease of the European Society of Cardiology. Eur Heart J. 2007;28:230–68.
10. Tribouilloy CM, Enriquez-Sarano M, Fett SL, et al. Application of the proximal flow convergence method to calculate the effective regurgitant orifice area in aortic regurgitation. J Am Coll Cardiol. 1998;32:1032–9.
11. Lancellotti P, Tribouilloy C, Hagendorff A, et al. European Association of Echocardiography recommendations for the assessment of valvular regurgitation. Part 1: aortic and pulmonary regurgitation (native valve disease). Eur J Echocardiogr. 2010;11:223–44.
12. Enriquez-Sarano M, Bailey KR, Seward JB, et al. Quantitative Doppler assessment of valvular regurgitation. Circulation. 1993;87:841–8.
13. Teague SM, Heinsimer JA, Anderson JL, et al. Quantification of aortic regurgitation utilizing continuous wave Doppler ultrasound. J Am Coil Cardiol. 1986;8:592–9.
14. Bonow RO. Chronic aortic regurgitation. Role of medical therapy and optimal timing for surgery. Cardiol Clin. 1998;16:449–61.
15. Borer JS, Hochreiter C, Herrold EM, et al. Prediction of indications for valve replacement among asymptomatic or minimally symptomatic patients with chronic aortic regurgitation and normal left ventricular performance. Circulation. 1998;97:525–34.
16. Tarasoutchi F, Grinberg M, Spina GS, et al. Ten-year clinical laboratory follow-up after application of a symptom-based therapeutic strategy to patients with severe chronic aortic regurgitation of predominant rheumatic etiology. J Am Coil Cardiol. 2003;41:1316–24.
17. Dujardin KS, Enriquez-Sarano M, Schaff HV, et al. Mortality and morbidity of aortic regurgitation in clinical practice. A long-term follow-up study. Circulation. 1999;99:1851–7.
18. Joint Task Force on the Management of Valvular Heart Disease of the European Society of Cardiology (ESC), European Association for Cardio-Thoracic Surgery (EACTS), Vahanian A, Alfieri O, Andreotti F, et al. Guidelines on the management of valvular heart disease (version 2012). Eur Heart J. 2012;33:2451–96.
19. Roy DA, Schaefer U, Guetta V, et al. Transcatheter aortic valve implantation for pure severe native aortic valve regurgitation. J Am Coll Cardiol. 2013;61:1577–84.
20. Wendt D, Kahlert P, Pasa S, et al. Transapical transcatheter aortic valve for severe aortic regurgitation: expanding the limits. J Am Coll Cardiol Intv. 2014;7:1159–67.
21. Wöhrle J, Rodewald C, Rottbauer W. Transfemoral aortic valve implantation in pure native aortic valve insufficiency using the repositionable and retrievable lotus valve. Catheter Cardiovasc Interv. 2016;87:993–5.
22. Seiffert M, Diemert P, Koschyk D, et al. Transapical implantation of a second-generation transcatheter heart valve in patients with noncalcified aortic regurgitation. J Am Coll Cardiol Intv. 2013;6:590–7.
23. Zhu D, Chen Y, Guo Y, et al. Transapical transcatheter aortic valve implantation using a new second-generation TAVI system - J-valve for high-risk patients with aortic valve diseases: initial results with 90-day follow-up. Int J Cardiol. 2015;199:155–62.
24. Barbanti M, Ye J, Pasupati S, El-Gamel A, Webb JG. The Helio transcatheter aortic dock for patients with aortic regurgitation. EuroIntervention. 2013;9(Suppl):S91–4.

25. Seiffert M, Bader R, Kappert U, et al. Initial German experience with transapical implantation of a second-generation transcatheter heart valve for the treatment of aortic regurgitation. J Am Coll Cardiol Intv. 2014;7:1168–74.
26. Wei L, Liu H, Zhu L, et al. A new transcatheter aortic valve replacement system for predominant aortic regurgitation implantation of the J-valve and early outcome. JACC Cardiovasc Interv. 2015;8:1831–41.